Other monographs in the series Major Problems in Clinical Pediatrics:

Altman and Schwartz: *Malignant Diseases of Infancy, Childhood and Adolescence*—1978

Avery and Fletcher: *The Lung and Its Disorders in the Newborn Infant*—Third Edition, 1974

Bell and McCormick: *Increased Intracranial Pressure in Children*—Second Edition, 1978

Bell and McCormick: *Neurologic Infections in Children*—1975

Brewer: *Juvenile Rheumatoid Arthritis*—1970

Cornblath and Schwartz: *Disorders of Carbohydrate Metabolism in Infancy*—Second Edition, 1976

Dubowitz: *Muscle Disorders in Childhood*—1978

Gryboski: *Gastrointestinal Problems in the Infant*—1975

Hanshaw and Dudgeon: *Viral Diseases of the Fetus and Newborn*—1978

Lubchenco: *The High Risk Infant*—1976

Markowitz and Gordis: *Rheumatic Fever*—Second Edition, 1972

Oski and Naiman: *Hematologic Problems in the Newborn*—Second Edition, 1972

Rowe and Mehrizi: *The Neonate with Congenital Heart Disease*—1968

Royer et al: *Pediatric Nephrology*—1974

Scriver and Rosenberg: *Amino Acid Metabolism and Its Disorders*—1973

Smith: *Recognizable Patterns of Human Malformation*—Second Edition, 1976

Smith: *Growth and Its Disorders*—1977

Solomon and Esterly: *Neonatal Dermatology*—1973

Forthcoming Monographs

Belman and Kaplan: *Urologic Problems in Pediatrics*

Bluestone and Klein: *Otitis Media in Infants and Children*

Drash: *Juvenile Diabetes*

Glader: *Anemia in Children*

Griffin: *Children's Orthopaedics*

Harrison and Harrison: *Disorders of Calcium and Phosphate Metabolism in Childhood and Adolescence*

Wannamaker: *Streptococcal Infections*

ADOLESCENT DERMATOLOGY

By
Lawrence M. Solomon, M.D.
Professor and Head, Department of Dermatology, College of Medicine,
Abraham Lincoln School, University of Illinois, Chicago, Illinois

Nancy B. Esterly, M.D.
Professor of Pediatrics and Dermatology,
Northwestern University Medical School,
Head, Division of Pediatric Dermatology,
Children's Memorial Hospital,
Chicago, Illinois

E. Dorinda Loeffel, M.D.
Associate Professor, Department of Dermatology, College of Medicine,
Abraham Lincoln School, University of Illinois, Chicago, Illinois

Volume XIX in the Series
MAJOR PROBLEMS IN
CLINICAL PEDIATRICS
ALEXANDER J. SCHAFFER
Consulting Editor
MILTON MARKOWITZ
Associate Consulting Editor

W. B. Saunders Company, Philadelphia, London, Toronto   1978

W. B. Saunders Company: West Washington Square
Philadelphia, PA 19105

1 St. Anne's Road
Eastbourne, East Sussex BN21 3UN, England

1 Goldthorne Avenue
Toronto, Ontario M8Z 5T9, Canada

Library of Congress Cataloging in Publication Data

Solomon, Lawrence Marvin, 1931–

Adolescent dermatology.

(Major problems in clinical pediatrics; v. 18)

1. Pediatric dermatology.   2. Youth – Diseases.   I. Esterly, Nancy B., 1935–   joint author.   II. Loeffel, E. Dorinda, joint author.   III. Title. [DNLM: 1. Skin diseases – In adolescence. W1 MA492N v. 18 / WS260 S689a]

RJ511.S64   616.5   77-78574

ISBN 0-7216-8492-0

Adolescent Dermatology   ISBN 0-7216-8492-0

© 1978 by W. B. Saunders Company. Copyright under the International Copyright Union. All rights reserved. This book is protected by copyright. No part of it may be reproduced, stored in a retrieval system, or transmitted in any form or by any means, electronic, mechanical, photocopying, recording, or otherwise, without written permission from the publisher. Made in the United States of America. Press of W. B. Saunders Company. Library of Congress catalog card number 77-78574.

Last digit is the print number: 9   8   7   6   5   4   3   2   1

CONTRIBUTORS

WILMA FOWLER BERGFELD, M.D.
Associate Professor and Head of Dermatopathology Section, Departments of Dermatology and Pathology, The Cleveland Clinic Foundation, Cleveland, Ohio.
Hair Disorders

RAYMOND V. CAPUTO, M.D.
Fellow, Pediatric Dermatology, University of Illinois Hospital, Chicago, Illinois.
Vascular Reactive Diseases

DAVID L. CRAM, M.D.
Associate Professor of Dermatology, University of California School of Medicine, San Francisco, California.
Common Diagnostic Procedures

ALEXANDER A. FONDAK, M.D.
Assistant Professor of Dermatology, New York University School of Medicine; Physician-in-charge, Division of Dermatology, Booth Memorial Medical Center, Flushing, New York.
Cutaneous Nevi

NANCY FUREY, M.D.
Assistant Professor of Dermatology, Northwestern University Medical School, Chicago, Illinois.
Lupus Erythematosus

JAY G. HIRSCH, M.D.
Professor of Psychiatry, The Abraham Lincoln School of Medicine, University of Illinois, Chicago, Illinois.
Understanding the Adolescent Patient

CLARK HUFF, M.D.
Assistant Professor of Dermatology, University of Colorado School of Medicine, Denver, Colorado.
Eczematous Dermatitis

GUINTER KAHN, M.D.
Director, Pediatric Dermatology Seminar, St. Francis Hospital, Miami Beach, Florida.
Photodermatoses

MILTON ORKIN, M.D.
Clinical Professor of Dermatology, University of Minnesota Medical School; Active Staff, North Memorial, Mt. Sinai, and Fairview Hospitals, Minneapolis, Minnesota.
Scabies and Pediculosis

CONTRIBUTORS

DAVID L. RAMSAY, M.D., M. Ed.

Assistant Professor and Head of Education Section, Department of Dermatology, New York University Medical Center, New York, New York.

Cutaneous Nevi

JAMES E. RASMUSSEN, M.D.

Assistant Professor of Dermatology and Assistant Professor of Family Medicine, State University of New York at Buffalo; Pediatric Dermatologist, The Children's Hospital of Buffalo, Buffalo, New York.

Acne

PRUDENCE B. STEWARDSON-KRIEGER, M.D.

Consultant Pediatric Infectious Diseases, Lutheran General Hospital, Park Ridge, Illinois.

Pyogenic and Fungal Infections

LOUISE E. TAVS, M.D.

Clinical Professor of Dermatology, The Abraham Lincoln School of Medicine, University of Illinois; Staff Physician, Chicago Health Department, Chicago, Illinois.

Syphilis and Other Venereal Diseases

ROSALYN WEINTRAUB, M.D.

Assistant Professor of Dermatology and Pediatrics, Wayne State University School of Medicine; Director of Dermatology Clinic, Children's Hospital of Michigan; Attending Physician, Department of Dermatology and Pediatrics, William Beaumont Hospital, Royal Oak, Michigan.

Viral Infections

WILLIAM L. WESTON, M.D.

Associate Professor of Dermatology and Pediatrics; Chairman, Department of Dermatology, University of Colorado School of Medicine, Denver, Colorado.

Eczematous Dermatitis

SOPHIE MARIE WOROBEC, M.D.

Clinical Assistant Professor of Dermatology and Assistant Professor of Occupational Medicine, The Abraham Lincoln School of Medicine, University of Illinois; Associate Attending Physician, Cook County Hospital, Chicago, Illinois.

Structure and Function of Skin

FOREWORD

Those of you who are regular subscribers to Major Problems in Clinical Pediatrics need not be introduced to Drs. Solomon and Esterly. You know them well from their first contribution to the series, *Neonatal Dermatology*. Stimulated by the enthusiastic acceptance of that offering, they themselves suggested that they tackle the other end of the pediatric spectrum in similar fashion. They proposed to concentrate their attention upon the cutaneous disorders of adolescence, that somewhat neglected age group, so different physically and emotionally from children on the one hand and adults on the other. In order to accomplish that task even more expeditiously, they enlisted the help of Dr. E. Dorinda Loeffel, an Associate Professor of Dermatology at the University of Illinois in Chicago, soon to succeed to the position of Professor and Chairman of the Department of Dermatology at the University of Illinois, Peoria, School of Medicine.

I am sure you will find, as I did, this monograph to be as useful, instructive, and broadly based (by which I mean as comprehensively directed toward the whole persona) as their monograph on the newborn.

ALEXANDER J. SCHAFFER, M.D.

PREFACE

In recent years adolescents have been receiving increased attention as a group of patients with special problems that require an informed and sympathetic approach to their management. Just as the teenager is neither child nor adult, his or her cutaneous problems also seem to overlap pediatric and adult dermatology. This book has several purposes: It is meant to draw the attention of pediatricians and dermatologists to the adolescent as a person with special needs; it is considered to be a vehicle for elaborating in greater detail the pathogenesis and management of certain diseases (such as acne and eczema) that are particularly important to the adolescent, diseases which of necessity receive cursory attention in general texts of dermatology and pediatrics; it is also designed to include brief discussions of disease entities, such as scleroderma, that are particularly pertinent to the adolescent but are adequately discussed in textbooks of adult medicine. We did not intend to produce a complete textbook of dermatology. We hope this focused approach will be educational and useful to pediatricians, dermatologists, internists, family practitioners, and others who grapple with the cutaneous problems of this physically and emotionally distinct group of patients. We hope also that the book reflects our genuine affection for the vulnerable teenager.

We are grateful to the many contributors of both words and pictures, to Marie Ehrlicher, Sue Hunter, Debby Smith, and Pat Thomas for their skills and advice, and to our families and pets who often suffered acute author insufficiency during preparation of the manuscript.

LAWRENCE M. SOLOMON
NANCY B. ESTERLY
E. DORINDA LOEFFEL

CONTENTS

Chapter 1
STRUCTURE AND FUNCTION OF THE SKIN.................................... 7
Sophie M. Worobec, M.D. and Lawrence M. Solomon, M.D.

Chapter 2
UNDERSTANDING THE ADOLESCENT PATIENT............................. 28
Jay G. Hirsch, M.D.

Chapter 3
COMMON DIAGNOSTIC PROCEDURES 39
David L. Cram, M.D.

Chapter 4
ACNE... 54
James E. Rasmussen, M.D.

Chapter 5
ECZEMATOUS DERMATITIS 86
J. Clark Huff, M.D. and William L. Weston, M.D.

Chapter 6
PHOTODERMATOSES... 123
Guinter Kahn, M.D.

Chapter 7
PSORIASIS IN ADOLESCENCE... 143
E. Dorinda Loeffel, M.D.

Chapter 8
PYOGENIC INFECTIONS 163
Prudence B. Stewardson-Krieger, M.D. and Nancy B. Esterly, M.D.

Chapter 9
VIRAL INFECTIONS 184
Rosalyn Weintraub, M.D.

Chapter 10
SCABIES AND PEDICULOSIS 209
Milton Orkin, M.D.

Chapter 11
SYPHILIS 222
Louise E. Tavs, M.D.

Chapter 12
OTHER VENEREAL DISEASES 257
Louise E. Tavs, M.D.

Chapter 13
FUNGAL INFECTIONS 293
Prudence B. Stewardson-Krieger, M.D. and Nancy B. Esterly, M.D.

Chapter 14
CUTANEOUS NEVI 326
Alexander A. Fondak, M.D. and David L. Ramsay, M.D., M.Ed.

Chapter 15
HAIR DISORDERS 347
Wilma F. Bergfeld, M.D.

Chapter 16
LUPUS ERYTHEMATOSUS 367
Nancy L. Furey, M.D. and Nancy B. Esterly, M.D.

Chapter 17
VASCULAR REACTIVE DISEASES 404
Raymond V. Caputo, M.D. and Lawrence M. Solomon, M.D.

Chapter 18
MISCELLANEOUS DERMATOSES 433
Lawrence M. Solomon, M.D.

INDEX 469

Illustrated Guide to the Structure of the Skin
Illustrations by Pat Thomas

FIGURE 1 Cutaneous embryogenesis

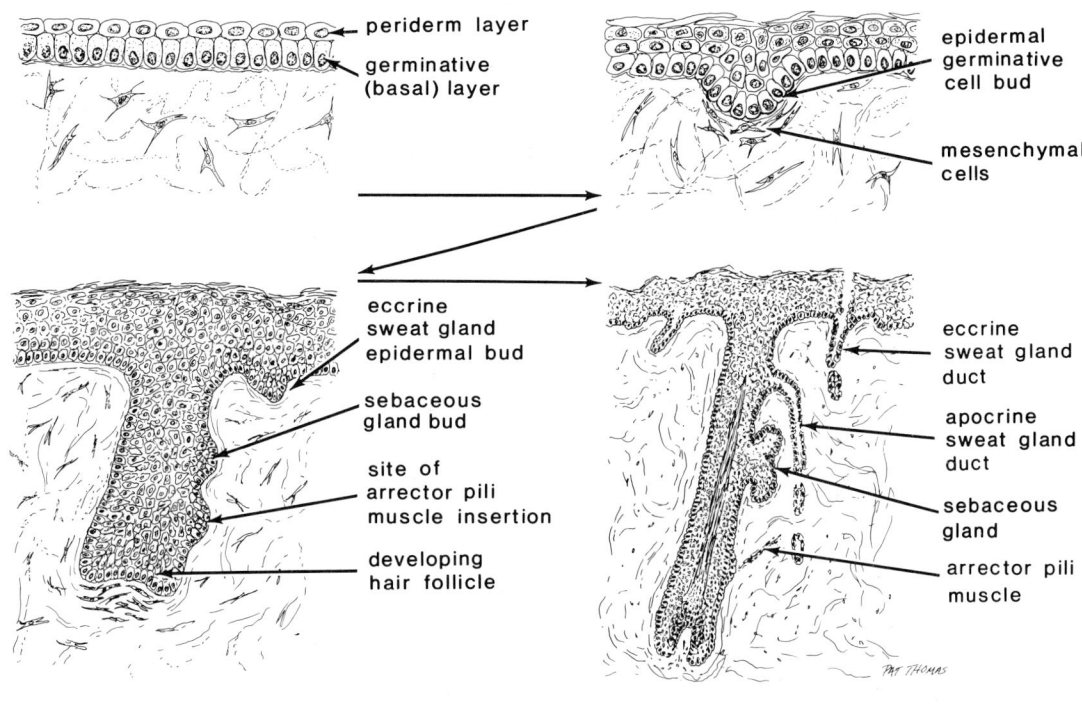

FIGURE II Origin and location of melanocytes

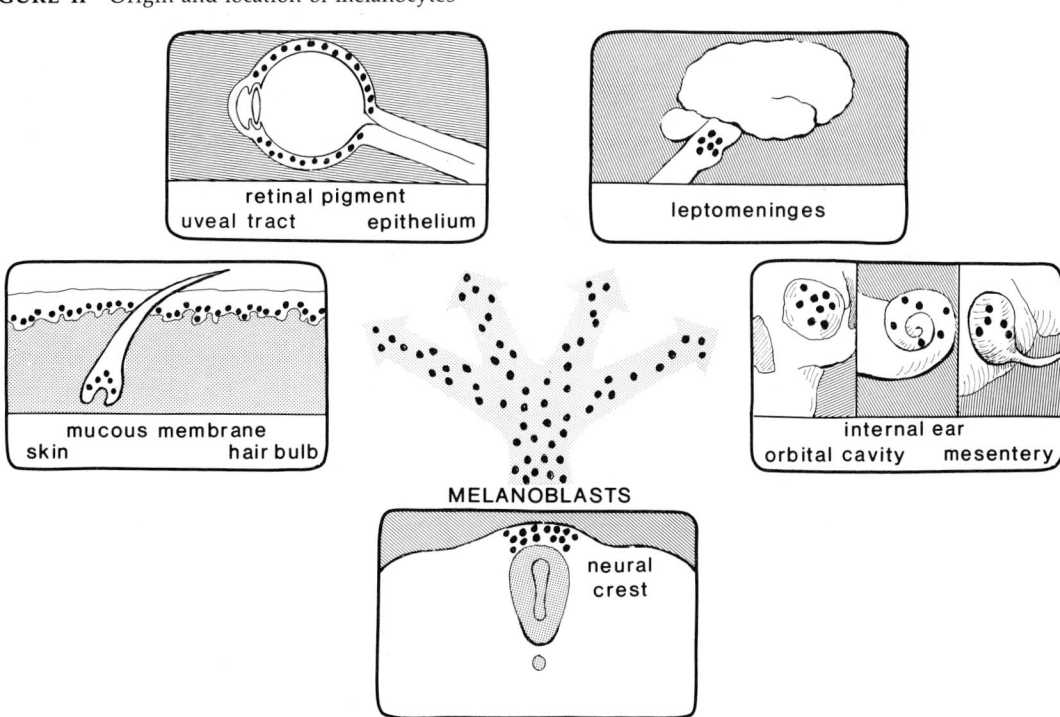

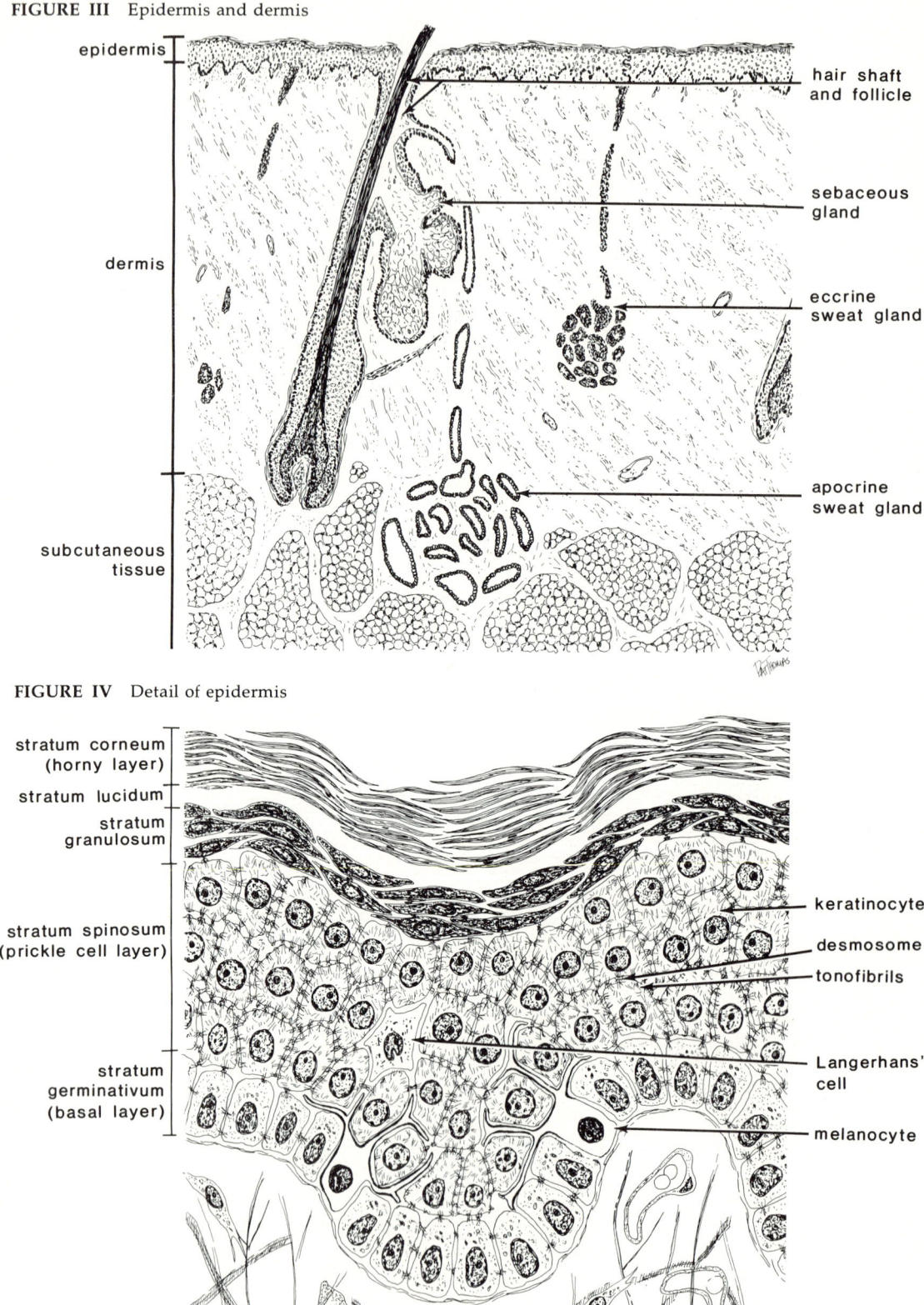

FIGURE III Epidermis and dermis

FIGURE IV Detail of epidermis

FIGURE V Connective tissue components of the dermis

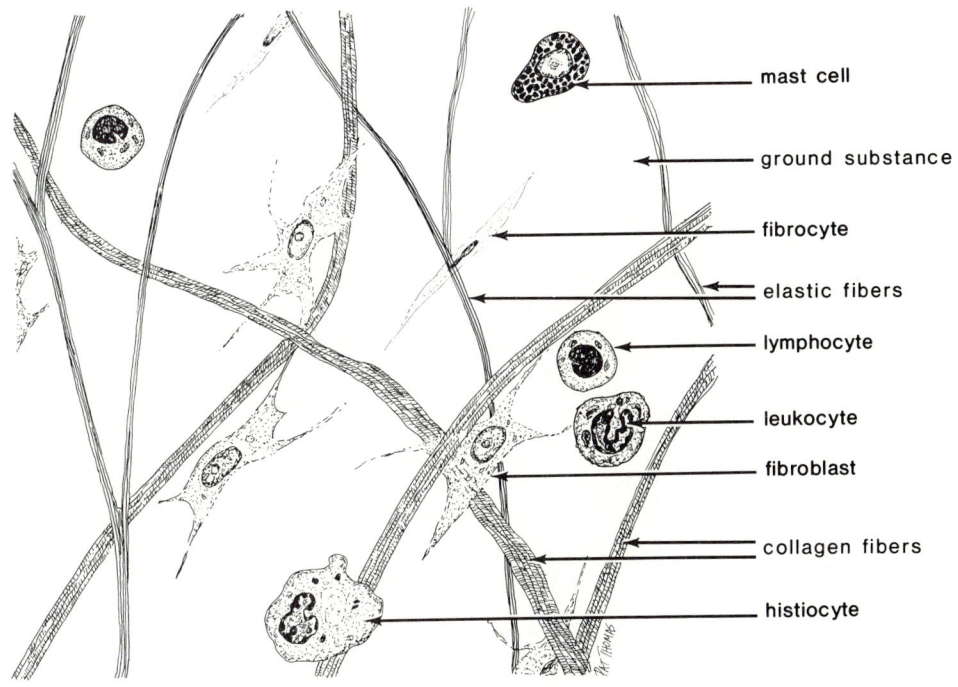

FIGURE VI Vascularization and innervation of the dermis

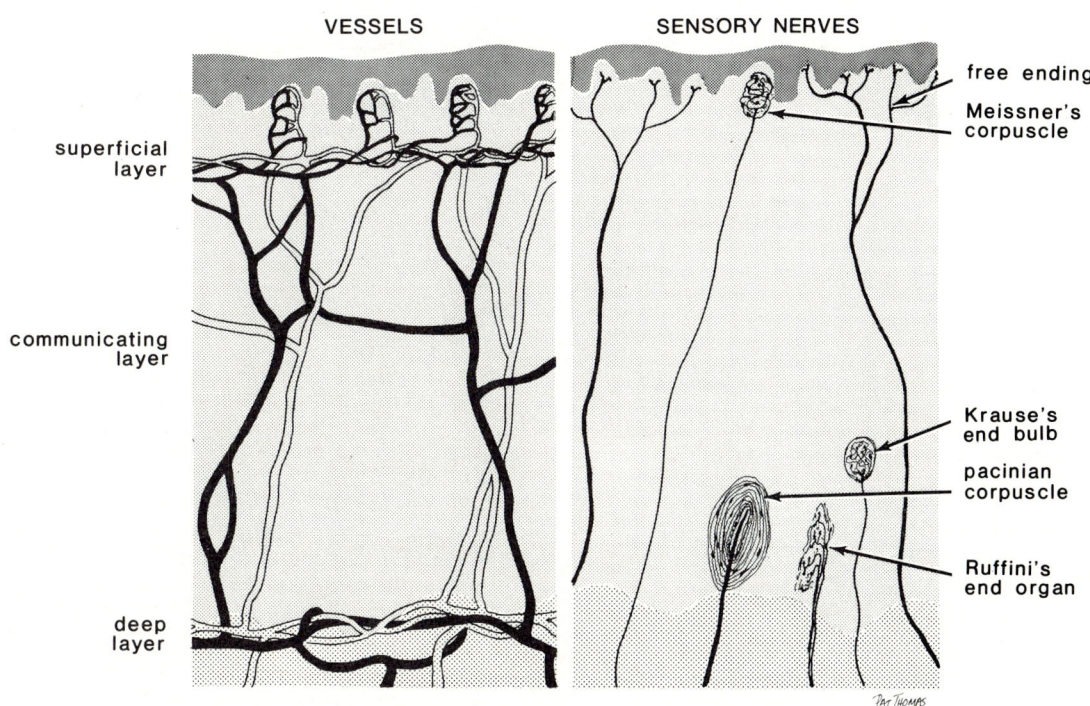

FIGURE VII Glands of the skin

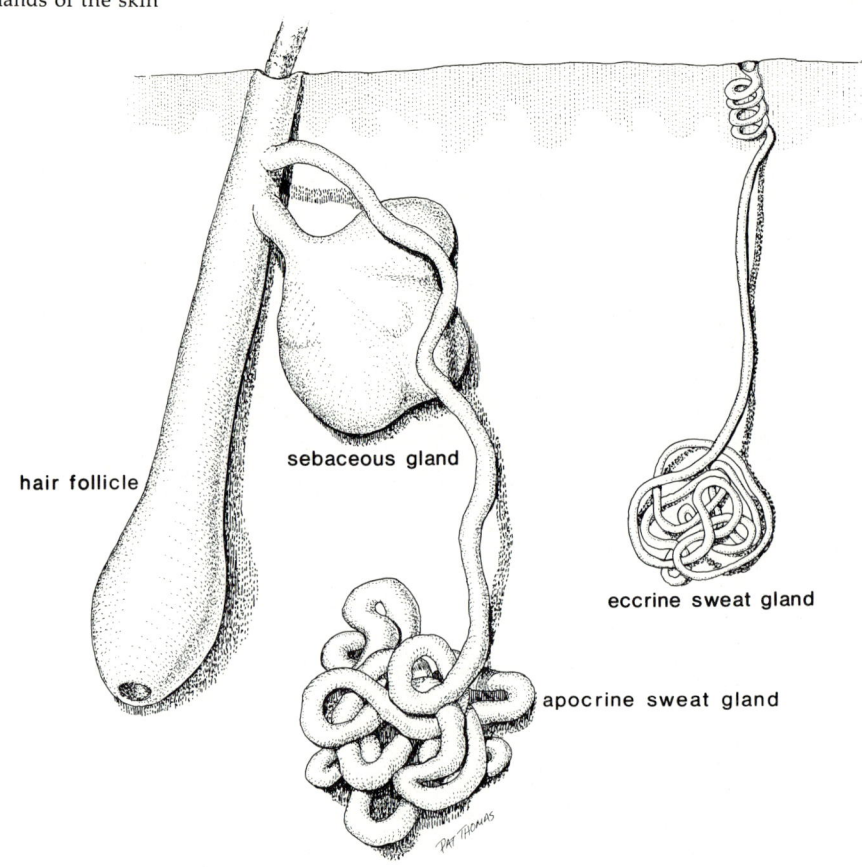

FIGURE VIII Glandular acini

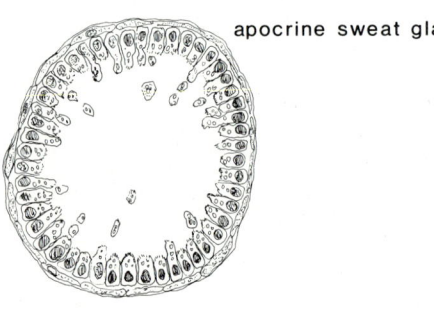
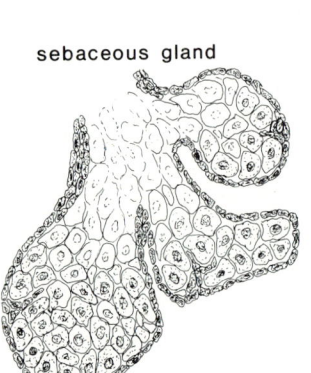
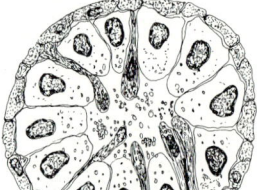

FIGURE IX Hair

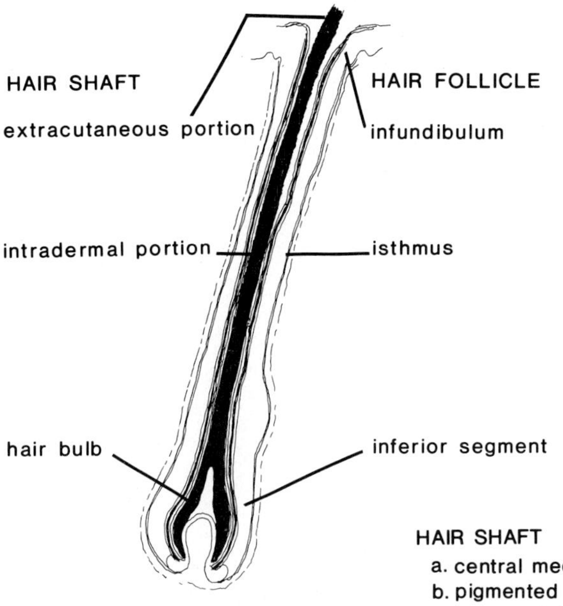

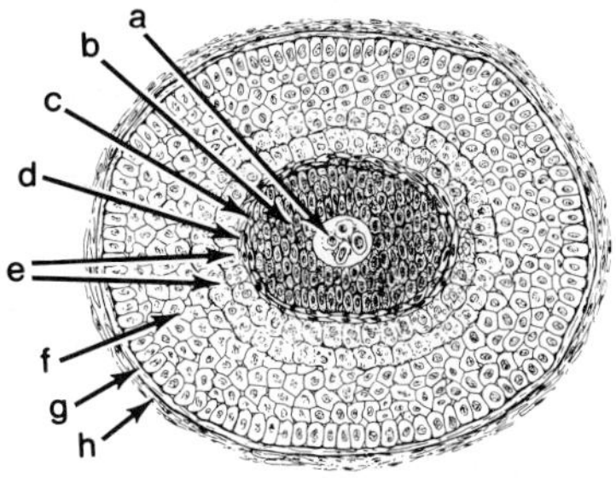

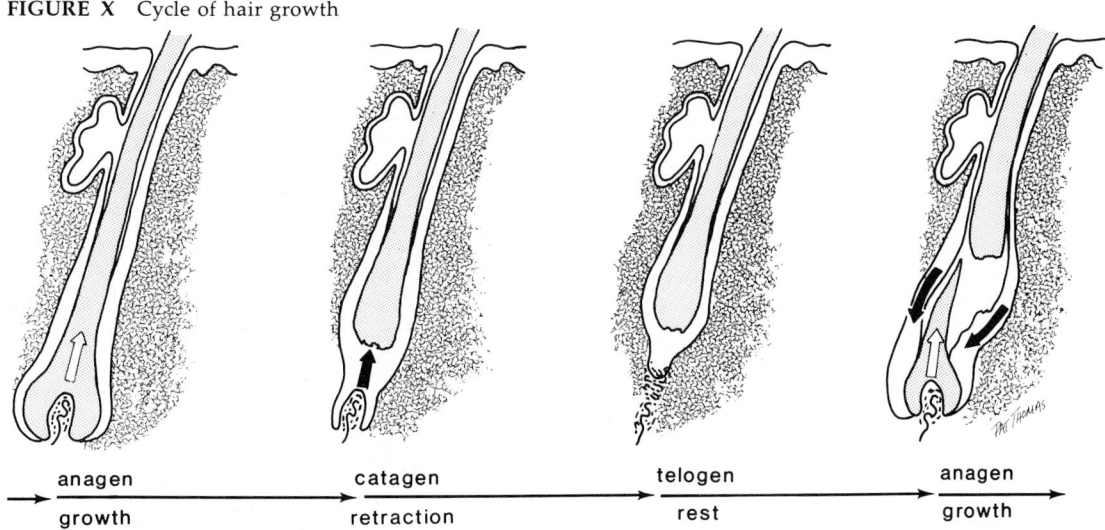

HAIR SHAFT
extracutaneous portion
intradermal portion
hair bulb
HAIR FOLLICLE
infundibulum
isthmus
inferior segment

a
b
c
d
e
f
g
h
i
j
PAT THOMAS

a
b
c
d
e
f
g
h

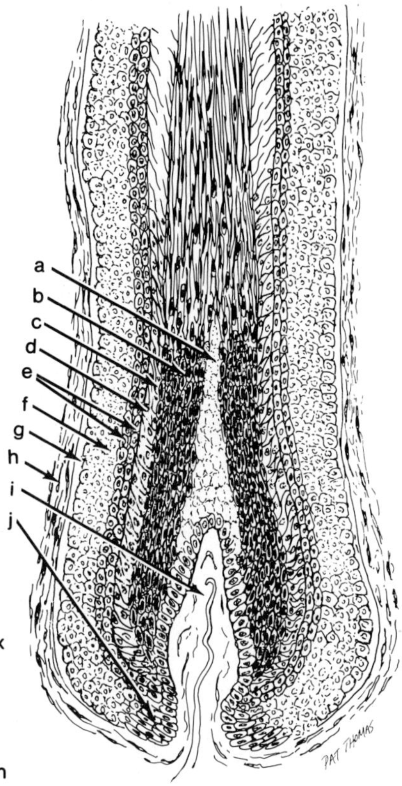

HAIR SHAFT
- a. central medulla
- b. pigmented cortex
- c. hair cuticle

HAIR FOLLICLE
- d. follicle cuticle
- e. inner root sheath
  - Henle's layer
  - Huxley's layer
- f. outer root sheath
- g. hyaline basement membrane
- h. fibrous sheath

- i. papilla
- j. germinative cells

FIGURE X Cycle of hair growth

PAT THOMAS
anagen
growth
catagen
retraction
telogen
rest
anagen
growth

FIGURE XI The nail and surrounding tissue

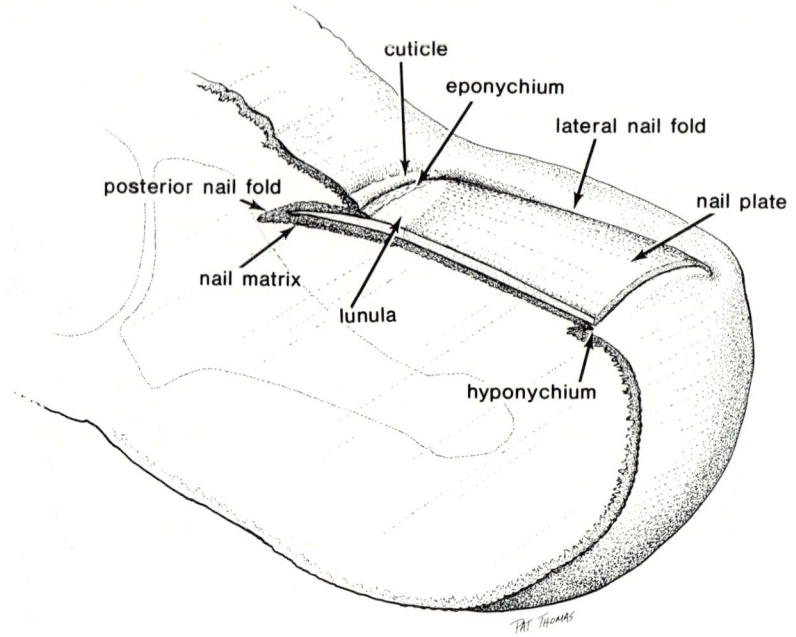

FIGURE XII Detail of nail matrix in longitudinal section

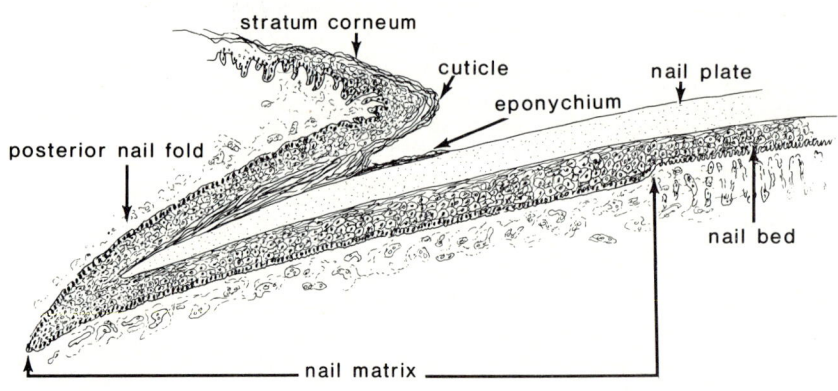

FIGURE XIII Cross section

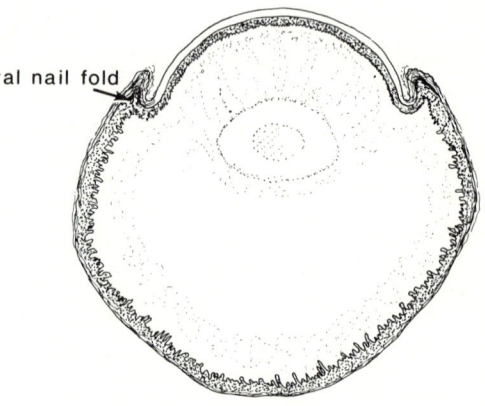

STRUCTURE AND FUNCTION OF THE SKIN

SOPHIE M. WOROBEC, M.D.
LAWRENCE M. SOLOMON, M.D.

INTRODUCTION

The human skin is a complex organ that acts as a barrier to the environment and helps to maintain homeostasis. The basic structural components of the skin are the epidermis and the dermis; however, the proportions of each component differ greatly from one part of the body to another. Within two areas of skin, one glabrous (non-hairy) and the other hairy, there are many variations. Glabrous skin is found only on the volar surfaces of hands and feet and probably evolved as an aid to grasping and walking.[1] It is characterized by a relatively thick epidermis, encapsulated sense organs, and lack of pilosebaceous units. Hairy skin, in contrast, lacks encapsulated sense organs but contains a complicated network of nerve endings around the lower hair follicle.

The surface of glabrous skin is grooved by ridges and sulci whose patterns form dermatoglyphics. The differentiation of dermatoglyphics occurs during the 13th through 19th weeks of fetal life. Dermatoglyphic patterns are so individual that imprints of finger patterns in adults are distinctive enough to furnish conclusive identification. Footprints can be used to identify neonates. Distinctive dermatoglyphic patterns have been associated with the following diseases: trisomy 21 or the Down syndrome, the Klinefelter syndrome, the Turner syndrome, certain congenital heart defects, some cases of schizophrenia, alopecia areata, and psoriasis.[2]

The size of both components of the pilosebaceous unit (sebaceous gland and hair follicle) varies on different parts of the body. The nipple area has some characteristics of glabrous skin, such as loosely encapsulated nerve endings, but also contains pilosebaceous structures.

Aging may profoundly affect the cutaneous structures because collagen can become thicker, terminal hair growth can revert to vellus growth, hair can lose pigment, sebaceous glands can hypertrophy, and eccrine glands can undergo cystic degeneration.

The skin then is a dynamic organ with structural changes occurring throughout intrauterine existence, childhood, puberty, adolescence, and adulthood.

THE EPIDERMIS

The human embryo of two to four weeks is covered by a single cell layer called the periderm, which resembles amniotic epithelium and permits the exchange of vital substances between the fetus and the amniotic fluid. At four weeks of life, a second layer of cells, known as the stratum germinativum, forms below the periderm. It is the stratum germinativum that gives rise to the epidermis and its appendages. At three months of fetal life, the epidermis is two to four cells thick. By the fifth month, there is active keratin formation in the epidermis, as evidenced by the appearance of keratohyaline granules in some of the cells. When a stratum corneum is formed, the periderm is shed into the amniotic fluid. By the sixth month, functioning epidermal melanocytes are present in the basal layer. These cells originate in the neural crest, then migrate to various tissues, including the basal ganglia and the epidermis.

The epidermis is a highly organized cellular structure containing two main divisions: the stratum corneum, consisting of anuclear keratinocytes (Fig. 1–1) and the stratum malpighii, consisting of basal cells, keratinocytes, melanocytes, and a scattering of two cells of unknown function, the Langerhans and Merkel cells. The stratum malpighii is further divided into: the basal cell layer, which is one cell layer thick and rests on the dermis; the prickle cell layer, lying superficial to the basal layer, which is several cell layers thick and has prominent intercellular connections; and the granular cell layer, with granules containing a substance called keratohyaline. In glabrous skin, there is an additional layer visible between the stratum corneum and the granular layer called the stratum lucidum.

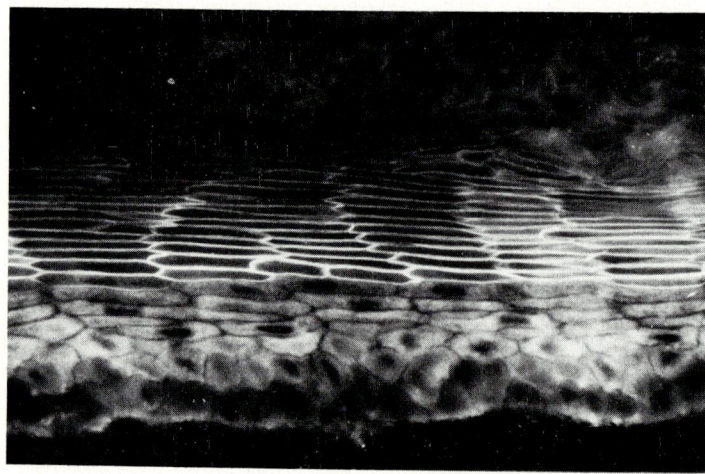

FIGURE 1–1 Cells in the cornified layer are arranged in vertical columns, resembling stacked pie plates. Cryostat section of guinea pig skin treated with 0.1 N sodium hydroxide. (Courtesy of Enno Christophers, M.D.)

KERATINOCYTES

The surface cells of the epidermis are continuously being shed. Therefore, the maintenance of the skin's integrity requires constant replication of keratinocytes followed by their upward migration to the cell surface. Replication occurs primarily in the basal layer, where one daughter cell migrates upward and undergoes profound change while the other remains in place. The keratinocyte in the basal layer is columnar in form. It contains an organelle-rich cytoplasm along with a few fibrils of keratin (called tonofibrils) and melanin transferred from adjacent melanocytes (Fig. 1–2). The basal cell is anchored to the basal lamina by means of a hemidesmosome. This modification of the cell wall consists of an intracytoplasmic attachment plaque to which tonofibrils are attached at one end, the other end lying free in the cytoplasm (Fig. 1–3). In the prickle cell layer, the cell becomes polyhedral and develops a network of tonofibrils connected at one end to attachment plaques of other keratinocytes, forming a multilayered desmosome (Fig. 1–4). As the keratinocyte matures, it moves through the granular cell layer toward the surface. Keratohyaline granule formation occurs as the result of the condensation of ribonucleoprotein around tonofilaments. Mature keratin is formed as the tonofilaments become ensheathed. Keratinocytes in the granular layer also produce membrane-coating granules (Odland bodies) within their Golgi regions, which are

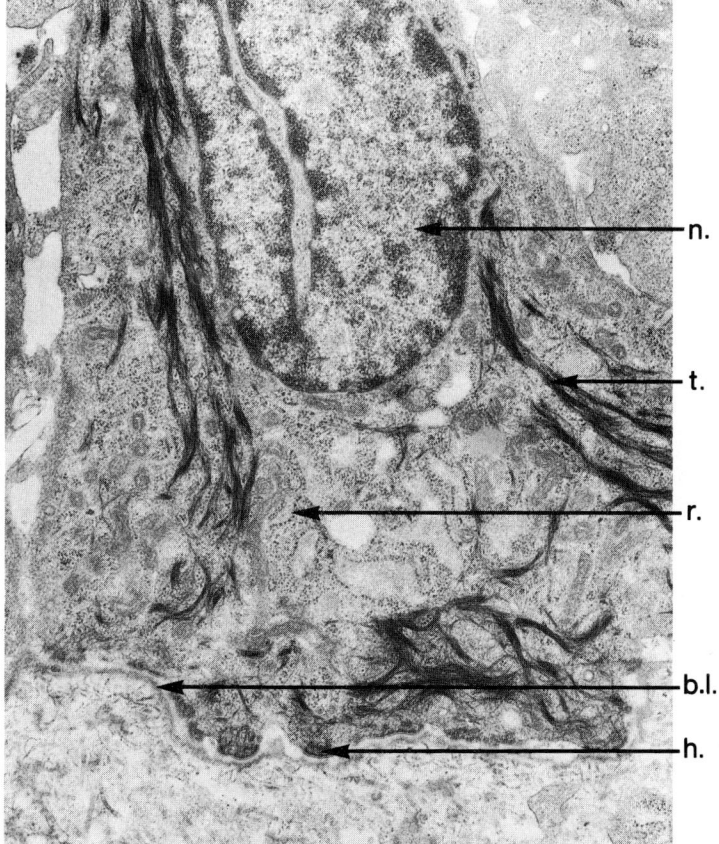

FIGURE 1–2 Basal cell cytoplasm contains abundant mitochondria and ribosomes and relatively few tonofibrils, the fundamental structure of all keratinocytes. A basal cell is situated upon the basal lamina and is connected to it by a number of hemidesmosomes. n., nucleus; t., tonofibrils; r., ribosomes; b.l., basal lamina; h., hemidesmosome. (× 25,000.) (Courtesy of Ken Hashimoto, M.D.)

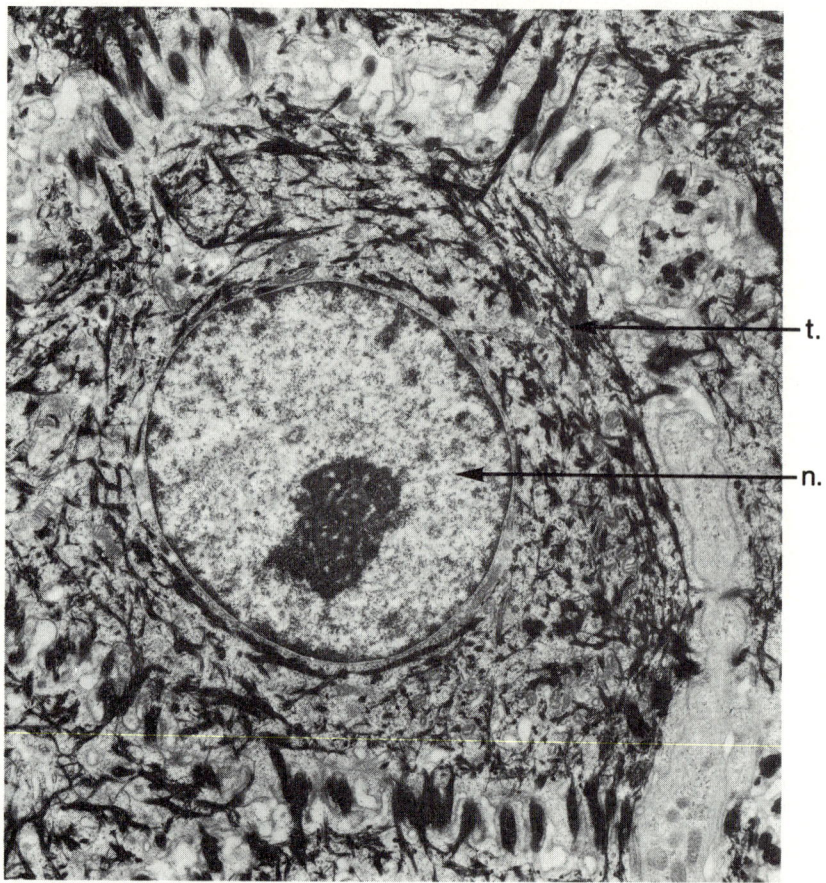

FIGURE 1–3 Spinous cell cytoplasm is almost entirely occupied by tonofibrils, except for a small number of mitochondria and scattered free ribosomes. The tonofibrils surround the nucleus and radiate toward the periphery, particularly converging upon desmosomes. *t.*, tonofibrils; *n.*, nucleus. (×9,500.) (Courtesy of Ken Hashimoto, M.D.)

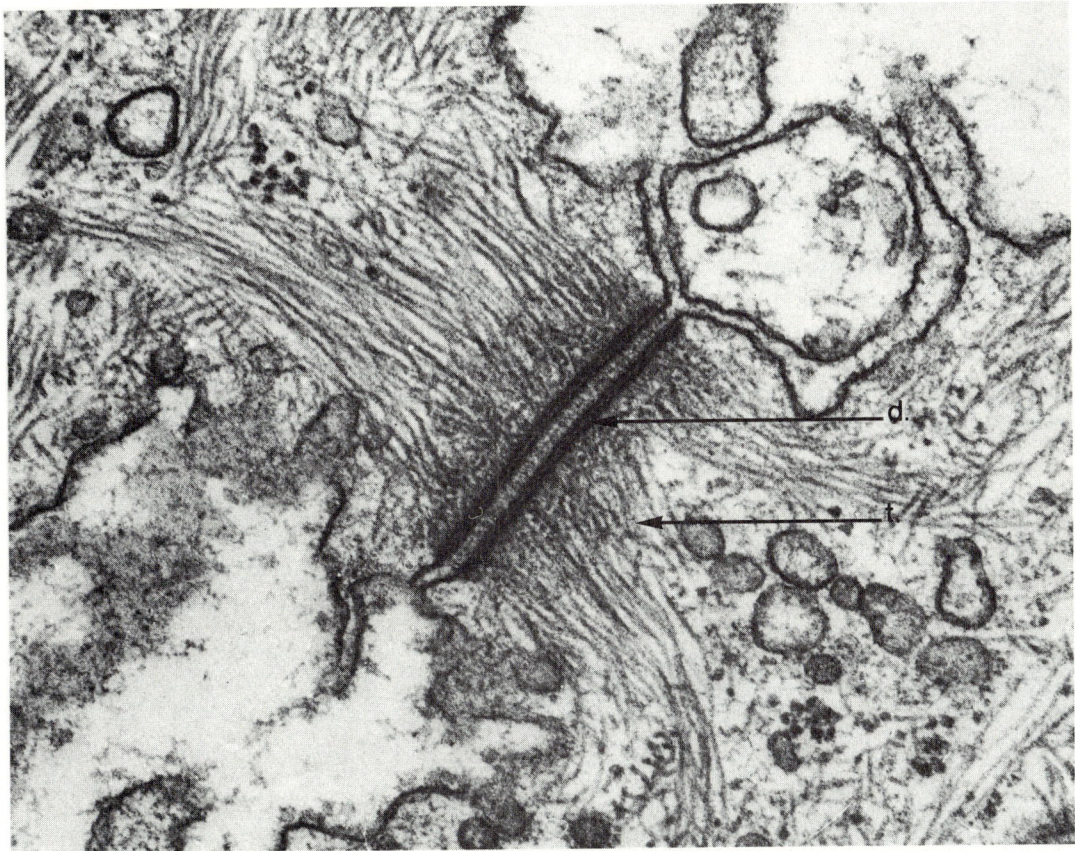

FIGURE 1–4 Looping of tonofibrils at the desmosomes between adjacent keratinocytes. *d.*, desmosome; *t.*, tonofilaments. (×132,300.) (Courtesy of Douglas E. Kelly, Ph.D.)

then extruded into the intercellular space. As Odland bodies disintegrate, they release phospholipids that probably contribute to the physiological barrier zone of the skin.[3] Keratinocytes in the stratum corneum lose their individuality as they undergo further marked changes, including disintegration of nuclei and organelles, thickening of cell membranes, engorgement with keratin, and rapid dehydration from 60 per cent to 10 per cent water. The transit time of keratinocytes from the basal layer to the stratum corneum is normally 26 to 28 days.[4, 5]

DENDRITIC CELLS OF THE EPIDERMIS

Melanocytes are dendritic cells that produce melanin. They are found interspersed among keratinocytes in the basal layer. Each melanocyte together with about ten neighboring keratinocytes forms an epidermal-melanin unit. The melanocyte transfers melanin through its dendrites to the keratinocytes for dispersion throughout the epidermis. In Caucasians, melanin is limited almost exclusively to the basal layer, whereas in people with darker skin, melanin predominates in the basal layer but can also be found throughout the epidermis in varying concentrations, depending on the depth of skin color. Melanocytes are more numerous in light-exposed and genital areas of the body. The number of melanocytes found in the basal layer is similar in both sexes and in all races; cell concentration is greatest in young adults. Caucasians not exposed to sunlight have melanocytes that vary in melanin-producing potential, while blacks have highly active melanin-producing melanocytes. Black skin also contains larger melanocytes with a greater number of dendrites (Figs. 1–5 and 1–6).

The melanocyte contains specialized organelles, known as melanosomes, for the production of melanin. The shape of the melanosomes varies with hair color, being ellipsoid with brown or black hair, and spherical with red and blond hair. In blacks, melanosomes are transferred singly to keratinocytes, but in Caucasians and Mongoloids, they form complexes.[6,7] Melanin is a polymer of indole quinones derived from tyrosine and dopa. The production of melanin is dependent on the presence of tyrosinase, a copper-containing enzyme. Within melanocytes, tyrosinase is manufactured in ribosomes, then transferred to Golgi complexes where it is incorporated into melanosomes. There it oxidizes both tyrosine and dopa, starting a series of reactions leading

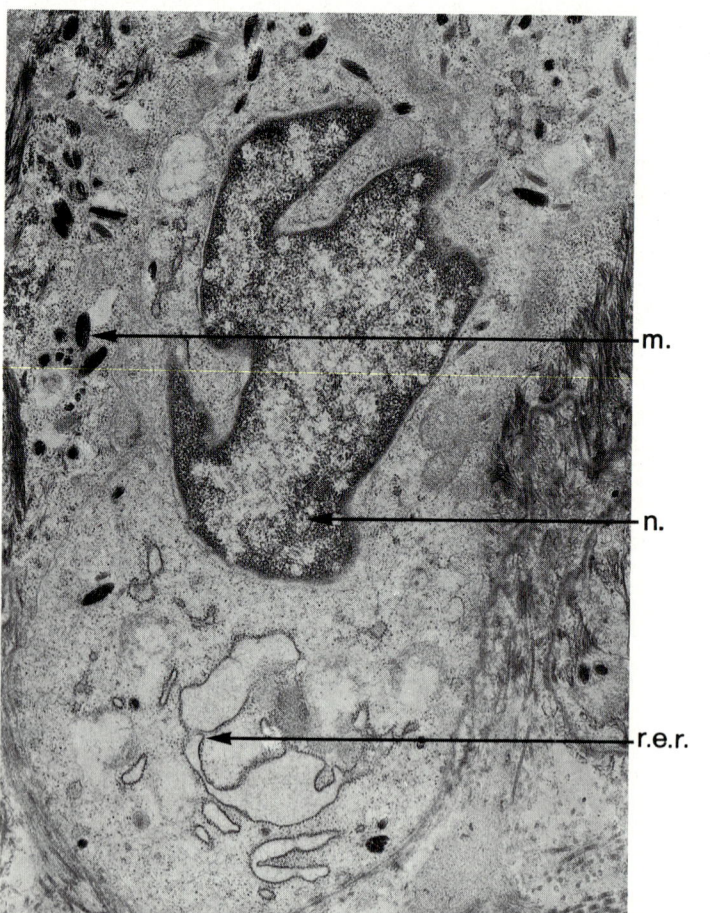

FIGURE 1–5 A melanocyte is distinguished by the presence of melanosomes and the absence of tonofibrils. *m.,* melanosome; *n.,* nucleus; *r.e.r.,* rough endoplasmic reticulum. (×17,000.) (Courtesy of Ken Hashimoto, M.D.)

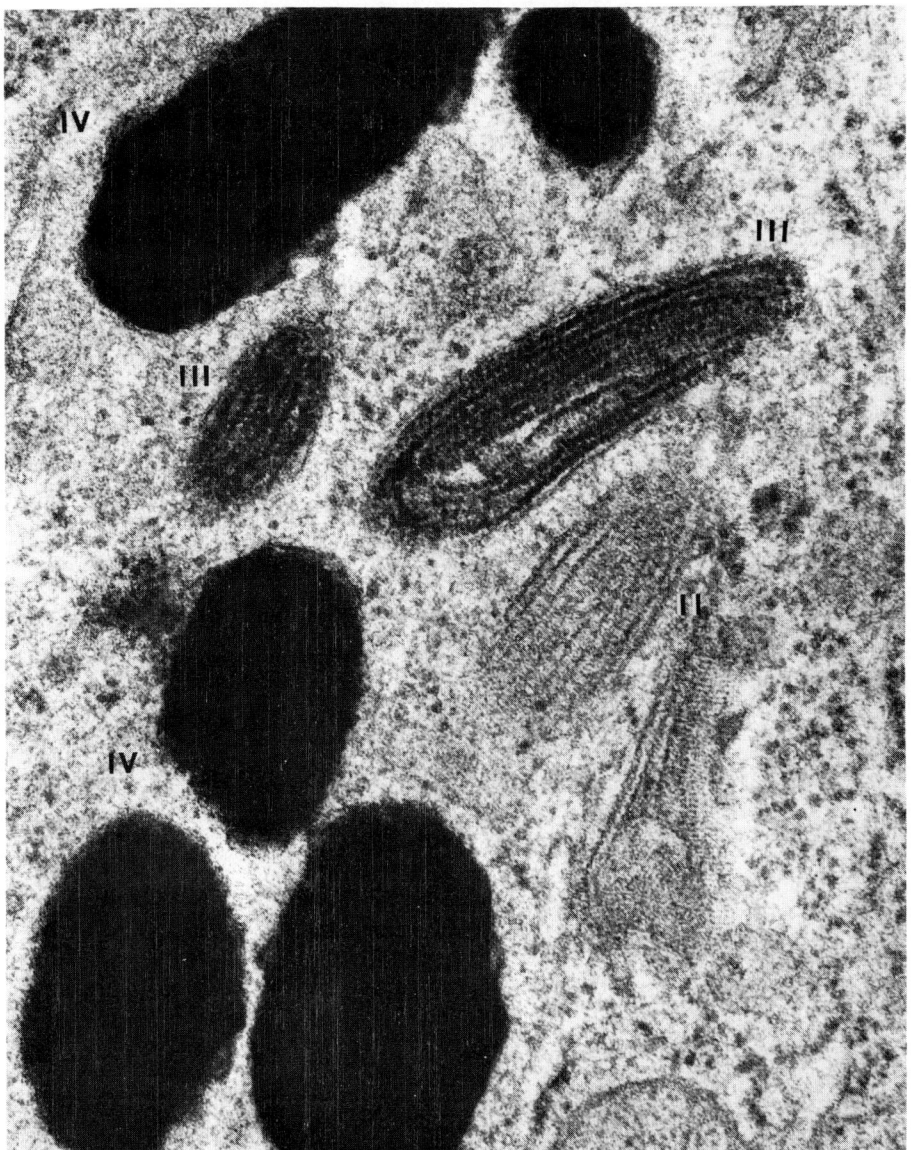

FIGURE 1–6 Medium-power electron micrograph depicting melanosomes in several stages of melanization within a normal melanocyte. Stages II, III, and IV are shown. (× 65,000.) (Courtesy of Dr. K. Jimbow.)

to the formation of the highly complex polymer, melanin. As melanin is formed, it is laid down on the inner membranes of the melanosome. Melanosomes are then dispersed within the cytoplasm of melanocytes for later transfer to keratinocytes. Such transfer occurs through the active phagocytosis of melanosome-laden dendrites by keratinocytes.

The Langerhans cell is a dendritic cell that contains racquet-shaped organelles (Fig. 1–7). Although its origin and purpose are still disputed, some authors believe it has a phagocytic or immunocytic function.[8] Indeterminate dendritic cells are also present in the epidermis. These Merkel cells have nei-

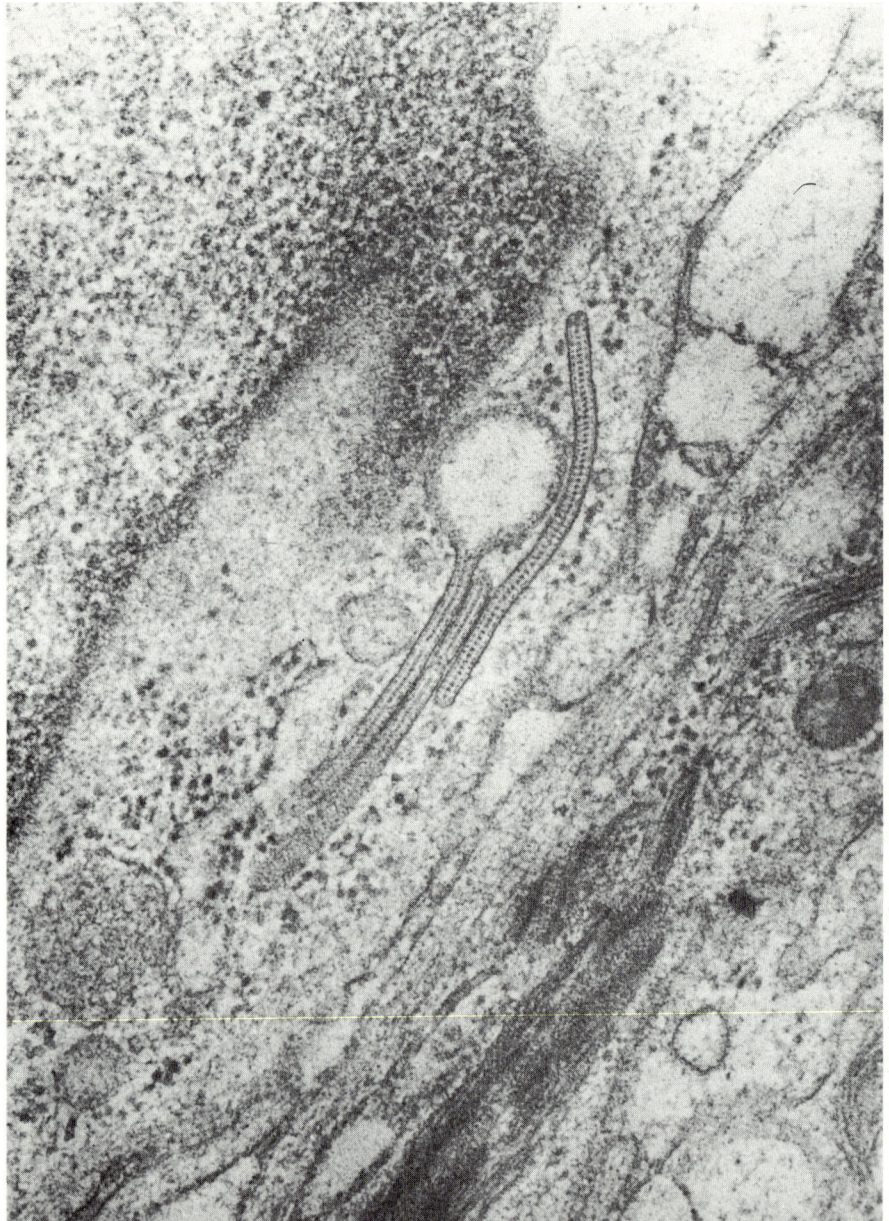

FIGURE 1–7 Langerhans' granules have a tennis-racquet configuration resulting from vesicular dilatation at one end of the organelle. (×82,600.) (Courtesy of Alvin Zelickson, M.D.)

ther melanosomes nor racquet-shaped organelles but may possibly be precursors of either melanocytes or Langerhans' cells.

THE APPENDAGES

The appendages of the skin include the hair, nails, sebaceous glands, and sweat glands. These structures are derived from an invagination or downgrowth of epidermal germinative buds into the dermis. The sebaceous and apocrine glands usually differentiate from the germinative buds that give rise to the hair follicle. The eccrine gland differentiates from a separate epidermal germinative bud.

HAIR

Hair begins to develop at about the third month of fetal life. A cylindrical invagination of epidermal cells called the follicle produces hair, a tubular structure of tightly cemented keratinized and pigmented cells. Melanin granules line up longitudinally in the cortex of pigmented hairs and are absent in white hairs. The cortex is the thickest part of the hair and is made up of keratinized cells. The medulla consists of loosely connected keratinized cells interspersed with air spaces. Color tones of hair are greatly influenced by the large air spaces found within the medulla.[1]

The hair follicle can produce either a fine, thin, unmedullated vellus hair (Fig. 1–8) or a long, coarse, medullated terminal hair. All follicles initially produce vellus hair and later, depending on body location, produce terminal hairs. Scalp hairs increase in diameter from birth until about 12 years of age. Axillary hair follicles produce vellus hair until adolescence and then change to making terminal hair. In male pattern baldness, the process is reversed as scalp follicles return to producing fine vellus hairs.

Hair grows in cycles that alternate with periods of rest. The growth phase is called anagen and the resting phase is called telogen. There is also a brief transitional period from anagen to telogen known as catagen. As a phase of anagen starts, a new hair either can grow alongside an existing hair within a follicle or can push it out. The greatest anagenic activity occurs during puberty. The number of resting hair follicles increases in the late teen years. Growth of chin and mustache hairs is influenced by androgens, which also play a role in male pattern baldness.[9]

The rate of human hair growth is about 0.4 mm per day.[10, 11] Short rest periods are generally followed by growth periods of about four or five years,

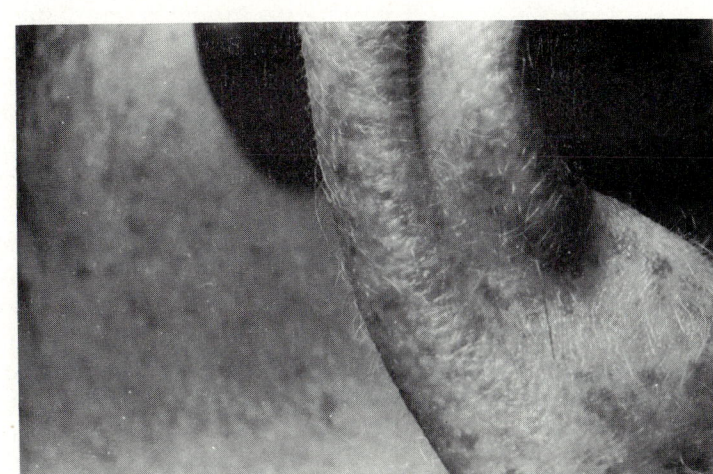

FIGURE 1–8 Vellus hair covers the pinna of the ear.

although some scalp follicles may remain in anagen for as long as eight years. Genetically determined properties of hair, such as waviness, curliness, and straightness, depend on the position of hair fibers in the follicle and on the angle of insertion of the hair bulb in the scalp.[1] Other properties of hair, such as luster, depend on anatomical changes in the hair, as discussed further on.

The terminal hair shaft consists of an outer cuticle, a cortex, and a central medulla (the medulla is lacking in vellus hair). Deep in the follicle the cuticle merges with the inner root sheath lining the follicle, firmly anchoring the hair shaft. The sheen of hair is determined by the degree of cuticular smoothness because cuticular cells are arranged like shingles on a roof, with one edge raised free. If the free cuticular cell edges are raised at a high angle, the hair looks dull, since light falling on the hair is broken up as if reflected from the surface of a choppy sea. If the free edges lie flat against the surface, light hits a smooth flat plane, giving the hair a high degree of luster. The hair cuticle also protects the cortex from fraying. "Split ends" are due to the absence of cuticle on the ends of long hair.

SEBACEOUS GLANDS

The sebaceous gland arises from an embryonic bulge on the side of the hair follicle. Embryonal hair follicles, even before they have started to form a hair, develop two lateral bulges. The upper one eventually differentiates into a sebaceous gland, and the lower one becomes the site of attachment for an arrector pili muscle. Since embryonic hair buds appear in a cephalocaudal sequence, sebaceous gland development proceeds similarly. Therefore, in the fetus at three and one-half months, sebaceous glands are well developed on the scalp and face but are not present elsewhere. At birth, sebaceous glands are well differentiated. Afterwards, they diminish rapidly in size and remain small until puberty. Their growth spurt at birth is probably due to stimulation by maternal androgens and possibly to fetal steroid production. At puberty, full development takes place, with sebaceous glands attaining a larger volume in boys than in girls. Increase in gland size and sebum secretion are under the control of testicular testosterone in men and of ovarian and adrenal androgens in women. All androgens probably exert their effect through a metabolite, dihydrotestosterone (DHT). Both cytoplasmic and nuclear receptors[12] for DHT have been found within sebaceous glands.[13] The pituitary gland appears to be necessary for maintenance of sebaceous gland function, perhaps through a sebotropic moiety on prolactin or growth hormone molecules.[14] Estrogens can diminish glandular size and sebaceous secretion, but their effects may be overcome by testosterone administration. Prednisone can decrease sebum production in women and eunuchs but not in normal men. Except in the meibomian glands of the eyelid, there is no neural regulation of sebaceous gland secretion. The control of sebaceous gland size and activity is entirely hormonal in nature, with androgens playing the dominant role.

Individual sebaceous glands consist of clusters of acini that develop from epidermal outpouchings on the upper third of hair follicles. The short excretory ducts most frequently empty into the pilary canal and only rarely directly into the epidermis. Development of individual sebaceous cells results in the intracellular synthesis and accumulation of lipid vacuoles, so that eventually the cell consists of a fine network of cytoplasm holding large lipid droplets. The nucleus is distorted, and when the cell bursts, releasing its lipid contents, the nucleus disintegrates. Sebaceous secretion is holocrine, that is, the whole cell dies and is excreted with its products. The lipid products in sebum consist of triglycerides, wax esters, squalene, cholesterol esters, and cholesterol. The function of sebum may be that of a vestigial pheromone (an odoriferous sexual attractant), as even fresh sterile sebum has a distinctive odor.[1]

The largest sebaceous glands are located on the forehead and face. Sebaceous follicles are gigantic sebaceous glands associated with tiny vellus hairs.[16] They have widely dilated follicular ducts, "patulous pores," to which sebaceous gland lobules are connected by their short ducts. When the follicular ducts become impacted with sebum, keratinous debris, and bacteria, a comedone results. An inflammatory lesion of acne is produced when a comedone ruptures, releasing its contents into the dermis.

APOCRINE GLANDS

Apocrine glands, like sebaceous glands, develop embryonically from an appendageal bud arising from the hair follicle. However, apocrine glands develop only after the hair is formed and the sebaceous glands have differentiated. The embryonic bud develops in the five- to six-month-old fetus, and at birth the apocrine gland is structurally complete but functionless. From age seven through adolescence, the glands become larger and begin to function. Gonadal hormones seem to be necessary for initiation but not for maintenance of the gland's functions. Both cholinergic and adrenergic stimuli result in apocrine gland secretion.[1]

The individual apocrine gland consists of a long, narrow, keratinizing duct and a coiled secretory unit. The duct leading from the coiled segment runs parallel to a hair follicle and opens into the pilary canal near the surface (above the entrance of the sebaceous gland duct). The coiled secretory units of small glands lie in the dermis, but those of larger glands may extend deeply into the subcutaneous fat. Many interluminal connections exist in the secretory portion of one gland and sometimes between adjacent glands. Individual secretory cells have one or two nuclei, and their cytoplasm is filled with granules of different sizes, shapes, and staining properties. The secretory unit contains one cell type, in contrast to the two cell types found in eccrine glands.[1] The function of the cellular granules is not well understood. Dark granules found above the nucleus have been described variously as "presumptive keratin granules,"[17] as lysosomes,[18] and as granules containing lipid, pigment, and iron.[19] Rarely, apocrine sweat may be green or blue, containing lipofuscin pigment granules found in the cytoplasm of secretory cells.[20] The secretory cells lie on regularly arranged contractile myoepithelial cells, which in turn rest on a thick basement membrane. The transition between the secretory unit and the duct is abrupt, and no myoepithelial cells are found around the duct.

Apocrine glands secrete small amounts of a viscous fluid containing protein, reducing sugars, and ammonia.[21] They cannot be called true sweat glands, as they seldom respond to heat stimuli.[1] Since their mode of secretion varies from merocrine through holocrine, they cannot be considered apocrine[7] with complete accuracy. However, the name "apocrine gland" has persisted because under the light microscope the top of the cell appears to be pinched off during secretion. The largest and most numerous glands are found in the axilla, where a single apocrine gland in association with a single eccrine gland forms "the axillary organ." The more watery secretion of the eccrine gland helps to spread the viscous apocrine secretions onto the axillary surface.[1] Axillary apocrine secretions become strongly malodorous when they are decomposed by bacterial flora. Axillary odor is strongest in adolescence and young adulthood and becomes weaker with maturity. The axillary odor may have served as a primordial pheromone and perhaps played a primitive role in sexual attraction. Apocrine glands may also occur in the mons pubis, perineum, genitalia, face, scalp, and abdomen.[22] The mammary glands, the ceruminous glands, and the glands of Moll on the eyelids are modified apocrine glands.

ECCRINE GLANDS

Eccrine glands develop directly from their own fetal epidermal buds. In the 16th fetal week, these buds are present on the palms and soles and by the 22nd week appear elsewhere on the body in a cephalocaudal sequence. Eccrine glands begin to function only 24 to 48 hours after birth, first on the palms and soles where function is continuous and then on the rest of the body. Palmar, axillary, and forehead glands respond sharply to emotional stimuli, whereas all the other eccrine glands respond mainly to environmental heat. The average adult at rest produces about 65 kilocalories (kcal) per hour while an adult working in heavy industry produces about 300 kcal per hour.

Body heat can be lost by irradiation and convection only when the temperature of the external environment is lower than that of the body. At warmer temperatures, heat may be lost by evaporation. Even evaporative heat loss through sweating may be limited by high humidity. At 40.88°C (105°F) and 15 per cent humidity, a person can feel comfortable, but as the humidity rises, his discomfort increases, and he begins to suffer heat exhaustion.[23] Although thermoregulation is an important function of eccrine sweat glands, the exact relationship between heat stress and sweat response is still poorly understood in many respects.

The individual eccrine gland is composed of a duct and a secretory unit. The duct consists of three parts: a spiral intraepidermal segment, an elongated helical dermal segment, and a supracoiled segment lying just above the secretory part of the gland. The portion of the duct closer to the surface has one layer of keratinizing cells, while the lower portion is made up of a double layer of cuboidal cells. The coiled secretory part of the gland consists of a cell layer containing two cell types: small, basophilic "dark cells" with a nucleus displaced toward the lumen and larger "clear cells" whose nuclei rest in mid-cell. Both cells have a truncated pyramidal shape and rest on a layer of contractile myoepithelial cells. The coil is surrounded by a basement membrane. A loose net of elastic fibers surrounds the secretory portion. Both the duct and secretory portions of the eccrine gland are richly vascularized. On stimulation by acetylcholine, secretions are formed in the secretory coil, then altered in passage through the duct. Normal sweat contains sodium chloride, potassium, lactate, urea, and small amounts of amino acids, calcium, phosphorus, proteins, and iron but is hypotonic to plasma.

Individual eccrine sweat glands are surrounded by a basket-like nerve network that originates from postganglionic fibers of the para-aortic ganglia. Acetylcholine is released by these nerve endings; therefore, physiologically these plexuses are cholinergic. Sweating responses to intradermal injections of acetylcholine can be produced at lower concentrations in men than in women. There is a great deal of unexplained individual variation in sweating responses, especially those on the palms and in the axillae. Eccrine sweat glands also respond to epinephrine. This adrenergic response is not blocked by atropine, so it cannot be mediated by acetylcholine release.

Adrenergic stimulation of eccrine sweating is prolonged, equal in both sexes, unaffected by changes in skin temperatures, and greatest on the palms. Cholinergic stimulation produces different responses, depending on skin temperature (greater at high temperatures), season (greater in summer), and acclimatization. Acclimatization, which occurs after days of prolonged heat exposure, refers to an increase in the sweating rate with a concurrent decrease in the sodium content of sweat. During acclimatization, sensitivity of the sweating response to acetylcholine remains unchanged. Therefore, the change may take place within the enzyme systems of the sweat gland.[1]

THE NAIL

The nail is a keratinous plate lying on top of a digit. Morphological features of the nail are best described diagrammatically (see page 6). The nail matrix is a wedge of epidermal tissue lying at an oblique angle to the skin surface at the level of the terminal interphalangeal joint. The nail plate is a flat, firm layer of dead keratinized cells extending distally over the epidermis from the nail matrix. The nail bed is the stratified epidermis lying below the nail plate and tightly adherent to it.

The nail bed consists of epidermal cells that do not form a stratum corneum and do not contribute to the growth of the nail plate. However, cornified cells produced by the nail bed are pushed forward by the distal growth of the nail plate and then appear as debris under its free edge.[25] The distal groove is the site of separation of the nail plate from the nail bed. The hyponychium is the epidermis found under the distal free edge of the nail plate. The proximal nail fold is the fold of skin covering the nail plate at its origin in the matrix. The lateral nail folds are the skin folds on both sides of the nail plate.

Differentiation of epidermis into nail matrix begins in the ninth week of fetal life, when a linear wedge of germinative cells originating in the primitive epidermis grows proximally into deeper tissues to give rise to the nail matrix.[24] The invagination of cells forms the nail matrix and develops into the overlapping proximal nail fold, which is continuous on its sides with the lateral nail folds. Nail growth proceeds in a distal direction from the matrix, forming a plate that slowly moves over the nail bed. A thin layer of cornified epidermal cells, the cuticle, grows from the proximal fold to cover the emerging nail plate. The lunula, an elliptical white crescent seen through the proximal part of the nail plate, is the part of the matrix first to actively produce the nail plate. Production of the nail plate occurs when the matrix cells mature, become filled with keratin, and eventually lose their nuclei. The cells then become transparent in the area known as the keratogenous zone. Injury to the nail matrix may result in imperfect keratinization, leading to nuclear retention. Imperfect keratinization may be seen as small white spots, nail "pitting," or nail deformity.

There is no subcutaneous tissue under the dermis of the nail, and the dermis adheres directly to the periosteal tissue. In the nail bed dermis, capillaries run in dermal ridges parallel to the length of the digit. Their disruption, therefore, results in splinter hemorrhages. Clubbing may result from fibrovascular hyperplasia of the dermis below the nail bed and matrix. Glomera are specialized arteriovenous shunts present in the nail bed and volar digit tips (see further on).

The keratinous substance of the nail plate is similar to that of hair, having a large protein component and a high sulfur content. The nail is a porous structure that readily absorbs water. The nail of infants suffering from cystic fibrosis has a high chloride content.[26] Calcium in the nail increases with age or after trauma. The normal rate of growth of fingernails is about 3.5 mm per month. Toenails grow much more slowly. Malnutrition adversely affects nail growth.

THE DERMIS

Lying between the epidermis and the subcutaneous fat, the dermis consists of fibrous elements, amorphous ground substance, free cells, nerves, blood vessels, and lymphatic vessels. Morphologically, the dermis is divided into the papillary and reticular layers. The papillary layer forms the upper part of the dermis and interdigitates with the epidermis. It is more cellular and more vascularized than the lower or reticular dermis. The reticular dermis is distinguished by a thick meshwork of collagen and elastic fibers. Smooth muscle is found in the arrectores pilorum muscle. Other smooth muscle fibers are found only in arterial vessels, the areola, nipple, penis, scrotum, and perineum, where they produce wrinkling by contraction.

Fetal dermis is free of fibrils in the first two to four months. By the 20th to 40th week of intrauterine life, a moderate number of elastic and collagen fibers are found. During this period, the fetal dermis also changes from an organ rich in water, sugar, and hyaluronic acid to one composed mainly of collagen and sulfated mucopolysaccharides.[27] Both dermis and epidermis probably exert inductive influences on each other during cutaneous morphogenesis.[28-30]

After birth, further changes occur. Collagen bundles continue to become thicker until 20 years of age, and elastic fibers increase in number and thickness throughout life. Hyaluronate and dermatan sulfate contents decrease during infancy until adolescence. Both the sulfated and total acidic glycosaminoglycans decrease by 50 per cent from birth to adult life. Two thirds of the polysaccharide in adult skin is dermatan sulfate.[31]

COLLAGEN

Over 90 per cent of the dry weight of dermal tissue consists of collagen. The basic tropocollagen molecule produced by fibroblasts consists of three polypeptide chains rich in proline and hydroxyproline. These form the alpha chains of a stable triple helix. Tensile strength is produced by opposing twists in the individual chains (right-handed) and in the helix (left-handed) and by intramolecular covalent bonds.

Tropocollagen molecules are assembled within fibroblasts and extruded after the hydroxylation of proline to hydroxyproline and lysine to hydroxylysine and glucose or after glucose-galactose units have been added to hydroxylysine residues.[32] Tropocollagen then forms cross-linkages with other tropocollagen molecules. As the collagen ages and the number of cross-linkages increases, it becomes less soluble.[33] Cross-linking results from the formation of alyllysine through the oxidative deamination of the alpha-amino groups of lysine and hydroxylysine residues. This process requires copper and is inhibited by penicillamine.

Several tropocollagen molecules thus combine to form a filament. Bundles of filaments form microfibrils, which align in a parallel order to become fibrils (Fig. 1–9). Fibrils are the smallest collagen unit to be seen under the light microscope. These fibrils show cross-striations with periodicity of 640 Å[34] and aggregate to form unbranched fibers. Reticulin fibers consist of fine collagen fibrils with 640 Å periodicity. They are argyrophilic and can be considered lipoglycoproteins, since they contain 11 per cent firmly bound fatty acid.[1]

Collagen fibers confer on skin its great tensile strength, and also limit the extent of deformation of skin caused by pulling on it. Tensile strength is the

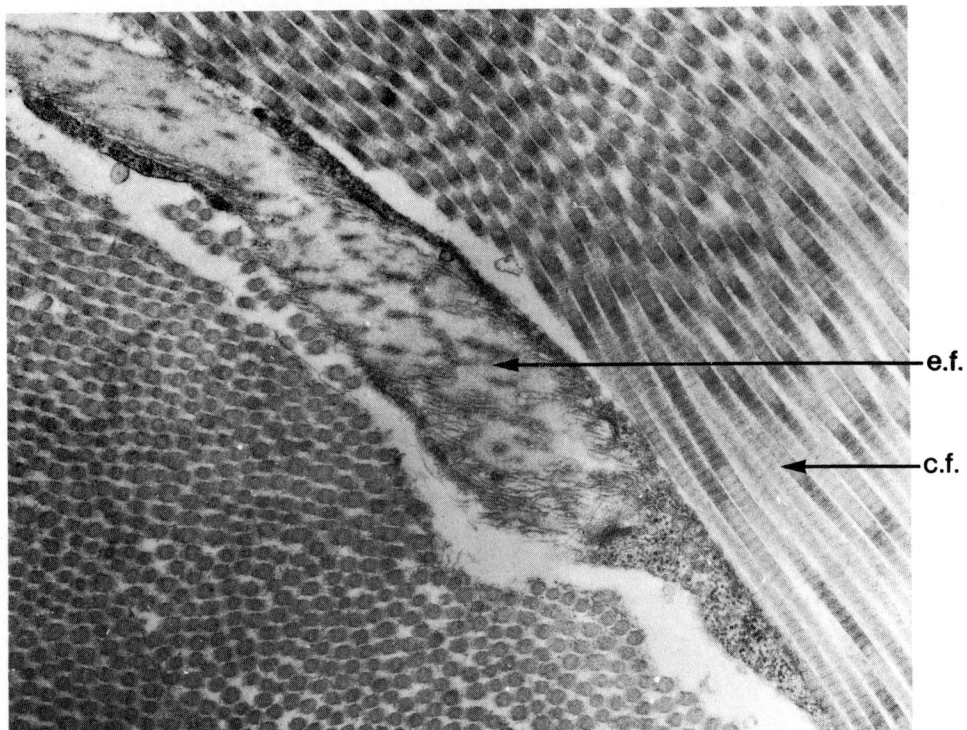

FIGURE 1–9 Longitudinally cut collagen fibrils have a width of about 1000 Å and a distinct cross-banding, 680 Å apart. An elastic fiber consists of non-collagenous fibrils embedded in homogeneous elastic. *e.f.*, elastic fiber; *c.f.*, collagen fibrils. (×55,000.) (Courtesy of Richard Wood, Ph.D.)

resistance to the amount of force exerted to pull a material apart. The arrangement of collagen fibers in a loose meshwork allows them to become aligned in the direction of stress and to absorb more stress as this aligning process proceeds.[35]

ELASTIC FIBERS

Elastic fibers impart to the skin the ability to resume its original shape after being stretched. They form perpendicular, palisading branching networks in the papillary dermis. In the reticular dermis, coarse elastic fibers intertwine with collagen fibers. Elastic fibers anchor the arrectores pilorum muscles to hair follicle bulbs and form supportive networks around the secretory portions of the sweat glands (Fig. 1–10). Elastic fibers appear in the fetus at 22 weeks, and an elastic network is present after 32 weeks.[36]

The elastic fiber consists of a branched fibrillar tube containing inner amorphous components. The protein components of both the tubular and amorphous parts differ from those of collagen. The amino acid composition

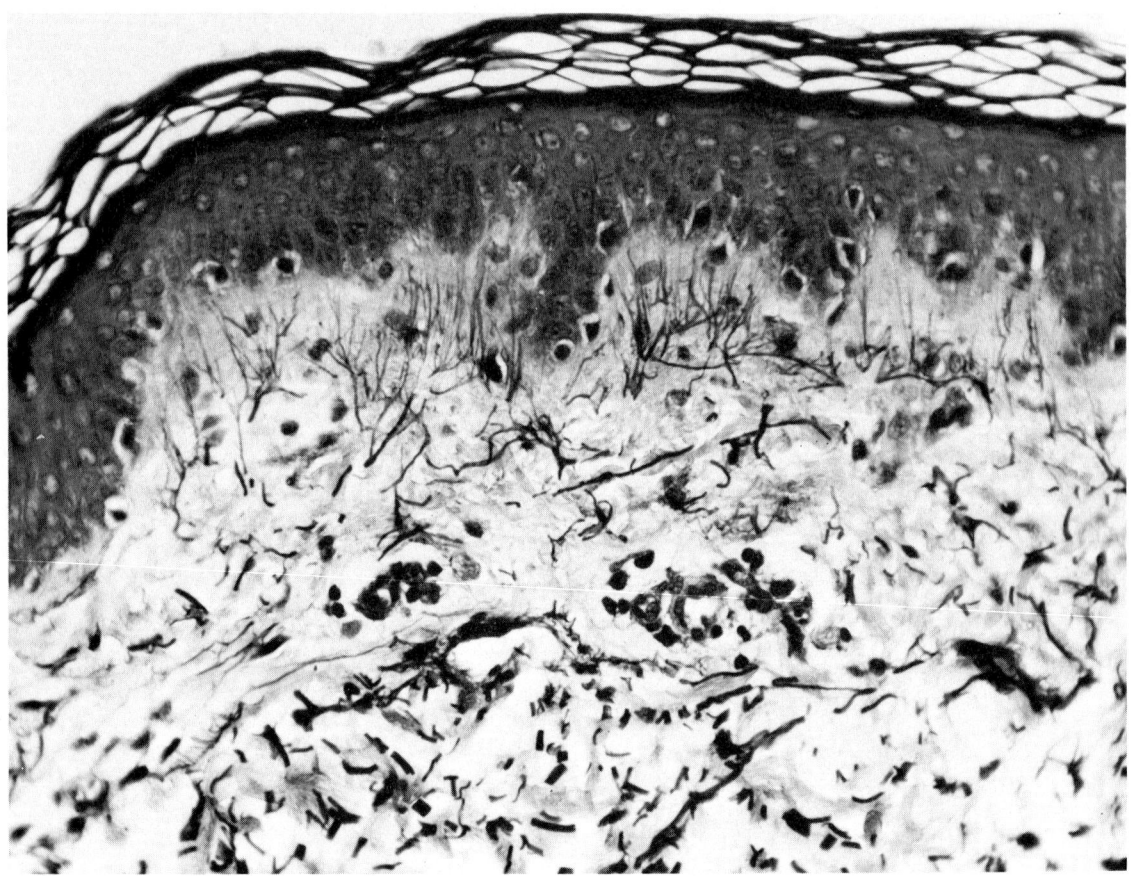

FIGURE 1–10 The thin elastic fibers in the papillary dermis appear to be mostly oriented perpendicular to the surface, whereas those in the reticular dermis are thicker and seemingly arranged mostly parallel to the skin surface. (×462.)

of the amorphous part is similar to that of the elastin precursor, tropoelastin, which requires the copper-dependent enzyme lysyl oxidase for its formation. This enzyme plays a role in the formation of the unique amino acids contained in elastin, desmosin, and isodesmosine. Newly synthesized elastin quickly enters a three-dimensional cross-linking process that renders it insoluble.[1]

GROUND SUBSTANCE

The dermal matrix consists of an amorphous ground substance that cushions and lubricates the dermal constituents, such as the collagen fibers, and helps nourish and support the epidermis and the vascular system. It contains metabolic products of parenchymal and connective tissue cells, the soluble precursors of fibrous proteins, and complexes of glycoproteins and proteoglycans.[37] Proteoglycans consist of a central protein core with polysaccharide side chains.[38] The major polysaccharide moieties consist of three glycosamino glycans: hyaluronate, dermatan sulfate (chondroitin sulfate B), and chondroitin sulfate A. These are hydrophilic substances that bind water in the dermis. As mucopolysaccharides decrease in the dermis with age, and as collagen increases, the hydration of the dermis decreases, and the diffusion characteristics of the ground substance change.

Lysosomal hyaluronidase may play a role in the degradation of dermal proteoglycans, although such a hyaluronidase has not been isolated.[1] Various hyaluronidases isolated from snake venom and several species of bacteria are capable of degrading chondroitin sulfates A and C but not chondroitin sulfate B.

CELLULAR COMPONENTS OF THE DERMIS

Fibroblasts derived from mesenchyme are the most numerous cells in the dermis and are responsible for the synthesis of both the fibrous components and the ground substance of the dermis. Other cells found in the dermis include: macrophages, mast cells, histiocytes, lymphocytes, neutrophils, plasma cells, and eosinophils.

Macrophages remove foreign material and dead cells from the dermis by digesting them with lysosomal enzymes. Macrophages process antigens, participate in both cellular and humoral immune responses, and also produce interferon.[39] Because macrophages also synthesize and metabolize lipids, lipid storage diseases may result if they malfunction.

Mast cells contain heparin and histamine. Heparin prevents blood clotting, inhibits hyaluronidase, and accelerates lipid clearance. In the skin, histamine mediates early inflammation, hyperemia, and pruritus.

CUTANEOUS VASCULATURE

The cutaneous vasculature controls body temperature, affects blood pressure, and carries nutrients to the skin. Blood flow in the skin may vary from

0.5 to 150 ml per 100 mg tissue per minute.[40] The vascular network is of mesodermal origin and varies from region to region, depending on dermal thickness, number and type of dermal appendages present, and the relationship of the dermis to the underlying structures. Cutaneous vessels arise from the perforator arteries of segmental arteries. Formerly, the dermis was believed to contain superficial and deep plexuses, but Winkelman[41] and Saunders[42] demonstrated interconnecting vessels at all dermal levels. In addition to widespread dermal anastomoses, there is also a rich periappendageal vascular network. In areas where the papillae are long and narrow, long capillary loops run perpendicular to the skin surface.

Cutaneous terminal arterioles end in metarterioles that have a muscular wall, form a preferential channel toward the venular circulation, and regulate flow to capillary beds through precapillary sphincters. Contraction of precapillary sphincters shunts blood through the preferential channel, bypassing the capillary bed. Venules also control capillary flow by their ability to dilate and constrict passively.[43]

Cutaneous vessels, especially in the reticular dermis of the fingertip and nail bed, also possess glomera (arteriovenous anastomotic shunts). The glomus originates as an arterial or arteriolar branch and terminates in an accompanying vein or venule. Glomera have a small lumen, are contractile, and are under autonomic control. They play a role in temperature regulation by increasing blood flow through the shunts and decreasing capillary bed flow, thereby decreasing oxygen supply to the target tissue.

Cutaneous vessels in various parts of the body are affected differently by the sympathetic system and circulating pressor agents. For example, after the inhalation of amyl nitrate, the skin of the blush area (head, neck, upper chest) undergoes a deep blush reaction as the cutaneous vessels on the extremities constrict.[44]

Lymphatic vessels are abundantly present in the dermis. Embryologically, they arise from primitive venous channels, but in the adult they can arise only from the ruptured ends of existing lymphatics. The lymphatics originate in large sinuses in the papillary dermis and then drain through a dermal network to subcutaneous lymphatic trunks. The most important function of the lymphatics is to reabsorb serum proteins that have left the arterial circulation because of high osmotic pressures but cannot directly reenter the venous circulation. If these proteins remain in tissue, edema results because their osmotic "pull" leads to fluid accumulation. Lymphatic vessels are also vital for carrying antigen-laden macrocytes and other immunocytes to and from the site of reaction in cell-mediated immunity.

CUTANEOUS INNERVATION

Cholinesterase-rich structures first appear in the dermis at about the fifth week of fetal life, well before epidermal appendages develop. Nerve trunks can be discerned in the second month. Specialized nerve endings form later. Meissner's corpuscles start forming in the fourth month, and pacinian corpuscles appear between the third and sixth months.

The cutaneous nerves are one of the body's main sensory accesses to its environment. Nerve fibers can be classified as type A, B, or C, according to their diameter and action potential. Type A fibers have the largest diameter, the shortest electrical spike potential, and the highest velocity of conduction. Type C fibers are narrower, have a wider based spike, and conduct more slowly. Mechanoreceptors seem to be largely type A fibers; pain, itch, cold, and warmth sensations seem to be carried by type C fibers. Type B fibers have characteristics between A and C. The specific sensation one experiences appears not to depend upon the position of morphological characteristics of the nerve fibers stimulated but instead on the spatial arrangements of these fibers within tissues,[45] the frequency and sequence of neural volleys fired, and the reception of these volleys by the spinal cord and brain. Sensation depends on the frequency of impulses, the number of fibers stimulated, and various inhibiting and reinforcing factors in the central nervous system.

There are several types of nerve endings in the skin: a superficial dermal nerve network, a hair follicle network, mucocutaneous end organs, Meissner's corpuscles, and Vater-Pacini corpuscles. The dermal nerve network, consisting of nerves of varying densities, is the chief sensory receptor. Nerve nets around hair follicles form more ordered patterns and serve as tactile receptors. In mucocutaneous tissues and erogenous zones, the nerve endings are rolled into coils and resemble the "basket" type of nerve networks found around hair follicles.

Meissner's corpuscles are similar in structure, except that the nerve endings are flattened and encapsulated. Meissner's corpuscles are found in the volar surfaces of hands and feet and serve some function in two-point discrimination. Pacinian corpuscles are the largest and most highly organized nerve endings. They are found deep in the dermis and are most numerous on the digits and the clitoris. The nerves entering a pacinian corpuscle are heavily myelinated and execute many lamellar turns within a fibrous, fluid-filled onion-like structure. Without the capsule, the nerve endings would greatly resemble those found in the dermal network. The pacinian corpuscle is at least partly responsible for the sensation of deep pressure, and also seems to play a role in regulating the arteriovenous shunts in the dermis by sensing the volume of local blood supply. Merkel-Ranvier corpuscles are disk-shaped touch receptors found on the distal parts of the limbs.

All cutaneous sensory nerve endings contain non-specific cholinesterases. Nerves of the dermal and hair follicle networks also contain specific cholinesterases. All effector nerves to the skin and its appendages are postganglionic fibers of the paravertebral chain ganglia and are therefore sympathetic. Yet some have acetylcholine as their neurotransmitter and therefore have a cholinergic function. Eccrine sweat glands respond to both acetylcholine and norepinephrine. Cutaneous blood vessels and arrector pili muscles respond to norepinephrine. The axon reflex is a phenomenon in which impulses initiated in sensory nerves are relayed antidromically down other branches of the sensory nerves. It helps to explain why a local stimulus causes reactive changes in an area of skin wider than that directly affected by the stimulus.

SUBCUTANEOUS TISSUE

Deep to the dermis lies the adipose tissue, which serves to cushion underlying structures against external trauma and to insulate them from rapid temperature change. Subcutaneous fatty tissue, metabolically distinct from adult fat, is first formed in the 14th week of fetal life from primitive mesenchymal cells.

Fibrous septa traverse the subcutaneous fat to anchor the dermis to the underlying periosteum or fascial planes. Contained in the subcutaneous adipose tissue are nerves, blood vessels, reticuloendothelial cells, and transient white blood cells.

REFERENCES

1. Montagna, W., and Parakkal, P. F.: The Structure and Function of the Skin. 3rd ed. New York, Academic Press, 1974.
2. Ebling, F. J.: The normal skin. In: Rook, A., Wilkinson, D. S., and Ebling, F. J. G. (eds.): Textbook of Dermatology. Philadelphia, F. A. Davis, 1968, pp. 4–14.
3. Lever, W. F., and Schaumberg-Lever, G.: Histopathology of the Skin. 5th ed. Philadelphia, J. B. Lippincott, 1975, pp. 13–15.
4. Rothberg, S., Crounse, R. G., and Lee, J. L.: Glycine-C^{14}-incorporation into the proteins of normal stratum corneum and the abnormal stratum corneum of psoriasis. J. Invest. Dermatol., 37:497, 1961.
5. Weinstein, G. D., and Frost, P.: Replacement kinetics. In Fitzpatrick, T. B., Arndt, K. A., Clark, W. H., et al. (eds.): Dermatology in General Medicine. New York, McGraw-Hill, 1971, pp. 78–87.
6. Szabo, G.: Photobiology of melanogenesis: Cytological aspects with reference to differences in racial coloration. In: Montagna, W., and Hu, F. (eds.): Advances in Biology of Skin. Vol. 8. The Pigmentary System. Oxford, Pergamon Press, 1968, pp. 379–396.
7. Mitchell, R. E.: The skin of the Australian Aborigine; a light and electron microscopical study. Aust. J. Dermatol., 9:314, 1968.
8. Shelley, W. B., and Juhlin, L.: Selective Uptake of Contact Allergens by the Langerhans Cell. Arch. Dermatol. 113:187, 1977.
9. Puche, R. C., Pecoraro, V., Astore, I., and Barman, J. M.: Relationships between the urinary 17-ketosteroids and some characteristics of the human scalp hair. Steroidologia, 2:121, 1971.
10. Myers, R. J., and Hamilton, J. B.: Regeneration and rate of growth of hairs in man. Ann. N.Y. Acad. Sci., 53:562, 1951.
11. Saitoh, M., Uzuka, M., Sakamoto, M., and Kobori, T.: Rate of hair growth. In: Montagna, W., and Dobson, R. L. (eds.): Advances in Biology of Skin. Vol. 9. Hair Growth. Oxford, Pergamon Press, 1969, pp. 183–201.
12. Takayasu, S., and Adachi, K.: Hormonal control of metabolism in hamster costovertebral glands. J. Invest. Dermatol., 55:13, 1970.
13. Fang, S., and Liao, S.: Androgen receptors. Steroid- and tissue-specific retention of a 17 beta-hydroxy-5 alpha-androstan-3-one protein complex by the cell of nuclei of ventral prostate. J. Biol. Chem., 246:16, 1971.
14. Ebling, F. J., Ebling, E., and Skinner, J.: The influence of pituitary hormones on the response of the sebaceous glands of the rat to testosterone. J. Endocrinol., 45:245, 1969.
15. Montagna, W., and Ford, D. M.: Histology and cytochemistry of human skin. XXXII. The eyelid. Arch. Dermatol., 100:328, 1969.
16. Kligman, A. M., and Shelley, W. B.: An investigation of the biology of the human sebaceous gland. J. Invest. Dermatol., 30:99, 1958.
17. Munger, B. L.: The cytology of apocrine sweat glands. II. Human. Z. Zellforsch., 68:837, 1965.
18. Biempca, L., and Montes, L. F.: Secretory epithelium of the large axillary sweat glands. A cytochemical and electron microscope study. Am. J. Anat., 117:47, 1965.
19. Ellis, R. A.: Eccrine, sebaceous and apocrine glands. In: Zelickson, A. S., Ultra Structure of Normal and Abnormal Skin. Philadelphia, Lea & Febiger, 1967, pp. 132–162.
20. Hurley, H. J.: Diseases of apocrine sweat glands. In: Fitzpatrick, T. B., Arndt, K. A., Clark, W. H., et al. (eds.): Dermatology in General Medicine. New York, McGraw-Hill, 1971, p. 389.
21. Shelley, W. B., and Hurley, H. J.: The physiology of the human axillary apocrine sweat gland. J. Invest. Dermatol., 20:285, 1953.
22. Pinkus, H.: Embryology of hair. In: Montagna, W., and Ellis, R. H. (eds.): The Biology of Hair Growth. New York, Academic Press, 1958, pp. 1–32.
23. Cage, G. W.: Eccrine and apocrine secretory glands. In: Fitzpatrick, T. B., Arndt, K. A., Clark, W. H., et al. (eds.): Dermatology in General Medicine. New York, McGraw-Hill, 1971, pp. 103–109.
24. Zaias, N.: Embryology of the human nail. Arch. Dermatol., 87:37, 1963.

25. Zaias, N.: The movement of the nail bed. J. Invest. Dermatol., *48*:402, 1967.
26. Kopito, L., Mahmoodian, A., Townley, R. R., et al.: Studies in cytstic fibrosis: Analysis of nail clippings for sodium and potassium. N. Engl. J. Med., *272*:504, 1965.
27. Odland, G. F., and Short, J. M.: Structure of the skin. *In*: Fitzpatrick, T. B., Arndt, K. A., Clark, W. H., et al. (eds.): Dermatology in General Medicine. New York, McGraw-Hill, 1971, pp. 39–48.
28. Flaxman, A. B.: Principles of skin development. *In*: Fitzpatrick, T. B., Arndt, K. A., Clark, W. H., et al. (eds.): Dermatology in General Medicine. New York, McGraw-Hill, 1971, p. 54.
29. Saunders, J. W.: The proximo-distal sequence of origin of the parts of the chick wing and the role of the ectoderm. J. Exp. Zool., *108*:363, 1948.
30. Trelstad, R. L., and Coulombre, A. J.: Morphogenesis of the collagenous stroma in the chick cornea. J. Cell. Biol., *50*:840, 1971.
31. Loewi, G., and Meyer, K.: The acid mucopolysaccharides of embryonic skin. Biochim. Biophys. Acta, *27*:453, 1958.
32. Pinto, J.: The dermis. *In*: Montagna, W., and Parakkal, P. F.: The Structure and Function of Skin, 3rd ed. New York, Academic Press, 1974, pp. 96–141.
33. Jackson, D. S., and Bentley, J. P.: On the significance of the extractable collagens. J. Biophys. Biochem. Cytol., *7*:37, 1960.
34. Zelickson, A. S.: Fibroblast development and fibrinogenesis. Arch. Dermatol., *88*:497, 1963.
35. Odland, G. F.: The Skin: A Description of the External Organ and its Common Afflictions. Seattle, University of Washington Press, 1971.
36. Deutsch, T. A., and Esterly, N. B.: Elastic fibers in fetal dermis. J. Invest. Dermatol., *65*.320, 1975.
37. Dorfman, A.: The effects of adrenal hormones on connective tissues. Ann. N.Y. Acad. Sci., *56*:698, 1953.
38. Mathews, M. B.: Biophysical aspects of acid mucopolysaccharides relevant to connective tissue structure and function. *In:* Wagner, B. M., and Smith, D. E. (eds.): The Connective Tissue Baltimore, Williams & Wilkins Co., 1967, pp. 304–329.
39. Acton, J. D., and Myrvils, Q. N., Production of interferon by alveolar macrophages. J. Bacteriol., *91*:2300, 1966.
40. Champion, R. H., and Wilkinson, D. S.: Disorders affecting blood vessels. *In*: Rook, A., Wilkinson, D. S., and Ebling, F. J. G. (eds.): Textbook of Dermatology. Philadelphia, F. A. Davis, 1968, p. 397.
41. Winkelman, R. K., Scheen, S. R. Jr., Pyka, R. A., et al.: Cutaneous vascular patterns in studies with injection preparation and alkaline phosphatase reaction. *In:* Montagna, W., and Ellis, R. A., (eds.): Advances in Biology of Skin. Vol. 2. Blood Vessels and Circulation. Oxford, Pergamon Press, 1961 pp. 1–19.
42. Saunders, R. L.: X-ray projection microscopy of the skin. *In:* Montagna, W., and Ellis, R. A., (eds.): Advances in Biology of Skin. Vol. 2. Blood Vessels and Circulation. Oxford, Pergamon Press, 1961, pp. 38–56.
43. Zweibach, B. W.: Structural aspects and hemodynamics of microcirculation in the skin. *In:* Rothman, S. (ed.): The Human Integument. Washington, D.C., American Association for the Advancement of Science, 1959.
44. Froese, G., and Burton, A. C.: The heat losses of the human head. J. Appl. Physiol., *10*:235, 1954.
45. Nafe, J. P.: Neural correlates of sensation. *In*: Kenshalo, D. R. (ed.): The Skin Senses. Springfield, Ill., Charles C Thomas, 1969, pp. 5–14.

2 | UNDERSTANDING THE ADOLESCENT PATIENT

JAY G. HIRSCH, M.D.

INTRODUCTION

Every circumstance in medicine can be viewed from three interrelated perspectives: the *biological,* the *psychological,* and the *social.* Of all the stages of the life cycle, adolescence best exemplifies the application of this truism to clinical practice. And of all the afflictions that occur in adolescence, the common cutaneous diseases best demonstrate these powerful interrelationships.

The other chapters in this book outline in considerable detail the biological aspects of adolescent skin development and the known relationships of endocrine, glandular, bacteriological, and other physiological factors in the occurrence of skin disease. In this chapter we will discuss the social and psychological variables that play a part in the teenager's response to a biological fact, his skin condition. These variables, in turn, impinge heavily on the patient's capacity for a therapeutic alliance with the doctor and ultimately have a major effect on treatment outcome.

For the purpose of this presentation we will not address the controversial question of primary psychological causation of skin disease. Biological factors will be treated as primary, while psychological and social consequences and correlates are in this context defined as secondary. We will nevertheless observe their great significance in a variety of clinical applications.

We must begin by viewing, from a developmental perspective, the psychological and social world of the adolescent. With this as a background, we can move to a description of the adolescent as a person, highly sensitive to changes taking place within himself and in the world around him. We can then speak of the impact of cutaneous disease on the life of the adolescent, and the myriad ways, both adaptive and maladaptive, he or she may respond to its presence.* And finally, we will consider the techniques of therapeutic inter-

---

*The masculine pronoun is used for convenience henceforth, but all of what is said applies to persons of both sexes without discrimination.

vention the medical practitioner can use to meet the psychological and social needs of the patient, as he deals with the physiological requirements of the clinical situation.

NORMAL ADOLESCENT DEVELOPMENT

For all humans, the skin is one of the major media of social exchange and pleasure, beginning no later than the first neonatal day. The softness, warmth, and smoothness of the baby's skin serve as a pleasurable focus for caretaking adults, while gentle manipulation, caressing, and tickling on the part of the adult evoke pleasure in the child. This pattern continues throughout childhood, with the child's being stimulated and pleased and communicating his pleasure through a smile or a laugh, which leads to more stimulation and more pleasure—a positive feedback loop. Conversely, if there is a break in the skin, or if there is eczema or other cutaneous lesions, a negative feedback loop is set up, wherein stimulation leads to pain, soon producing a cessation of stimulation. In addition, the observing adult is often repelled by the infant with a rash and cannot be so loving to the baby whose "beauty" is dependent (in Western culture, at least) upon blemish-free skin. For example, mothers of babies with eczema describe the shame that attends taking the baby for a walk or showing him to friends who respond less than enthusiastically to the sight of a child with blemishes.

Within modern American culture, there is an implicit system of values that makes beauty, attractiveness, and self-confidence dependent on blemish-free skin. Not only is this communicated early in life through parent–child interactions, but it is explicitly reinforced by advertisements and television commercials showing people with unusually attractive natural endowments extolling the virtues of soaps, creams, lotions, and cosmetics as "beauty aids." A large proportion of these advertisements is directed to teenagers, who represent a lucrative market for these products.

The adolescent population that must endure this perpetual bombardment is a diverse group, with varied interests, orientations, life styles, and values. As a developmental stage, we usually think of adolescence as a transitional period between childhood and adulthood. As such, in the United States and other Western cultures, adolescence spans a relatively long time, from age 12 to 18 at least, and for many (perhaps most) individuals extends well into the twenties. Because of this long time span, some authors have divided adolescence into three sub-stages: early, middle, and late adolescence.[1]

During early adolescence, puberty is the biological event of greatest importance. There are great variations in its time of onset and in the rapidity of the resulting changes in physical and psychological characteristics, with girls being ahead of boys by as much as two years on the average.[2, 3] The individual variations in the timing of puberty have many psychological and social consequences. Who among us can forget the teasing and embarrassment experienced by the girl who blossomed "too early" and the boy or girl who bloomed "too late"? Through the adult's retrospective we wonder why "minor things" meant so much, and how such sensitivity could be manifested over something that "would work itself out in time." But how many adults would want to be

14 again? Is there anyone without some painful memories of those awkward years?

Variations in physical characteristics serve as the biological substrate for diverse social phenomena and psychological processes. Physical prowess for boys and attractiveness for girls serve as major underpinnings for shaky adolescent self-esteem and for emergent heterosexual explorations. Complex networks of peer relationships rest upon, and to some extent determine the outcome of, the emergence of a positive self-image. The fragility of the adolescent's self-evaluations and the daily risk-taking that takes place in school and in other activities intensify concern about social standing. The first two sub-stages of adolescence encompass years when appearances *do* count. When one has little else to fall back on, a pleasing personal appearance can buttress an otherwise shaky self-image. Conversely, a minor physical difference can be magnified in the mind's eye so as to threaten or topple even the firmest of positive self-images.

The peer group is an important reference point and a crucial source of messages about the self. A chance remark by an acquaintance can cause preoccupation for weeks or even years. A chiding comment meant in good-natured jest and taken calmly in public can constitute a serious threat to self-esteem in private reflections later. Conversely, positive messages from peers can be highly reassuring and self-affirming.

During the sub-stage of late adolescence, issues relative to "who do I want to be" and "what do I want to do" gain ascendency. Erikson has referred to this as the stage of identity crisis.[4, 5] At this time, the teenager begins to see himself as an emerging adult, ready to take on a new set of social roles in work, with members of the opposite sex, with friends, and with his family.

By this time, doubts about body image and self-esteem should have given way to positive personal self-definition. With this new-found confidence, the young person is ready to risk the travails of the adult world and is less vulnerable to negative messages emanating from within himself or from his environment.

THE SOCIAL AND PSYCHOLOGICAL IMPACT OF CUTANEOUS DISEASE IN ADOLESCENCE

The presence of a skin eruption during the adolescent years is to be expected in perhaps over 90 per cent of the population.[6] Some form of acne, however mild, is the rule rather than the exception. In addition, of course, other forms of cutaneous disease make their appearance at this time. Among the most frequent are seborrhea and eczematous dermatitis, and less frequently, psoriasis.

Most of these skin lesions are mild in nature, seldom coming to the attention of medical practitioners, and even less often to the attention of dermatologists. However, severity of lesion interacts with socioeconomic status to determine patterns of service demands and delivery. Very severe disease is likely to demand care across the whole socioeconomic spectrum. At higher socioeconomic levels, milder forms of skin lesions are more likely to be brought to the physician's attention earlier in their course and when symptoms are not yet full-blown.

Although in a large series of patients there may be some statistical trend that correlates severity of skin disease with degree of emotional and behavioral response, in individual patients there may be no correlation whatever. A few adolescents with severe skin disorders will have no apparent psychological or social fallout; others with mild lesions will be greatly affected emotionally. "The smallest skin lesion, if it concerns the feelings, concerns the whole personality."[7] "The spots of acne are magnified in any mirror. The patient and the dermatologist see two different images. It is the patient's that must be treated."[8]

A high proportion of adolescent patients with skin disease will have a significant degree of anxiety and depression as part of their presenting picture. These emotional reactions are manifest in a variety of thoughts, feelings, and behaviors. Adolescents can feel "unclean," sinful, angry, excessively self-conscious, and preoccupied with how they look; they can feel unworthy, have a low opinion of themselves, blame themselves, demonstrate excessive fears, and have hypochondriacal symptomatology.

They also demonstrate in their behavior a wide variation in adaptive and maladaptive defenses. It is not uncommon to see withdrawal from social contacts and a serious decline in school achievement; school attendance may suffer because of phobic fears resulting in elective truancy. Because of increased irritability, episodes of family conflict become more frequent; temper outbursts or social withdrawal are common manifestations within the family. Heterosexual relationships which, prior to the appearance of the skin disorder, were moving along a good developmental trajectory, now may undergo exaggeration in the form of hyperaggressiveness or promiscuity or total withdrawal from involvement. Self-destructiveness in several forms can appear, either as overt suicidal behavior or in the less extreme form of self-laceration, scratching, or picking at the skin lesions. Group delinquency or even individual criminal behavior may be seen; behavioral evidence of "giving up" can be seen in a deterioration in dress, grooming, and hygiene; even runaway episodes or psychotic reactions to the stress of the situation are not unusual.

The medical practitioner facing patients with such reactions can easily discern stereotypes (singly or in combination) that could be labeled: the Depressed Adolescent, the Uncooperative Adolescent, the Missing Adolescent, the Hyperaggressive Adolescent, the Excessively Dependent Adolescent, the Crazy Adolescent, the Unreachable Adolescent, the Anxious, Self-conscious Adolescent, and finally—the Untreatable Adolescent.

The management of each of these sub-types of adolescent patients can be extremely difficult, frustrating, and unrewarding. For the physician with a busy schedule, the range of symptoms and behaviors constitutes a formidable list of impediments to successful treatment. On the other hand, to effectively reach such patients, despite the initial problems of establishing a therapeutic alliance, can be one of the most gratifying experiences a practitioner can have.

ESTABLISHING THE THERAPEUTIC ALLIANCE

The first contact with the physician usually takes place in the office or clinic outpatient setting. The patient is never a casual arrival; he has already sifted through the pros and cons of whether to seek medical help for the skin problem, both in his own thoughts and in his interaction with his parents and other family members. Sometimes he will arrive in great embarrassment or under duress, but secretly he will be very relieved to be there. At other times he will be overtly cooperative and friendly, but passively resistive. Probably in most instances he is willing to take a "wait and see" attitude toward the first visit to the physician. He is likely to feel some anxiety because of the strangeness of the new situation, in addition to his concern about the seriousness of his skin condition. He certainly wants help and wants to believe it will be forthcoming.

He will have anticipatory concerns about the physician, whom he has not yet met, but will usually assume he is a competent professional. He will want to like him; attitudes toward the doctor will largely depend on the quality of the first encounter. The adolescent will want to be recognized as a worthwhile individual whose complaints justify proper attention. The physician should demonstrate by his demeanor the appropriate combination of interest, friendliness, competence, and caring. Just as he has learned to pick up subtle cues regarding what a patient is feeling, patients also pick up subtle messages from doctors in their initial meeting. These unspoken messages influence the tone of their involvement together.

Accordingly, an *unhurried, private* talk with the patient on the first visit is the sine qua non for establishing the level of rapport that will be required. It is probably best not to jump directly to the skin problem, but rather, after an initial friendly greeting, to direct the conversation at getting to know the patient by asking questions about where he lives, what school he attends, and about his family, his interests, and his activities. This might lead to a discussion of music, athletics, after-school jobs, social life, neighborhood activities, or future educational plans. The clinician will have abundant cues as to where to begin by observing the patient's grooming, dress, and general manner of relating. Some positive comment about an aspect of the patient's life or his appearance will encourage the patient to see the doctor as a giving person and as one who will communicate respect and concern.

The conversation may proceed relatively quickly to a careful history of the current problem. Often, the adolescent will be either too voluble in his description or will speak in monosyllables and with great reluctance. The physician should try to avoid communicating impatience with these adolescent styles and gently lead or chide the patient into offering the needed information. At this time the practitioner may call upon the parent or accompanying adult for information. Although there may be some disagreement on this point, I believe in establishing a therapeutic alliance first with the patient and subsequently with the family. Both will be needed. The reason for this sequential approach is that sometimes the adolescent will be locked in a struggle with his parents, and the physician must avoid appearing to take sides with the parents against the child. If the medical care is to be free of the negative family dynamics that may be operating, the primary alliance must be between the practitioner and his adolescent patient. The physician also must avoid being used by one camp against the other and always must maintain his primary interest in the patient's welfare. Consequently, individual involvement with the adolescent, followed by contact with the family, is the preferred sequence of necessary relationships.

The examination, which usually follows the period of initial history-taking, bears discussion. Boys most likely will prefer to be examined privately by the physician, whether male or female. Girls most likely will be reassured by the presence of a female nurse or aide in the room during an examination by a male physician. In public clinics or university facilities, the dermatology clinic can easily be turned into a spectacle or a voyeur's paradise. This is greatly to the detriment of the patient's feelings about himself and may interfere with obtaining his trust and cooperation. The patient's skin problem is a sensitive and private matter that warrants the most delicate and respectful handling. At the time of the first examination, it is important for the clinician to show sympathetic concern, even for minor lesions, and to inhibit overreaction to severe disease. These subtle, often non-verbal, messages to the patient communicate better than words the doctor's interest and hope regarding the patient's condition.

If the clinician is able to make a diagnosis, even a tentative one, on the basis of this first examination, the patient will be eager to hear what it is. It is important to give not only the medical name (which often is very formidable and makes even the simplest lesion sound serious) but also a popular name with which the patient might be more familiar. This should be followed by some information regarding its causation, its natural history, and the various forms of treatment that are available. There should be some clear statement and a step-by-step explanation of what the physician wants to do, and what that will mean in terms of the patient's participation. The patient will then want to know what he can reasonably expect and may or may not openly seek prognostic information. He will want the physician to be straightforward without being blunt, to deliver what he has promised, and to not promise what he cannot deliver. He will want him to be warm, cheerful, and hopeful.

One of the most useful ways a dermatologist or other non-psychiatric physician can reassure the adolescent with a skin problem is to comment on the common feelings experienced by young people with skin problems. This helps the patient to appreciate that he is not the only one who has ever felt that way, and also indicates to him that the practitioner's experience can be helpful to him. For example, the physician might say something like this: "Often when young people have blemishes on their skin they have all kinds of confusing feelings. This may not be the way you feel but let me share some of those feelings with you. Sometimes they mistakenly feel dirty, or guilty, and blame themselves for their skin disease; sometimes they mistakenly blame other people; sometimes they've heard other kids tease about skin disease being caused by sexual activity or by masturbation, or by V.D.—that is absolutely not true and is not true for the problem you have; sometimes they think that it might get so bad that they are going to die from it—that is also not true; sometimes they think that if they touch someone or are touched by someone else they will transmit the disease to the other person—that is also not true because skin disease is not contagious in that way. Often they want to know such things as: Why does it spread? When will it stop? What did I do to get it? How long will I have it? Will I have scars? What can I do about it? I will try to answer all of these questions for you as best I can. Which of these questions do you want me to begin with?"

Such an approach will usually open up the discussion with the adolescent so that he knows the clinician wants to talk candidly with him and will help him adapt to his skin problem during the course of treatment.

If the parents have not yet had contact with the physician, it may be necessary to repeat for them (preferably, in most instances, in the presence of the patient) all the discussion regarding diagnosis, treatment, and prognosis that had previously been covered with the patient alone. This is not a waste of time; it will give the patient a chance to integrate a lot of information that was missed the first time. In more severe cases, in which the treatment may be complex and may cause considerable disruption in the life of the patient or the family, the aid of the family will be needed. If the patient is to be hospitalized, complex arrangements will have to be made. If, as is the case with all but a few adolescents, the patient is to remain at home and be seen as an outpatient, arrangements may have to be worked out for the administration of compresses or salves or other treatments that require the aid of others. In each instance, it is important for the practitioner to spell out in detail who will be responsible for which aspect of the care, and how its administration is to be recorded, so that there is some assurance that the recommendations will be carried out. Perhaps a simple charting on graph paper can serve as an organizer for the treatment plan. The patient simply checks off the appropriate box, brings the chart to the physician's office at the subsequent visit, and is rewarded by the doctor's praise. With less cooperative patients whose families might be in conflict over compliance with the prescribed therapeutic measures, a behavioral checklist can be used effectively to motivate both the patient and his family to carry out their respective responsibilities. A prearranged set of rewards can be established to help motivate the patient and to avert sabotage of the plan by conflict within the family.

In selected cases, the physician also may have to contact various social agencies, such as welfare and rehabilitation facilities, and speak with school personnel to work out special arrangements regarding school attendance, assignments, homebound tutoring, and the like. In many instances in which the disease is relatively mild, it is important to work with the school and family in keeping the child at school.

For children with significant morbidity from their skin disease who are seen in a clinic, hospital, or busy dermatologist's office, there are sufficient numbers of such adolescents to establish discussion groups that serve a health education function as well as a group support function. It is very reassuring to meet with other people who have the same or similar problems, to share concerns and feelings with them, and to learn from others how they cope with their circumstances. For many disabilities (e.g., hemophilia, leukemia, mental retardation), parent groups held concomitant with groups for children have proved very successful in increasing the level of family and patient comfort with their disease, as well as their ability to cooperate in its treatment. With adolescent skin problems, a group approach would seem advisable because of the natural tendency for groups to form during adolescence and for young people to coalesce for purposes of mutual support and problem-solving.

COMPLICATING EMOTIONAL FACTORS

Just because the two conditions happen to coexist in the same individual, skin disease is not necessarily the *cause* of emotional disturbance or social maladjustment. As pointed out earlier in this chapter, the stresses and strains on the adolescent's psychic economy are myriad. The presence of a skin problem is only one of those stresses. Other loci of problems in adaptation may be the school, the family, peers, the neighborhood, or conflicts with the self.

Often a youngster appears for treatment of a relatively mild dermatological problem, rather than presenting himself to a psychiatrist for treatment of a more obvious, debilitating, and serious coexisting emotional disorder. The physician called upon to treat the skin problem is in a unique position to observe the patient and to take note of salient psychological and social aspects of his current adjustment. In many instances the physician can help the patient in working out some of the conflicts by engaging him in a discussion of the stresses he is under and by suggesting ways to lessen his tension. He also might be available as advocate for the patient in a meeting with one or both parents to help sort out current family issues and to reduce parent–child misunderstanding and conflict. He could suggest other community resources, such as community centers, athletic facilities, social clubs, and part-time jobs. As stated earlier, there may be specific indications for contacting the school in cases in which the physical or emotional problems lead to the avoidance of school or to academic or behavioral problems in school; here, communication with the school guidance counselor, psychologist, or social worker may be indicated.

In circumstances where the youngster's difficulty seems extremely deep, has been longstanding, or affects several areas of his life (e.g., home and school, or school achievements and peer relationships), a psychiatric evaluation may be warranted. The best way of making such a referral is to speak directly with a psychiatric colleague about the patient, tell him of your findings, and indicate your concerns and questions. If the psychiatrist agrees to accept the patient, he should be ready to meet the young person and his family within a short time. It is reasonable for the referring physician to expect a call from the psychiatrist, who should want to communicate his findings and outline his recommendations for further treatment. Often in these circumstances there is good rationale for dividing the labor. The physical aspects of the problem can be managed by a general physician or dermatologist, while the emotional and social aspects can be managed by a mental health professional. Telephone contact between the two professionals can help coordinate their respective efforts.

When a referral is to be made to a psychiatrist, the referring physician can help pave the way for acceptance by reassuring the patient and his family that this procedure is often the most direct way of obtaining help, by telling them something about the psychiatrist if he knows him personally, and by describing some positive past experience with psychiatric treatment in similar circumstances.

Conditions certainly warranting such a referral would be instances in which the adolescent is judged to be dangerous to himself or to others; in such circumstances, psychiatric hospitalization would have to be considered. The possibility of suicide during adolescence demands that adequate precautions be taken when signs of the patient's discomfort warrant such care.

In the large majority of adolescents, outpatient evaluation and treatment will suffice. Instances of mild-to-moderate depression, school phobia, truancy, group delinquency, and borderline or impending psychotic states would all fall into this category.

Less severe adolescent problems also can benefit from the involvement of a psychiatrist or of other mental health personnel. A trusting relationship between dermatologist and patient can set the stage for referral of the patient for such help.

Available treatment options cover the gamut of social and psychological interventions, such as individual, family, and group therapy, as well as biological interventions, usually in the form of pharmacotherapy.

PSYCHOTROPIC MEDICATION AND THE ADOLESCENT SKIN PATIENT

One question often asked by dermatologists of psychiatrists is: "Should the dermatologist use tranquilizers for adolescent patients?" This question can be expanded to include all psychotropic medication.

Unfortunately, the answer cannot be clearly affirmative or negative. Obviously, specific aspects of the adolescent and his family, the social context in which he finds himself, and the particular styles and predispositions of the responsible physician must be taken into account. The nature of the relationship between doctor and patient is central here.

It is my impression that non-psychiatric physicians often prescribe psychotropic medication for their patients as a substitute for talking to them. If this is the basis for the prescription, there will be little therapeutic benefit accruing to the patient and it is better not to prescribe anything. The medications usually prescribed are the minor tranquilizers, which supposedly have an anti-anxiety effect. Examples of this class of medication are meprobamate (Miltown, Equanil), chlordiazepoxide (Librium), and diazepam (Valium). These medications are relatively ineffective for children and adolescents, and are rarely, if ever, indicated. The major tranquilizers do have an effect on behavior by both their antipsychotic and their sedative actions. If the youngster is in need of those medications, he probably ought to be under the care of a psychiatrist, whose experience in their use for behavioral change is likely to be greater than that of the primary physician or dermatologist. Examples of these types of medication are chlorpromazine (Thorazine), thioridazine (Mellaril), haloperidol (Haldol), and fluphenazine (Prolixin).

A growing number of adolescents receive stimulant drugs, such as dextroamphetamine (Dexedrine), methylphenidate (Ritalin), and pemoline (Cylert), which have been prescribed for hyperactivity, learning disability, perceptual handicap, or minimal brain dysfunction syndrome. It is important for the clinician evaluating the skin lesion to discuss with the physician prescribing the stimulant medication the rationale for its continuance. There is no indication for prescribing these medications for the skin problems per se, but no contraindication to their usage with skin disease, unless the skin condition is possibly allergic in nature.

One major class of medications that has been found to be a useful adjunct in the treatment of skin problems is the tricyclic antidepressants, exemplified by imipramine (Tofranil), amitriptyline (Elavil), desipramine (Norpramin), and doxepin (Sinequan). These medications must be given with careful attention to dosage and side effects, and require close follow-up on the part of the prescribing physician.

ON SQUEEZING PIMPLES

A particular problem during adolescence is the tendency for teenagers to pick at or squeeze their skin lesions. In acne, in which comedones are a major part of the problem, it may not always be antitherapeutic if the squeezing is done gently, cleanly, and infrequently. There are times, though, when such picking and squeezing becomes habitual or even compulsive. It is almost as if the patient wishes to obliterate his skin problem by "getting it all out." Often he is disappointed to find that his efforts result in additional excoriation of his skin and, not infrequently, worsening of his lesions. The squeezing activity has been subject to a wide variety of symbolic and deep psychological interpretations which imply masochistic tendencies and masturbatory imagery. These actions are seen as means of coping with the narcissistic blow of having the skin disorder.

The physician should be alert to the presence of picking and squeezing, and should try to communicate his understanding of their significance in the patient's *skin* disease. *No* deep psychological interpretations should be made; rather, this behavior can be interpreted as the patient's efforts to make himself look better, although, paradoxically, in most instances he is making his skin problem worse. Without provoking guilt, and without blaming the patient, the doctor should explain the medical reasons for not picking the skin. Sometimes he can offer to remove the most offensive blackheads when the patient is in the office on his regular visits. Often the youngster will welcome the restraint that comes from having limits set on this activity. Sometimes he will need the added incentive of a behavioral checklist which can help make him responsible for decreasing the frequency and intensity of squeezing. The physician can help the patient and his family devise a system of small rewards for continued progress in this direction.

THE VERY SERIOUS OR "HOPELESS" CASE

In a small minority of skin problems during adolescence, we are dealing with disease that may either be lifelong and very extensive, or that may be life-threatening.

Very serious, chronic skin disease of adolescence is almost invariably accompanied by severe impairment of body image and concomitant depression, regression, hostility, frustration, and anxiety. The youngster who has to be hospitalized because of the seriousness of his skin condition, who must remain away from friends and family for long periods of time, and who is unable to return to his usual activities, is an unhappy person. He will often reflect this unhappiness in his relationships with hospital staff and to other patients and visitors. He will sometimes demonstrate a stubborn refusal to cooperate in his own care or a passive resistance to his own management. He may throw tantrums or withdraw completely from outside contact. He may demonstrate signs of impending psychotic withdrawal, with paranoid tendencies, hallucinatory or delusional experiences, and other signs of impairment in reality-testing.

In such instances, it is most important to establish primary responsibility for the patient's management with a relatively small group of medical and nursing staff and to make the hospital surroundings as supportive as possible. Consultation with the liaison psychiatrist is certainly indicated. He might be able to arrange for changes in the routine of the hospital or in the distribution of personnel to mitigate a difficult situation.

Often, no matter what, the patient will remain unhappy about his skin condition. He may need psychotherapeutic support in order to mourn the loss of his good health and normal body image, and he may need time to adjust to his permanently changed health status. A directional shift in career or educational plans may be required. His need to spend time and energy in the adjustment to the chronic nature of his disease is paramount.

SUMMARY

This chapter has presented a frame of reference with which to approach adolescent patients with skin disease. To be most effective, the physician must understand the complexities of adolescent development and the various biological, social, and psychological circumstances and reactions with which young people must cope. Suggestions are made regarding approaches to the management of the adolescent skin patient, in the wish to maximize the usefulness of the physician–patient relationship as a resource for helping young people to health and happiness.

REFERENCES

1. Blos, P.: On Adolescence: A Psychoanalytic Interpretation. Glencoe, Ill. The Free Press, 1962, pp. 75–158.
2. Nicolson, A. B., and Hanley, C.: Indices of physiological maturity: Derivation and interrelationships. Child Dev. 24:3, 1953.
3. Tanner, J. M.: Growth at Adolescence. Philadelphia, F. A. Davis, 1962, p. 80.
4. Erikson, E. H.: Childhood and Society. New York, W. W. Norton, 1950.
5. Erikson, E. H.: Identity: Youth and Crisis. New York, W. W. Norton, 1968.
6. Rook, A., Wilkinson, D. S., and Ebling, F. J. G.: Textbook of Dermatology. 2nd ed., Vol. 2, Philadelphia, F. A. Davis, 1972, p. 1545.
7. Winnicott D. W.: Trans. St. John's Hosp. 1938, 62.
8. Rook, A., Wilkinson, D. S., and Ebling, F. J. G.: Textbook of Dermatology. 2nd ed., Vol. 2, Philadelphia, F. A. Davis, 1972, p. 1825.

3

COMMON DIAGNOSTIC PROCEDURES*

DAVID L. CRAM, M.D.

INTRODUCTION

The skin is the most accessible organ of the body for direct examination. Nevertheless, the same basic principles of data gathering should be applied to the detection of disorders of the skin as are used to determine the presence of disease in any other organ. Before a diagnosis is made, an adequate history should be obtained and a thorough physical examination performed. Whenever possible, the clinical impression based on physical examination and history should be verified by appropriate laboratory studies.

Examination of the skin should be performed in a well-lighted room, preferably in natural light. The patient with a dermatological disorder should disrobe completely for complete examination of the skin, including the scalp, nails, and mucosae, unless the problem is obviously a local one, such as a wart. Transillumination or side lighting may help to visualize the surface configuration of some lesions.

Close examination of a skin lesion can be performed with a magnifying hand lens (Fig. 3–1). The lens may be held close to the eye to magnify a large field or held close to the lesion to obtain maximum enlargement. Magnification is especially helpful in examining the topography of a lesion or in searching for parasites.

In addition to direct examination, other techniques are useful in the diagnosis of skin disorders. Special techniques are particularly helpful in documenting fungal or viral infections and in searching for mites or insects. Allergic disorders due to externally applied agents (contactants) may be iden-

---

*The figures are from the sound-slide program, "Techniques for Examination of the Skin," produced and distributed by the Institute for Dermatologic Communication and Education, San Francisco, California.

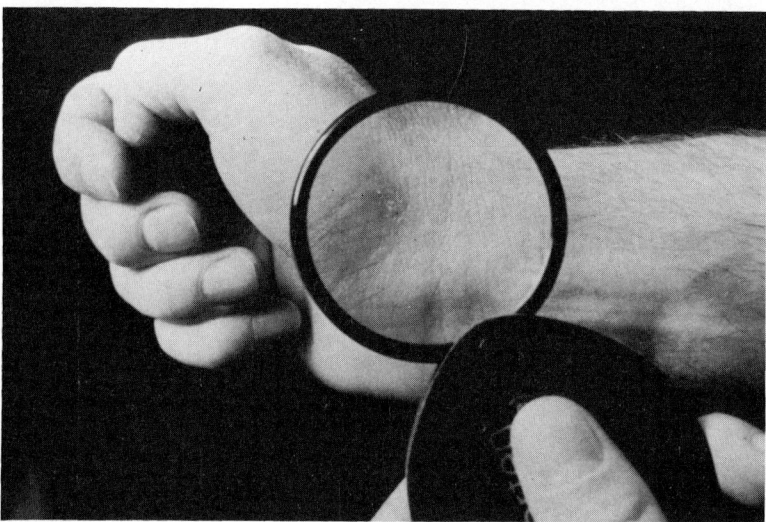

FIGURE 3–1 The hand lens.

tified by patch testing with appropriate materials. Biopsy of the skin can be readily effected with minimal discomfort, using specialized instruments. We will enlarge upon all of these procedures in the paragraphs and illustrations to follow.

EXAMINATION FOR FUNGUS AND YEAST

Superficial fungal infections are relatively uncommon in infants and young children in the United States. It is not until adolescence that tinea pedis and tinea cruris begin to appear with significant frequency. Superficial fungal infections (tineae) are caused by various species of dermatophytes, which can affect all areas of the skin. They often are classified according to their location on the body. They may affect the face (tinea faciale), the scalp (tinea capitis), the groin (tinea cruris), the glabrous skin (tinea corporis), the nails (tinea unguium or onychomycosis), or the feet (tinea pedis). Correct identification of the species of fungus causing an infection may be difficult at times on clinical grounds alone. However the *direct* examination of infected hair, skin, and nails under the microscope is the best means for identifying the specific fungus involved in the disease being studied. The infected tissue should be examined under the microscope and cultured to demonstrate the presence of a dermatophyte.

Specimens for mycological study may be obtained in a variety of ways, depending upon the type and location of the infection. Specimens of horny skin needed for examination should be obtained by scraping from the edge of a scaly area toward the surrounding normal skin, using a rounded scalpel blade. The skin lesion should be cleaned with a 70 per cent alcohol solution before taking the specimen, in order to remove any topical medication that may be present. To secure specimens from vesicular or bullous lesions, the tops of the blisters should be cut off with a small scissors (Fig. 3–2). Speci-

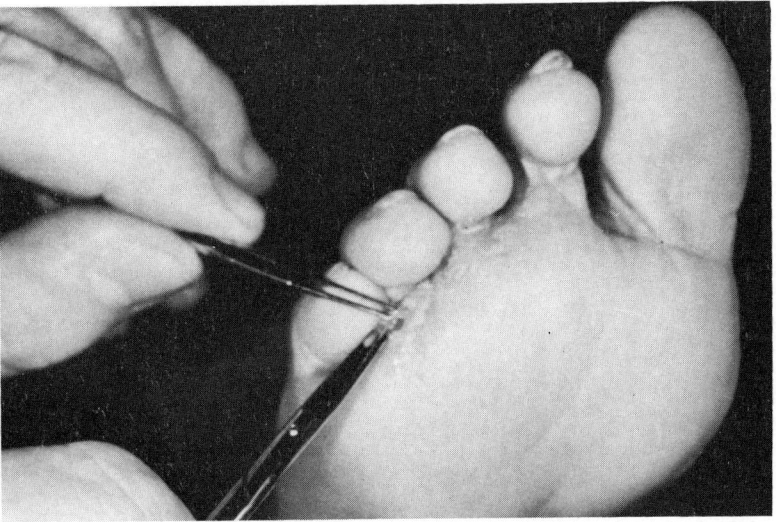

FIGURE 3-2 Clipping off top of fungus blister.

mens of infected hairs can be cut or removed from the scalp, using depilating forceps. Infected hairs are usually easy to pluck because they are loose within the follicle. To obtain material from infected nails, friable or discolored areas should be selected for scraping with the edge of a microscopic slide or a scalpel (Fig. 3-3). The initial superfical nail scrapings should be used for potassium hydroxide (KOH) examination and only the sub-surface material should be used for culture. Debris removed from under thick hyperkeratotic nails also should be examined with KOH.

Material for direct examination is placed on a microscopic slide and covered with a glass coverslip. One or two drops of 10 to 40 per cent KOH are added to the edge of the coverslip and permitted to flow between the coverslip

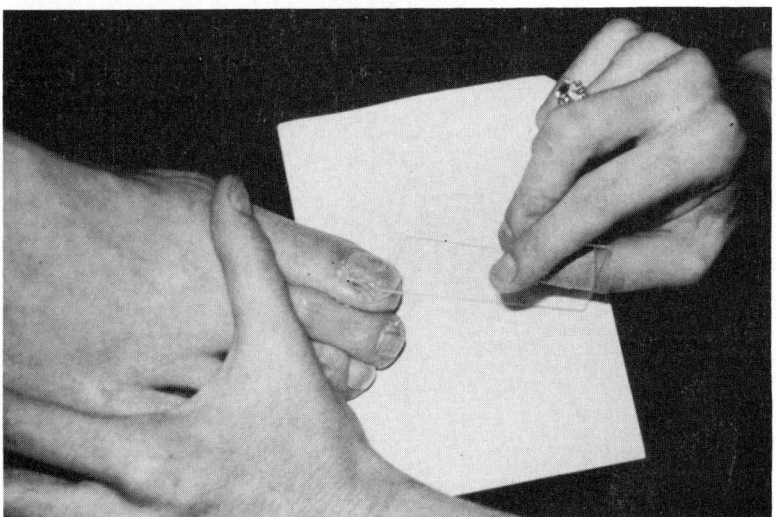

FIGURE 3-3 Scraping infected nail with glass slide.

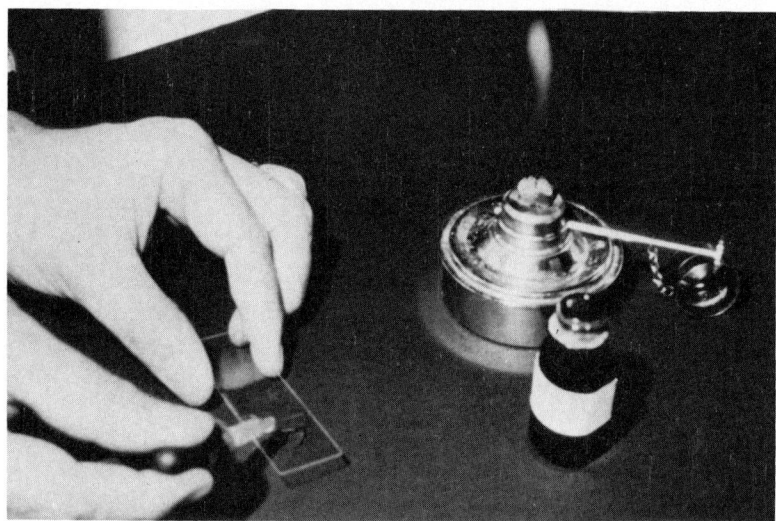

FIGURE 3-4 Adding KOH to slide for fungal identification.

and the slide by capillary action (Fig. 3-4). Small, thin pieces of tissue are the easiest to study because they are dissolved more quickly by KOH. Gentle pressure is applied to the top of the coverslip to flatten the specimen and to eliminate excess potassium hydroxide and air bubbles. The specimen is next examined microscopically under low power and low illumination. If no fungus is seen, the preparation is heated gently over a low flame and the microscopic examination is repeated (Fig. 3-5). It is important to prevent the preparation from boiling in order to avoid crystallization of the KOH. To the inexperienced eye, the identification of fungal structures may be difficult, but they usually appear as segmented, branching, threadlike elements called mycelia or

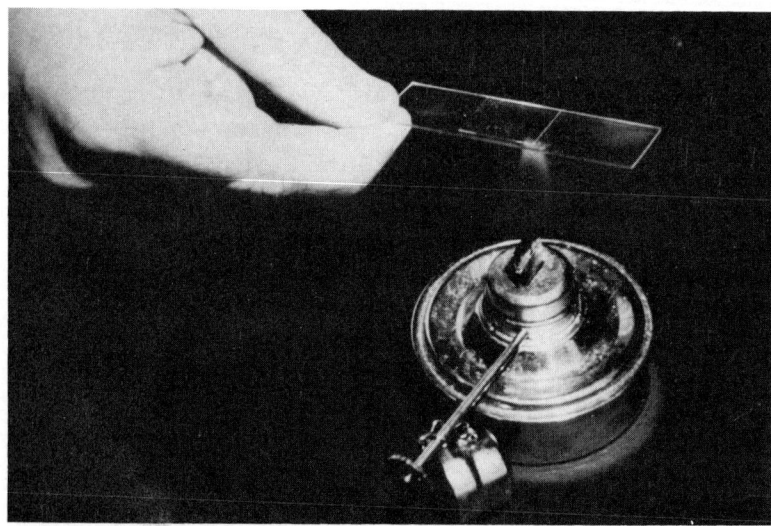

FIGURE 3-5 Gently heating slide for KOH preparation.

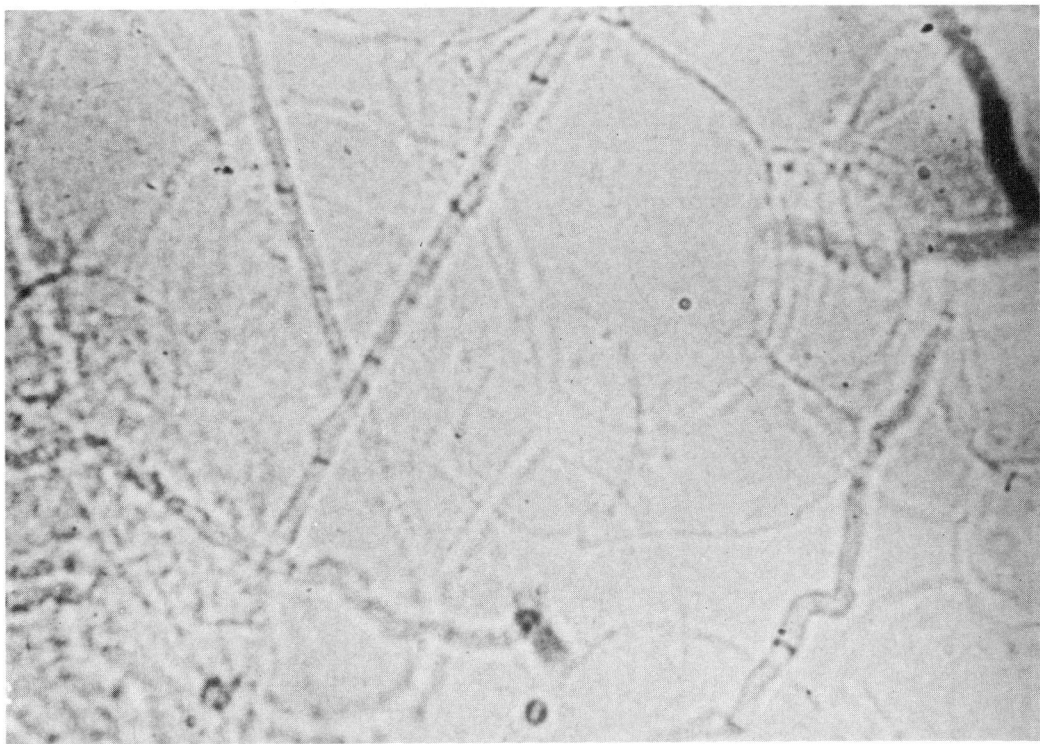
FIGURE 3–6 Hyphae of tinea by KOH technique.

hyphae (Fig. 3–6). These mycelia are transparent and are best seen under low illumination, achieved by adjusting the iris diaphragm of the substage condenser. Such artifacts as "mosaic particles," unlike mycelia, tend to follow the outline of the cells. Infected hairs may reveal the presence of fungal spores either outside or inside the hair shaft. Those species causing ectothrix infections arrange their spores in rows outside the hair shaft (Fig. 3–7). Species causing endothrix infections arrange their spores inside the hair shaft. Nail material may not contain organisms visible under the microscope, despite clinical evidence of infection, so that culturing the scrapings may be the only means of confirming the diagnosis.

Infected hairs and scrapings can be transferred directly from the lesions to Sabouraud's glucose agar, which contains antibiotics that prevent bacterial contamination and overgrowth by non-pathogenic mold. For best results, two or three culture tubes should be inoculated and the tissue fragments partially embedded in the medium. All cultures for superficial fungi are kept at room temperature for at least three weeks and examined frequently. Dermatophytes often produce typical growth patterns on culture media, but further species identification may require additional procedures, including slide mounts and subcultures.

The KOH technique is particularly useful for the diagnosis of superficial infections caused by some yeasts, including tinea versicolor and candidiasis.

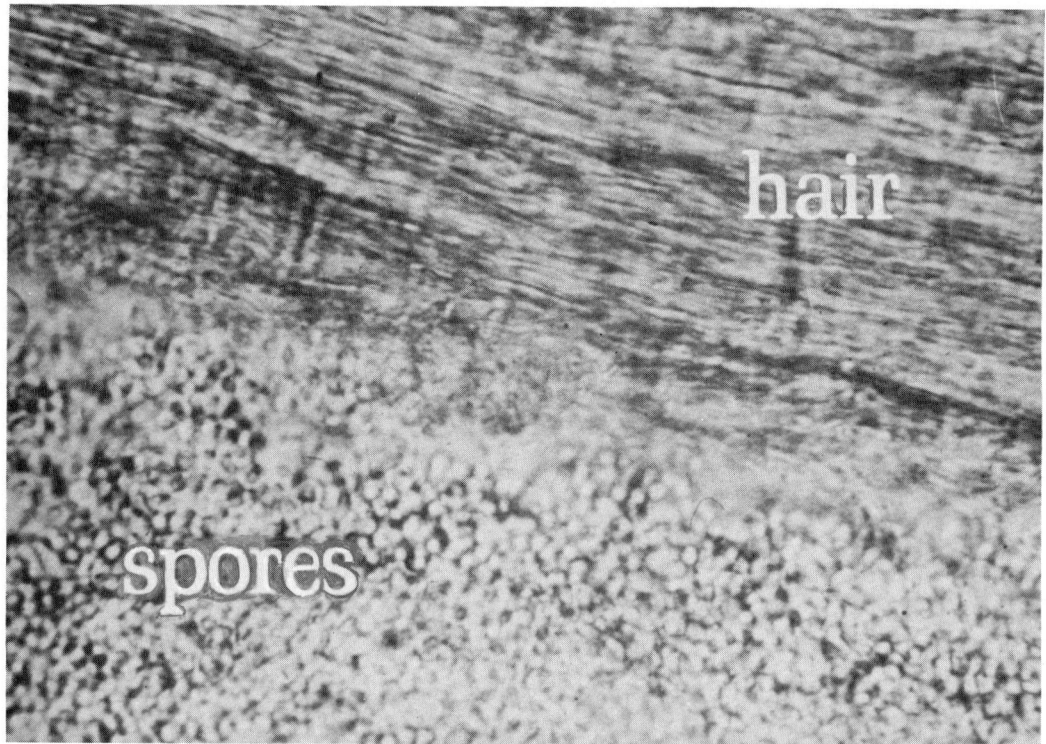
FIGURE 3–7 Ectothrix fungal hair infection.

Tinea versicolor is a chronic disease characterized by fawn- or brownish-colored scaly macules on the trunk. It occurs frequently in adolescents, and is most common in hot, humid environments. Under the microscope, the yeast of tinea versicolor appears as clusters of thick-walled round and budding spores surrounded by tangled short fragments of mycelia (Fig. 3–8). The KOH preparation is the most important procedure for making the diagnosis of tinea versicolor, since the organism cannot be cultured by standard techniques.

Candidiasis, caused by the yeast *Candida albicans* appears as an acute or subacute infection of the mouth, the moist intertriginous areas of the skin, the nails, and the paronychial areas. Infections with *Candida albicans* in the adolescent occur most frequently in diabetics, immunosuppressed patients, and patients receiving high doses of antibiotics or corticosteroids. Skin and nail scrapings should be obtained and examined with potassium hydroxide in the manner previously described. *Candida albicans* is a dimorphic organism which may be found in infected tissue in both the yeast (round spore) and pseudo-mycelial (filamentous) forms. The pseudo-mycelia of Candida species are wider and less regular than those of the true mycelial dermatophytic fungi. The yeast buds appear as clusters of spherical blastospores. The culture of *Candida albicans* on Sabouraud's agar usually produces a moist, creamy growth in two to four days. Cultures on cornmeal agar media reveal an additional characteristic of *Candida albicans*: the production of rounded thick-walled macroconidia or chlamydospores at the tips of the hyphae.

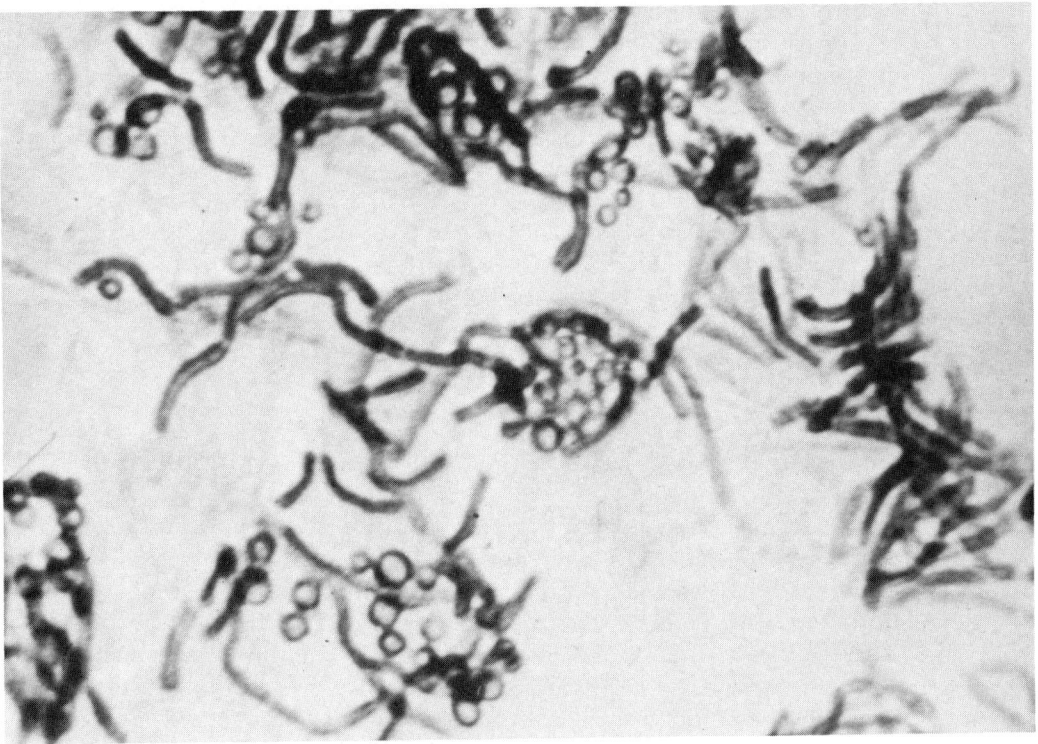
FIGURE 3–8 Grouped spores and short hyphae of tinea versicolor by KOH technique.

THE WOOD'S LIGHT

The Wood's light, often called "black light," is a source of ultraviolet radiation of around 3650 Angström units (360 nm). It is a useful device in the diagnosis of several cutaneous disorders[1] and is inexpensive, safe, and easy to use. Certain lesions of the skin and mucous membranes can be seen only poorly in natural light. Sometimes a heightened contrast can be achieved by using Wood's light illumination, which permits a clearer view of the eruptions. It is best to use a Wood's lamp in a darkened room in order to visualize colors adequately.

The Wood's light is most useful in the diagnosis of common forms of tinea capitis, caused by fungi of the genus *Microsporum*. These fungi fluoresce a bright blue-green color, which not only suggests the diagnosis but also helps the examiner to locate infected hairs for mycological examination (Plate I–A). Scalp infections due to other fungi, such as *Trichophyton tonsurans,* usually fluoresce poorly or not at all. The nature of the fluorescent substance in infected hairs is not completely understood. Bits of lint, horny material, and some topically applied agents will also fluoresce but the "color" tends to be brighter, weaker, or different from that produced by fungi. Infection with *Microsporum audouini* is seen less frequently today than in the past, but when it occurs, it occurs primarily in the under 10-year-old group. *Microsporum canis* infections, in contrast, are seen both in younger children and in adolescents.

The Wood's light is also employed in the diagnosis of erythrasma.[2]

Erythrasma is a superficial bacterial infection of the skin that is often mistaken for fungal infection. It usually involves intertriginous areas of the body and occurs more frequently in the adult than in the adolescent. Yet, in one study, 14 per cent of adolescent boys had erythrasma of the toe webs.[3] The *Corynebacterium* responsible for the eruption produces a porphyrin which fluoresces a bright orange-pink color under the Wood's light. The presence of this typical fluorescence is usually all that is necessary to confirm the diagnosis of erythrasma. Since the fluorescing material is soluble in water, it may be washed away if the area has been cleaned recently (Plate I–B).

The Wood's light is also useful in detecting the presence of uroporphyrin, which imparts a pink fluorescence to the urine of patients suffering from porphyria cutanea tarda.

EXAMINATION FOR SCABIES (See also Chapter 10)

Scabies is a contagious, highly pruritic, parasitic infestation that has a rather typical distribution on the body. It usually involves the webs of the fingers and toes, the flexor aspects of the wrists, the axillary folds, the umbilicus, the female nipple, and glans penis. The diagnostic lesion of scabies is the burrow, which can be identified as a serpiginous track on the skin (Fig. 3–9). Burrows are not always easily detectable in scabies, especially in persons who keep themselves fastidiously clean. The diagnosis of scabies may be confirmed by finding the causative mite, which has four pairs of legs. The female of the species is illustrated in Figure 3–10. Examination for scabies begins with obtaining material from a papule or burrow that has not been excoriated. The papules and burrows most likely to provide a good preparation are often barely visible but may be detected with a hand lens. Selected areas should be scraped vigorously with a sharp, sterile scalpel and the material placed on a glass slide for examination under the microscope. Some examiners

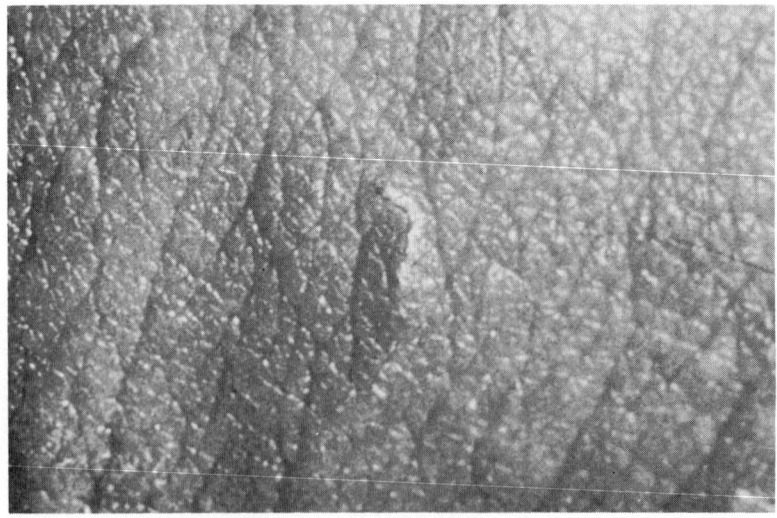

FIGURE 3–9 Scabies burrow.

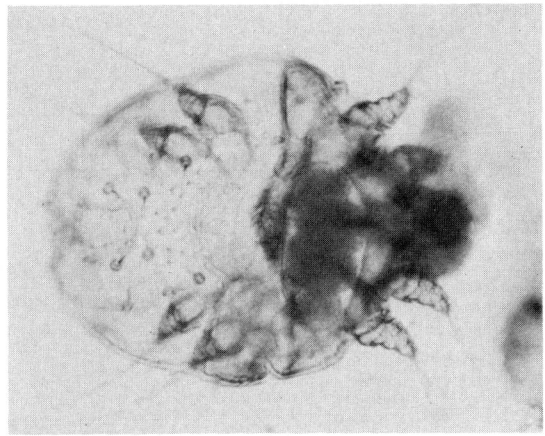

FIGURE 3–10 Adult scabies mite.

mount the tissue in 10 per cent KOH, while others prefer to place a drop of mineral or immersion oil on the skin, on the scalpel, or on the slide.[4] The oil adheres to the mite, which is thus not readily fragmented. A coverslip is then placed on the slide and the entire field is microscopically examined under low power. This technique often yields a higher percentage of positive scrapings, but the procedure may have to be repeated several times before the parasite is discovered. At times, a fresh burrow can be neatly decapitated with a scalpel, revealing the fertilized female with her eggs and feces (Fig. 3–11).[5] This last procedure is done with a No. 15 blade and requires no anesthesia.

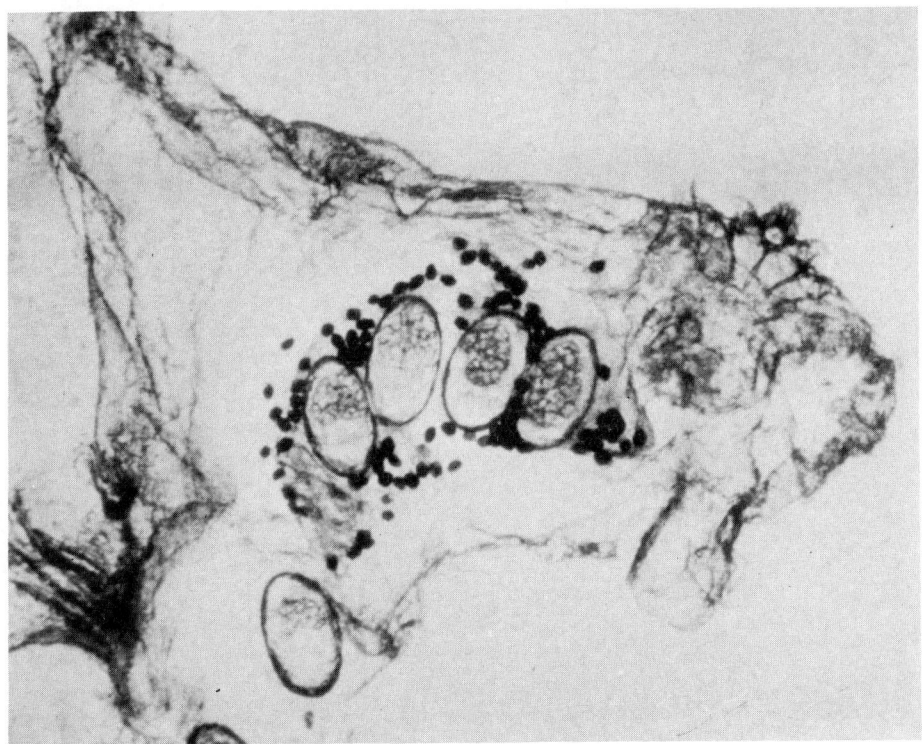

FIGURE 3–11 Adult scabies mite trailed by eggs and feces.

THE TZANCK SMEAR

The Tzanck smear is a cytological technique primarily used in dermatology for diagnosis of some bullous diseases of the skin, including several viral eruptions.[6,7] The technique is easy to perform and once interpretation of the smears is mastered, a clinical diagnosis often can be suggested long before results of a skin biopsy or laboratory identification of a virus becomes available.

If the presence of herpes simplex, herpes zoster, or varicella is suspected, the top of a fresh vesicle should carefully be removed with scissors or a scalpel and the fluid contents blotted away, without touching the base of the lesion. The base of the lesion is then scraped with a sharp curette or scalpel and the scrapings spread on a clean glass slide (Fig. 3–12). The slide is air dried, fixed in a 95 per cent alcohol solution for five minutes, and stained with Giemsa, Wright, or methylene blue stain. The presence of bizarre, multinucleated giant cells visible under low power of the light microscope is indicative of either herpes simplex, herpes zoster, or varicella (Fig. 3–13). The more definitive diagnosis must depend of course on the detection of the causative virus by culture or immunological means. Viral-induced giant cells often contain six or more nuclei which show great variation in size and shape. Multinucleated giant cells do not commonly occur in vaccinia or smallpox, a useful point to remember in the differential diagnosis.[8]

A Tzanck smear may be used to establish the diagnosis of molluscum contagiosum, a viral disease whose lesions contain very large, rounded molluscum bodies, which are groups of virus-laden cells. Molluscum bodies are

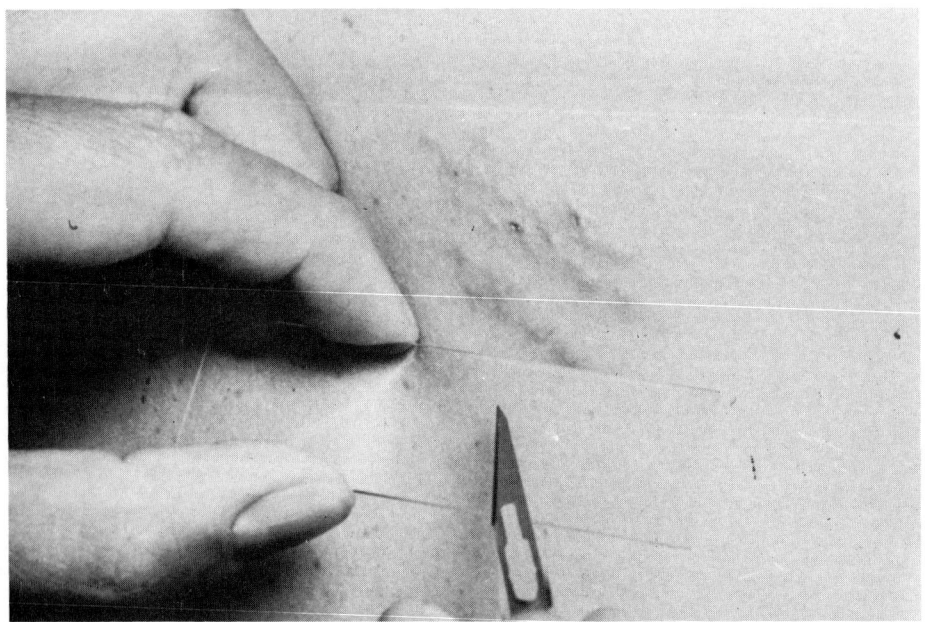

FIGURE 3–12 Tzanck smear for herpes simplex.

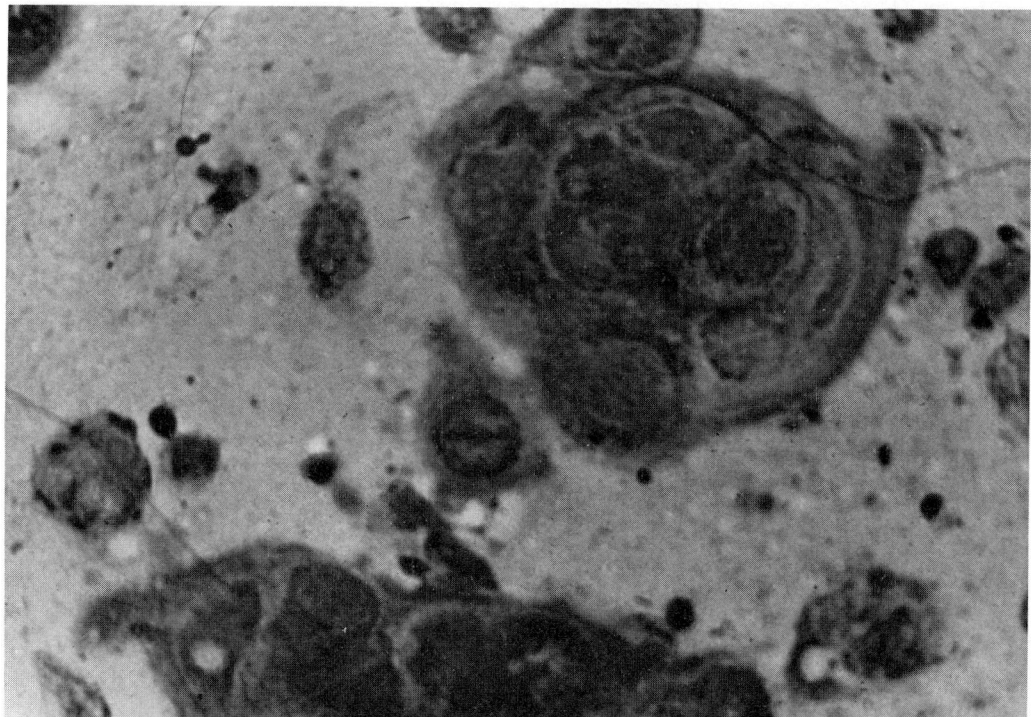
FIGURE 3-13 Multinucleated giant cell of herpesvirus infection by Tzanck smear.

found in the cheesy material expressed from the center of a characteristic button-like lesion.

The Tzanck smear can also demonstrate the presence of acantholytic cells in pemphigus, a disease that is extremely rare in adolescents. Acantholytic cells are rounded epidermal cells with dark staining nuclei. These cells have lost their normal attachment sites to other epidermal cells and may indicate the presence of an autoimmune phenomenon in the skin. Acantholytic cells are not pathognomonic of the presence of pemphigus, since they are also found in other conditions, such as pyoderma.

DIASCOPY

The diascope is a piece of clear plastic or glass that can be firmly pressed against a skin lesion. Diascopy is a very simple but useful technique for determining if an erythematous lesion is caused by vascular dilatation or bleeding into the skin (petechiae). Under pressure, lesions caused by hemorrhages in the skin do not blanch (Fig. 3-14), whereas most lesions containing dilated blood vessels do. Diascopy is also useful in the detection of the glassy, yellow-brown papules found in some granulomatous diseases of the skin, such as lupus vulgaris.

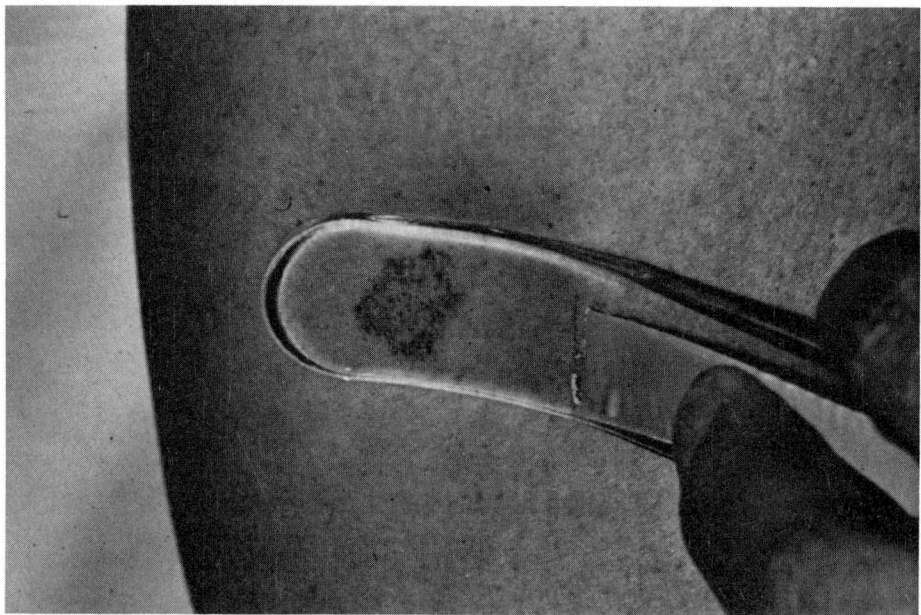

FIGURE 3–14 Diascopy over an area of hemorrhage (petechiae).

PUNCH BIOPSY

The punch biopsy is a technique for obtaining tissue from the skin for histopathological diagnosis.[9] It is a reasonably simple procedure which is safe, causes little pain, and results in minimal scarring. Biopsy of a skin lesion often becomes necessary when the diagnosis is in doubt or when the possibility of malignancy has been raised. With the punch biopsy, a small, cylindrical plug of skin can be removed quickly with minimal inconvenience to the patient.

The equipment needed to perform a punch biopsy includes a syringe containing local anesthetic, a small forceps, an iris scissors, and a circular punch measuring from 2 to 6 mm in diameter (Fig. 3–15). The lesion selected for biopsy should be fully matured and typical of the eruption. After the patient has been questioned about possible allergic sensitivity, the area for biopsy should be carefully marked with a pen (Fig. 3–16) and injected with a local anesthetic. The skin about the lesion is spread apart between the fingers so that, following removal of the punch specimen and release of the tissues, the round excision site will be elliptical in shape. The elliptical wound tends to heal with more acceptable scarring. The circular punch is applied perpendicularly to the skin surface with downward pressure and rotated until it cuts to the depth desired, usually into the subcutaneous fat (Fig. 3–17). The punch is then removed and the specimen gently and carefully teased from the biopsy site with forceps so as not to damage the tissue. The specimen is snipped off at the base with iris scissors to include the deepest portion of the biopsy specimen (Fig. 3–18). Placing the specimen on a small piece of blotting paper with the subcutaneous tissue oriented downward helps the pathologist identify the ex-

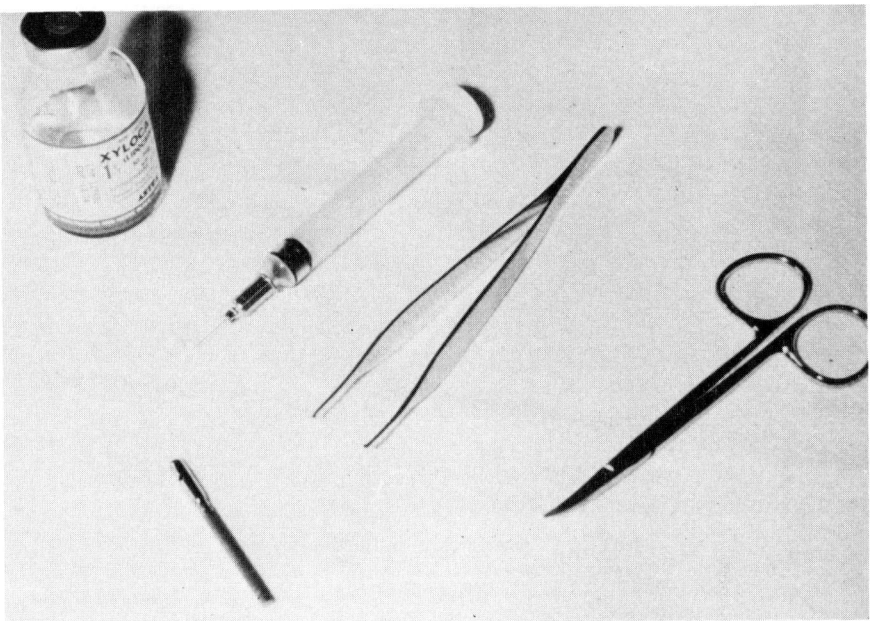

FIGURE 3–15 Equipment needed for punch biopsy.

terior surface of the specimen. Biopsy specimens meant for routine processing are placed in a 10 per cent solution of formalin.

For special techniques, such as histochemical staining or electron microscopy, other tissue fixatives may be required. The wound site is treated with a mild coagulating compound, such as Monsel's solution, followed by the application of pressure over the site to control bleeding. The wound is initially covered with a small bandage for 24 hours, after which the biopsy site can be cleaned once daily with rubbing alcohol until healing is complete. The biopsy

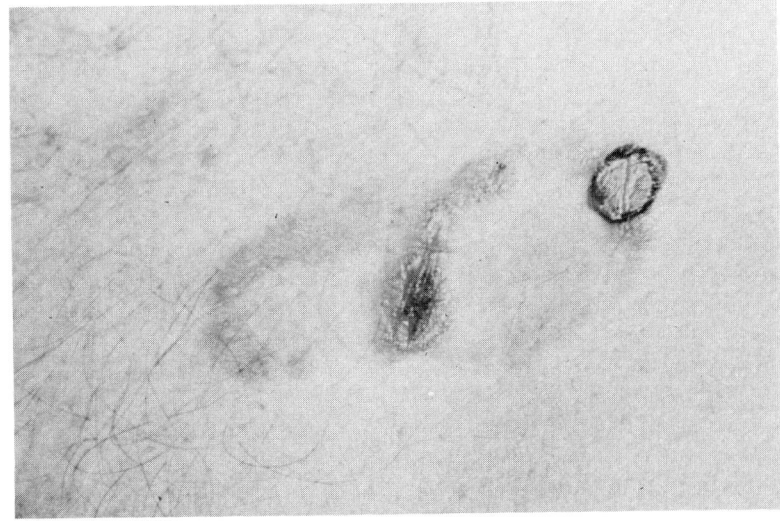

FIGURE 3–16 Marking of biopsy site for punch biopsy.

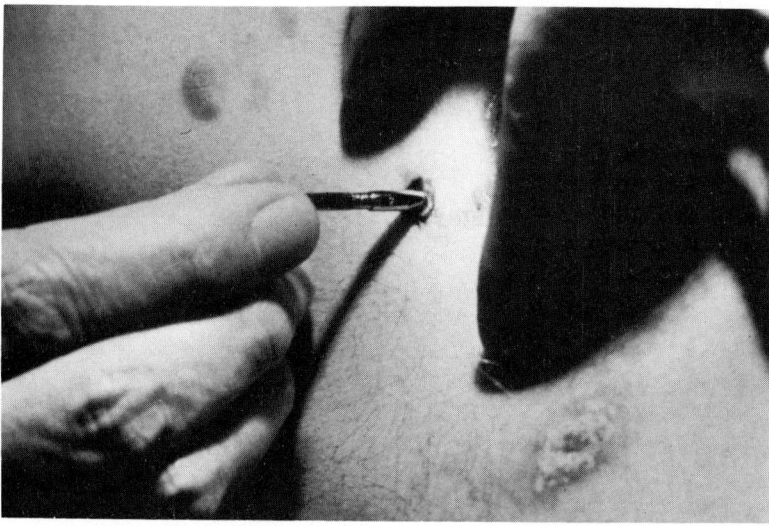

FIGURE 3–17 Performance of punch biopsy.

site does not require suturing unless a 4 mm or larger punch is used. Cosmetic considerations require that the smallest useful specimen be taken from the face. If a particularly large specimen of skin is needed, or if the subcutaneous tissue is of primary interest, an excisional biopsy by scalpel is indicated, followed by the placement of sutures. The biopsy specimen is then submitted to a pathologist for examination. The pathologist will need to know the name and age of the patient, the duration of the lesion, the site of biopsy, and the physician's clinical impression.

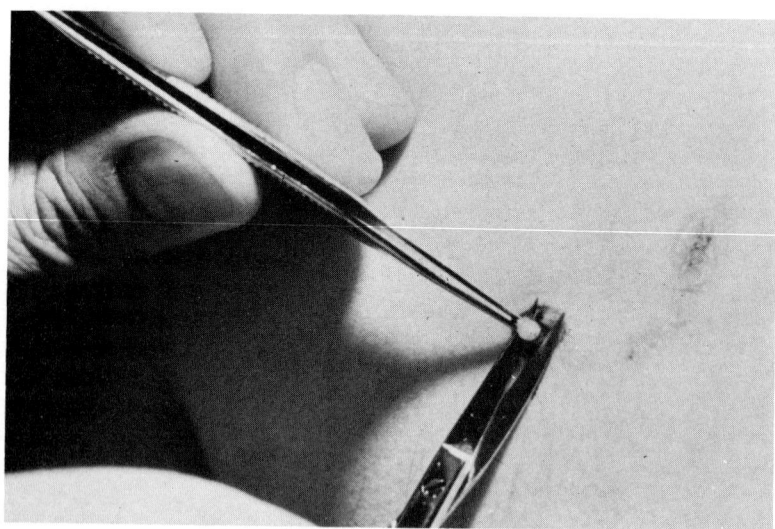

FIGURE 3–18 Removal of tissue from punch biopsy.

THE PATCH TEST

The patch test is used to determine the possible course of allergic contact dermatitis, a cutaneous eczematous process mediated by cellular immunity (see Chapter 5). Although the cause of the dermatitis is sometimes obvious, the use of the patch test may still be necessary to secure the diagnosis.[10] The patch test procedure consists of applying the suspect chemical substances to the uninvolved skin in the hope of reproducing the original condition in miniature and under controlled conditions. The suspect hapten must be brought into intimate contact with normal skin in order for it to penetrate the epidermis, and thus participate in the formation of the complete antigen. Commercial patch test kits are now available and permit multiple simultaneous tests to be performed. The positive test reaction develops within 24 to 48 hours. It reveals varying degrees of redness and swelling and the presence of papules, vesicles, or bullae. Patch testing should never be done on inflamed skin and should be delayed until the acute stage has subsided for fear of aggravating the inflammation. Since difficulties can arise in the application and interpretation of patch tests, some experience is necessary to interpret the results correctly.

REFERENCES

1. Caplan, R. M.: Medical uses of the Wood's lamp. JAMA, *202*:1035, 1967.
2. Michaelides, P., and Shatin, H.: Erythrasma fluorescence under the Wood light. Arch. Dermatol. *65*:614, 1952.
3. Munro-Ashman, D., Wells, R. S., and Clayton, Y. M.: Erythrasma in adolescence. Br. J. Dermatol., *75*:401, 1963.
4. Muller, G., Jacobs, P. H., Moore, N. E.: Scraping for human scabies. Arch. Dermatol., *107*:70, 1973.
5. Hoke, A. W.: Scabies scraping. Arch. Dermatol., *108*:424, 1973.
6. Blank, H., Burgoon, C. F., Baldridge, C. D., et al.: Cytologic smears in diagnosis of herpes simplex, herpes zoster and varicella. JAMA, *146*:1410, 1951.
7. Goldman, L., McCabe, R. M., and Sawyer, F.: The importance of cytology technic for the dermatologist in office practice. Arch. Dermatol., *81*:359, 1960.
8. Wilson Jones, E.: Cytodiagnosis. *In* Rook, A., Wilkinson, D. S., and Ebling, F. J. G. (eds.): Textbook of Dermatology. 2nd ed., Vol. 1, Philadelphia, F. A. Davis, 1972, pp. 73–76.
9. Lever, W. F., and Schaunberg-Lever, G.: Histopathology of the Skin. Philadelphia, J. B. Lippincott, 1975, pp. 1–2.
10. Shelley, W. B.: The patch test. JAMA, *200*:874, 1967.

4 ACNE

JAMES E. RASMUSSEN, M.D.

This chapter deals with the most common cutaneous problem of adolescence — acne. Although the subject needs no introduction, I will begin by defining my objectives. Clinicians and researchers have compiled a great mass of facts about acne. Although there are large gaps in our knowledge, it has become popular to gather a related group of facts and mold them into a specific hypothesis about the pathogenesis of acne. In each hypothesis, the greatest attention is devoted to one major area — the sebaceous gland and the factors that influence the composition of sebum and its rate of excretion. Other aspects of sebaceous gland structure and function have been given little notice. The belief that there is one completely valid theory to explain the etiology of acne is probably a satisfying self-delusion. Yet without the ability to pinpoint the basic defect in the pilosebaceous apparatus, treatment of acne remains empirical, erratically successful, and unscientific.

In this chapter, I will describe the cast of players: the sebaceous gland with its secretions, the pilosebaceous canal, and the bacteria. The roles they play will be related to the clinical aspects of acne and to its response to treatment, and each theory of the pathogenesis of acne will be examined.

THE SEBACEOUS GLAND[1,2]

The holocrine sebaceous gland is distributed widely throughout the human skin. The greatest concentration of glands is on the face and scalp (900/cm^2).[1] In most areas (except on or near mucous membranes), the duct of the gland empties into the midportion of a hair follicle, so that sebum escapes to the surface through the follicular pore. Each gland is composed of several lobules which converge on the sebaceous duct. The anatomical junction of the sebaceous duct, the hair follicle lining, and the external epidermis forms a complex zone which is sheltered enough to provide a suitable medium for the growth of anaerobic organisms. This zone is also influenced by the surface environment. It represents an area in which three separate cell types evolve in transit and are shed, each in a different manner. The result is a complex biological column that exudes sebum onto the surface.

The sebaceous gland is rimmed with a thin layer of small, undifferentiated basal cells. As individual cells mature, they come to lie closer to the center of the lobule. Individual droplets of sebum form in the cytoplasm of the sebaceous cells, become larger, and finally coalesce around the centrally placed nucleus, forming a reticulated cytoplasm. Disintegration of the cell wall, which is itself secreted, exposes the raw sebum to degradation by lipases. This mixture of lipids, debris, and keratin which has been shed from the follicular wall eventually reaches the surface of the skin through the hair pore.

The control of sebum production is complex; androgens are the prime movers, but other hormones play "permissive" roles.[3-9] Estrogens suppress the function of the sebaceous gland at least in part because they inhibit gonadal and adrenal androgen synthesis.[3] Although most glands have recognized feedback control mechanisms, such a control system is only conjectured for the sebaceous glands.[10] In utero and during the first few weeks of life, the sebaceous glands are stimulated by maternal androgens, but during the next eight to ten years they remain relatively dormant.

Early in puberty, the production of adrenal and gonadal androgens begins to increase and these androgens become primary stimulants to the sebaceous glands. The glands enlarge greatly, and the production of sebum increases five to ten fold.[11] Most of the pituitary hormones act indirectly on the sebaceous gland (adrenocorticotropic hormone or ACTH through the adrenals, follicle-stimulating hormone or FSH through the gonads), but growth hormone acts directly. Some investigators have suspected the presence of a pituitary sebotrophic hormone, since pituitary extracts free of ACTH, TSH (thyroid-stimulating hormone), FSH, and LH (luteinizing hormone) activity can stimulate the sebaceous gland in animals.[12,13] This agent has never been identified in human beings. Recently, there has been an interest in β-MSH (a melanocyte-stimulating hormone) as a possible sebotrophic hormone in animals, but levels of this hormone do not increase in patients with acne and β-MSH has not been shown to be sebotrophic in man.[14]

It is probable that adrenal and gonadal androgens are metabolized locally by the sebaceous glands. The enzyme 5α-reductase is capable of producing dihydrotestosterone (DHT), a potent but short-lived androgen.[15,16] This enzyme is contained in sebaceous glands and may account for the oily seborrhea usually associated with acne. High rates of conversion of testosterone to DHT are associated with severe acne in women but, paradoxically, not in men.[15,17] These studies obviously need expansion and confirmation.

Figures for the rate of turnover of the maximally stimulated sebaceous gland have ranged from 7 to 21 days.[18,19] This range may be due to the difference in techniques used to study turnover time or may be an indication that each lobule of a sebaceous gland acts individually. Whether either extreme of this time period or their average fairly represents the turnover time, it is obvious that the sebaceous gland can not demonstrate an immediately visible response to any stimulus.

Innervation. In spite of a perilobular supply of cholinergic nerves, described by Montagna and Ellis,[20] the sebaceous gland does not respond to stimulation with acetylcholine or epinephrine, or to blockade with propranolol.[21-23]

Feedback. The repeated removal of sebum leads to an apparent local increase in sebum production which may represent a feedback mechanism.[4, 10] This may be important because most people remove facial sebum each day by washing.

SEBUM

Sebum is a viscous, complex mixture of cytoplasmic lipids and cell fragments. When isolated from adult sebaceous glands, it contains 60 per cent triglycerides, 20 per cent wax esters, 10 per cent squalene, and 10 per cent minor components, such as steroids, phospholipids, and diglycerides.[25, 26] Before puberty, the concentration of squalene is lower but more sterols (e.g., cholesterol) are present.[11] Because it is technically not feasible, the rate of production and concentration of sebum components usually is not measured inside the gland itself. When lipid samples are collected from the skin surface, the specimens reflect changes that have occurred in transit through the pilar canal as well as contamination from epidermally derived lipids. The most obvious change in the composition of sebum is due to the hydrolysis of triglycerides with the release of free fatty acids (FFA). As a result, 30 per cent of skin surface lipids are FFA.[25, 27] These FFA have chain lengths of from 4 to 30 carbon atoms, but the most frequently occurring chain is C–16, palmitic acid, which constitutes 25 per cent of the FFA.[28] The FFA are branched and unbranched, saturated and unsaturated. Octa-deca-5, 8-dienoic acid (seboleic acid) has been the only FFA found in patients with acne but not found in individuals free of acne.[29, 30] The concentration of FFA is about the same in prepubertal children[11] as in adults with acne,[31-36] without acne, or with a past history of acne.[35] A decreased concentration of FFA in many patients with acne[25] has also been described.

Quantification of the epidermal contribution to surface lipids is difficult and is based mainly on observation of those cutaneous areas with few sebaceous glands, such as the back of the hand.[37, 38] Observations of this kind have led to the presumption that some sterol esters, cholesterol, phospholipids, and triglycerides originate in the epidermis. Artifacts that may alter FFA concentrations on the surface include topically applied lipids, such as those contained in cosmetics, hair dressings, and bacterial cell wall components.

The sebaceous gland and epidermis synthesize sterols, triglycerides, and wax esters from fatty acids. After injecting ^{14}C acetate as a tracer around sebaceous glands, Summerly and Woodbury detected labeled squalene, triglycerides, wax esters, and small amounts of FFA.[2, 39] From this and other studies, it may be concluded that dietary lipids are not incorporated directly into the complex lipid mixture known as sebum. Gross dietary manipulation can, however, affect the composition of sebum and the rate of its production in both mice[23] and humans,[40] but the mechanism of these changes is not known. Certain lipophilic substances, such as tetracycline, may selectively be concentrated in the sebaceous gland.[41]

SAMPLING OF SEBUM[43, 44]

There are numerous methods available for the collection and analysis of surface sebum, each with its advantages and sources of error.[44] Early attempts to quantify sebum production consisted of ether extraction and identification of lipids accumulated in full-length underclothing (long johns) after overnight wear. The most frequently used methods today are modifications of the older absorption technique. Strauss and Pochi have used several layers of cigarette paper applied to the forehead and left in place for several hours.[45] The absorbed lipid is extracted with ether, which is then evaporated to leave a residue that can be weighed. The result is expressed as ug sebum/cm^2/min. The "normal" adult values are mcg/cm^2/min in males and 0.7 mcg/cm^2/min in females.

Sebum can also be collected by scrubbing the skin with a sponge soaked in solvent or by placing a glass cylinder filled with ether directly on the skin. The paper technique of Strauss and Pochi tends to produce more constant results than either the cylinder or sponge methods. A more recent method uses infrared spectroscopy for analysis of sebum and FFA.[46,47]

Many factors, both technical and physiological, can affect both the measurable rate of production and the content of sebum.[42] These factors include: site of sampling;[48] duration of storage of samples (prolonged storage leads to increased FFA);[49] time of day (? diurnal rhythm);[50] menstrual cycle (? increased triglycerides);[51] pregnancy and lactation (increased sebum production);[52] age (decreased sebum production in men and women after age 40);[53] change in skin temperature (increased sebum production with increased temperature);[54] topical and systemic anti-acne therapy (decreased FFA,[55-57] decreased sebum with estrogens);[5] diet (decreased sebum with decreased intake of calories);[40] and emotional stress (increased FFA and sebum).[58,59] It is important to recognize that different methods of collecting and analyzing sebum, as well as choice of controls and time of year, may impart such differences as to make any two studies virtually incomparable.

FUNCTION OF SEBACEOUS GLANDS

Those who have studied sebum and acne tend to assign a biological function to sebaceous glands and sebum.[2] Although in certain animals modified sebaceous glands produce a water-repellent oil that plays a role in sexual attraction, their function in humans is uncertain. Little controlled work has been done on the antibacterial and antifungal qualities of sebum. However, Kligman[2] has shown that the FFA of sebum are incapable of arresting fungal growth when stratum corneum is used as a substrate. It seems rather odd that glands so widespread, so numerous and so strategically placed on the body, and so functional at critical developmental stages (in utero and at puberty), could be considered a "living fossil with a past but not a future."[2]

THE PILOSEBACEOUS UNIT

The sebaceous gland empties into the middle third of the canal. Above the gland, the follicular canal, or infundibulum, has epidermal (acro-infundibulum) and dermal (infra-infundibulum) components. Cells derived from the gland, and those derived from the two parts of the hair follicle, appear to have separate and distinct mechanisms for adhesion and lysis. The mature sebaceous cells appear to follow a simple and quite visible path of rupture and disintegration. In contrast, cells of the acro-infundibulum (epidermal component) resemble cells of the surface epithelium and form a granular layer and a compact, adherent stratum corneum. In the dermal portion of the infundibulum (infra-infundibulum), keratinizing cells gradually lose their ability to form a thick, stable, granular layer and stratum corneum. At the junction of the sebaceous gland, the infundibulum is represented by only one or two poorly adherent cells.[60] It is in this narrow area (the dermal infundibulum) that the initial lesion of acne begins.

However, not all follicles develop lesions; those containing terminal (adult-type) hairs seem particularly immune. In addition, other factors seem to affect susceptibility to the disease. Certain areas of the body rarely develop acne, suggesting that there may be limiting forces, possibly related to androgen receptors, critical mass of sebum or bacteria, pore size, surface temperature, sebum viscosity, biochemical composition of sebum, or some other unknown factor. Although most of these factors have not been adequately studied, it is known that the pores in the most acne-prone areas of the face are smaller than those of the back, which in turn are smaller than those of the chest.[1] Thus, decreasing poral diameter apparently closely parallels regional susceptibility to acne.

ECOLOGY[61-65]

The ecology of acne-prone areas of the skin has been intensively investigated. The results are often difficult to interpret and compare because of the wide variety of sampling sites, methods, and culture media used.[66] The data have also been subject to criticism because in almost all the sampling methods used, specimens have been obtained from the external epidermis instead of from the depths of the hair pore, which is the presumed target zone of sebum, FFA, and bacteria.

Three main groups of microorganisms have been incriminated[63] at some time in the pathogenesis of acne and each will be discussed briefly.

Corynebacterium Acnes. FFA are generally accepted as playing an important role in causing acne. FFA are derived almost entirely from the hydrolysis of triglycerides by lipases, which are produced mainly by C. acnes.[67-70] C. acnes is an anaerobic gram-positive rod and is one of the principal microflora of the face and other sebaceous areas. The concentration of these organisms increases considerably at the onset of puberty.[71, 72] In stationary, sheltered loci, such as comedones, they may clump to form large masses. Several subgroups of C. acnes including Types 1 and 2 have been isolated on the basis of colony morphology and biochemical differences.[73] The different growth and enzyme patterns have been until now mainly of academic interest, but it is possible that certain C. acnes subgroups may turn out to be associated with certain clinical varieties of acne.

Patients with acne have a greater number of surface C. acnes present than those without acne and the number of organisms increases even more in patients with inflammatory varieties of acne.[74] Open and closed comedones have more C. acnes than any other type of bacterium.[62] Papules and pustules also contain C. acnes, but in small numbers.[74, 75] Only one third of acne nodules contain *C. acnes*,[75] perhaps because of the bactericidal effects of the inflammatory response.

Of all the enzymes *C. acnes* produces, only lipases have received much attention. There is some evidence that patients with acne harbor strains of *C. acnes* that hydrolyze triglycerides more efficiently than do strains isolated from controls. However, these findings may result from the exposure of the bacteria to greater amounts of sebum.[73] Voss[76] has suggested that protease, lecithinase, neuramidinase, and hyaluronidase may also be contributing factors in acne. In partial support of this theory there is evidence that *C. acnes* isolated from patients with inflammatory acne produce more hyaluronidase than do those organisms isolated from control subjects without acne.[76]

Micrococcaceae. The Micrococcaceae are aerobic gram-positive cocci. This large group of organisms can be subdivided according to the Baird-Parker classification into staphylococci, micrococci, and sarciniae.

Staphylococcus epidermidis (S. albus) is the most frequently found bacterium of the family Micrococcaceae in the acne-prone areas of the body but occurs less frequently than *C. acnes* in most patients.[77, 78] The Micrococcaceae are the most common microorganisms found in cysts.[75] *S. epidermidis* also produces lipases,[79] but probably contributes in only a minor way to the formation of FFA in sebum, since selective eradication of this organism with agents that do not destroy *C. acnes* causes little change in the composition of sebum.[69] What role, if any, *S. epidermidis* plays in the etiology of acne is not known at this time. Vaccines using an extract of this organism have been rightly abandoned by most physicians as a treatment for acne.

Pityrosporum. This genus contains at least two lipophilic, yeast-like organisms. Both *P. ovale* and *P. orbiculare* are commonly found in areas afflicted by acne. Because they are fairly difficult to culture and quantify,[61-65] they have not been studied as thoroughly as the less fastidious *C. acnes* and *S. epidermidis*. *P. ovale* is the more common organism of the two, but both are found in comedones and pustules. Although this group of organisms can produce lipase,[80] the FFA concentration in an area such as the scalp does not decrease when *P. ovale* is inhibited with antibiotics.[69, 81] Although Weary[82] has described an unusual pustular eruption associated with *P. ovale* which recurred regularly when antibiotics were taken systemically, there does not seem to be much evidence to support a causative relationship between *P. ovale* and acne vulgaris.

Other Microorganisms

GRAM-NEGATIVE ORGANISMS. *Proteus, Klebsiella, Aerobacter* species, and *E. coli* have only rarely been isolated from the exposed skin of normal patients or those with acne.[62, 75, 83] They are most commonly found in the nasopharynx, the axillae, and in the perianal area.[84] Small numbers of gram-negative organisms may also be found in some of the inflammatory lesions of acne, but are usually isolated only in a rare group of patients with gram-negative folliculitis, a disease that simulates acne.

Patients with gram-negative folliculitis were initially described by Fulton and his colleagues as falling into two groups, both of which had received long-term, broad-spectrum antibiotics.[83, 85] *Klebsiella-Aerobacter* species were found in patients with numerous small pustules located in the midface and

Proteus in those with nodular cystic acne.[86] The authors felt that a short, intensive course of ampicillin might benefit some patients with this condition, but most of those studied required a continuous course of broad-spectrum antibiotic drugs.

MITES. *Demodex folliculorum* is a mite which inhabits the hair follicles of the face of the human adult. On occasion in the past it has been indicted in the pathogenesis of acne, but its relationship to acne remains a controversial subject.

ETIOLOGY

No theory about the cause of acne has yet been offered that accounts for all that is known about the disease. Although each hypothesis may explain one or more of the clinical and experimental observations, each has a serious weakness. Most of the prominent theories of causation have centered around poral obstruction, increased sebum excretion rate, irritation by FFA, and the role of the lipases produced by *C. acnes*.

THEORIES

Existing etiological theories include the following: excessive production of sebum, irritation by FFA or other components of sebum; infection by *C. acnes*; hormonal abnormality; pilar obstruction as a result of the first three factors; dietary deficiency; psychological disorder; and allergy.

Many patients with acne have a high sebum excretion rate (SER), but 10 to 30 per cent do not, and some studies show little deviation from the normal rate.[31, 34, 96-98, 233] An increase in SER may be genetically determined, but the supposition needs to be confirmed. A higher flow rate within a gland, coupled with a modest reduction in the size of the orifice, could produce a considerable increase in intraductal or glandular pressure, making the wall of the follicle more susceptible to rupture or "blowout." Whether or not the size of the sebaceous gland is increased in acne remains uncertain, but there may be an increase in the number of glands present.[233] A greater number of glands could account for an increase in SER without an increased flow rate being evident at the mouth of the individual follicle. In a retrospective study,[97] SER was found to remain high when acne was in remission and was also elevated in conditions such as Parkinson's disease, a disorder not usually associated with acne.[236]

With the exception of estrogens, most topical and systemic drugs that modify acne, such as retinoic acid, benzoyl peroxide, and tetracycline, do not change the SER.[55, 57, 181] An increase in SER alone, therefore, cannot account for many of the features of acne.

When human sebum was induced into the external ear canal of the rabbit, FFA[106] and squalene[76, 96] proved to be comedogenic. However, the production of comedones in human skin is a more complex process.[235-237] Patients with acne do not have a higher concentration of FFA than normal adults or prepubertal children,[30-36] yet most effective anti-acne agents lower FFA.[55, 56, 57, 184, 238, 239] In fact, most studies have shown a lower *concentration* of FFA in the sebum of patients with acne than in that of individuals without acne. A greater output of sebum would cause a greater amount of FFA to come into contact with the skin. Unfortunately, surface studies do not test the FFA hypothesis adequately, since acne begins in the follicles, and the concentration of FFA in the depths of comedones far exceeds that present on the skin.[103, 240] It is quite possible that a sudden change in the intrafollicular concentration of FFA could cause irritation and stimulate rapid production of cells,[101] with resulting microcomedo formation. In some individuals, this microcomedo could continue to enlarge to the size of a clinically visible lesion, and in others it could become a pustule. The effects of FFA (or other components of sebum) might also explain the early stages of comedo formation as elaborated by Knutson.[60]

The study of intrafollicular concentration of FFA and its relationship to the dynamics of comedo formation is a highly promising area of acne research, but because of technical difficulties success remains elusive.

The role of the acne bacillus also remains unclear. It is doubtful that the organism is truly pathogenic. Its effects are probably related to its lipases, which release FFA through the hydrolysis of triglycerides. The effects of these and other enzymes on the wall of the follicle are virtually unknown, and how they contribute to the formation of the comedo and subsequent inflammation has yet to be studied.

The significance of the morphological and biochemical variants of *C. acnes*[62, 73] in acne is not clear. Certain antibiotics reduce the *C. acnes* population, but induce other organisms to rapidly increase in number.[191] Infection, therefore, cannot explain all we know about this disease.

Since normal subjects, as well as those who have inactive acne, harbor great numbers of *C. acnes,* it is doubtful that allergic hypersensitivity to the organism alone can account for the spectrum of disease seen in acne. However, patients with the disease may be more sensitive to the enzymes of cellular components of *C. acnes,*[241] with increased skin reactivity to the organisms and their products, which may be related to the demonstrated suppressive effects of corticosteroids on the inflammatory process. Patients with acne also have increased antibodies to *C. acnes,*[106, 242, 243] and skin tests with extract of *C. acnes* produce a more severe reaction in patients with acne than they produce in controls.[241] However, the formation of antibodies may result from the disease rather than cause it. Tetracycline may have more than an antibacterial effect in acne; it may also impair the function of leukocytes and subsequently reduce inflammation.[246]

Strauss and Pochi[16] reviewed the role of androgens in acne. Sansone and Reisner[17] were the first to demonstrate an abnormal local metabolism of androgens in the sebaceous gland. Other researchers[34] have looked in vain for an increase in plasma or in urinary androgenic steroids. Using very sensitive assays, several investigators have documented unusually high plasma levels of 17-β-hydroxysteroids (androgens) in some (less than 25 per cent) women with acne.[244] Their assay results did not correlate with the extent or severity of acne, although hirsute females with acne have been found to have increased production of androgens.[245]

The abnormal local metabolism of testosterone by the acne-prone sebaceous gland is difficult to interpret. Sansone and Reisner's experiments indicated that the enzyme 5α-reductase (which produces dihydrotestosterone, a very potent androgen) is present in abnormally high concentrations in the dermis of acne patients. The correlation held only for women, and the levels were not increased in those with the most severe acne. Hay and Hodgins[15] similarly reported an increased rate of production of dihydrotestosterone in the skin of acne patients but correlation between sex and severity of acne was low.[15] At present, therefore, there is only an indication that patients with acne either have more androgens or metabolize them in an abnormal way. No other hormonal defects have been consistently identified in acne patients.[14] They are neither hypo- nor hyperthryoid. The "sebotrophic" hormone has not been found in human beings,[14] and its significance remains elusive.

It is possible that faulty cellular control contributes to abnormal intercellular adherence in the pilar canal. This mechanism could be mediated by androgens, and it would be interesting to study the effects of androgens on the process of pilar keratinization in acne-prone areas.

Since none of the previously mentioned theories alone can explain all that is known about acne, one must consider the possibility that it is a multifactorial disease. It is possible that a patient predisposed by heredity could develop abnormally high SER, mediated by abnormal androgen metabolism at the glandular level. A heavy growth of *C. acnes* then could develop in the follicle, splitting triglycerides into FFA. The FFA and androgens, plus other irritating enzymes, produced by the bacteria, could cause the wall of the follicle to form abnormally adherent keratin,[60] leading to the formation of microcomedones. If the process is rapid, the wall of the follicle could be ruptured by chemical or physical action. The type of lesion that develops papule, pustule, or nodule might depend on the depth of the process. For the present, however, a multifactorial theory must remain entirely speculative.

There is considerable opinion favoring an association between psychic tension and exacerbation of acne. FFA's may be increased during periods of stress,[58] but flares of acne have not correlated well with emotional stress in at least one prospective controlled study. Patients with acne tend to have more personality disorders than do controls,[135] but treatment with tranquilizers has little effect on their skin condition.[138]

CLINICAL ACNE

Acne is the most common cutaneous disease of adolescents and young adults. Because it is so common, especially in its milder forms (comedones), it is often not considered to be a disease. Nearly all teenagers have a few blackheads, which may appear as early as seven or eight years of age.[87, 88] Starting at this age, the number and severity of lesions gradually increase to a peak incidence at 14 to 16 years in girls and at 16 to 19 years in boys.[89] Males usually have more severe inflammatory acne than females,[88] but a persistent form of late-arising acne occasionally plagues the older woman.

There are few data that can be used to compare the incidence of acne in different races, cultures, and societies. Wilkins and Voorhees,[90] in a study of a prison population, found that blacks had much less cystic acne than Caucasians. Most studies, however, have not carefully considered the obvious variables, such as diet, exposure to sunlight, topical care, degree of urbanization, and patient selection that should be considered in such comparisons.[91, 92]

Many patients with early-appearing or severe acne have parents or other relatives with a similar history, but supporting evidence for this observation has never been accumulated prospectively. However, several retrospective studies have suggested that such an association is a real one.[93] There is also an association between an XYY genotype and severe cystic acne.[94] Although the incidence of the XYY genotype is greater in patients with cystic acne than in the general population, it is still less than 2 per cent. Severe acne may also be seen in the Apert form of craniofacial synostosis with syndactyly.[95]

THE LESIONS

Acne is a polymorphous disease with lesions that vary from open and closed comedones to papules, pustules, nodules, and cysts. Although the complete panorama of lesions can occur in a single patient, most individuals with acne have one type of lesion predominantly.

Patients with acne generally have an increased production of sebum,[31, 34, 96, 97, 98] but not all patients with excessive sebum production have acne. Increase in sebum production is most noticeable in severe acne. An oily complexion does not necessarily reflect seborrhea, since patients with acne may apply hair dressings or greasy cosmetics to treat acne or to combat the dryness induced by topical acne therapy. The clinical lesions of acne are most frequently found on the face, especially on the chin, cheeks, perioral area, and forehead. Lesions are seldom found in areas where hair is coarsest—the beard area, the scalp, and the eyebrows, or in some areas of the body with fewer sebaceous glands, such as the eyelids, the posterior surface of the ears, the midaxillary line, and the distal portions of the upper and lower extremities. Some patients have lesions in all of the common areas, but in many others the disease is concentrated in one anatomical zone.

Comedones (singular: comedo). Formed within the follicles of vellus hairs, comedones are plugs of keratin, sebum, and bacteria. Those that lie flush with the poral opening (open comedones) contain melanin pigment in their upper portions, delivered from the surrounding epidermis,[99, 100] and are commonly called "blackheads." When removed atraumatically, they are seen to be cylindrical in shape. A second type of comedo (closed) is shaped more like an upright flask with its narrow neck pinched tight. These contain little pigment. They are more difficult to extract because of their tight epidermal collar. Neither open nor closed comedones darken on exposure to air (Fig. 4–1).[100]

Both open and closed comedones may persist for months, but neither is biochemically quiescent during this time. Plewig and his associates,[101] have shown an uptake of tritiated glycine, histidine, and thymidine by both types of comedones. In open comedones, excretion of the ^{3}H label eventually appears on the surface. In fact, the cells of the basal layer around comedones were found to be more active in metabolizing ^{3}H than was normal skin. The label was discharged into the keratinized mass of the open comedones in a U-shape and was subsequently carried into the center of the comedones and toward the surface. In closed comedones, the label was quickly surrounded by more recently desquamated cells and seemed to be compressed toward the center of the mass. It is obvious from these and other studies that both open and closed comedones are biologically active and still may produce keratin.

The clinical fate of comedones is poorly defined. It is distinctly unusual to

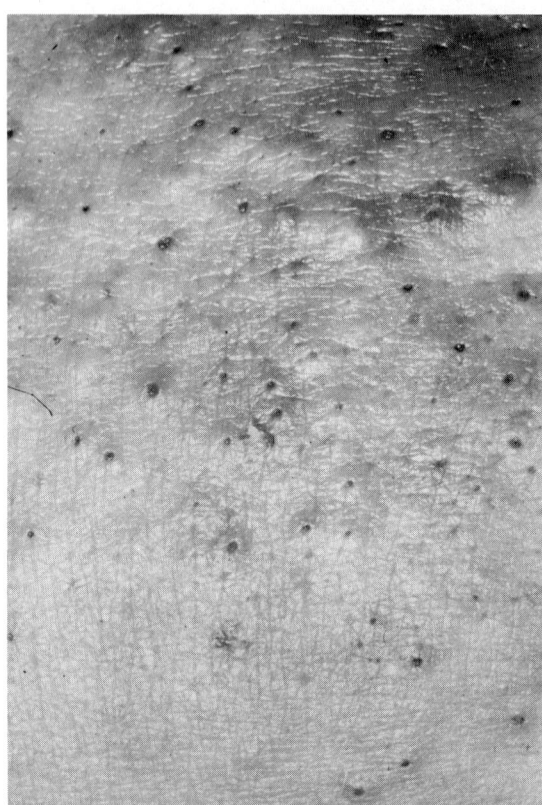

FIGURE 4–1 Open and closed comedones.

see pustules developing at the site of unmolested open comedones, but Orentreich has documented that this may occur, although rarely.[102]

The contents of very early pustules, surgically removed, do not show easily recognizable blackheads, but frequently contain a white ovoid mass similar to the contents of a closed comedo. Kligman and others believe these obstructed follicles (closed comedones) are the "time bombs" of acne. Rupture of the follicular wall and ensuing inflammation may occur as a result of an increase in internal pressure or a change in the concentration of FFA.[103] Knutson has shown that keratin may sometimes extrude through the wall of a follicle into the dermis without generating an inflammatory cellular response,[60] but most of the lesions he studied contained a comedo too small to be detected clinically. It is still not certain then, if the mechanical removal of open or closed comedones prevents their progressing to inflammatory lesions. In my opinion, most pustules do evolve from closed comedones but usually from those that are too small to be noticed clinically.

Papules and Pustules. Papules and pustules are inflammatory lesions that frequently develop in the same locations as comedones (Figs. 4–2A and 4–2B). They are also the types of lesion that involve the chest and back, where comedones are less often seen. It is not unusual to see papules and pustules clustered in one or two sites on the face. Premenstrual exacerbations and postmenstrual temporary remission may be seen frequently in women. However, exacerbation and remission may also be seen in men since this is the natural course of the disease.

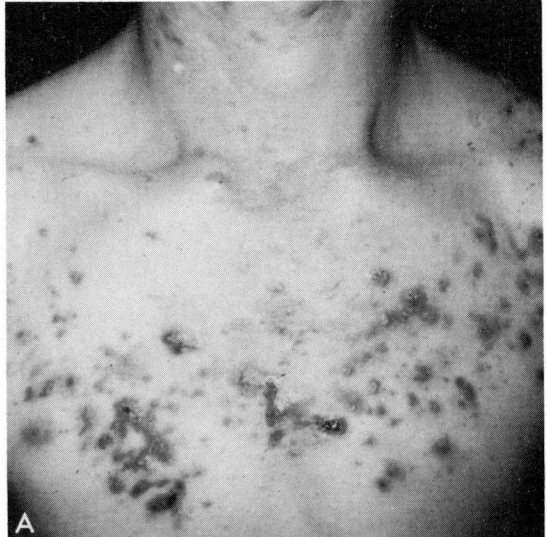
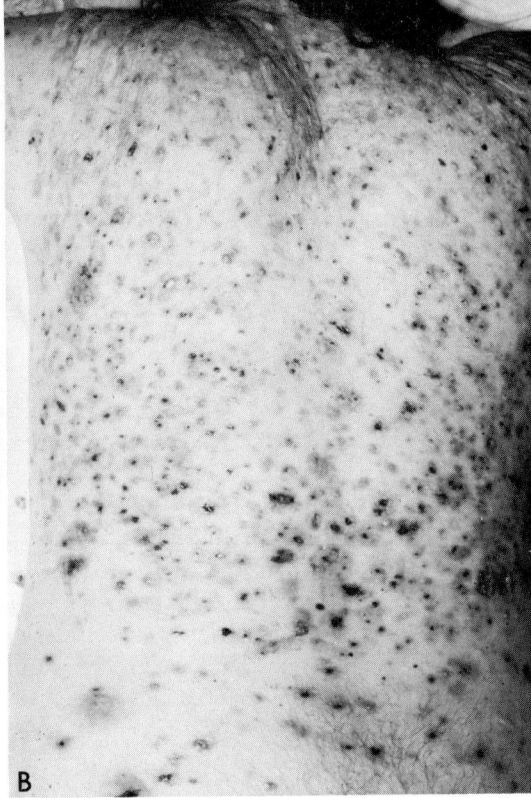

FIGURE 4–2 Chest and back of patient with pustules, nodules, cysts, and scars. This patient also had fever, arthralgia, and leukocytosis.

The inflammatory component may be superficial or relatively deep in relation to the hair follicle.[104] Most papules and pustules resolve spontaneously or rupture through the poral opening in 5 to 12 days. The more superficial the inflammation, the quicker and more benign the resolution. In dark-skinned individuals, however, even minor inflammatory lesions may produce long-lasting hyperpigmentation, which may be more disturbing than the acne itself.

The genesis of inflammation in inflammatory acne is not fully understood. Sebum and comedones produce a definite reaction when injected into the skin, but injection is hardly a physiological phenomenon.[105] FFA are definitely irritating, but how they gain access to the dermis is unknown.[106]

Nodules and Cysts. These are the least common expressions of acne. They may accompany pustular acne or, less commonly, may dominate the clinical picture. It is not too unusual to see many of these lesions in a single area of the body, such as the back, while other areas are spared. Multiple cysts, interconnected by sinuses, may also form. When mature, most large nodular lesions contain thick yellow-green pus and, frequently, blood.[107] The lesions are tender and appear as 1 to 2 cm red-blue inflammatory nodules. Spontaneous drainage may take place through the overlying necrosed epidermis and the lesion may resolve with scarring and fibrosis. Partial resolution also occurs subject to repeated episodes of swelling and discoloration. Some lesions may calcify,[108] while others may become pseudocysts with thick fibrous walls surrounding fragments of hair; the latter regularly discharge small quantities of pus through an overlying sinus tract. True cysts lined with epidermis may require surgical removal.

Scars. Small, flat, or pitted scars are a not uncommon consequence of inflammatory acne, especially on the face, back, and shoulders. Hypertrophic and keloidal scars may occur in patients who are not disposed to such scarring on other parts of the body. The back and shoulders may develop a distinctive small (1 to 3 mm in diameter), sharply marginated, subepidermal, yellow-tan scar that may simulate millia or epidermal cysts.

COURSE

Most patients with acne initially develop their disease during the second decade of life. Comedones appear first and this phase may remain relatively stationary for two to seven years, punctuated occasionally by an erythematous papule or pustule. Inflammatory lesions sometimes arise or become predominant on apparently normal skin. Some patients may continue to have small numbers of papules and pustules for five to ten years, and these may persist well into the third and fourth decades of life. A smaller group, usually male, may have a rapid progression of pustules, nodules, and cysts with very few visible comedones. A smaller group of these severely affected individuals may also show a decrease in serum gamma-globulin.[109]

Some women may develop unusual acne lesions late in the second decade, with a moderate number of deep-seated papules and pustules progressing to scars. These women may or may not have had moderate acne as teenagers.

FACTORS CONSIDERED TO EXACERBATE ACNE

Diet. It is commonly believed that certain foods exacerbate acne.[110, 111] Chocolate, nuts, fried foods, tomatoes, cola drinks, and shellfish are most often incriminated, with exacerbation said to occur from one to three days after the suspected agent has been eaten. Most of these beliefs have been implanted in impressionable teenage patients by their parents or by the lay literature. The current belief that "we are what we eat" has given further impetus to the idea that greasy foods produce greasy complexions.

Many dermatology texts discount the effect of diet on acne, citing several sources. One study suggests that fats in the diet will not be excreted unchanged by the sebaceous gland,[2, 39] since in animals ^{14}C-labeled acetate was rapidly incorporated into the products of the sebaceous gland, whereas lipids per se (cholesterol, FFA, triglycerides) were not. Animals fed chocolate or other fats in moderate amounts exhibited little change in sebum or FFA.[35] Nor did reduction of sugar in the diet improve an acne condition.[112] Fulton and his

TABLE 4–1 FACTORS CONSIDERED TO "EXACERBATE" ACNE

Diet and iodine	Topical agents (ointments and makeup)	Picking at lesions
Heat	Seasonal change	Sexual habits
Menses	Tension	Drugs

colleagues[113] studied the effect of chocolate on the number of acne lesions, on sebum excretion, and on FFA production. Control subjects ate a placebo chocolate bar, and after both groups had been followed for one month, the routine was switched. At the end of the study, the authors concluded that "there was no difference between the bars" in causing acne.

A more recent study on the effect of diet in acne came from the University of Missouri.[114] Patients with acne were selected who, by their own histories, were sensitive to chocolate, cola drinks, nuts, milk, and fish. The members of each group agreed to challenge themselves with the suspected food by drinking a quart of cola drink, a quart of milk, and so on, daily for one week. There was no change in either the type or number of lesions as evaluated by the patient and the physician.

In contrast, there is significant evidence from studies of animals and humans that diet may influence sebum production, concentration of FFA, and acne itself.

1. Major dietary manipulation can increase sebum production rates in animals and humans fed fats or carbohydrates.[23, 115, 116, 117]

2. An abrupt reduction in calories can cause a 40 per cent reduction in sebum excretion rates and FFA.[40]

3. The chocolate and acne study of Fulton appears to contain some weaknesses in methodology. Some of the author's conclusions may not have been based on the evidence obtained.*

4. An increase in dietary sucrose causes an increase in FFA.[117]

5. Obese patients may have more acne than their slimmer peers.[118]

6. Some chlorinated hydrocarbons, when accidentally ingested with food, can cause severe acne.[119, 120, 121] This indicates that at least some ingested products can cause acne. Who knows what effect trace amounts of artificial preservatives, flavorings, and colors may have on a complexion?

At present, it seems reasonable to accept a patient's history of exacerbation after eating certain foods and to agree to their elimination from his diet. Imposed dietary restrictions are probably of no value, since compliance is extremely difficult to obtain. It is best to attempt to gain a patient's compliance with the use of the more accepted and effective topical and antibiotic agents.

Heat. "Tropical acne" is characteristically associated with residence in a warm, humid climate. The eruption is usually very inflammatory and located primarily on the back. Similarly, it is believed that acne may be exacerbated by working near a stove, grill, or fire. It is postulated that an elevated environmental temperature may either increase sebum excretion[50] or cause shrinkage of pilar orifices owing to hydration of the epidermis by sweat and environmental moisture.

---

*The patients given chocolate bars versus placebos were evaluated by counting "lesions" in the generic sense. Comedones, pustules, nodules, and cysts were each given the unit number 1. A patient who developed ten new pustules on an original base of 50 comedones would have been considered "unchanged" in this investigation, since an increase or decrease of 30 per cent in the number (not type) of lesions was required in order to be considered "worse" or "improved." Yet a patient who developed ten new pustules would be considered "worse" if no pustules were present to begin with. In addition, the authors reported that patients eating the chocolate bars had "no change in sebum," yet their own statistics indicate that 60 per cent of these individuals had an increase in sebum and FFA.

Menses. Some women experience acne flares during the ten days preceding the onset of menses.[122, 123] This phenomenon could possibly result from an increase in sebum excretion rate,[124] a change in skin pH,[125] a decrease in pore size,[122] a change in sebum composition,[51] or an increase in the number of functioning sebaceous glands.[123] Yet, unfortunately, each of the studies leading to these suppositions is only loosely supported by the evidence or is subject to other interpretations. The exact mechanism of premenstrual acne is unknown, but changing balance between estrogen, progesterone, and perhaps pituitary stimulatory factors may be involved in the process.

Many women with acne will undergo remission during the last half of pregnancy. But nearly as many experience exacerbation of the disease during this time. It is difficult to predict accurately how each patient will respond. It is not known whether those women who flare premenstrually are those who will have more acne during pregnancy.

Strauss and Pochi have determined that at least 0.1 mg of the common estrogens (ethinyl estradiol, diethylstilbestrol) will suppress both the rate of sebum excretion and the development of acne in many women.[126] This indicates that either progesterone or pituitary trophic hormones might be responsible for premenstrual acne and acne exacerbation during pregnancy. The exact effect of progesterone on the human sebaceous gland has not been fully determined.[127] Unfortunately, estrogens are associated with many side effects and the current trend is to reduce their concentration in birth control pills. Attempts to reduce premenstrual edema through treatment with diuretics have not been found to modify the course of acne.[128, 129]

Topical Agents.[130] Some popular over-the-counter remedies for dry skin and "blemishes" contain acnegens (ingredients that cause acne) of moderate potency. Certain cosmetic creams and ointments used by black patients for hair grooming may also exacerbate acne.[131] Pomades,[131] topical fluorinated corticosteroids, moisturing cosmetics, and even therapeutic sulfur[132] have also been incriminated in the pathogenesis of acne.[133] There has also been an attempt to subclassify these different clinical presentations as acne cosmetica, pomade acne, and so forth.

Seasonal Change. About 75 per cent of all patients with acne notice improvement during the summer. Increasing exposure to sunlight is usually given as the cause of this improvement, but there are no controlled studies to document this assumption. In fact, no changes have been noticed in sebum after weekly exposures to ultraviolet light (UVL).[4] Possibly other seasonal changes (environmental, biological, or hygienic) may explain the beneficial effects of summer for some patients.

Tension. Anxiety and tension ("nerves") have been felt in the past to play a major role in exacerbating acne. Controlling these emotions has often been one of the major therapeutic goals. Patients with acne appear to have more emotional problems than do those who do not,[135] but this might be related to the severity of the acne, rather than to its cause. Treatment with tranquilizers is not usually helpful for acne,[136] although one rather unusual study claims the opposite.[137] Emotional stress may increase the production of sebum and the concentration of FFA but this consequence may be the indirect result of sweating.[58, 59]

Picking at Lesions. The sight of a fresh pustule frequently incites an irresistible urge to squeeze and pick. If the manipulations are gentle and not repeated, open comedones and superficial pustules are easily removed and heal rapidly. Closed comedones, inflammatory papules, deeper pustules, nodules, and cysts cannot be dealt with so simply, and the patient will usually do more harm than good if he attempts to squeeze these lesions. A well-motivated patient, instructed as to which lesions may be removed, can usually be given a comedo extractor, sparing the physician or nurse the tedium of time-consuming acne surgery.

Picking becomes a problem when real or imaginary lesions are badly traumatized. Repeated attacks on deeply situated lesions may result in spreading infection, delayed healing, and scarring. One of the most distressing situations occurs in young women who repeatedly pick at early or imagined lesions. This so-called acne excoriée des jeunes filles is tied to a nervous habit and cannot be treated as ordinary acne. Possible sources of tension in the patient's life need to be discussed and the patient helped to realize that picking is actually aggravating the acne. Some of these patients have significant behavioral problems and may require appropriate psychiatric counseling. For others, treatment with mild tranquilizers may be effective.[138]

Sexual Habits. There is no proof that virginity, promiscuity, sadism, masochism, sodomy, masturbation, or any other form of sexual activity is in any way related to the causes of acne.

Drugs. In rare instances, several drugs have been reported to cause acneiform eruptions.[139-145] These include isoniazid, corticosteroids, chloral hydrate, and even tetracycline. Iodine and its salts have been implicated as aggravating factors in acne, but most of the evidence does not substantiate this claim. Oral iodine in fairly large quantities has even been used to treat acne, with good results;[146] in a large field survey, low iodine intake was not associated with a greater number or degree of inflammatory lesions.[147] Sulzberger,[255] however, did use iodine in massive quantities (grams) and found exacerbations of acne in his patients. This evidence does not warrant removing small quantities of iodine (as in iodized table salt) from the diet.

The effects of hormonal drugs, such as estrogens, progesterones, and androgens, should always be closely observed. Although estrogens are used as a treatment for acne, not all women who use oral contraceptives will benefit from this treatment. The concentration of estrogen and the androgenic effects of the progesterone component appear to be crucial variables in the acnegenic potential of the birth control pills.

SPECIAL FORMS OF ACNE

Special forms of acne and the conditions with which they may be intimately associated include the following: hidradenitis suppurativa, acne with fever and arthralgia, dissecting cellulitis of the scalp, acne excoriée des jeunes filles, gram-negative acne, steroid acne, acne rosacea, acne necrotica, Mallorca acne, and neonatal acne (Figs. 4–3 and 4–4).

Acne excoriée and gram-negative acne have been mentioned earlier. In some individuals, acne vulgaris is associated with hidradenitis suppurativa. This furuncle-like condition is caused by staphylococcal infection resulting from obstruction of the apocrine glands. Acne vulgaris may also be associated with dissecting cellulitis of the scalp. The facial lesions of acne are fortunately

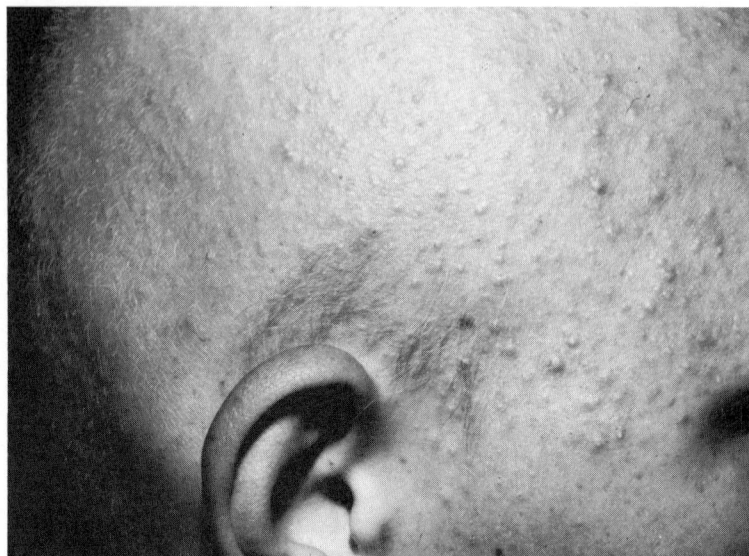

FIGURE 4–3 Steroid acne. This patient had alopecia universalis which was treated with systemic corticosteroids. He now has numerous inflammatory papules but no comedones.

not as severe as either of these other complications, which are often quite resistant to treatment.

A few patients may develop a serious constitutional reaction to severe nodular acne consisting of arthralgia, malaise, and fever.[247, 248] The few patients with this syndrome who have been studied did not have septicemia, nor did they improve after the administration of large amounts of antibiotics. Parenteral corticosteroid therapy, however, did improve their condition.

Prolonged systemic administration of corticosteroids may cause a florid eruption of papules and pustules, but without comedones.[141] This drug-induced, or "steroid," acne does not usually result in scarring. It has a more widespread distribution on the back, chest, and arms than conventional acne vulgaris (Fig. 4–3). There are very few published studies of the efficacy of treatment for this condition, but topically applied retinoic acid is said to be helpful.[249]

Acne rosacea superficially resembles acne vulgaris. Only the lack of comedones and scarring separates it from acne vulgaris on morphological grounds. Acne rosacea occurs more frequently in women from 30 to 50 years of age and is always confined to the face. Fortunately, tetracycline is an effective treatment for both acne vulgaris and acne rosacea, so little harm is done by confusing the two.

Acne necrotica is a disease in which small pustules occur around the hairline and throughout the scalp (acne necrotica miliaris). This is presumed to result from a bacterial infection that produces episodes of pruritus and burning. Individual papules and pustules are quickly excoriated and dominate the clinical picture. Systemic antibiotics are usually helpful in alleviating the condition.

Keratotic papules seen in the summer or after a vacation in the sun have been called "Mallorca" acne.[250] Blackheads are not seen and pustules are rare in this unusual eruption.

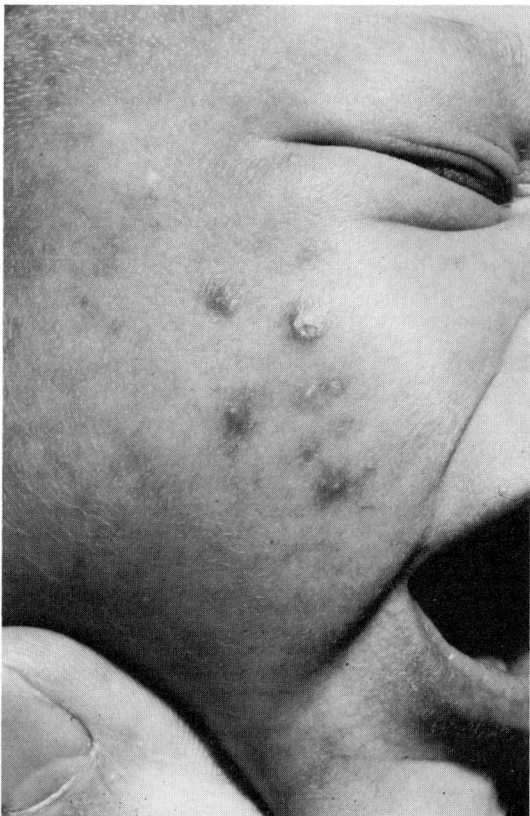

Figure 4-4 Neonatal acne—papules, pustules, and closed comedones.

Neonatal acne (Fig. 4-4) most often appears in the first three to five months of life. This disease looks exactly as it does in adults but usually is not as severe or widespread. Comedones, papules, and pustules are the rule, nodules the exception. Treatment must be modified by the patient's age, avoiding tetracycline or harsh topical remedies. It is usually not necessary to undertake an endocrine investigation of such patients, since very few of them show other signs of virilization. The cause of infantile acne is unknown. These children may be the progeny of parents with severe acne, but no prospective study has been made of the course of the disease through puberty and adolescence in these infants.

DIFFERENTIAL DIAGNOSIS

The differential diagnosis of acne includes a number of conditions that only superficially resemble acne vulgaris. These include: keratosis pilaris, bacterial and fungal infections of the face, flat warts, and adenoma sebaceum.

Keratosis pilaris (KP) usually results from a predisposition to the development of keratotic follicular papules on the extensor surfaces of the arms and legs. Occasionally these papules occur on various areas of the face and are designated accordingly, e.g., keratosis pilaris faciei, keratosis pilaris vermiculata, and so on. Follicular pustules may appear in cases in which keratosis pilaris is extensive. This condition is usually easy to differentiate from acne vulgaris. Acne begins later and has a more widespread distribution. KP lacks true blackheads, has firm adherence of follicular plugs, and has no tendency to form inflammatory nodules.

Bacteria and fungi,[250] including the Trichophyton group, *Candida albicans,* and Staphylococcus, may infect the superficial portions of the epidermis and follicles. Acne-like lesions with asymmetrical or annular configurations, unusual distribution, and absence of comedones, or those that fail to respond to treatment that is usually effective in acne, should suggest further studies. Bacterial and fungal cultures, along with a Gram-stain and KOH preparation, may be in order.

Verrucae plana (flat warts) appear as red or flesh-colored papules, which at a distance may mimic acne. Close inspection will disclose flat-surfaced, sharply marginated papules, pink-to-tan in color. Retinoic acid used to the point of brisk desquamation will usually cause the lesions to subside. Skin color is an important fact to consider (see Chapter 9).

The red papular angiofibromas of adenoma sebaceum occur at a much earlier age than acne. They tend to concentrate about the nose, never become pustular, and are usually associated with mental retardation, oblong white spots, and epilepsy. They form part of the tuberous sclerosis spectrum of lesions.

TREATMENT

No other cutaneous disease has attracted so many therapists with such differing points of view as acne. Several hundred over-the-counter[148] and prescription items claim to benefit acne, yet fewer than five compounds have been proved effective in controlled studies. The successful treatment of acne can usually be accomplished with one or two agents, so that the physician's pharmacopoeia for combating acne should be adequate if it contains 10 to 12 items. Ideally, all products should carry scientific proof, not merely enthusiastic endorsement. It makes no sense to use the latest scrub, soap, or tinted complexion aid only because it is new.

In order to evaluate the efficacy of the drugs in this cluttered and competitive field, one should rely on controlled and comparable studies.

TABLE 4–2 TREATMENT OF ACNE

Local (Topical)
  Benzoyl peroxide, retinoic acid, sulfur, resorcinol, corticosteroids
  Antiandrogens, estrogens, anticholinergics
  Soap and water
  Physical: gritty scrubs, facial masks, acne surgery, treatment with ultraviolet light

Systemic
  Antibacterial agents: tetracycline, erythromycin, clindamycin, ampicillin
    trimethoprim-sulfamethoxazole
    dapsone
  Hormones: corticosteroids, estrogens, antiandrogens, thyroid
  Diet
  Others: vitamins, diuretics, enzymes, tranquilizers, clofibrate,
    nicotine, vaccines, psychotherapy

Patients who participate in such studies should preferably have lesion counts documented by photography. Comedones, papules, cysts, and nodules should be evaluated in separate groups. These precautions are necessary because some drugs may be effective in treating only one type of acne lesion. A study evaluating the efficacy of tetracycline would prove little if the patients studied had only non-inflammatory comedones, no matter how numerous, since tetracycline is not effective with non-inflammatory lesions. Patients who believe certain foods aggravate their acne complain of new papules and pustules, not comedones, so that a count of comedones is an inappropriate measure of the effect of diet on acne.

In studying efficacy, therapy should not be changed from week to week, since a therapeutic lag time may exist. Several studies of tetracycline have failed to show any significant effect on acne, perhaps because the study period was too short.[149]

GENERAL RECOMMENDATIONS

Acne cannot be cured, only suppressed. It is probably wise to tell every patient at the initial visit that even the best result may still leave a few lesions or that solitary inflammatory papules may continue to arise from time to time. Emphasizing this point during the first meeting will help keep the patient from developing unrealistic expectations.

Acne responds slowly. Patients frequently expect treatment to result in the immediate clearing of acne. Because they are aware that antibiotics clear impetigo and "strep throat" within a few days, they may expect acne to respond equally quickly. Offering a realistic time frame in which to expect improvement will improve compliance and help establish confidence in the treatment. The physician may wish to point out that tetracycline does not even appear on the surface of the skin until four to six days after the initiation of systemic therapy,[150] so that the expectation of instant improvement is unrealistic.

Do only a few things, but do them well. I doubt seriously if one can achieve compliance with a program of restrictive diet, gritty soap, drying lotion, medicated makeup, oral antibiotic, and sun lamp, each used on a different daily or weekly schedule. It is better to offer only a few effective medications, such as a topical agent and a systemic antibiotic, suggesting to the patient that other forms of therapy may be added later, as necessary.

Local (Topical) Therapy. Most physicians who treat acne employ topical therapy on nearly all their patients,[151, 153-158] although a few feel that it only aggravates already inflamed skin. There is no experimental support for the latter view.

Benzoyl peroxide,[152] retinoic acid, and resorcinol are frequently prescribed for acne. They are irritants that dry and peel the skin, but this may not be the basis of their efficacy. It is important to remember that each patient will react differently to these topical products, and in order to achieve therapeutic benefit, the symptomatic end point of treatment (slight dryness) should be identified for each individual. There is a fine line between unacceptable irritation and effective treatment with these agents. Of this group, retinoic acid is the most difficult to use, but it is also perhaps the most rewarding in the long run.[151, 157]

For fair-skinned patients, one initial application of retinoic acid for two to three hours a night is not too cautious a beginning. The patient can then increase or decrease the duration of the application, depending on the response.

Sulfur in its many forms has also been widely used and accepted. There is nothing to indicate its superiority over other topical products, and recently it has even been incriminated as an acnegen.[132] There are no controlled studies demonstrating its effectiveness when used alone.

Corticosteroids have no real place in the topical management of acne.[159, 160] Products that combine steroids with irritating agents usually offer the patient little benefit, and they have a higher prescription cost. If applied before warm compresses, corticosteroids may help resolve large inflammatory nodules, but at the same time may aggravate small papules and pustules.[161, 162] Prolonged use of topical steroids can produce cutaneous atrophy and a rosacea-like eruption of the face.

There are many combinations of agents intended for use in the treatment of acne.[159, 163] Sulfur, resorcinol, and alcohol are commonly mixed and reported to be effective in uncontrolled clinical studies. The effectiveness of sodium thiosulfate has been demonstrated in a blind and controlled study.[164]

Other Topical Agents. Antiandrogens,[165] estrogens,[166] glucuronidase inhibitor,[167] anticholinergics,[22] antiperspirants (aluminum hydroxychloride, zirconium), ethyl lactate,[168] salt solutions, and drugs to inhibit lipid synthesis[21, 169, 170] have all been used to treat acne. All of these medications suffer at present either from lack of effectiveness data, unacceptable side effects, or unavailability. Topical erythromycin has recently been studied and may prove to be an effective and acceptable form of therapy.[132] However, it is not yet available for commercial use, and making a stable product from erythromycin tablets or capsules is difficult.

The frequent removal of superficial skin oils with soap and water or other solvents is often advised by parents and peers. There is little to document the effectiveness of washing, and it is certain that neither open nor closed comedones can be simply washed out. If the sebaceous gland is controlled by a surface feedback mechanism, as suggested by Shuster,[4, 10] the removal of sebum could lead to an increase in seborrhea. The patient with acne may sometimes feel dirty because he has blackheads, so that a medicated wash may diminish the unpleasant "greasy" feeling and help him feel he is actively contributing to his treatment.[172]

The use of gritty and abrasive scrubs, bars, or pads may also seem to be a logical approach, but it does not reduce sebum excretion rate (SER) or remove comedones. While these products may unroof superficial pustules and promote mild irritation of the skin, vigorous use of a washcloth is a cheaper and equally effective method of accomplishing the same purpose.

Increased ultraviolet light exposure is usually given credit for acne improvement in the summertime, although SER has not been changed by UVL therapy.[134] Improvement may be related to changes in spring or summer temperature, humidity, diet, or clothing.

Acne surgery, performed in the office, is often included in the management of acne. It has been used to open large cysts for purposes of drainage, but it is best used to treat open comedones and superficial pustules. One study[102] has demonstrated its effectiveness for this purpose, and it is certainly faster than using chemical agents to remove visible lesions. However, acne surgery probably does not change the number of developing inflammatory lesions, since most originate in subclinical comedones. Chemical agents appear to offer a more logical method of prophylaxis. The incision and drainage of nodules and cysts is helpful. However, fluctuation in a nodule is frequently misleading, and if there is doubt about the "ripeness" of a lesion, incisions should be avoided to reduce the possibility of scarring. Many nodules will resolve promptly after the injection of a corticosteroid, but the cysts require surgical removal. It should be recognized that prolonged intralesional use of soluble steroids may suppress the adrenal gland.[173]

Cryotherapy is used by some practitioners and is probably an effective (and certainly a dramatic) means of dealing with pustules, papules, and nodules.[174] Dry ice, taken from a block or collected in a chamois bag from a tank of pressurized carbon dioxide or liquid nitrogen,[175] is applied briefly to the skin. However when cryotherapy is applied to dark-complected individuals, it often causes unacceptable or even permanent changes in pigmentation.[176]

Systemic Therapy. A wide variety of antibacterial agents,[177] including tetracycline, erythromycin, clindamycin, ampicillin, trimethoprim-sulfamethoxazole, and a sulfone, is frequently administered as treatment for inflammatory acne, usually in conjunction with topical therapy. These agents are effective primarily against inflammatory lesions; a prospective study on their usefulness in inhibiting the development of new comedones has not been published. The antimicrobials all reduce the concentration of fatty acids and the number of C. acnes on the surface of the skin and presumably in the lumen of the follicle as well.[61, 154, 178] Those agents that are effective are usually concentrated in the sebaceous gland, so that they become components of sebum as it proceeds toward the skin's surface.

Tetracycline combined with topical care should usually be the first choice for the untreated patient with inflammatory acne.[158, 179-184] No particular type of tetracycline has been shown to be more effective than any other type in the treatment of acne,[185] although demethylchlortetracycline is apparently most effective in reducing the concentration of FFA. However, this drug also has a high incidence of side effects, including phototoxicity, so that the less expensive and safer tetracycline HCl is a better prescription choice. Tetracycline is best taken with water on an empty stomach, since most tetracyclines are chelated by cations in milk, antacids, and iron pills.[186] Some physicians advocate 1 to 2 gm a day for an initial period of two to four weeks, followed by maintenance therapy at 250 to 500 mgm/day[187] in divided doses.

Even with prolonged use, tetracyclines appear to be safe.[188-190] Extensive examinations have disclosed no consistent ill effects on either the hematological or hepatic systems.[186] An inability to concentrate the urine fully is probably a common consequence of tetracycline therapy but is rarely of clinical significance.[195, 196] Tetracyclines should be used with great caution in patients with renal disease. Bacteria resistant to tetracyclines commonly emerge on the skin[84, 191] and in the gut,[61, 193, 194] but secondary infection with these organisms is exceptional with the low doses usually employed. Women may develop monilial vaginitis as a side effect of tetracycline therapy.[189] This class of drugs should not be used in the second or third trimester of pregnancy or with lactating women, since it may cause discolored teeth in the infant. Rare and unusual side effects of tetracycline therapy include onycholysis[197] and an acneiform reaction[130] due to secondary bacterial overgrowth.

If no beneficial effect is noted after two to three months of tetracycline administration, erythromycin is a good therapeutic second choice.[177, 184] Although systemic clindamycin[198] is also an effective treatment, the incidence of complications (pseudomembranous colitis) sharply limits its use for acne.[199] In this litigious age, it would seem most prudent to avoid clindamycin, even though it has been used extensively in acne and has been listed as safe by the Acne Task Force of the National Program for Dermatology.[200] In one series of 60 acne patients treated with clindamycin, none had serious side effects and only two (3.4 per cent) developed diarrhea.[201] A combination of trimethoprim and sulfamethoxazole (Bactrim, Septra) is also reported to be effective.[56, 57, 202] Ampicillin has particular application for those unfortunate enough to develop gram-negative acne.[83]

As a rule, those antimicrobial drugs that are prescribed less frequently than tetracycline and erythromycin are reserved for the rare patient, not because they are less effective (although some are), but because of their greater side effects or higher cost. Dapsone particularly should be reserved for the exceptional patient with severe cystic acne.

Hormones. A short course of daily or alternate day therapy with corticosteroids is safe and effective in suppressing severe inflammatory acne.[203, 204] Corticosteroids should not be administered for long periods or prescribed for patients with contraindications. They should be given only to the exceptional patient.[77] Corticosteroids exert their beneficial effect by suppressing inflammation or adrenal androgens.[9]

Estrogens are used to treat acne only in women.[5, 6, 205] They are usually prescribed in the form and manner used for contraception, but Strauss and Pochi[126] have demonstrated that the response to these agents is variable and difficult to predict. Since the estrogenic component of the oral contraceptive can apparently promote vascular complications, this component of the pill has been reduced in concentration. This also reduces the therapeutic effect of the estrogen, while increasing the progestins, some of which have acnegenic androgen effects.[127] Before placing any woman on oral contraception, the physician should arrange for a gynecological examination with periodic follow-up care. The patient should also be fully cognizant of the risks and benefits of this therapeutic approach.[206] A careful choice should be made of the estrogen-containing compound to best suit the therapeutic need of each patient.

Patients with acne vulgaris have no particular tendency to hormonal defects. Thus the use of thyroid extract for acne is not justified and is placebo therapy at its worst. Antiandrogens seem to be promising agents of the future[207, 208] but are of no practical importance now.

Diet. Restrictive diets are of no value, perhaps because they are never followed strictly. It is logical and does no harm, however, to ascertain which foods, if any, the patient believes offends his complexion and to agree with restriction of only this small group. Even this advice is probably based on poorly founded data, since challenges with the suspected foods usually produce nothing but chagrin.[114] It does no good, however, to insist that a patient *may* eat a food he believes aggravates his acne.

Other Therapy. Patients with acne do not, as a group, have low serum or tissue vitamin A levels.[209-211] Although there are many advocates of the oral forms of this drug for acne,[212] controlled studies have failed to show any significant difference between the treated group and those patients who used a placebo.[213-215] The route of administration, either oral or intramuscular, made no difference.[216] Also, vitamin A may produce toxicity if taken in large quantities.[217]

Diuretics have been offered as agents to relieve premenstrual edema. Several studies have demonstrated their inability to modify acne and they should not be used for this disease.[128, 129]

One study has indicated that the oral enzymes, chymotrypsin and trypsin, can help reduce the inflammatory lesions of acne, but this has not been confirmed elsewhere.[218] It would seem to be a study worth repeating.

Tranquilizers have no place in the routine therapy of acne.[136] Acne patients with serious emotional problems may be referred to a psychiatrist; simple counseling is usually quite satisfactory for others.[219]

X-ray therapy will suppress acne and sebum production.[134, 230] The effect is usually short-lived, but may be long enough to permit more lasting control of acne by other means. Appropriate safeguards for shielding and dosage control are essential to prevent overdosage. Grenz rays are not effective.[231, 232]

Vaccine therapy with extracts of *C. acnes* and staphylococci seems illogical but is still used.[220-222] A variety of other agents, some reasonable and others not, are also advocated for the treatment of acne.[207, 223-227] Nearly all of them have been carefully reviewed by Frank[228] in his carefully referenced work.

For post-acne scarring, dermabrasion has been widely used, but many consider it to be of questionable benefit.[229] Careful patient selection and education are extremely important prior to dermabrasion. Some physicians believe that a promising, but still unapproved and unavailable, method of dealing with scars will be the injection of silicone or a gelatin foam to elevate them. Post-inflammatory hyperpigmentation is often very difficult to eradicate, but keloidal scars may respond to surgery or to the injection of corticosteroids.

REFERENCES

1. Cunliffe, W. J., and Cotterill, J. A.: The acnes: Clinical features, pathologenesis and treatment. *In* Rook, A. (ed.): Major Problems in Dermatology. Vol. 6. Philadelphia, W. B. Saunders, 1975.
2. Kligman, A. M.: The sebaceous gland. *In* Montagna, W., Ellis, R. A., and Silver, A. F. (eds.): Advances in Biology of Skin. Vol. 4. New York, Pergamon Press, 1963.
3. Strauss, J. S., Kligman, A. M., and Pochi, P. E.: The effect of androgens and estrogens on human sebaceous glands. J. Invest. Dermatol., *39*:139, 1962.
4. Ebling, F. J.: The action of testosterone and oestradiol on the sebaceous glands and epidermis of the rat. J. Embryol. Exp. Morphol., *12*:38, 1957.
5. Pochi, P. E., and Strauss, J. S.: Sebaceous gland suppression with ethinyl estradiol and diethylstilbestrol. Arch. Dermatol., *108*:210, 1973.
6. Strauss, J. S., and Pochi, P. E.: Systemic estrogen therapy of acne. Prog. Derm., *2*:7, 1967.
7. Wilde, P. F., and Ebling, F. J.: Preliminary observations on the composition of skin surface fat from rats treated with testosterone and estradiol. J. Invest. Dermatol., *52*:362, 1969.
8. Thody, A. J., and Shuster, S.: Control of sebum secretion by the posterior pituitary. Nature, *237*:346, 1972.
9. Pochi, P. E., Strauss, J. S., and Mescon, H.: The role of adrenocortical steroids in the control of human sebaceous gland activity. J. Invest. Dermatol., *41*:391, 1963.

10. Burton, J. L.: Factors affecting the rate of sebum excretion in man. J. Soc. Cosmet. Chem., 23:241, 1972.
11. Felger, C. B.: The etiology of acne. I. Composition of sebum before and after puberty. J. Soc. Cosmet. Chem., 20:565, 1969.
12. Thody, A. J., and Shuster, S.: Sebotrophic activity of β-lipotrophin. J. Endocrinol., 50:533, 1971.
13. Lasher, N., Lorincz, A. I., and Rothman, S.: Hormonal effects on sebaceous glands in the white rat. III. Evidence for the presence of pituitary sebaceous gland tropic factor. J. Invest. Dermatol., 24:499, 1955.
14. Thody, A. J., et al.: Plasma β-MSH levels in acne vulgaris. Br. J. Dermatol., 92:43, 1975.
15. Hay, J. B., and Hodgins, M. B.: Metabolism of androgens by human skin in acne. Br. J. Dermatol., 91:123, 1974.
16. Strauss, J. S., and Pochi, P. E.: Recent advances in androgen metabolism and their relation to the skin. Arch. Dermatol., 100:621, 1969.
17. Sansone, G., and Reisner, R. M.: Differential rates of conversion of testosterone to dihydrotestosterone in acne and in normal human skin — possible pathogenic factor in acne. J. Invest. Dermatol., 56:366, 1971.
18. Epstein, E. H., and Epstein, W. L.: New cell formation in human sebaceous glands. J. Invest. Dermatol., 46:453, 1966.
19. Plewig, G., and Christophers, E.: Renewal rate of human sebaceous glands. Acta Derm. Venereol., 54:177, 1974.
20. Montagna, W., and Ellis, R. A.: Histology and cytochemistry of human skin. XII. Cholinesterases in the hair follicles of the scalp. J. Invest. Dermatol., 29:151, 1957.
21. Cunliffe, W. J., and Cotterill, J.: The effect of propranolol on acne vulgaris and the rate of sebum excretion. Br. J. Dermatol., 83:550, 1970.
22. Cartlidge, M., Burton, J. L., and Shuster, S.: The effect of prolonged topical applications of an anticholinergic agent on the sebaceous glands. Br. J. Dermatol., 86:61, 1972.
23. Nikkari, T.: Composition and secretion of the skin surface lipids of the rat; effects of dietary lipids and hormones. Scand. J. Clin. Lab. Invest. (Suppl.), 16:4, 1964–1965.
24. Burton, J. L., and Shuster, S.: Effect of L-dopa on seborrhoea of Parkinsonism. Lancet, 2:19, 1970.
25. Cunliffe, W. J.: The relationship between surface lipid composition and acne vulgaris. Br. J. Dermatol., 85:86, 1971.
26. Kellum, R. E.: Human sebaceous gland lipids. Analysis by thin-layer chromatography. Arch. Dermatol., 59:218, 1967.
27. Shalita, A. R.: Genesis of free fatty acids. J. Invest. Dermatol., 62:332, 1974.
28. Kellum, R. E.: Acne vulgaris. Studies in pathogenesis: Relative irritancy of free fatty acids from C_2 to C_{16}. Arch. Dermatol., 97:722, 1968.
29. Krakow, R., Downing, D. T., Strauss, J. S., and Pochi, P. E.: Identification of a fatty acid in human skin surface lipids apparently associated with acne vulgaris. J. Invest. Dermatol., 61:286, 1973.
30. Kellum, R. E., and Strangfeld, K.: Acne vulgaris. Studies in pathogenesis: Fatty acids of human surface triglycerides from patients with and without acne. J. Invest. Dermatol., 58:315, 1972.
31. Powell, E. W., and Beveridge, G. W.: Sebum excretion and sebum composition in adolescent men with and without acne vulgaris. Br. J. Dermatol., 82:243, 1970.
32. Runkel, R. A., Wurster, D. E., and Cooper, G. A.: Investigation of normal and acne skin surface lipids. J. Pharm. Sci., 58:582, 1969.
33. Freinkel, R. K.: Pathogenesis of acne vulgaris. N. Engl. J. Med., 280:1161, 1969.
34. Pochi, P. E., and Strauss, J. S.: Sebum production, casual sebum levels, titratable acidity of sebum, and urinary fractional 17-ketosteroid excretion in males with acne. J. Invest. Dermatol., 43:383, 1964.
35. Boughton, B., MacKenna, R. M. B., Wheatley, V. R., and Wormall, A.: The fatty acid composition of the surface skin fats (sebum) in acne vulgaris and seborrheic dermatitis. J. Invest. Dermatol., 33:57, 1959.
36. Cotterill, J. A., Cunliffe, W. J., Williamson, B., and Bulusu, L.: Further observations on the pathogenesis of acne. Br. J. Dermatol., 3:444, 1972.
37. Wilkinson, D. I.: Variability in composition of surface lipids. The problem of the epidermal contribution. J. Invest. Dermatol., 52:339, 1969.
38. Greene, R. S., Downing, D. T., Pochi, P. E., and Strauss, J. S.: Anatomical variation in the amount and composition of human skin surface lipid. J. Invest. Dermatol., 54:240, 1970.
39. Summerly, R., and Woodbury, S.: The in vitro incorporation of 14 C-acetate into the isolated sebaceous glands and appendage-freed epidermis of human skin. A technique for the study of lipid synthesis in the isolated sebaceous gland. Br. J. Dermatol., 85:424, 1971.
40. Pochi, P. E., Downing, D. T., and Strauss, J. S.: Sebaceous gland response in man to prolonged total caloric deprivation. J. Invest. Dermatol., 55:303, 1970.

41. Marks, R., and Davies, M. J.: The distribution in the skin of systemically administered tetracycline. Br. J. Dermatol., *81*:448, 1969.
42. Cunliffe, W. J., and Shuster, S.: The rate of sebum excretion in man. Br. J. Dermatol., *81*:697, 1969.
43. Hodgson-Jones, I. S., MacKenna, R. M. B., and Wheatley, V. R.: The study of human sebaceous activity. Acta Derm. Venereol., *32*:155, 1952.
44. Cotterill, J. A., Cunliffe, W. J., and Williamson, B.: Variations in skin surface lipid composition and sebum excretion rate with different sampling techniques II. Br. J. Dermatol., *86*:356, 1972.
45. Strauss, J. S., and Pochi, P. E.: The quantitative gravimetric determination of sebum production. J. Invest. Dermatol., *36*:293, 1961.
46. Pablo, G. M., and Fulton, J. E.: Sebum: Analysis by infrared spectroscopy. II. The suppression of fatty acids by systemically administered antibiotics. Arch. Dermatol., *111*:734, 1975.
47. Anderson, A. S., and Fulton, J. E.: Sebum: Analysis by infrared spectroscopy. J. Invest. Dermatol., *60*:115, 1973.
48. Anderson, R. L., Bozeman, M. A., Voss, J. G., and Whiteside, J. A.: Individual and site variation in composition of facial surface lipids. J. Invest. Dermatol., *58*:369, 1972.
49. Downing, D. T.: Lipolysis by human skin surface debris in organic solvents. J. Invest. Dermatol., *54*:395, 1970.
50. Burton, J. L., Cunliffe, W. J., and Shuster, S.: Circadian rhythm in sebum excretion. Br. J. Dermatol., *82*:497, 1970.
51. MacDonald, I., and Clarke, G.: Variations in the levels of cholesterol and triglyceride in the skin surface fat during the menstrual cycle. Br. J. Dermatol., *83*:473, 1970.
52. Burton, J. L., Shuster, S., and Cartlidge, M.: The sebotrophic effect of pregnancy. Acta Derm. Venereol., *55*:11, 1975.
53. Cotterill, J. A., Cunliffe, W. J., Williamson, B., and Bulusu, L.: Age and sex variation in skin surface lipid composition and sebum excretion rate. Br. J. Dermatol., *87*:333, 1972.
54. Williams, M., Cunliffe, W. J., Williamson, B., et al.: The effect of local temperature changes on sebum excretion rate and forehead surface lipid composition. Br. J. Dermatol., *88*:257, 1973.
55. Beveridge, G. W., and Powell, E. W.: Sebum changes in acne vulgaris treated with tetracycline. Br. J. Dermatol., *81*:525, 1969.
56. Strauss, J. S., and Pochi, P. E.: The effect of sulfisoxazole-trimethoprim combination on titratable acidity of human sebum. Br. J. Dermatol., *82*:493, 1970.
57. Cotterill, J. A., Cunliffe, W. J., and Williamson, B.: The effect of trimethoprim-sulphamethoxazole on sebum excretion rate and biochemistry in acne vulgaris. Br. J. Dermatol., *85*:130, 1971.
58. Kraus, S. J.: Stress, acne and skin surface free fatty acids. Psychosom. Med., *32*:503, 1970.
59. Wolff, H. G., Lorenz, T. H., and Graham, D. T.: Stress, emotions and human sebum: Their relevance to acne vulgaris. Trans. Assoc. Am. Physicians., *64*:435, 1951.
60. Knutson, D. D.: Ultrastructural observations in acne vulgaris: The normal sebaceous follicle and acne lesions. J. Invest. Dermatol., *62*:288, 1974.
61. Goltz, R. W., and Kjartansson, S.: Oral tetracycline treatment on bacterial flora in acne vulgaris. Arch. Dermatol., *93*:92, 1966.
62. Marples, R. R., McGinley, K. J., and Mills, O. H.: Microbiology of comedones in acne vulgaris. J. Invest. Dermatol., *60*:80, 1973.
63. Scheimann, L. G., Knox, G., Sher, D., and Rothman, S.: The role of bacteria in the formation of free fatty acids on the human skin surface. J. Invest. Dermatol., *34*:171, 1960.
64. Marples, R. R.: The microflora of the face and acne lesions. J. Invest. Dermatol., *62*:326, 1974.
65. Smith, M. A., and Waterworth, P. M.: The bacteriology of acne vulgaris in relation to its treatment with antibiotics. Br. J. Dermatol., *73*:152, 1961.
66. Williamson, P., and Kligman, A. M.: A new method for the quantitative investigation of cutaneous bacteria. J. Invest. Dermatol., *45*:498, 1965.
67. Kellum, R. E., and Strangfeld, K.: Acne vulgaris: Studies in pathogenesis: Fatty acids of *Corynebacterium acnes*. Arch. Dermatol., *101*:337, 1970.
68. Kellum, R. E., Strangfeld, K., and Ray, L. F.: Acne vulgaris studies in pathogenesis: Triglyceride hydrolysis by *Corynebacterium acnes* in vitro. Arch. Dermatol., *101*:41, 1970.
69. Marples, R. R., Downing, D. T., and Ligman, A. M.: Control of free fatty acids in human surface lipids by *Corynebacterium acnes*. J. Invest. Dermatol., *56*:127, 1971.
70. Reisner, R. M., Silver, D. Z., Puhvel, M., and Sternbert, T. H.: Lipolytic activity of *Corynebacterium acnes*. J. Invest. Dermatol., *51*:190, 1968.
71. Henning, D. R., Dixon, R., and Akers, W. A.: Isolation of *Corynebacterium acnes* from the foreheads of prepubertal children. J. Military Derm., *6*:64, 1972.
72. Matta, M.: Carriage of *Corynebacterium acnes* in school children in relation to age and race. Br. J. Dermatol., *91*:557, 1974.
73. Voss, J. G.: Differentiation of two groups of *Corynebacterium acnes*. J. Bacteriol., *101*:392, 1970.

74. Smith, M. A., and Waterworth, P. M.: The bacteriology of acne vulgaris in relation to its treatment with antibiotics. Br. J. Dermatol., *73*:152, 1961.
75. Shalita, A. R., and Rosenthal, S. A.: Tetracycline-resistant staphylococci in acne vulgaris. Acta Derm. Venereol., *52*:64, 1972.
76. Voss, J. G.: Acne vulgaris and free fatty acids: A review and criticism. Arch. Dermatol., *109*:894, 1974.
77. Becker, F. T.: Treatment of tetracycline-resistant acne vulgaris. Cutis, *14*:610, 1974.
78. Osment, L. S., Noojin, R. O., and Winkler, C. H.: Comparative antibiotic sensitivity studies in pustular acne vulgaris, 1954 and 1962. Southern. Med. J., *59*:85, 1966.
79. Reisner, R. M., and Puhvel, M.: Lipolytic activity of *Staphylococcus albus*. J. Invest. Dermatol., *53*:1, 1969.
80. Weary, P. E.: Comedogenic potential of the lipid extract of *Pityrosporum ovale*. Arch Dermatol., *102*:84, 1970.
81. Marples, R. R., Downing, D. T., and Kligman, A. M.: Influence of *Pityrosporum* species in the generation of free fatty acids in human surface lipids. J. Invest. Dermatol., *58*:155, 1972.
82. Weary, P. E., Russell, C. M., Butler, H. K., and Hsu, Y. T.: Acneform eruption resulting from antibiotic administration. Arch. Dermatol., *100*:179, 1969.
83. Fulton, J. E., McGinley, K., Leyden, J., and Marples, R.: Gram-negative folliculitis in acne vulgaris. Arch. Dermatol., *98*:349, 1968.
84. Marples, R. R., Fulton, J. E., Leyden, J., and McGinley, K. J.: Effect of antibiotics on the nasal flora in acne patients. Arch. Dermatol., *99*:647, 1969.
85. Leyden, J. J., Marples, R. R., Mills, O. H., and Kligman, A. M.: Gram-negative folliculitis—a complication of antibiotic therapy in acne vulgaris. Br. J. Dermatol., *88*:533, 1973.
86. Paver, K.: Complications from combined oral tetracycline and oral corticoid therapy in acne vulgaris. Med. J. Aust., *1*:1059, 1970.
87. Hinrichsen, J., and Ivy, A. C.: Incidence in the Chicago region of acne vulgaris. Arch. Dermatol., *37*:975, 1938.
88. Bloch, B.: Metabolism, endocrine glands and skin diseases, with special reference to acne vulgaris and xanthoma. Br. J. Dermatol., *43*:61, 1931.
89. Burton, J. L., Cunliffe, W. J., Stafford, I., and Shuster, S.: The prevalence of acne vulgaris in adolescence. Br. J. Dermatol., *85*:119, 1971.
90. Wilkins, J. W., and Voorhees, J. J.: Prevalence of nodulocystic acne in white and Negro males. Arch. Dermatol., *102*:631, 1970.
91. Hazen, H. H.: Personal observations upon skin diseases in the American Negro. J. Cutan. Dis., *32*:705, 1914.
92. Hamilton, J. B., Terada, H., and Mestler, G. E.: Greater tendency to acne in white American than in Japanese populations. J. Clin. Endocrinol. Metab., *24*:267, 1964.
93. Hecht, H.: Hereditary trends in acne vulgaris. Dermatologica, *121*:297, 1960.
94. Voorhees, J. J., Wilkins, J. W., Hayes, E., and Harrell, E. R.: Nodulocystic acne as a phenotypic feature of the XYY genotype. Arch. Dermatol., *105*:913, 1972.
95. Solomon, L. M., Fretzin, D., and Pruzansky, S.: Pilosebaceous abnormalities in Apert's syndrome. Arch. Dermatol., *102*:381, 1970.
96. Cunliffe, W. J., Cotterill, J. A., and Williamson, B.: Skin surface lipids in acne. Br. J. Dermatol., *85*:585, 1971.
97. Cunliffe, W. J., and Shuster, S.: Pathogenesis of acne. Lancet, *1*:685, 1969.
98. Burton, J. L., and Shuster, S.: The relationship between seborrhoea and acne vulgaris. Br. J. Dermatol., *84*:600, 1971.
99. Kaidbey, K. H., and Kligman, A. M.: Pigmentation in comedones. Arch. Dermatol., *109*:60, 1974.
100. Blari, C., and Lewis, C. A.: The pigment of comedones. Br. J. Dermatol., *82*:572, 1970.
101. Plewig, G., Fulton, J. E., and Kligman, A. M.: Cellular dynamics of comedo formation in acne vulgaris. Arch. Dermatol. Forsch., *242*:12, 1971.
102. Orentreich, N., and Durr, N. P.: The natural evolution of comedones into inflammatory papules and pustules. J. Invest. Dermatol., *62*:316, 1974.
103. Gershbein, L. L., Haeberlin, J. B., and Singh, E. J.: Composition of human comedone lipids. Dermatologica, *140*:264, 1970.
104. Lynch, F. W.: Acne vulgaris. Review of histologic changes observed in early lesions. Arch. Dermatol., *42*:593, 1940.
105. Strauss, J. S., and Pochi, P. E.: Intracutaneous injection of sebum and comedones. Arch. Dermatol., *92*:443, 1965.
106. Ray, T., and Kellum, R. E.: Acne vulgaris. Studies in pathogenesis: Free fatty acid irritancy in patients with and without acne. J. Invest. Dermatol., *57*:6, 1971.
107. Leyden, J. J., and Mills, O. H.: Cystic acne as a source of bleeding in hemophilia. Arch. Dermatol., *107*:465, 1973.
108. Basler, R. S. W., Taylor, W. B., and Peacor, D. R.: Postacne osteoma cutis. Arch. Dermatol., *110*:113, 1974.

109. Warshaw, T.: Conglobate acne vulgaris associated with low levels of serum gamma globulin. J. Med. Soc. N.J., 64:218, 1967.
110. Hoehn, G. H.: Acne and diet. Cutis, 2:389, 1966.
111. Glickman, F. S., and Silvers, S. H.: Dietary factors in acne vulgaris. Arch. Dermatol., 106:129, 1972.
112. Cornbleet, T., and Gigli, I.: Should we limit sugar in acne? Arch. Dermatol., 83:968, 1961.
113. Fulton, J. E., Plewig, G., and Kligman, A. M.: Effect of chocolate on acne vulgaris. JAMA, 210:2071, 1969.
114. Anderson, P. C.: Foods as the cause of acne. Am. Fam. Physician, 3:102, 1971.
115. MacDonald, I.: Effects of a skimmed milk and chocolate diet on serum and skin lipids. J. Sci. Food Agric., 19:270, 1968.
116. Wilkinson, D. I.: Psoriasis and dietary fat: The fatty acid composition of surface and scale (ether-soluble) lipids. J. Invest. Dermatol., 47:185, 1966.
117. MacDonald, I.: Dietary carbohydrates and skin lipids. Br. J. Dermatol., 79:119, 1967.
118. Goodman, H.: Acne vulgaris: Relation of weight, age, height and religious faith (Jewish and non-Jewish). Am. Med., 40:258, 1934.
119. Crow, K. D.: Chloracne: A critical review including a comparison of two series of cases of acne from chlornaphthalene and pitch fumes. Trans. St. Johns Hosp. Dermatol. Soc., 56:79, 1970.
120. Chloracne. Comment. Br. J. Dermatol., 83:599, 1970.
121. May, G.: Chloracne from the accidental production of tetrachlorodibenzodioxin. Br. J. Ind. Med., 30:276, 1973.
122. Williams, M., and Cunliffe, W. J.: Explanation for premenstrual acne. Lancet, 2:1055, 1973.
123. Kalz, F., and Scott, A.: Cutaneous changes during the menstrual cycle: A clinical and experimental study under physiological condition and after therapy. Arch. Dermatol., 74:493, 1956.
124. Burton, J. L., Cartlidge, M., and Shuster, S.: Variations in sebum excretion during the menstrual cycle. Acta Derm. Venereol., 53:81, 1973.
125. Freinkel, R. K., and Shen, Y.: The origin of free fatty acids in sebum II. J. Invest. Dermatol., 53:422, 1969.
126. Strauss, J. S., and Pochi, P. E.: Effect of cyclic progestin-estrogen therapy on sebum and acne in women. JAMA, 190:815, 1964.
127. Strauss, J. S., and Kligman, A. M.: The effect of progesterone and progesterone-like compounds on the human sebaceous gland. J. Invest. Dermatol., 36:309, 1961.
128. Jelinek, J. E.: Hydrochlorothiazide and the control of premenstrual exacerbation of acne. Arch. Dermatol., 105:79, 1972.
129. Riley, K. A.: Failure of treatment of acne vulgaris with hydrochlorothiazide. Arch. Dermatol., 84:186, 1961.
130. Crocker, H. R.: Comedones in children. Lancet, 1:704, 1884.
131. Plewig, G., Fulton, J. E., and Kligman, A. M.: Pomade acne. Arch. Dermatol., 101:580, 1970.
132. Mills, O. H., and Kligman, A. M.: Is sulphur helpful or harmful in acne vulgaris? Br. J. Dermatol., 86:620, 1972.
133. Kligman, A. M., and Mills, O. H.: "Acne Cosmetica." Arch. Dermatol., 106:843, 1972.
134. Prose, P. H., Baer, R. L., and Herrmann, F.: Studies of the ether-soluble substances on the human skin. J. Invest. Dermatol., 19:227, 1952.
135. Wright, E. T., Kyle, N. I., and Gunter, R.: Personality test configurations in acne vulgaris. Percept. Mot. Skills, 30:191, 1970.
136. Lester, E. P., Wittkower, E. D., Kalz, R., and Azima, H.: Phrenotropic drugs in psychosomatic disorders (skin). Amer. J. Psychiat., 19:136, 1962.
137. Ellerbroek, W. C.: Hypotheses toward a unified field theory of human behavior with clinical application to acne vulgaris. Perspect. Biol. Med., 16:240, 1973.
138. Segal, A. E., and Rogin, J. R.: Management of the psychogenic factors in dermatoses by use of chemotherapy. Med. Times, 92:113, 1964.
139. Lantis, S. H.: Acneform eruptions. JAMA, 24:305, 1969.
140. Bean, S. F.: Acneiform eruption from tetracycline. Br. J. Dermatol., 85:585, 1971.
141. Sullivan, M., and Zeligman, I.: Acneform eruption due to corticotropin. A.M.A. Arch. Dermatol., 73:133, 1956.
142. Christianson, H. B., and Perry, H. O.: Reactions to chloral hydrate. Arch. Dermatol., 74:232, 1956.
143. Behrman, H. T., and Goodman, J. J.: Skin complications of cortisone and ACTH therapy. JAMA, 144:218, 1950.
144. Brunner, M. J., Riddell, J. M., and Best, W. R.: Preliminary and short reports. Cutaneous side effects of ACTH, cortisone and pregnenolone therapy. J. Invest. Dermatol., 16:205, 1951.
145. Cohen, L. K., George, W., and Smith, R.: Isoniazid-induced acne and pellagra. Occurrence in slow inactivators of isoniazid. Arch. Dermatol., 109:377, 1974.
146. Gaul, L. E., and Underwood, G. B.: Oral iodine therapy in acne vulgaris. Failure of iodine, or

the equivalent of iodized salt, to produce pustular exacerbations. Arch. Dermatol., *58*:439, 1948.
147. Hitch, J. M., and Greenburg, B. C.: Adolescent acne and dietary iodine. Arch. Dermatol., *84*:898, 1961.
148. Hopponen, R. E.: O-t-c- anti-acne aids. J. Am. Pharm. Assoc., *6*:466, 1966.
149. Smith, M. A., Waterworth, P. M., and Curwen, P.: A controlled trial of oral antibiotics in the treatment of acne vulgaris. Br. J. Dermatol., *74*:86, 1962.
150. Rashleigh, P. L., Rife, E., and Goltz, R. W.: Tetracycline levels in skin surface film after oral administration of tetracycline to normal adults and to patients with acne vulgaris. J. Invest. Dermatol., *49*:611, 1967.
151. Kligman, A. M., Fulton, J. E., and Plewig, G.: Topical vitamin A acid in acne vulgaris. Arch. Dermatol., *99*:469, 1969.
152. Vasarinsh, P.: Benzoyl peroxide—sulfur lotions: A histologic study. Arch. Dermatol., *98*:183, 1968.
153. DeBersaques, J.: Topical vitamin A acid. Review of the literature and results of a clinical trial in acne. Arch. Belg. Dermatol., *28*:315, 1972.
154. Gunther, S.: Vitamin A acid in acne vulgaris: Association between peeling effect and improvement. Dermatol. Monatsschr., *160*:215, 1974.
155. Peachey, R. D. G., and Connor, B. L.: Topical retinoic acid in the treatment of acne vulgaris. Br. J. Dermatol., *85*:462, 1971.
156. Quarterly Review: Therapeutics XVI. Retinoic acid. Br. J. Dermatol., *85*:500, 1971.
157. Christiansen, J. V., Gadborg, E., Ludvigsen, K., et al.: Topical tretinoin, vitamin A acid (Airol) in acne vulgaris: A controlled clinical trial. Dermatologica, *148*:82, 1974.
158. Christiansen, J. V., Gadborg, E., Ludvigsen, K., et al.: Topical vitamin A acid (Airol) and systemic oxytetracycline in the treatment of acne vulgaris: A controlled clinical trial. Dermatologica, *149*:121, 1974.
159. Ede, M.: A double-blind, comparative study of benzoyl peroxide, benzoyl peroxide-chlorhydroxyquinoline, benzoyl peroxide-chlorhydroxyquinoline-hydrocortisone, and placebo lotions in acne. Curr. Ther. Res., *15*:624, 1973.
160. Juhlin, L., Michaelsson, G., and Ohman, S.: Topical triamcinolone acetonide and chlorhydroxyquinoline in acne. Acta Derm. Venereol., *48*:255, 1968.
161. Tye, M. J., and Leibsohn, E.: Acne treated with wet compresses followed by corticosteroid cream. Ariz. Med., *25*:38, 1968.
162. Wexler, L.: Two controlled studies of a topical steroid preparation in the treatment of acne vulgaris. Appl. Ther., *10*:455, 1968.
163. Frank, L., and Petrou, P.: Active oxygen plus chlorhydroxyquinoline in acne and pyodermas, including in vitro and in vivo bacteriological studies. Cutis, *3*:256, 1967.
164. Hall, J. H., and Lupton, E. S.: Topical acne therapy: A double-blind study. Cutis, *9*:545, 1972.
165. Cunliffe, W. J., Shuster, S., and Smith, A. J. C.: The effect of topical cyproterone acetate on sebum secretion in patients with acne. Br. J. Dermatol., *81*:200, 1969.
166. Kuhn, B.: The role of topical hormone therapy acne vulgaris—An evaluation of two decades of topical diethylstilbestrol therapy. Cutis, *5*:1124, 1969.
167. Ohkubo, T., and Sano, S.: Mechanism of the action of β-glucuronidase inhibitor upon apocrine sweat and sebaceous glands and its dermatological application. Acta Derm. Venereol., *53*:85, 1973.
168. Swanbeck, G.: A new principle for the treatment of acne. Acta Derm. Venereol., *52*:406, 1972.
169. Burton, J. L., and Shuster, S.: Topical tetraynoic acid and sebum excretion. Br. J. Dermatol., *82*:626, 1970.
170. Haroon, T. S., Hall, J., and Haroon, A.: Effect of topical tetraynoic acid on sebum excretion. Br. J. Dermatol., *86*:64, 1972.
171. Lennihan, R.: A salt lotion for the treatment of acne vulgaris. Arch. Dermatol., *105*:761, 1972.
172. Cunliffe, W. J., Cotterill, J. A., and Williamson, B.: The effect of a medicated wash on acne, sebum excretion rate and skin surface lipid composition. Br. J. Dermatol., *86*:311, 1964.
173. Potter, R. A.: Intralesional triamcinolone and adrenal suppression in acne vulgaris. J. Invest. Dermatol., *57*:364, 1971.
174. Moseley, J. C., and Katz, S. I.: Acne vulgaris: Treatment with carbon dioxide slush. Cutis, *10*:429, 1972.
175. Goette, D. K.: Liquid nitrogen in the treatment of acne vulgaris: A comparative study. South. Med. J., *66*:1131, 1973.
176. Kenney, J. A.: Management of dermatoses peculiar to Negroes. Arch. Dermatol., *91*:126, 1965.
177. Wansker, B. A.: Antibiotics and pustulocystic acne: A long-term, double-blind evaluation. Arch. Dermatol., *84*:146, 1961.
178. Marples, R. R.: Comparison of the effects of four tetracyclines and ampicillin on the normal flora of human forehead and axilla. Arch. Dermatol., *103*:148, 1971.
179. Puhvel, S. M., and Reisner, R. M.: Tetracyclines in the treatment of acne. Arch. Dermatol., *106*:923, 1972.

180. Lane, P., and Williamson, D. M.: Treatment of acne vulgaris with tetracycline hydrocholoride: A double-blind trial with 51 patients. Br. Med. J., 2:76, 1969.
181. Fry, L., and Ramsay, C. A.: Tetracycline in acne vulgaris. Clinical evaluation and the effect on sebum production. Br. J. Dermatol., 78:653, 1966.
182. Witkowski, J. A., and Simons, H. M.: Objective evaluation of demethylchlortetracycline hydrochloride in the treatment of acne. JAMA, 196:111, 1966.
183. Plewig, G., Petrozzi, J. W., and Berendes, U.: Double-blind study of doxycycline in acne vulgaris. Arch. Dermatol., 101:435, 1970.
184. Strauss, J. S., and Pochi, P. E.: Effect of orally administered antibacterial agents on titratable acidity of human sebum. J. Invest. Dermatol., 47:577, 1966.
185. Juhlin, L., and Liden, S.: A quantitative evaluation of the effect of oxytetracycline and doxycycline in acne vulgaris. Br. J. Dermatol., 81:154, 1969.
186. Hagermark, O., and Hoglund, S.: Iron metabolism in tetracycline-treated acne patients. Acta Derm. Venereol., 54:45, 1974.
187. Friedman-Kien, A., Shalita, A. R., and Baer, R. L.: Tetracycline therapy in acne vulgaris. Arch. Dermatol., 105:606, 1972.
188. Verbov, J. L.: Tetracyclines in dermatology. Trans. St. Johns Hosp. Dermatol. Soc., 55:78, 1969.
189. Bjornberg, A., and Roupe, G.: Susceptibility to infections during long-term treatment with tetracyclines in acne vulgaris. Dermatologica, 145:334, 1972.
190. Ashton, H., Beveridge, G. W., and Stevenson, C. J.: Quarterly Review. Therapeutics VII: Tetracyclines in Dermatology. Br. J. Dermatol., 81:637, 1969.
191. Marples, R. R., and Kligman, A. M.: Ecological effects of oral antibiotics on the microflora of human skin. Arch. Dermatol., 103:148, 1971.
192. Marples, R. R., and Williamson, P.: Effects of systemic demethylchlortetracycline on human cutaneous microflora. Appl. Microbiol., 18:228, 1969.
193. Schmidt, H., From, E., and Heydenreich, G.: Bacteriological examination of rectal specimen during long-term oxytetracycline treatment for acne vulgaris. Acta Derm. Venereol., 53:153, 1973.
194. Datta, N., Faiers, M. C., Reeves, D. S., et al.: R factors in Escherichia coli in faeces after oral chemotherapy in general practice. Lancet, 1:312, 1971.
195. Singer, I., and Rotenberg, D.: Demeclocycline-induced nephrogenic diabetes insipidus. In-vivo and in-vitro studies. Ann. Intern. Med., 79:679, 1973.
196. Hayek, A., and Ramirez, J.: Demeclocycline-induced diabetes insipidus. JAMA, 229:676, 1974.
197. Kestel, J. L.: Tetracycline-induced onycholysis unassociated with photosensitivity. Arch. Dermatol., 196:766, 1972.
198. Cunliffe, W. J., Cotterill, J. A., and Williamson, B.: The effect of clindamycin in acne—a clinical and laboratory investigation. Br. J. Dermatol., 87:37, 1972.
199. Tedesco, F. J., Stanley, R. J., and Alpers, D. H.: Diagnostic features of clindamycin-associated pseudomembranous colitis. N. Engl. J. Med., 290:841, 1974.
200. Ad Hoc Committee Report: Systemic antibiotics for treatment of acne vulgaris. Efficacy and safety. Arch. Dermatol., 111:1630, 1975.
201. Dantzig, P. I.: The safety of long-term clindamycin therapy for acne. Arch. Dermatol., 112:53, 1976.
202. Hersle, K.: Trimethoprim-sulphamethoxazole in acne vulgaris: A double-blind study. Dermatologica, 145:187, 1972.
203. Danto, J. L.: Effect of adrenocortical steroids on cystic and papular acne. J. Invest. Dermatol., 29:315, 1957.
204. Farber, E. M., and Claiborne, E. R.: Acne conglobata: Use of cortisone and corticotropin in therapy. California Med., 81:76, 1954.
205. Palitz, L. L., Milberg, I. L., and Kantor, I.: Enovid for acne in the female. Skin, 3:243, 1964.
206. Catalano, P. M.: Contraceptive conundrum I. Arch. Dermatol., 106:571, 1972.
207. Pria, S. D., Greenblatt, R. B., and Mahesh, V. B.: An antiandrogen in acne and idiopathic hirsutism. J. Invest. Dermatol., 52:348, 1969.
208. Dorfman, R. I.: Biological activity of antiandrogens. Br. J. Dermatol., 82:3, 1970.
209. Mier, P. D., and VanDenHurk, J. J. M. A.: Plasma vitamin A levels in the common dermatoses. Br. J. Dermatol., 91:155, 1974.
210. Leitner, Z. A., and Moore, T.: Vitamin A and skin disease. Lancet, 2:262, 1946.
211. Cornbleet, T., Popper, H., and Steigmann, F.: Blood vitamin A and cutaneous diseases. Arch. Dermatol., 49:103, 1944.
212. Straumfjord, J. V.: Vitamin A: Its effect on acne. Northwest. Med., 42:219, 1943.
213. Dalderup, L. M., Vermeulen, C. W., and Verbeek, A.: Vitamin A and acne vulgaris. Int. Z. Vitaminforsch., 38:451, 1968.
214. Report by the South-east Scotland Faculty of the College of General Practitioners. Vitamin A in acne vulgaris. Br. Med. J., 5352:294, 1963.

215. Lynch, F. W., and Cook, C. D.: Acne vulgaris treated with vitamin A. Arch. Dermatol., 55:355, 1947.
216. Mitchell, G. H., and Butterworth, T.: Results of treatment of acne vulgaris by intramuscular injections of vitamin A. Arch. Dermatol., 64:428, 1951.
217. Restak, R. M.: Pseudotumor cerebri, psychosis, and hypervitaminosis A. J. Nerv. Ment. Dis., 155:72, 1972.
218. Spencer, M. C.: Oral enzyme therapy in treatment of acne. Arch. Dermatol., 92:688, 1965.
219. Coles, R. B.: Group treatment in the skin department. Trans. St. Johns Hosp. Dermatol. Soc., 53:82, 1967.
220. Vymola, F., Buda, J., Lochmann, O., and Pillich, J.: Successful treatment of acne by immunotherapy. J. Hyg. Epidemiol. Microbiol. Immunol., 14:135, 1970.
221. O'Driscoll, B. J.: Acne: An allergic disease? Br. J. Clin. Pract., 23:225, 1969.
222. The vaccine treatment of acne. Lancet, 1:1056, 1909.
223. Burton, J. L., Libman, L. J., Hall, R., and Shuster, S.: Levodopa in acne vulgaris. Lancet, 2:370, 1971.
224. Burton, J. L., and Goolamali, S. K.: Zinc and sebum excretion. Lancet, 1:1448, 1973.
225. Cotterill, J. A., Cunliffe, W. J., and Williamson, B.: Sebum excretion rate and biochemistry in patients with acne vulgaris treated by oral fenfluramine. Br. J. Dermatol., 85:127, 1971.
226. Cotterill, J. A., Cunliffe, W. J., and Williamson, B.: Sebum excretion rate and skin-surface lipid composition in Parkinson's disease before and during therapy with levodopa. Lancet, 1:1271, 1971.
227. Cunliffe, W. J., and Shuster, S.: The effect of inhibitors of cholesterol synthesis on sebum secretion in patients with acne. Br. J. Dermatol., 81:280, 1969.
228. Frank, S. B.: Acne Vulgaris. Springfield, Ill., Charles C Thomas, 1971.
229. Epstein, E.: Dermabrasion for cosmetic purposes: A long-time evaulation by patients. Arch. Dermatol., 97:335, 1968.
230. Strauss, J. S., and Kligman, A. M.: Effect of X-rays on sebaceous glands of the human face: Radiation therapy of acne. J. Invest. Dermatol., 33:347, 1959.
231. Jelliffe, A. M., Soutter, C., and Meara, R. H.: An investigation into the treatment of acne vulgaris with Grenz x-rays. Br. J. Dermatol., 81:617, 1969.
232. Wright, W. L.: Grenz ray in the treatment of acne vulgaris: Controlled study. Arch. Dermatol., 89:417, 1964.
233. Powell, E. W., and Beveridge, G. W.: Sebum excretion and sebum composition in adolescent men with and without acne vulgaris. Br. J. Dermatol., 82:243, 1970.
234. Burton, J. L., and Shuster, S.: Effect of L-Dopa on seborrhea of Parkinsonism. Lancet, 2:311, 1970.
235. Kligman, A. M., Wheatley, V. R., and Mills, O.: Analysis of comedogenic constituents of human sebum. Arch. Dermatol., 102:267, 1970.
236. Kligman, A. M.: Pathogenesis of acne vulgaris. II. Histopathology of comedones induced in the rabbit ear by human sebum. Arch. Dermatol., 98:58, 1968.
237. Kligman, A. M., and Katz, A. G.: Pathogenesis of acne vulgaris. 1. Comedogenic properties of human sebum in external ear canal of the rabbit. Arch. Dermatol., 98:53, 1968.
238. Cunliffe, W. J., Forster, R. A., Greenwood, N. D., et al.: Tetracycline and acne vulgaris: A clinical and laboratory investigation. Br. Med. J., 4:332, 1973.
239. Freinkel, R. K., Strauss, J. S., Yip, S. Y., and Pochi, P. E.: Effect of tetracycline on the composition of sebum in acne vulgaris. N. Engl. J. Med., 273:850, 1965.
240. Nicolaides, N., Ansari, M. N. A., Fu, H. C., and Lindsay, D. G.: Lipid composition of comedones compared with that of human skin surface in acne patients. J. Invest. Dermatol., 54:487, 1970.
241. Puhvel, S. M., Hoffman, I. K., Reisner, R. M., and Sternberg, T. H.: Dermal hypersensitivity of patients with acne vulgaris to *Corynebacterium acnes*. J. Invest. Dermatol., 49:154, 1967.
242. Puhvel, S. M., Hoffman, I. K., and Sternberg, T. H.: *Corynebacterium acnes*. Arch. Dermatol., 93:364, 1966.
243. Puhvel, S. M., Barfatani, M., and Sternberg, T. H.: Study of antibody levels to *Corynebacterium acnes*. Arch. Dermatol., 90:421, 1964.
244. Lim, L. S., and James, V. H. T.: Plasma androgens in acne vulgaris. Br. J. Dermatol., 91:135, 1974.
245. Ettinger, B., Goldfield, E. B., Burrill, K. C., et al.: Plasma testosterone stimulation-suppression dynamics in hirsute women: Correlation with long-term therapy. Am. J. Med., 54:195, 1973.
246. Schoeff, L., and Plewig, G.: Data presented at the European Society of Dermatological Research, 1974.
247. Strom, S., Thyresson, N., and Bostrom, H.: Acute febrile ulcerative conglobate acne with leukemoid reaction. Acta Derm. Venereol., 53:306, 1973.
248. Kelly, A. P., and Burns, R. E.: Acute febrile ulcerative conglobate acne with polyarthralgia. Arch. Dermatol., 104:182, 1971.

249. Mills, O. H., Leyden, J. J., and Kligman, A. M.: Tretinoin treatment of steroid acne. Arch. Dermatol., *108*:381, 1973.
250. Frank, S. B.: Uncommon aspects of common acne. Cutis, *14*:817, 1974.
251. Danto, J. L., Maddin, W. S., Stewart, W. D., and Nelson, A. J.: A controlled trial of benzoyl peroxide and precipitated sulfur cream in acne vulgaris. Appl. Ther., *8*:624, 1966.
252. Arundell, F. D.: Acne Vulgaris. Pediatr. Clin. North Am., *18*:853, 1971.
253. Reisner, R. M.: Acne vulgaris. Pediatr. Clin. North Am., *20*:851, 1973.
254. Mills, O. H., Kligman, A. M., and Stewart, R.: The clinical effectiveness of topical erythromycin in acne vulgaris. Cutis, *15*:93, 1975.
255. Sulzberger, M. G., Rostenberg, A., and Sher, J. J.: Acneiform eruptions with remarks on acne vulgaris and its pathogenesis. N.Y. J. Med., *34*:899, 1934.

5

ECZEMATOUS DERMATITIS

J. CLARK HUFF, M.D.
WILLIAM L. WESTON, M.D.

INTRODUCTION

"Eczema" is a term used to denote a pattern of inflammation in the skin. Derived from a Greek word meaning "boiling out," eczema was originally reserved for a vesicular or weeping eruption. However, the term as it is currently used describes superficial cutaneous inflammation, with the features of acute, subacute, or sometimes chronic dermatitis (see pages 102–116). Rather than being a precise scientific term, eczema is poorly defined and has no etiological significance. Despite its imprecise definition, eczema is a better descriptive term than "dermatitis," which implies any inflammatory process in the skin. Nevertheless, eczema and dermatitis are often used interchangeably in clinical medicine today.

No single classification of eczema is entirely satisfactory. Because eczema represents a type of reaction pattern, its etiology often is multifactorial or unknown. Only in allergic contact dermatitis do we have some insight into the mechanism of pathogenesis. Eczematous eruptions that cannot be classified by etiology are frequently given names that describe the clinical morphology (nummular eczema) or specify the location (hand eczema). For an eczematous eruption without apparent cause, labeling the problem "eczema" is preferable to using a diagnostic term that may falsely imply a known etiology. Like other descriptive diagnoses, such as purpura and alopecia, eczema may have many causes. The skin is a major boundary between man and his environment, and probably all eczematous dermatoses are generated by the interplay of a number of factors. Even in contact dermatitis, in which the external contactant is paramount, internal factors may alter the clinical presentation.

The eczematous dermatoses of adolescence resemble those of adulthood more than those of infancy or childhood. We will exclude from our discussion of the eczematous eruptions of adolescence those dermatoses that are not usually eczematous in appearance, such as polymorphic light eruption and drug eruption, as well as those eczematous dermatoses that are rare in adolescence (stasis dermatitis). This discussion is divided into the following subjects: (1) clinical and histological features of eczema; (2) atopic dermatitis; (3) contact dermatitis; (4) other eczematous processes; and (5) topical therapy.

CLINICAL AND HISTOLOGICAL FEATURES OF ECZEMA

The clinical and histological appearances of eczema make up a spectrum; the place an eczematous eruption has in this spectrum depends primarily on the duration and intensity of the inflammatory process. The appearance may also be influenced by the area of the body where the eruption occurs.[1] An acute eczematous dermatitis is characterized clinically by the presence of erythema, edema, papules, vesicles, oozing (representing ruptured vesicles), and crusting. The histological correlates of the clinical features include dilation of subepidermal capillaries, edema fluid between epidermal cells (spongiosis), intraepidermal vesicles, a perivascular, largely mononuclear cell inflammatory infiltrate, and inflammatory cells within the epidermis (exocytosis). Vesicles may be larger and more persistent on the palms and soles where the stratum corneum is thick. The picture of an acute eczematous dermatitis is most frequently seen in acute allergic contact dermatitis.

A subacute eczematous dermatitis is less erythematous and has less tendency to vesiculate than the acute form but has more scaling and fissuring and results in thickening of the epidermis. Histologically, in subacute eczema, spongiosis, vesicle formation, and exocytosis are less marked; acanthosis (elongation of the rete ridges), hyperkeratosis (increased thickness of the stratum corneum), and parakeratosis (retention of nuclei in the stratum corneum) become prominent. Nummular eczema usually contains clinical and histological features of a subacute dermatitis.

Once it has become chronic, a superficial cutaneous inflammatory process differs from acute or subacute eczematous dermatitis in several aspects. The clinical appearance is dominated by scaling and epidermal thickening, which represent the histological features of hyperkeratosis and acanthosis. A perivascular lymphocytic infiltrate is usually present. Atopic dermatitis and lichen simplex chronicus are characterized by the features of a chronic dermatitis.

Obviously, there is no single feature that allows one to describe a dermatitis as eczematous. The most important clue is the epidermal involvement in the inflammatory process. This epidermal reaction may be recognized by the presence of superficial vesicles, oozing, fissuring, or scaling. Itching is prominent in most of the eczematous dermatoses, but itching is not an essential feature of these and certainly is not specific for eczema. Although the histological appearance of an eczematous dermatosis reflects the clinical appearance nicely, the diagnosis of eczema is made primarily from the clinical features; rarely is a biopsy necessary except to exclude the presence of some other rare disease process that may have a distinctive histological appearance.

ATOPIC DERMATITIS (Atopic Eczema)

Atopic dermatitis is a common chronic or recurrent pruritic dermatitis of unknown etiology that occurs in individuals with a constitutional predisposition to atopy. Although the primary defect in atopic dermatitis is hereditary, environmental factors may be responsible for exacerbations as well as for the peculiar distribution of the dermatitis on the body surface.

Atopy ("unusualness") was first used in the 1920's by Coca and Cooke to denote inherited human hypersensitiveness, as exemplified by asthma and hay fever. Atopic dermatitis was used by Hill and Sulzberger to describe the dermatitis that accompanies the atopic state.[3]

Studies of atopic dermatitis are clouded by the fact that the diagnosis is a clinical one; a specific marker for the disorder has not been identified. The clinical appearance of atopic dermatitis may represent a phenotype, resulting from many different mechanisms. Indeed, dermatitis resembling atopic dermatitis can be associated with other disorders, such as the Wiskott-Aldrich syndrome, phenylketonuria, Netherton's syndrome, and ichthyosis vulgaris[4] (Table 5-1).

A variety of terms have been used in the literature to name the condition we call atopic dermatitis. However, in the United States, atopic eczema, allergic eczema, eczema, Besnier's prurigo, and generalized neurodermatitis are less acceptable and less widely used terms than atopic dermatitis.

FEATURES OF ATOPIC DERMATITIS

Hereditary Predisposition. Studies have demonstrated a family history of atopy (asthma, allergic rhinitis, atopic dermatitis) in two thirds of individuals with dermatoses that are morphologically compatible with atopic dermatitis.[5, 6] A strongly positive history of atopy in close relatives is clinically useful, despite the difficulties of determining what constitutes such a history and the frequent occurrence of atopic disorders in the families of normal patients.[7] More convincing evidence of the importance of genotype in determining the occurrence of atopic dermatitis is the concordance of the disorder in identical twins (50 per cent) as compared with the 4 per cent prevalence in fraternal twins (Fig. 5-1).[8]

The inheritance of atopy does not follow a simple mendelian pattern but appears to involve a number of factors. The explanation proposed most frequently is that the inheritance of atopy is polygenic and the expression of the atopic genotype is determined by a complex interplay of genetic and environmental factors.

Association with Other Atopic Disorders. Up to 50 per cent of patients with atopic dermatitis also have respiratory manifestations of atopy, including

TABLE 5-1 DISORDERS WITH AN ATOPIC-LIKE DERMATITIS

Phenylketonuria
X-linked agammaglobulinemia (Bruton's disease)
Wiskott-Aldrich syndrome
Job's syndrome
Hurler's syndrome
Histidine deficiency
Ataxia-telangiectasia
Netherton's syndrome
Ichthyosis vulgaris

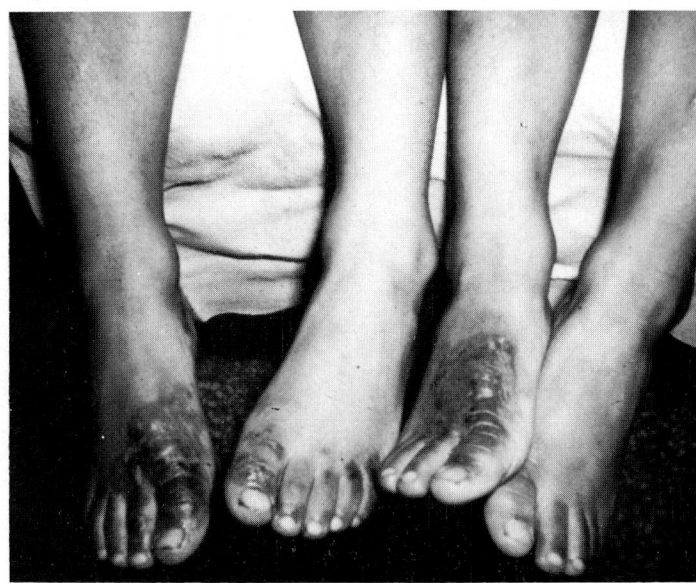

FIGURE 5–1 Atopic dermatitis in identical twins.

extrinsic asthma or allergic rhinitis.[5-7] The dermatitis is usually associated with one or the other; infrequently a patient will have all three aspects of the atopic triad (asthma, allergic rhinitis, and atopic dermatitis). Most individuals who develop asthma in association with atopic dermatitis have done so by early adolescence; over 50 per cent of those who develop allergic rhinitis do not do so until adolescence or early adulthood.[6] Atopic dermatitis and associated respiratory manifestations of atopy not only may begin at different ages but also may follow independent clinical courses.

Chronic Fluctuating Clinical Course. Atopic dermatitis has its onset during the first year of life in 60 per cent of cases and affects both sexes equally.[6] The majority of those who do not develop atopic dermatitis in infancy develop it by early childhood. About 90 per cent of those who develop atopic dermatitis have already done so by adolescence. Less than 6 per cent of individuals with atopic dermatitis develop the disorder during adolescence. In this last group, a history of either infantile or childhood eczema can be elicited. Atopic dermatitis may have a chronic persistent course from onset, but in most cases the problem runs a fluctuating course marked by remissions and exacerbations (Fig. 5–2).

Itching. Itching has long been recognized as a significant aspect of atopic dermatitis, as suggested by such early names as prurigo and neurodermatitis. Itching in atopic dermatitis is severe and often paroxysmal.[3] In most patients itching is more severe in the evening. The threshold for itching is lowered in atopic dermatitis patients, and the itch sensation is more prolonged than in normal individuals subjected to similar stimuli. The propensity for itching and the resultant trauma from scratching are central to the genesis of atopic dermatitis.[9]

Distribution of Dermatitis. The distribution of dermatitis on the body is a helpful clue in the diagnosis of atopic dermatitis, but this distribution is largely age-dependent (Fig. 5–3A and B). *Infantile* atopic dermatitis mainly involves the cheeks, forehead, scalp, limbs, and trunk. It evolves into the

90 CHAPTER 5—ECZEMATOUS DERMATITIS

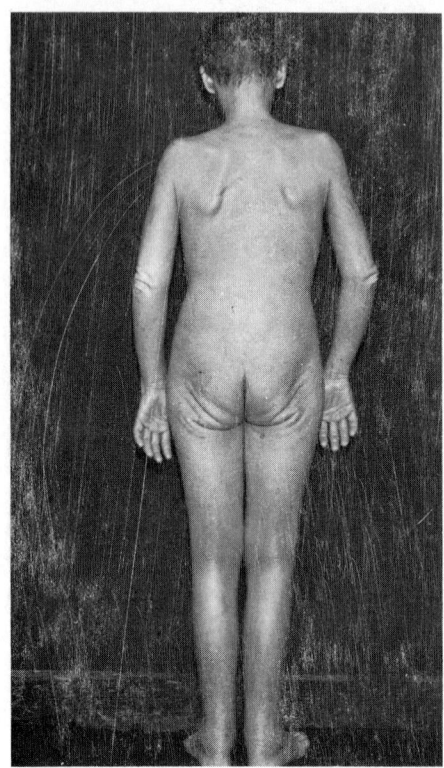

FIGURE 5-2 Diffuse erythroderma in atopic teen-ager. Generalized lymphadenopathy. Edema of lower legs.

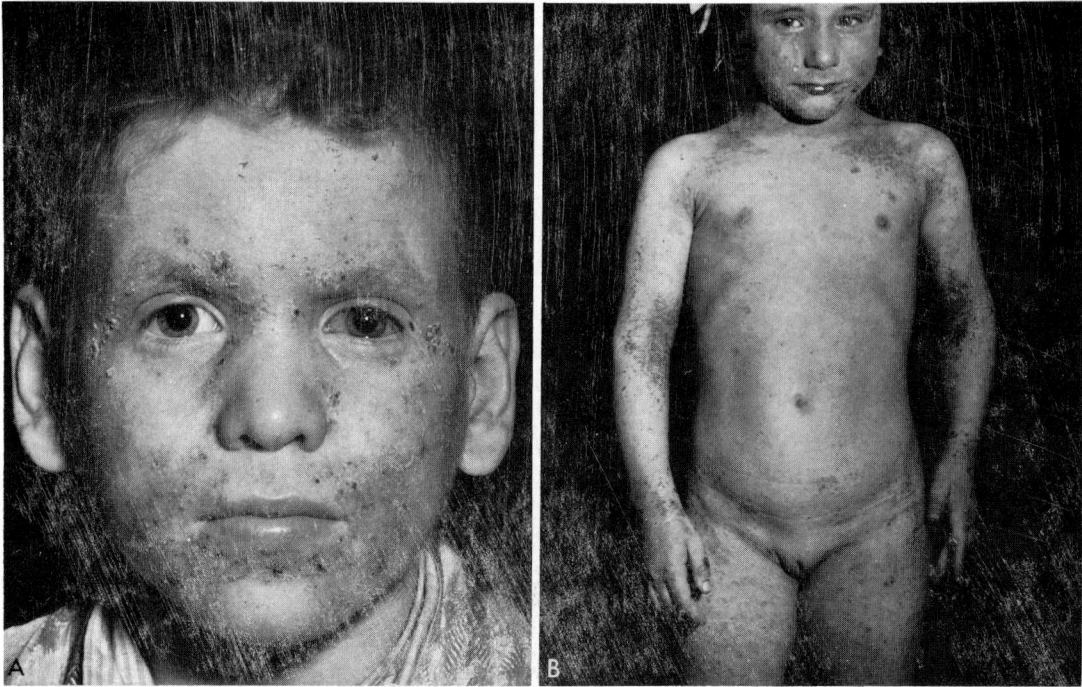

FIGURE 5-3 Atopic dermatitis. *A*, Characteristic facial appearance, chronic excoriated dermatitis, and "sad" and "strained" look. *B*, Female child with characteristic facies and predominantly flexural involvement.

childhood phase, with dermatitis primarily affecting the feet and flexural areas, such as the antecubital fossae, popliteal fossae, and neck. By *adolescence,* the distribution is characteristic of the adult phase, with bilateral involvement of flexural areas and hands. When adult-phase atopic dermatitis affects areas besides these, the condition frequently is accentuated in flexural areas as well as the hands (Fig. 5–4A, B, and C). Involvement of the eyelids is common to all phases of atopic dermatitis and may help to confirm the diagnosis. Foot involvement has recently been recognized as a feature of atopic dermatitis and may occur as a predominant characteristic in adolescents.[10]

Morphology of Skin Lesions. The primary clinical lesion of atopic dermatitis has not been defined; in fact, many clinicians believe that all visible skin lesions in atopic dermatitis are secondary to scratching. Vesicles are not usual in uncomplicated atopic dermatitis, although papules with focal spongiosis have been considered by some to be possible primary lesions.[11] In most cases, adolescent patients with flexural atopic dermatitis have thickened, dry, sometimes scaly, excoriated plaques with accentuated skin folds or lichenification (Fig. 5–5A and B). Intense erythema and oozing usually are absent, except in the presence of secondary bacterial infection. During exacerbations, many patients have follicular papules, especially on the trunk. The borders of the involved areas are usually indistinct, merging gradually with surrounding normal skin. Scaling of the scalp may be a prominent sign in some patients. In black skin, hyperpigmented lichenified nodules are frequently found in flexural areas and on the lower parts of the arms and legs.

Dry Skin. There is a strong association between dry skin and atopic dermatitis. In 50 per cent of patients with ichthyosis vulgaris, there is an atopic-like dermatitis.[3, 12] However, patients with atopic dermatitis may also have depressed secretion of sebum,[13] resulting in dry scaly skin and horny follicular papules (keratosis pilaris), particularly on the extensor surfaces. Microscopic fractures of the stratum corneum lead to loss of integrity of the epidermal barrier, increasing its susceptibility to irritation. There is little doubt that dry skin, which is most common during the winter in cold climates, is a significant factor in exacerbations of atopic dermatitis.[9]

Pityriasis Alba. Hypopigmented macules with indistinct borders and fine scaling (pityriasis alba) may be found on the face and upper arms of children with atopic dermatitis. This condition, particularly prominent in dark skin, probably represents low-grade chronic dermatitis. Although it is considered to be a variant of atopic dermatitis,[14] it may also be found in some patients who exhibit no other evidence of atopic dermatitis.

Abnormal Sweating. Many patients with atopic dermatitis complain of increased itching under conditions that induce sweating. In those parts of the body affected by atopic dermatitis, sweat secretion is not diminished. However, sweat duct occlusion by keratin plugs at the surface does occur, sometimes resulting in hypohidrosis and extravasation of sweat into the dermis. This phenomenon may account for the exacerbation of itching experienced by some patients.[15]

Seasonal Changes. Patients with atopic dermatitis may experience seasonal variation in the activity of their dermatitis.[9] In temperate climates, about 50 per cent of patients experience exacerbation in winter. Low humidity in a heated indoor environment and rapid changes in skin temperature have been suggested as explanations for this pattern of exacerbation. Fewer patients (ap-

92 CHAPTER 5—ECZEMATOUS DERMATITIS

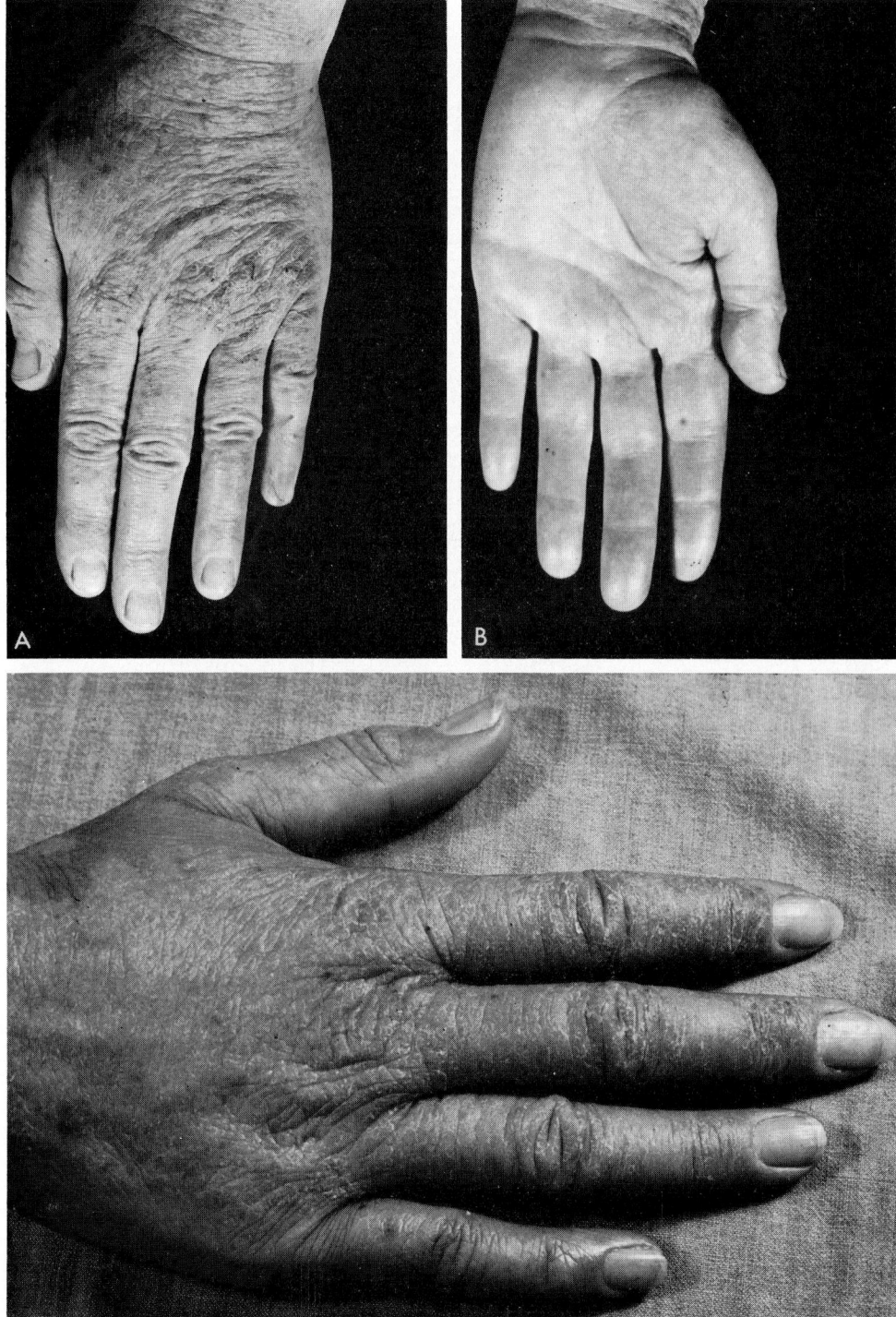

FIGURE 5–4 Chronic eczematous dermatitis. "Housewives' hands." *A* and *B* show the absence of involvement of the palm seen early in this dermatitis. *C,* Thickening, scaling, and fissuring in chronic phase.

ATOPIC DERMATITIS (ATOPIC ECZEMA)

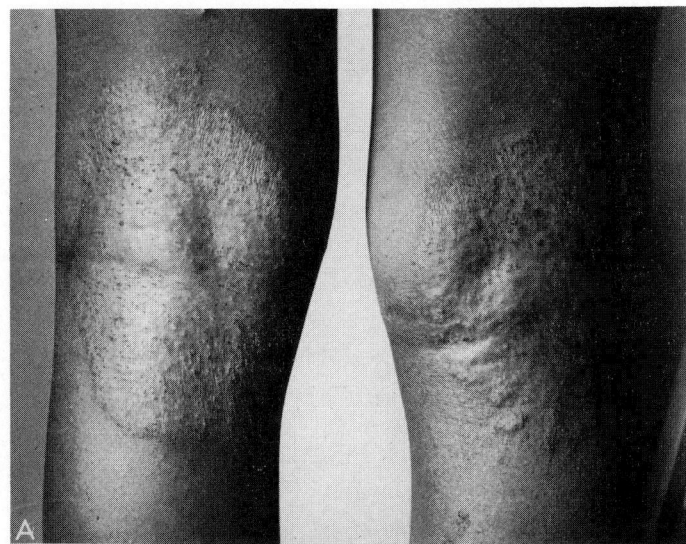
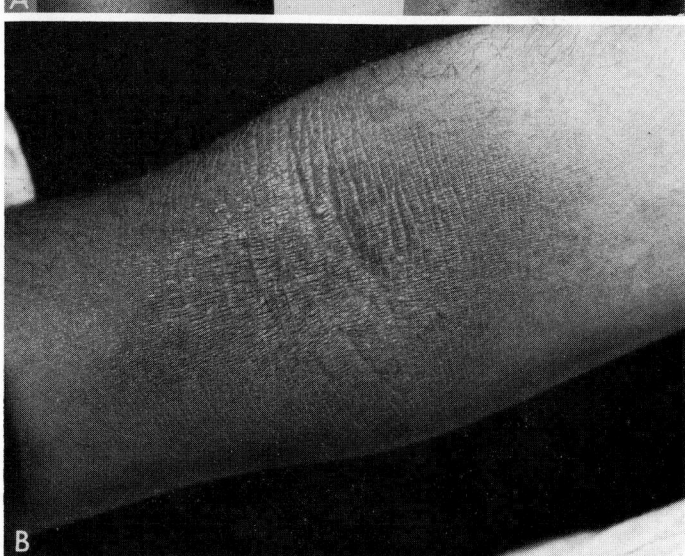

FIGURE 5–5 Atopic dermatitis—characteristic lesions. A, Sharply marginated excoriated lesions of popliteal spaces. B, Lichenification and thickening—antecubital fossa.

proximately 30 per cent) suffer exacerbation in the spring and summer. Only about 10 per cent of patients have no seasonal itching pattern.

Abnormal Vascular Phenomena. A variety of vasomotor reactions, including facial pallor, suggest that patients with atopic dermatitis have a tendency to vasoconstriction in the skin. Their peripheral extremities remain cooler than normal and react to cold with marked vasoconstriction. When the erythematous skin is stroked with a blunt instrument, a white line surrounded by blanching (white dermatographism) is the usual response (Fig. 5–6). This is in contrast to the expected triple response of Lewis, consisting of erythema, flare, and wheal.[16] The blanching phenomenon is thought to represent vasoconstriction, although some evidence suggests that it might instead represent edema.[17]

Abnormal Cutaneous Reactions to Pharmacological Agents. The most convincing evidence documenting the unusual reactions found in atopic der-

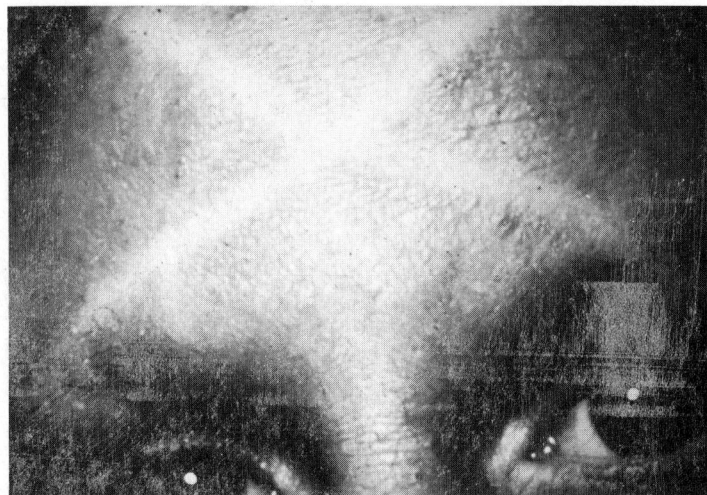

FIGURE 5-6 The white line response.

matitis is the paradoxical delayed blanching reaction to intradermally injected acetylcholine, an agent that normally causes a vasodilation. In the skin of individuals with atopic dermatitis, the response is an ephemeral wheal and flare reaction, followed by pallor which develops at the site within 3 to 30 minutes and persists for more than an hour (Fig. 5-7).[18] The vasoconstrictive reaction may also be found in asymptomatic relatives of individuals with atopic dermatitis. As a result, many practitioners consider this phenomenon a clinical marker of atopic dermatitis. Similar reactions may occur with other cholinergic agents and nicotinic acid esters.[17] Another unexpected reaction of atopic skin is a diminished response to the intradermal injection of histamine,[19, 20] with failure to exhibit the expected cutaneous flare.

Sensitivity to Contactants. The skin of an individual with atopic dermatitis is extremely sensitive to certain contactants. Wool and irritant chemicals, such as detergents,[9, 21] may induce bouts of itching and subsequent exacerbation of the dermatitis. Mechanical and chemical irritation, rather than allergic

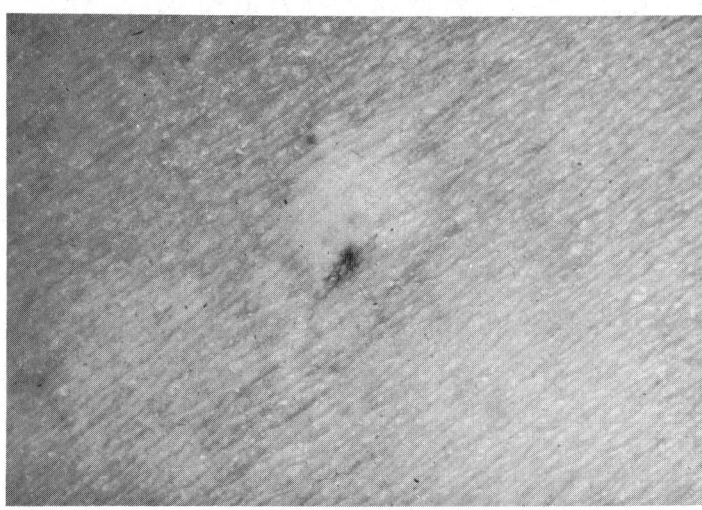

FIGURE 5-7 The delayed blanch phenomenon.

mechanisms, is responsible for increased itching in such cases; the skin appears to be innately more susceptible to itching stimuli. Contrary to former belief, the true incidence of allergic contact dermatitis in atopics is actually lower than in individuals with normal skin.[22-24] Primary irritation by contactants may partly explain the localization of dermatitis to the hands and feet in some cases.

COMPLICATIONS

Infections. Individuals with atopic dermatitis appear to have an increased susceptibility to certain cutaneous infections (Table 5–2). It is not clear whether this apparent susceptibility is due to a local abnormality of the cutaneous barrier or to a systemic immune defect. Recent evidence suggests the existence of a defect in cell-mediated immunity in these patients (see pages 97–99).

A generalized cutaneous infection with either vaccinia virus (eczema vaccinatum)[25, 26] or herpes simplex virus (eczema herpeticum)[27-29] is a dread and sometimes fatal complication of atopic dermatitis. These viral complications are grouped under the designation of Kaposi's varicelliform eruption and consist of a widespread vesiculopustular eruption accompanied by high fever. Eczema herpeticum may be differentiated from eczema vaccinatum by making a Giemsa stain on material scraped from a blister base (Tzanck smear). Multinucleated giant cells are found in smears from patients with herpes virus infections, but not in smears from those with poxvirus infections. With the cessation of routine smallpox vaccination, eczema vaccinatum has become rare. Nevertheless, atopic dermatitis in a patient or a member of his family remains a contraindication to smallpox vaccination. Analysis of eczema vaccinatum in Wales[26] indicates that this complication occurs in one out of 800 eczema patients and shows a familial pattern. Moreover, it may occur when the dermatitis has been quiescent for a long period.

Any site of dermatitis, where the normal barrier function of the epidermis has been lost, harbors large numbers of bacteria. Ninety per cent of patients with atopic dermatitis harbor excessive numbers of *Staphylococcus aureus* on the skin.[30] It is not known whether overgrowth of these bacteria plays a part in perpetuating atopic dermatitis. Secondary bacterial infection may develop, with marked erythema, edema, vesicles, pustules, oozing, and crusting[31]; these features are not usually seen in individuals with uncomplicated atopic dermatitis. Small erythematous papules, particularly on the palms, may also represent secondary staphylococcal infections of atopic dermatitis.[32] Although

TABLE 5–2 CUTANEOUS INFECTIONS TO WHICH ATOPIC DERMATITIS PATIENTS HAVE INCREASED SUSCEPTIBILITY

Vaccinia virus
Herpes simplex virus
Staphylococcal pyodermas
Trichophyton rubrum

Staphylococcus aureus may be present in infected lesions, beta-hemolytic streptococci are often the more significant culprits in secondarily infected atopic dermatitis. A small group of patients with atopic-like dermatitis also have a marked tendency to develop persistent or recurrent cutaneous and systemic bacterial infections. One such group of patients with atopic-like dermatitis, hyperimmunoglobulinemia E, and recurrent staphylococcal abscesses demonstrate altered immune function because of a defect in the directional movement of phagocytic leukocytes[31, 33-35] (Table 5–3).

Recent reports indicate that individuals with atopic dermatitis may have a higher than normal prevalence of chronic dermatophyte infections.[36, 37] A demonstrable lack of delayed hypersensitivity to dermatophyte antigens suggests that defective cell-mediated immunity may account for such fungal infections. Evidence supporting a susceptibility to other fungal infections in individuals with atopic dermatitis is lacking.

Eye Complications. The most frequent serious ocular complication in individuals with atopic dermatitis is cataract formation, which typically occurs in young adults. Cataracts in atopic individuals usually are bilateral and located in the anterior subcapsular area. They must be differentiated from posterior subcapsular cataracts, which occur in individuals who have received long-term systemic corticosteroid therapy. Atopic cataracts may begin in adolescence and, although as many as 16 per cent of patients have been found to have such ocular lesions, the actual prevalence is probably much lower.[13] Other less common but serious eye complications include keratoconus and retinal detachment.[38] The pathogenesis of these ocular complications in atopic patients is not well understood. However, years of rubbing the eyes, evidenced by double folds on the lower lids (Dennie's fold), may play a significant role.

Exfoliative Erythroderma. Adolescents with bronchial asthma and extensive atopic dermatitis may develop a generalized acute or chronic exfoliative dermatitis.[39] Without treatment, metabolic consequences may ensue, including excessive protein loss, hypoproteinemia, faulty temperature regulation, and high-output cardiac failure. Hair and nails may be lost. Although this complication of atopic dermatitis is rare,[39] exfoliative erythroderma is a serious complication of atopic dermatitis that should be recognized early and treated vigorously (Fig. 5–2).

TABLE 5–3 ATOPIC DERMATITIS, HYPERIMMUNOGLOBULINEMIA E, AND RECURRENT STAPHYLOCOCCAL PYODERMAS

Associated Findings	Leukocyte Random Mobility	Leukocyte Chemotaxis
Chronic mucocutaneous candidiasis, eosinophilia[33]	Normal	Decreased
Staphylococcal abscesses[34]	Normal	Decreased
Red hair, hyperextensible joints, "cold" staphylococcal abscesses (Job's syndrome)[35]	Normal	Decreased
Urticaria with/without asthma[31]	Normal	Decreased

PATHOGENESIS

The underlying cause of atopic dermatitis remains unknown. Since an atopic-like dermatitis can be associated with several distinct inborn errors of metabolism, multiple biochemical mechanisms could be involved. Since most, if not all, atopic dermatitis may be the result of chronic rubbing and scratching, the production of itching may be the path common to a number of different etiological mechanisms. We wish to discuss two theories of the pathogenesis of dermatitis associated with the atopic state: the immunological theory and the beta-blockade theory. Although they have certain similarities, each theory postulates a different basic defect.

IMMUNOLOGICAL THEORY

The hereditary pattern associating atopic dermatitis with allergic rhinitis and asthma has led investigators to seek a common underlying mechanism that would account for both the dermatitis and the respiratory symptoms. Theories postulating both overactivity and deficiency of the immune system (Table 5–4) have been put forth, but none of these is entirely satisfactory.

Overactivity of the Immune Response. When immunoglobulin E (IgE) was discovered and characterized,[40] many investigators were led to hope that it would represent a chemical marker of atopic dermatitis. However, the role of IgE in atopic dermatitis remains complex and uncertain. IgE has been identified as an antibody (reagin) with the ability to transfer urticarial reactions from a sensitized to a non-sensitized individual.[41] It is species-specific and demonstrates activity only in human skin. After IgE is injected into the skin, there is a delay of about 50 to 80 hours before urticaria can be produced by a specific antigen. This time represents the period of sensitization. The minimal sensitizing dose is 10^{-5} mcg. Once the dosage is fixed in the skin the potential for reaction persists for about one month. IgE does not fix complement and its activity is destroyed by heating to 56°C for 30 minutes. IgE demonstrates an electrophoretic mobility of 8 and is not transferred across the placenta.[41]

It may be interesting to examine some of the inconsistencies engendered by the notion that IgE causes atopic dermatitis. At the site of injection or production, IgE is rapidly bound to mast cells. There, IgE and its antigen induce structural changes in the mast cell which lead to histamine release.[40] Under controlled conditions, injection of IgE into the skin, followed by exposure to its specific antigen, causes a wheal and flare response, but not an eczematous dermatitis.

IgE may also be bound to lymphocytes. IgE-bearing lymphocytes are normally found in the respiratory and gastrointestinal tracts, but not in the skin

TABLE 5–4 IMMUNOLOGICAL DEFECTS IN ATOPIC DERMATITIS

Hyperimmunoglobulinemia E
Defective cell-mediated immunity
Defective neutrophil and monocyte chemotaxis
Increased susceptibility to infection

or subcutaneous lymph nodes.[40] One investigator, however, has found IgE-bearing lymphocytes in the skin of some patients with atopic dermatitis.[42] Yet, intradermal skin tests with anti-IgE antibody result in the same urticarial response in both atopic and non-atopic subjects, indicating there is not more IgE bound in the skin of patients with atopic dermatitis.[43]

Serum IgE levels may be elevated in patients with severe atopic dermatitis but often not in those with moderate or mild dermatitis.[43-48] Nor do the levels of IgE in the serum correlate positively with changes in the activity of atopic dermatitis.[44] Furthermore, IgE levels in the serum fluctuate considerably throughout the year in patients with atopic dermatitis but less so in patients with allergic rhinitis or hay fever.[49] Finally, treatment with corticosteroids or azathioprine does not affect serum IgE levels, although it may improve atopic dermatitis.[50]

The presence of IgE in the serum does not satisfactorily explain the pathogenesis of atopic dermatitis. Results of immediate skin tests (prick tests) also have been of little use in the evaluation of atopic dermatitis.[22] The presence in the serum or skin of IgE, directed against specific antigens, may correlate better with the presence of atopic dermatitis than does the total serum IgE, which represents antibodies against numerous antigens.

Immune Deficiency

FAULTY REGULATION OF IgE. It has been postulated that elevated serum IgE levels may result from faulty regulation of IgE-producing B-lymphocytes. Overactivity of the B cell immune system (hyperimmunoglobulinemia E) could result from T cell or regulatory cell deficiency. In laboratory animals, a population of thymic-derived T-lymphocytes regulates the production of reaginic antibody,[51-53] and there is some evidence for similar regulation in man. For example, T-lymphocyte regulation of specific IgE occurs in humans with ragweed antigen sensitivity.[54] In an infant with congenitally suppressed T-lymphocyte function (thymic alymphoplasia), levels of IgE in the serum were found to be quite high and correlated with an atopic-like eczema occurring at four weeks of age.[55] In this case, at least, elevated serum IgE apparently served as a marker of immunodeficiency.[55]

CELL-MEDIATED IMMUNODEFICIENCY. The true prevalence of suppressed cell-mediated immunity among atopic dermatitis patients is unknown, but some of the following studies provide evidence of qualitative changes in this biological property in patients with atopic dermatitis. Some patients with atopic dermatitis were found to have depressed cell-mediated immunity;[56] several were found to have cutaneous anergy, recurrent infections, and suppressed T-lymphocyte function;[37] some had little or no ability to become sensitized to dinitrochlorobenzene (DNCB);[57] and still others were found to have suppressed lymphocyte transformation[37, 56, 58, 59] as well as decreased numbers of circulating T-lymphocytes.[56, 60]

IMMUNOGLOBULIN A DEFICIENCY. A transient deficiency of immunoglobulin A (IgA) during infancy (age three months) has been postulated as a possible cause of atopic dermatitis.[61] Deficiency of IgA on mucous surfaces could increase the number of antigens entering the blood by ingestion during a vulnerable period of infancy, thus stimulating greater IgE production. However, this theory has not been confirmed. In one study, 43 of 641 atopic patients had suppressed serum levels of IgA, but only one of the 43 had atopic dermatitis.[62]

DEFECTIVE PHAGOCYTE FUNCTION. Several reports have recently described patients (Table 5–3) with atopic dermatitis who have associated recurrent staphylococcal pyodermas, hyperimmunoglobulinemia E, and defective neutrophil and monocyte chemotaxis.[31, 33, 35, 59] Such patients also may have chronic oral and nail candidiasis, as well as urticaria. One group of patients, said to have Job's syndrome, have red hair, fair skin, hyperextensible joints, atopic-like dermatitis, and "cold" staphylococcal abscesses.[35] In these patients, excessive serum IgE apparently does not interfere with neutrophil chemotaxis. However, histamine may alter neutrophil cell movement.[34] Neutrophil phagocytosis may also be suppressed during acute flares of atopic dermatitis.[63] Neutrophil chemotaxis was found to return to normal function during remissions of atopic dermatitis.[59, 63] The syndrome of hyperimmunoglobulinemia E, faulty neutrophil chemotaxis, and staphylococcal abscesses may also be seen in patients with skin diseases other than atopic dermatitis (Table 5–3), such as chronic urticaria[31] and incontinentia pigmenti.[64]

Certain patients with atopic dermatitis may have functional defects in T-lymphocytes, neutrophils, and monocytes, thus accounting for increased susceptibility to infection. Even though these phenomena may not provide a satisfactory explanation of the mechanism of this disease, the immunological status of an adolescent with atopic-like dermatitis who suffers persistent or recurrent infections should be investigated.

BETA-BLOCKADE THEORY

The beta-blockade theory was postulated by Szentivanyi to explain the cause of bronchial asthma and the atopic state in general. It takes into account both the vascular phenomena and the immunodeficiencies associated with atopic dermatitis. This theory postulates a deficiency in beta-adrenergic receptors on the cell membrane (either adenyl cyclase or its associated receptors) in atopic patients.[65] It further postulates that as a result of depressed beta-receptor function, catecholamines (epinephrine and norepinephrine) activate alpha-receptors excessively and thus cause increased vasoconstriction in the skin. This theory therefore attempts to explain the abnormal cutaneous vascular responses often found in patients with atopic dermatitis. Furthermore, defective beta-receptors on neutrophil and T-lymphocyte membranes could explain the faulty functioning of their immunocytes.

In support of this theory, it has been demonstrated that atopic dermatitis patients have decreased beta-adrenergic sensitivity in the epidermis.[66] Concentrations of substances in the epidermis that mediate beta-adrenergic responses, such as cyclic AMP (adenosine 3':5'-cyclic phosphate), adenyl cyclase, and phosphodiesterase, appear to be not significantly different in atopic dermatitis patients than in normal subjects or in those with other dermatoses. Lymphocytes from patients with atopic dermatitis have a suppressed cyclic AMP response to a beta-agonist (isoproterenol), while the response to prostaglandin E is normal.[67] Although the beta-blockade theory has not been proved by available scientific evidence, it is a promising attempt to explain the many abnormalities found in atopy by postulating a common biological defect.

DIAGNOSIS AND DIFFERENTIAL DIAGNOSIS

There is no single criterion for diagnosing atopic dermatitis; a combination of features must be considered. The following major features are useful in the diagnosis of atopic dermatitis in the adolescent: dry skin with itching and lichenification; personal history of asthma or allergic rhinitis; family history of asthma, eczema, or allergic rhinitis; elevated IgE in the serum; itching stimulated by sweating; and paradoxical vasoconstrictive cutaneous responses (Table 5–5). It is helpful to know the bodily distribution of the dermatitis. A history of remissions and exacerbations or of eczema in infancy or childhood is also useful. Although many other indications, such as facial pallor, Dennie's folds, intolerance to wool or occlusive clothing, associated ichthyosis, cataracts, and eosinophilia, may be found in some patients, they are less specific or less frequent than the primary features enumerated.

The differential diagnosis of atopic dermatitis in adolescence may include any type of dermatitis. Irritant and allergic contact dermatitis, seborrheic dermatitis, nummular eczema, tinea corporis, and scabies constitute the major diagnoses to be considered (Table 5–6). Differentiation between atopic dermatitis and other dermatoses may not be easy in the adolescent. For example, a person with atopic dermatitis since infancy may also develop seborrhea and facial dermatitis. Scabies also may be quite confusing because of the intense itching it engenders and the resulting excoriations and dermatitis. Patch testing (see pages 113–114) may help to exclude allergic contact dermatitis. An examination of skin scrapings with potassium hydroxide (KOH) will help discover tinea corporis and differentiate it from atopic dermatitis. Scabies may be found by mineral oil examination of a scraping (see Chapter 3). Nummular eczema and irritant contact dermatitis are often difficult to distinguish from atopic dermatitis. Nummular lesions may in fact occur in atopic dermatitis; some authors consider atopic dermatitis fertile ground in which nummular patches of eczema may develop. Irritants may cause exacerbations of atopic dermatitis, resulting in confusion and difficult management problems. In a patient thought to have atopic dermatitis, consideration should be given to the role played by irritants and special attention paid to their avoidance.

THERAPY OF ATOPIC DERMATITIS

Adolescents and their parents often seek immediate cause and effect relationships in atopic dermatitis. It is tempting for the physician to focus on one or several factors as "causes" and their elimination as "cures." However,

TABLE 5–5 MAJOR DIAGNOSTIC FEATURES OF ATOPIC DERMATITIS

Itching
Family or personal history of allergic rhinitis or asthma
Dry skin with increased itching with sweating
Hyperimmunoglobulinemia E
Paradoxical vasoconstrictive cutaneous reactivity

TABLE 5–6 DIFFERENTIAL DIAGNOSIS OF ATOPIC DERMATITIS IN ADOLESCENTS

Diagnosis	Identifying Features
Seborrheic dermatitis	Greasy scale Distribution in "seborrheic areas," such as scalp, brow, and behind ears
Nummular eczema	Round shape of areas of dermatitis Distribution on extremities Negative KOH examination
Irritant contact dermatitis	Scaling and fissuring Location on exposed skin (hands) or in occluded sites History of contactant Negative patch tests
Allergic contact dermatitis	Sudden onset Vesiculation Location on exposed skin or in occluded sites History of contactant Positive patch tests
Tinea corporis or tinea pedis	Scaling Blistering (tinea pedis) Sharp margins of involved skin (tinea corporis) Positive KOH examination
Scabies	Intense itching History of itching in personal contacts Distribution (hands, buttocks, groin) Mites and eggs in skin scrapings

without scientific evidence for the pathogenesis of atopic dermatitis, it is impossible to postulate or effect a "cure." Patients and their parents should be instructed that, although there is no permanent cure for atopic dermatitis, the disorder can be controlled by therapy until a spontaneous remission occurs.

Relief of itching is the cornerstone of therapy for atopic dermatitis. Careful attention to the common circumstances aggravating itching will be most helpful to the patient.[68] Dry skin with consequent breaks in the epidermal barrier will result in itching. Dry skin is corrected by hydration. Methods of hydration include humidifying the environment with room humidifiers, soaking the skin in tepid water and applying a lubricant to the hydrated skin, and using wet dressings (see pages 118–119). Excessive soaping of the skin results in further drying and may induce an irritant contact dermatitis, so that elimination of soaps as much as possible is helpful. Avoidance of wool garments and tight occlusive clothing is also advisable. Similarly, excessive sweating and drastic changes in temperature should be avoided. Itching in most cases can be controlled by the use of topical steroids. Generally, potent topical steroids are not necessary, for the absorption of low potency topical steroids through inflamed skin is quite adequate. One per cent hydrocortisone cream or ointment applied four to five times a day is often sufficient for the first week of therapy. When the skin is extremely dry, the 1 per cent hydrocortisone is best supplied in an ointment base; in intertriginous or moist areas, a cream base is preferable. After the itching has been relieved, topical steroids may be discontinued and lubricants substituted. Patients vary considerably in their tolerance to creams and ointments, and the choice of a suitable vehicle must be adjusted to the individual patient's preference. Lubrication after proper hydration of the skin is essential to optimal therapy.

Generalized or acute weeping dermatitis is best treated by the use of wet dressings (see pages 118–119). The application of topical steroid creams, 1 per cent hydrocortisone, or 0.01 per cent fluocinolone under wet dressings every four to five hours for 48 hours will bring about dramatic improvement in even the most severe dermatitis. This form of therapy may be successfully accomplished at home with careful instruction or during a two to three day hospitalization. In cases with multiple excoriations and crusting, secondary bacterial infection is often present. Appropriate cultures and treatment with systemically administered antibiotics are necessary. Treatment of such patients without resorting to antibiotics may be difficult. Hospitalization as a therapeutic "environmentectomy" may result in improvement even without topical or systemic therapy.[9] The hospital is also an excellent setting for patient education.

Tar preparations have traditionally been successful in treating atopic dermatitis. They are cosmetically inferior to topical steroids because of their odor and staining properties. However, in recalcitrant cases they are quite useful.[69]

Antihistamines are widely used in the treatment of atopic dermatitis.[70] We believe with other authors[68] that significant sedation must be achieved before relief of pruritus occurs. The placebo effect[70] is quite significant in antihistamine therapy, and individual patients vary considerably in their response to antihistamines. Hydroxyzine hydrochloride has been demonstrated to be more effective than other oral antihistamines in suppressing histamine wheals[71] and often is our preferred agent.

Emotional stress undoubtedly leads to increased scratching, either from greater awareness of itching or from habit. Atopic dermatitis often worsens during stress. It is important for the patient to recognize that scratching the skin is a means of expressing anxiety. Removing the patient from a stressful environment can be therapeutic when it is feasible.[9] The relief of anxiety states is obviously quite difficult. Controlled studies on the value of psychotherapy and the use of tranquilizers are lacking. The emotional support of the physician and the family is an important tool for the patient in controlling atopic dermatitis.

CONTACT DERMATITIS

An inflammatory response in the skin induced by substances that contact the skin surface is called contact dermatitis. Most forms of contact dermatitis are eczematous, in the sense that epidermal involvement with vesiculation, oozing, and fissuring is present. Certain unusual forms of contact dermatitis, however, may be characterized predominantly by atypical patterns of inflammation in the dermis or around hair follicles. General features that are helpful in the diagnosis of contact dermatitis are presented in Table 5–7. Especially helpful clues include the configuration of the lesions, their surface character-

TABLE 5-7 CHARACTERISTICS OF A CONTACT DERMATITIS

Sites involved	Skin exposed to contactant
Confluency	Tendency for dermatitis to be confluent
Borders	Lesions have relatively sharp borders and a tendency to form straight lines or sharp angles.
Usual morphology	Eczematous (vesiculation or oozing, fissuring or scaling)
Involvement of skin creases	Minimal if contactant is a solid object; accentuated if contactant is a fluid substance
Susceptible sites	Exposed skin, tops of hands and feet, eyelids, occluded sites (groin)
Resistant sites	Palms and soles

istics, and the distribution. In most instances, contact dermatitis involves a localized area, with borders formed by straight lines and sharp angles. Involvement of certain predisposed sites, such as the dorsum of the hand or the eyelids, also suggests a contact dermatitis. These characteristics are helpful in distinguishing contact dermatitis from a dermatitis generated by a systemic process, such as a drug eruption. In contrast to contact dermatitis, a systemically generated dermatitis is characterized by symmetrical, multiple, discrete round or oval lesions.

Two types of contact dermatitis may be distinguished (Table 5-8): irritant contact dermatitis, with non-specific damage to the skin caused by the contactant; and allergic contact dermatitis, caused by specific hypersensitivity to the contactant. The general characteristics of both types of contact dermatitis are summarized in Table 5-7. The following discussion will compare the two varieties of contact dermatitis and emphasize their occurrence in adolescence.

TABLE 5-8 CHARACTERISTICS OF IRRITANT AND ALLERGIC CONTACT DERMATITIS

	Irritant	Allergic
Occurrence	In all individuals if exposure is long enough and contactant is in high enough concentration	In individuals specifically sensitive to the contactant
Prior exposure	Not required for development of dermatitis	Necessary for sensitization
Mechanism	Structural damage to the skin due to destructive properties of contactant	Delayed hypersensitivity to contactant (hapten) plus carrier molecule
Hereditary predisposition	Atopic	None
Examples	Hand dermatitis due to detergents	Poison ivy dermatitis, nickel dermatitis

IRRITANT CONTACT DERMATITIS

Irritant contact dermatitis is an inflammatory response induced by a substance that disturbs the normal structure of the skin. No specific or allergic hypersensitivity to the substance is involved. Dermatitis caused by irritant substances is frequently accentuated by disturbances of water content in the skin.

Pathogenesis

An irritant contact dermatitis will occur in all normal individuals if the contactant is of sufficient strength and if it acts upon the skin for a sufficiently long period of time. The amount of exposure required depends primarily upon the innate destructive properties of the contactant and its concentration. Exposure to a potent irritant, such as a strong alkali, may induce intense inflammation within hours, while exposure to a mild irritant, such as a detergent, may require weeks to induce a dermatitis

Although irritant contact dermatitis is not the result of specific hypersensitivity, certain individuals may be constitutionally more susceptible than others to the effects of irritants. The atopic individual is particularly susceptible to irritant contact dermatitis. Such patients have a lower threshold to itching and develop dermatitis more readily when exposed to detergents or wool.[9]

The individual's constitutional predisposition and the nature of the contactant are the primary factors in inducing irritant contact dermatitis. However, once the epidermis is damaged and the normal barrier function of the skin is lost, many factors may become involved in producing the subsequent inflammation. Damaged skin has increased susceptibility to many additional irritants, including minor irritants that have little effect upon intact skin. There frequently occurs, therefore, a "snowball" effect. Rubbing, scratching, and bacterial overgrowth are factors that may further contribute to and exacerbate the inflammation.

The mechanism by which an irritant substance damages the skin depends upon its specific characteristics. Some agents, such as strong acids or alkalis, cause epidermal necrosis. Others, such as detergents or hot water, alter the chemical structure and hydration of the stratum corneum only after repeated exposure. Certain agents, such as oils, may penetrate pilosebaceous units and produce a primarily perifollicular dermatitis.

Clinical Characteristics

The severity of irritant contact dermatitis may vary with the nature of the contactant, its concentration, the duration of the dermatitis, and its location on the body. Such a dermatitis may occasionally appear as an acute eczematous process, with erythema, vesiculation, and oozing. More often, it resembles a chronic dermatitis, with scaling and fissuring. In unusual cases, perifollicular papules may be seen.

TABLE 5–9 EXAMPLES OF IRRITANT CONTACT DERMATITIS IN ADOLESCENCE

Contactant	Distribution	Specific Features of Dermatitis
Alkalis (detergents)	Exposed surfaces (dorsum of hand)	Common in atopic individuals. Accentuated with occlusion (under jewelry) Erythema and fissuring
Acids (vitamin A acid)	Sites where acid applied (face)	Erythema and scaling
Wool	Skin in contact with wool clothing (neck)	Common in atopic individuals, owing to mechanical irritation by coarse wool fibers Erythematous papules and itching
Fiberglass	Exposed skin (arms) Areas of skin exposed to clothing that has been impregnated with fiberglass during laundering	Itchy papules
Oils and tars	Exposed surfaces (hairy areas)	Accentuated around hair follicles

Specific Causes

Some typical examples of irritant contact dermatitis seen in adolescence are outlined in Table 5–9. In addition to the causes cited, other factors may predispose the skin to the effect of irritants. These include defects in hydration of the stratum corneum, which may disrupt the epidermal barrier.

Dry Skin. Contact with a dry environment under certain circumstances may lead to structural alterations in the skin and eventually to a dermatitis that resembles an irritant contact dermatitis. In order to maintain its barrier function, the stratum corneum requires a minimum water content of approximately 10 per cent.[72] Under conditions of extremely low atmospheric humidity (less than 60 per cent), this protection may be lost, resulting in a more permeable, superficially fissured cutaneous surface. Such changes are especially likely to occur during the winter, when people spend more time in dry indoor environments. Frequent hot baths or showers with soap may further impair the water-holding capacity of the stratum corneum. Once the stratum corneum has lost its intact protective function, the underlying portions of the skin are exposed to a variety of environmental irritants. The dermatitis that results, often called asteatotic eczema, or "winter itch," is characterized by erythema, scaling, and superficial fissures, located primarily on the extensor surfaces. Although dry skin is the predisposing factor, the actual development of such a dermatitis involves other irritant factors. This chain of events commonly occurs in elderly people and in atopic individuals, who seem to have an exaggerated response to a dry environment.

Excessive Moisture. The stratum corneum is hygroscopic and can hold large quantities of water, but prolonged excessive exposure to water produces maceration, with wrinkling and fissuring, loss of barrier function, and overgrowth of bacteria. Chronically overhydrated skin ceases to have an effective epidermal barrier and becomes more susceptible to environmental irritants, which further damage the skin and add to the inflammation. Maceration is most strikingly seen in the clinical picture of "immersion foot," which occurs following prolonged immersion of the feet in warm water. Maceration may also develop in skin occluded under plastic dressings or in moist intertriginous areas, such as the toe webs.

Diagnosis and Differential Diagnosis

The diagnosis of irritant contact dermatitis involves identification of the general characteristics of contact dermatitis (Table 5–7) and exclusion of allergic causes. Irritant contact dermatitis is a clinical diagnosis, based on data acquired from the patient's history and physical examination; there usually is no specific method to confirm the diagnosis. In acute irritant contact dermatitis caused by a potent irritant, the diagnosis is often readily apparent because the onset of symptoms occurs within hours of a single exposure. However, the appearance of the usual irritant contact dermatitis following repeated exposures to a weak irritant over a long period of time ("wear and tear" dermatitis) may suggest a list of diagnostic possibilities. Once contact dermatitis is suspected, a careful history of all agents that may have contacted the involved skin should be elicited. Particular attention should be focused upon occupational and household exposures, hobbies, and over-the-counter remedies or other substances being applied by the patient in an attempt to treat the dermatitis. Consideration should be given the possibility that alteration in water content may be damaging the skin. Dry skin (xerosis) should be suspected as a predisposing factor during winter, particularly if the patient who takes frequent showers with soap has skin lesions distributed over extensor surfaces and extremities and has other evidence of dry skin, such as keratosis pilaris. In contrast, overhydration is suggested by a history of prolonged exposure of the involved skin to moisture, white, wrinkled appearance of the skin surface, and confinement of the dermatitis to the feet and intertriginous areas.

The differential diagnosis of irritant contact dermatitis includes allergic contact dermatitis, atopic dermatitis, seborrheic dermatitis, photodermatitis, pityriasis rosea, tinea, and candidiasis. Atopic dermatitis is particularly difficult to exclude, since it is frequently exacerbated by irritants. If an atopic predisposition is present in a patient with an irritant dermatitis, atopic dermatitis is probably the more significant diagnosis.

In the special case of fiberglass dermatitis, a form of irritant dermatitis caused by fiberglass spicules, the differential diagnosis may also include insect bites, scabies, and dermatitis herpetiformis. Microscopic examination of skin scrapings may confirm the diagnosis of fiberglass dermatitis, by revealing fiberglass spicules.

Seborrheic dermatitis is defined primarily by its characteristic distribution and is easily diagnosed in most cases. An eczematous photodermatitis, such as polymorphic light eruption, is suggested by the distribution of lesions on light-exposed areas and a history of exacerbations after light exposure. Pityriasis rosea is easily distinguished in most cases by the characteristic herald patch and oval papulosquamous lesions distributed symmetrically along skin lines of cleavage. Tinea is characterized by sharp, active, scaly borders and may be diagnosed by examination with KOH. Candidiasis usually consists of confluent areas of erythema with satellite lesions and may also be diagnosed by examination of skin scrapings with KOH. A distinction between nummular eczema and irritant dermatitis is often not possible, since with dry skin, irritant dermatitis may contain areas of nummular eczematous dermatitis.

The most difficult distinction to be made is that between irritant contact dermatitis and allergic contact dermatitis. Most forms of irritant contact dermatitis have the appearance of a chronic dermatitis, with erythema, scaling, and fissuring, whereas allergic contact dermatitis frequently begins as an acute vesicular dermatitis. If a suspect cause of a contact dermatitis can be identified by history, the probable underlying mechanism can usually be identified. For instance, most detergents cause irritant contact dermatitis, while "caine" drugs (derived topical anesthetics) usually cause allergic contact dermatitis. Patch testing may also help identify the underlying mechanism (see pages 113–114).

Complications

As in other eczematous eruptions, loss of the barrier function of the epidermis facilitates overgrowth of bacteria, particularly *Staphylococcus aureus* and *Streptococcus pyogenes*. The point at which overgrowth represents infection rather than colonization is often unclear, since eczema and infection can cause similar morphological changes and significant bacterial overgrowth may occur before gross purulence is noted. Signs of secondary infection include intense erythema, pain, edema, pustules, and crusting. If large numbers of *Streptococcus pyogenes* are found on culture, a significant infection is probably present.

The loss of barrier function in irritant contact dermatitis also predisposes to development of a superimposed allergic contact dermatitis, particularly to sensitizing medications, such as neomycin or topical anesthetics, applied as treatment for dermatitis. If an irritant contact dermatitis flares acutely, a superimposed allergic contact dermatitis to medication should be suspected.

Treatment

For proper management of an irritant contact dermatitis, identification and removal of possible irritants are essential. Often, a less irritating substance (such as a milder soap) or mechanical protection from the irritant (such as special clothing or gloves) will be beneficial. Proper hydration of the skin is essential for irritant dermatitis characterized by dry, scaly, fissured skin. Humidification of the home, infrequent tepid showers, and avoidance of drying soaps and detergents will help to restore hydration. Most beneficial, however, is daily immersion of the involved skin in tepid water (without added soap) for 15 to 20 minutes followed by gentle removal of the excess moisture and application of a bland lubricating ointment or lotion. Many individuals prefer to add a lubricant to the bath water in the form of a bath oil. Creams containing urea may also be useful for lubrication, although some individuals find they cause further irritation to the skin.

The mainstay of therapy for irritant contact dermatitis remains topical corticosteroids, although some patients respond to elimination of the irritant followed by hydration of the skin. An acute irritant dermatitis will respond best to corticosteroid creams covered with wet dressings applied three or four times a day (see pages 118–119). More chronic irritant dermatitis may be treated by the application of a corticosteroid ointment following hydration or by the application of a corticosteroid cream under an occlusive covering, such as Saran wrap.

Systemic corticosteroids should not be used as therapy for most irritant dermatitis. Oral antipruritic agents, such as hydroxyzine, may be useful, particularly if taken at bedtime, when their sedative effects may cause less difficulty. The routine administration of antibiotics is unnecessary, but if secondary infection appears likely, erythromycin in divided doses (1.0 gm per day) is usually adequate therapy. In the instance of secondary infection with penicillin-resistant *Staphylococcus aureus,* therapy with an oral penicillinase-resistant synthetic penicillin, such as dicloxacillin, is necessary.

ALLERGIC CONTACT DERMATITIS

Allergic contact dermatitis is a specific type of delayed hypersensitivity reaction of the skin to a contactant, which is usually expressed as an acute eczematous dermatitis. Although it is relatively infrequent in infancy or childhood, allergic contact dermatitis is common in adolescence. This discrepancy is probably explained by the years of exposure to environmental chemicals accumulated by the second decade rather than by the maturation of the immune system.

PATHOGENESIS

Our current concept of the evolution of allergic contact dermatitis involves two phases: the induction or sensitization phase, in which specific sensitivity to a chemical antigen is acquired; and an elicitation phase, in which the sensitivity is expressed as a dermatitis.

Sensitization Phase. The development of contact allergy begins with cutaneous exposure to the allergen (antigen), although not all exposures to a potential sensitizer will induce contact sensitivity. For sensitization to take place, the offending substance must be able to penetrate the protective stratum corneum, the substance must be chemically reactive, and it must combine with normal body components, such as free proteins or biological membranes (Table 5–10).

Most potent contact sensitizing substances possess significant in vivo chemical reactivity. The chemical itself does not act as the complete antigen, but must first combine with a "carrier" molecule in the skin, thereby serving as a hapten. The conjugation of the hapten with a carrier molecule produces a large (complete) antigen which is recognized by the body as foreign. The exact nature of carrier molecules is unknown. However, both the hapten and the carrier molecule determine the antigenic sites, so that the resulting delayed hyper-

TABLE 5–10 CHARACTERISTICS OF SENSITIZING CHEMICALS

Penetration of the Stratum Corneum
High concentration per surface area
Low molecular weight
Lipid solubility
Prolonged contact with skin
Contact with damaged skin (eczematous, burned) or occluded skin
Chemical Reactivity

sensitivity response is specific for the carrier molecule. The delayed hypersensitivity reaction is not expressed to the hapten alone or to the combination of hapten and different carrier molecule. Allergic contact dermatitis is also not completely specific for the hapten, since an individual sensitized by the application of one contactant to the skin may have a subsequent reaction to a chemically similar contactant. Such cross reactivity of contactants is of considerable clinical significance in dealing with allergic contact dermatitis.

Recognition of the complete antigen (hapten plus carrier molecule) as foreign is the task of uncommitted small lymphocytes. The competence of such lymphocytes in reacting to an antigen is determined by their previous exposure to a functioning thymus. In most cases, the sensitization process occurs in the regional lymph nodes where macrophages present the antigen to immunocompetent T-lymphocytes. The antigen reaches the regional lymph nodes within a few hours after exposure. Much of the sensitization process occurs distant from the site where the contactant and the skin react. Even if the skin where the sensitizer was applied is excised 12 to 24 hours after application, sensitization can develop.[73] After the application of a potent sensitizer, large pyroninophilic "transformed" lymphocytes proliferate in the thymus-dependent paracortical areas of regional lymph nodes, reaching a maximum number about four days after application of the contactant.[74] If the regional lymph nodes are removed within five days after application, sensitization will not occur.[73] After four or five days, the proliferating lymphocytes in regional lymph nodes give rise to "educated" small lymphocytes that can recognize the foreign antigen. Onset of contact sensitivity occurs as these lymphocytes enter the circulation. This has been demonstrated by applying the strong sensitizer, dinitrochlorobenzene (DNCB), to human skin, after which there is evidence of circulating reactive lymphocytes by the seventh day. These lymphocytes reach a maximum number at two to three weeks, approximating the developmental period of specific cutaneous reactivity to the antigen.[75]

Elicitation Phase. The elicitation phase involves the development of an allergic contact dermatitis by interaction of specifically reactive lymphocytes with the sensitizing antigen. Elicitation of dermatitis may occur at the site of initial sensitization after 10 to 14 days if the antigen still remains there, or it may occur at any new site within 12 to 24 hours after application of the contactant to the new site. The delayed response of a reaction after cutaneous application of a chemical to which an individual has been sensitized is typical of delayed hypersensitivity. The actual timing and intensity of the skin reaction are influenced by the concentration of the applied chemical, its penetration into the skin, and competence of the individual's immune system.

When the contactant chemical combines with its carrier molecule, the complete antigen is detected by previously sensitized circulating small T-lymphocytes, which then react by releasing lymphokines into the tissue. These soluble mediators initiate an inflammatory response by attracting other inflammatory cells with chemotactic factors, by preventing the movement of cells out of the area through migration-inhibition factor, and by activating the inflammatory cells with macrophage-aggregating factor. Many lymphokines probably represent a single factor with multiple actions. Through lymphokines, a small number of sensitized lymphocytes can amplify a response and generate inflammation. Thus, only a small number of inflammatory cells in the final delayed hypersensitivity response are sensitized lymphocytes;[76] most of the cells bear no specificity for the antigen that initiated the process. The sites of reaction in allergic contact dermatitis are in the upper dermis and the epidermis where presumably the sensitized lymphocytes meet the antigen. Neutrophils may be present early in the reaction, but later, lymphocytes and macrophages predominate in most inflammatory processes.

The exact manner in which the foreign antigen (hapten plus carrier molecule) is recognized by the T-lymphocyte is unknown. The specificity for recognizing the antigen, however, resides in the lymphocytes since contact sensitivity can be transferred from one animal to another by cells but not by serum.[77] Presumably, the receptor is associated with the cell membrane of the T-lymphocyte. However, we still do not know the exact nature of the complete antigen nor how the antigen is recognized.

Clinical Characteristics

The general characteristics of a contact dermatitis (Table 5–7) are equally applicable to an allergic contact dermatitis. Most forms of allergic contact dermatitis are eczematous and begin with an acute dermatitis characterized by vesicles, weeping, and intense itching. If the dermatitis is prolonged for weeks or months, it may become subacute or chronic, with fissuring, scaling, and thickening of the skin. The specific characteristics of allergic contact dermatitis depend not only on its duration but also on the nature of the responsible contactant and the area of the body affected. In unusual cases, an allergic contact dermatitis may have only erythema and edema with minimal epidermal involvement, so that it cannot be qualified as eczematous. Such dermal contact dermatitis is likely to be caused by a few specific contactants, such as neomycin and nickel.

It is characteristic of allergic contact dermatitis that it does not clear immediately, even though there is no further exposure to the contactant. An acute allergic contact dermatitis due to a single exposure to a contactant may require up to two or three weeks for resolution. Certain forms of allergic contact dermatitis are characteristically chronic. One chronic allergic contact dermatitis is caused by dichromates found in cement. The eruption may undergo extremely slow resolution after exposure to the contactant has been stopped.

Specific Causes

To list all possible causes of allergic contact dermatitis would be impossible, for almost any chemical is a potential candidate. Fortunately, a relatively small number of contactants account for most episodes of allergic contact dermatitis, because of their innate sensitizing properties and their presence in the environment. Fifteen substances that commonly cause allergic contact dermatitis are listed in Table 5–11 in estimated decreasing order of frequency.[78] Figures documenting the exact frequency of allergic contact dermatitis due to specific agents are unavailable. Rhus antigen or poison ivy antigen (3-pentadecylcatechol) is assumed to be the commonest cause; the frequency of allergic contact dermatitis from other contactants is extrapolated from studies of the prevalence of positive patch tests. The sensitizing potential of topical medications is apparent; seven of the 15 most common sensitizers (Table 5–11) may be found in these preparations. The two greatest causes of allergic contact dermatitis, 3-pentadecylcatechol and nickel, will be discussed in some detail.

TABLE 5–11 MOST COMMON CAUSES OF ALLERGIC CONTACT DERMATITIS

Contactant	Common Source
3-Pentadecylcatechol (Rhus antigen)	Poison ivy, poison oak, poison sumac, mango rind, cashew nut shells
Nickel	Jewelry (earrings, rings, necklaces, watches), metal eye glass frames, belt buckles, zippers, snaps
Caine drugs	Topical medications, lozenges, suppositories
Dichromate	Cement, tanned leather, match heads
Fragrances and flavorings (balsam of Peru — a screening mixture)	Topical medications, perfumes, cosmetics, toothpastes
Thimerosal (Merthiolate)	Germicides, topical medications
Paraphenylenediamine	Hair dyes, fur dyes, rubber
Ethylenediamine	Stabilizer in topical medications, dyes, rubber
Neomycin	Topical medications
Ammoniated mercury	Topical medications
Thiuram	Rubber
Parabens	Preservatives in topical medications and cosmetics
Formaldehyde	Shampoos, nail polish, permanent press clothing
Mercaptobenzothiazole	Rubber
Epoxy resin	Glue

Allergic contact dermatitis to 3-pentadecylcatechol (Rhus antigen) occurs most often in the spring and summer but can be acquired at any time of year. The most common sources of Rhus antigen in the United States are poison ivy and poison oak vines. The antigen is present in the resin of the plant and characteristically produces linear groups of vesicles on cutaneous surfaces exposed to vine or leaves. The resin may also be deposited on clothing, tools, or animal fur, or even in smoke from burning plants.

Nickel is ubiquitous in our environment, but the high incidence of nickel sensitivity in women suggests that sensitization may be acquired from jewelry, especially from earrings inserted into pierced ears. The occurrence of a dermatitis in any localized area where metal in jewelry or clothing fasteners contacts the skin strongly suggests sensitivity to nickel. Dermatitis due to nickel sensitivity is more likely to occur where the skin is moistened with sweat, presumably because under such conditions the nickel is dissolved and penetrates the skin more easily.[79]

Certain areas of the body, such as the scalp and palms, are unusual sites for allergic contact dermatitis, whereas other sites, including the eyelids and scrotum, are especially vulnerable. Areas of skin where allergic contact dermatitis frequently occurs are listed in Table 5–12, along with possible causes of the dermatitis.

Diagnosis and Differential Diagnosis

Once the diagnosis of a contact dermatitis is suspected on the basis of history and physical examination, a careful inquiry must be made into all substances that may have contacted the involved areas. Because of the high incidence of allergic contact dermatitis to ingredients found in medications, a detailed list should be made of those substances the patient has been applying to his skin. The development of an acute dermatitis, characterized by vesiculation and oozing, is more indicative of an allergic contact dermatitis than of a typical irritant contact dermatitis. Knowledge of the characteristics of the suspected contactant that may have caused the dermatitis may help in determining the pathogenesis. Some contactants generally cause irritant contact dermatitis, while others cause allergic contact dermatitis. When a distinction cannot be made between allergic and irritant contact dermatitis, patch testing may be helpful (see pages 113–114).

Besides irritant contact dermatitis, the differential diagnosis of allergic contact dermatitis includes atopic dermatitis, seborrheic dermatitis, dermatophyte infections, and candidiasis. Atopic dermatitis can usually be distinguished by the presence of atopy in personal and family histories, the chronicity of the eruption and the distribution of the lesions. Seborrheic dermatitis may be identified by its chronicity, distribution, and characteristic scaling. Dermatophyte infections (tinea) are identified by examination with KOH of the characteristic sharp scaly borders. In any case of an acute vesicular dermatitis on the feet of an adolescent, an examination with KOH should be performed. In intertriginous areas, either candidiasis or an allergic contact dermatitis may cause an acute weeping dermatitis. The presence of satellite lesions and the identification of *Candida* in skin scrapings by examination with KOH or use of the Gram stain allow differentiation between the two processes.

TABLE 5-12 COMMON AREAS OF INVOLVEMENT AND CAUSES OF ALLERGIC CONTACT DERMATITIS

Area	Causes
Earlobes	Earrings (nickel)
Postauricular area	Hair dye (paraphenylenediamine) Shampoos (formalin) Hearing aids or glasses (nickel or plastic)
Ear canal	Medications
Face	Hair dye (paraphenylenediamine) Poison ivy Cosmetics Sprays or any airborne contactant
Eyelids	Sprays or any airborne contactant Cosmetics Eyelash curlers (rubber accelerators or nickel) Any contactant on the hands (topical medications, formalin in nail polish)
Perioral area	Lipstick Toothpaste
Neck	Jewelry (nickel) Perfumes Sprays or other airborne contactants
Axilla	Deodorants Clothing (formalin)
Chest	Brassieres (rubber accelerators) Metal objects carried in pockets (nickel)
Back	Metal fasteners (nickel)
Waist	Belt buckles or snaps (nickel) Waist bands or girdles (rubber accelerators)
Extremities	Poison ivy Airborne contactants
Wrists	Jewelry (nickel)
Hands	Rings (nickel) Gloves (rubber accelerators)
Feet	Components of shoes (rubber accelerators, dichromates in leather)
Scrotum	Any contactant on the hands or agent applied in the groin (topical medications)

Patch Testing

Patch testing is a standardized procedure for identification of contact sensitivity which entails the application of suspect agents to small areas of the skin. A positive reaction represents an experimentally induced miniature version of the disease, allergic contact dermatitis confined to a small area. This test procedure may be used to identify contact sensitivity to common sensitizing environmental antigens contained in a screening tray or to test suspect contactants from the patient's environment which may not be on the screening tray. Screening trays contain agents that have proved to be most frequent offenders in allergic contact dermatitis. Most of the agents listed in Table 5–11 are included. The concentrations of the agents contained in the tray are such that the likelihood of a positive response, representing allergy, is maximized, and the likelihood of an irritant reaction is minimized. When suspect contactants from the environment are used for patch testing, there is a greater probability of both false positive and false negative reactions. Certain potent sensitizers, such as 3-pentadecylcatechol and dinitrochlorobenzene, are not routinely used for patch testing, since there is a significant risk of sensitizing a previously non-reactive individual.

The preferred site for most patch testing is the upper back. The agents to be tested are applied to specially prepared aluminum-backed patch test strips which are then placed on the upper back and secured with non-irritating tape. The patch tests are left in place for 48 hours. The results are best read several hours after the patch tests have been removed. The reactions are recorded in the following manner: negative; 1+, a slightly erythematous reaction; 2+, a markedly erythematous, edematous, or vesicular reaction; and 3+, an intense bullous or ulcerative reaction. Significant positive reactions may also be characterized by intense itching, spread beyond the borders of the patches, persistence for several days after removal of the patches, and flare of the patient's original contact dermatitis at a site remote from the patch. Very weak reactions (1+) often are of no clinical significance. Some positive patch tests elicited from a screening tray may be incidental and bear no relationship to the patient's dermatitis. Other patch test reactions may not represent true contact sensitivity but denote non-specific irritant reactions. An irritant reaction is usually weak (1+), does not spread beyond the borders of the patch, and persists for only a short period after removal of the patch. Certain metals may cause a pustular patch test, which also has no clinical significance. Such a reaction is common in atopic individuals who are patch tested with nickel.[80]

Patch testing is best performed by physicians experienced in the procedure. The interpretation of positive patch tests requires knowledge of cross reactions between various contactants. Some of the agents on a patch test tray are particularly useful as screening agents for groups of chemicals that cross react. For instance, balsam of Peru is a useful screening mixture for contact sensitivity to a number of flavorings and fragrances. Further details of patch testing and interpretation of reactions and cross reactions may be found in Fisher's text.[79]

COMPLICATIONS

Allergic contact dermatitis is subject to the same complications as irritant contact dermatitis. The point at which overgrowth of bacteria in an area of allergic contact dermatitis represents secondary infection is imprecise, but such infection is suggested by the presence of fever, tenderness in the involved area, purulent exudation, and large numbers of *Streptococcus pyogenes* found on culture. Loss of an intact stratum corneum may lead to further damage by a variety of irritants. In addition, multiple contact sensitivities may develop as a result of other substances that contact the eczematous skin, particularly medications.

A complication occasionally seen in allergic contact dermatitis is autoeczematization, with the development of a more generalized dermatitis far removed from the original site of sensitization. The mechanisms underlying this phenomenon are not yet understood. Patients who develop this complication first have a localized area of allergic contact dermatitis which persists for some time and then suddenly develop a generalized eruption characterized by vesicles and papules distributed symmetrically over the body. This acute generalized dermatitis may require several weeks to resolve.

Allergic contact dermatitis involving large portions of the cutaneous surface may evolve into a generalized scaly erythema known as exfoliative erythroderma. Although allergic contact dermatitis is only one cause of erythroderma, it should rank high as a possible cause in an adolescent.[39]

A complication of contact sensitivity now being widely recognized is the development of a dermatitis following ingestion of a substance to which the patient is contact-sensitive. This dermatitis is usually eczematous and more generalized than the usual allergic contact dermatitis, with accentuation in the original sites of contact dermatitis. For example, nickel-sensitive patients were found to develop exacerbations of hand eczema when they were administered nickel orally.[81] Such "internal contact dermatitis" may help to explain some eczematous eruptions not previously understood.

TREATMENT

All treatment of an allergic contact dermatitis must include eliminating exposure to the agent to which the patient is sensitive. In certain cases, such as poison ivy dermatitis, the allergen is usually contacted outside the patient's ordinary environment, so that no attempt at environmental manipulation is necessary. Allergic contact dermatitis caused by a substance common in the patient's environment (such as nickel) requires identification of the sources of the chemical and prevention of exposure to them. Occasionally, major changes in activities or life styles are required to achieve relief and prevent recurrence of the dermatitis. Therapy for the allergic contact dermatitis itself depends upon its severity. If the patient is relatively comfortable, symptomatic therapy for the purpose of controlling itching may be sufficient. Oral antipruritic medications, such as hydroxyzine taken at bedtime, and topical measures that are soothing and drying, including moist compresses, tepid baths, and calamine lotion, may be adequate. If there is no further exposure to the contactant, the dermatitis will resolve.

For an allergic contact dermatitis of greater severity, topical corticosteroid preparations are extremely helpful, particularly when applied under wet compresses or wet dressings (see pages 118–119). For an acute weeping dermatitis, a topical corticosteroid agent in a cream base is preferred. Once the condition has assumed the characteristics of a chronic dermatitis, with fissuring and scaling, a similar agent in an ointment base becomes more appropriate, especially if the ointment is applied to hydrated skin.

For a patient who is made extremely uncomfortable by autoeczematization or an extensive or rapidly spreading dermatitis, a short course of systemic corticosteroids given in decreasing daily doses is effective therapy. Orally administered prednisone, 40 to 60 mg per day, will decrease the intensity of the dermatitis and alleviate the itching in three or four days. The doses of prednisone should then slowly be decreased during the subsequent two to three weeks. An acute allergic contact dermatitis initially controlled with prednisone may still flare after the medication is discontinued. We prefer the oral administration of prednisone to intramuscular injections of corticosteroid preparations because it permits more effective day-to-day control of the dosage.

Routine administration of antibiotics is unnecessary in allergic contact dermatitis. If secondary infection develops, therapy with erythromycin or a penicillinase-resistant synthetic penicillin may be necessary. Topical antibiotics, such as neomycin, should not be used because of their sensitizing potential.

OTHER ECZEMATOUS PROCESSES

Certain common patterns of eczema are given names that are morphologically descriptive but do not imply knowledge of the pathogenesis of the eruption. These five common patterns—nummular eczema, dyshidrotic eczema, seborrheic dermatitis, lichen simplex chronicus, and hand and foot eczema—will be discussed briefly.

NUMMULAR ECZEMA

Nummular eczema (nummular dermatitis, discoid eczema) is a reaction pattern of the skin characterized by round to oval (coin-shaped) areas of eczema. The lesions are intensely itchy and are typically found on the extremities, especially the dorsal surface of the hands. In most cases, this pattern of eczematous dermatitis has a chronic course, marked by remissions and exacerbations.

The etiology of nummular eczema is unknown. In many cases it appears to be related to dry skin and contact with irritants, with a peak incidence in the winter. It is usually confined to the extensor surfaces of the extremities.[82] The association of nummular eczema with the atopic state is a matter of controversy. Certainly, not all individuals who develop this pattern of dermatitis are atopic, but some patients with nummular eczema may have an atopic diathesis, marked by a positive atopic history and elevated IgE levels.[46] The lesions of nummular eczema are often markedly exudative and crusted and contain staphylococci. However, the part played by bacterial infection in the genesis of the lesions is unknown. Since most cases of nummular eczema resemble a fungus infection, an examination with KOH should be performed to exclude tinea corporis. Differentiation of a nummular eruption from other skin conditions including the herald patch of pityriasis rosea, discoid lupus erythematosus, and psoriasis may be difficult.

Treatment of nummular eczema is similar to treatment of irritant contact dermatitis or atopic dermatitis. Hydration of the skin and application of topical steroids are the most useful modalities. Use of tar preparations in a cream or bath oil may increase the efficacy of topical therapy. Oral antibiotics (erythromycin) may also enhance the therapy, particularly for patients with exudative, crusted lesions.

DYSHIDROTIC ECZEMA

Dyshidrotic eczema (pompholyx) is a pattern of vesicular dermatitis of the palms and soles. This pattern is distinctive because of its location, as any acute dermatitis in the hyperkeratotic palms and soles will tend to produce large clear vesicles. The lesions are usually recurrent, with acute episodes that require several weeks for resolution.

Although the name suggests a disorder of sweating, this etiology is not uniformly accepted.[83] Dyshidrotic eczema is probably best regarded as a pattern of eczema on acral skin that may bear a relationship to sweating but may also have multiple other causes. Dyshidrotic eczema may be found in atopic individuals, presumably as a manifestation of atopic dermatitis.[46] In other cases, it may represent an acute allergic contact dermatitis. Dyshidrotic eczema may also be precipitated in individuals contact-sensitive to nickel by the oral administration of nickel.[81]

The term "dyshidrotic eczema" may be misleading because this diagnosis often deters the physician from further investigation into the etiology of the dermatitis. A careful history for atopy and possible contactants should be recorded. Patch testing should be performed in patients with chronic or recurrent dermatitis. In all instances of vesicles on the feet, a blister top should be removed, treated with KOH, and examined microscopically for hyphae.

Dyshidrotic eczema may be treated in the same way as other forms of hand or foot eczema. Topical corticosteroid creams under wet dressings (cotton gloves) may be helpful during the acute vesicular stage. Topical corticosteroid creams or ointments under occlusion with vinyl gloves may be appropriate when fissuring and scaling ensue.

SEBORRHEIC DERMATITIS

Dermatitis limited to areas of excessive sebaceous activity has been termed "seborrheic dermatitis."[84] Erythema is characteristic of this problem, with greasy scales occurring on the scalp, eyebrows, forehead, nasal folds, and mid-chest. The pathogenesis of seborrheic dermatitis is not understood.[85] Although it may become most manifest in adolescence, at the time of increased sebaceous activity, overproduction of sebum (seborrhea) may occur in the absence of dermatitis.[86] Seborrheic dermatitis is sometimes distinguished only with great difficulty from atopic dermatitis, irritant contact dermatitis, and psoriasis. In most cases, seborrheic dermatitis responds to the topical measures (topical corticosteroids, tar preparations) that are useful in atopic dermatitis.

LICHEN SIMPLEX CHRONICUS

Lichen simplex chronicus (localized neurodermatitis) is an intensely pruritic, chronic dermatitis. The precipitating cause is unknown in most cases, but trauma from constant rubbing is believed to perpetuate the process. Atopic individuals may be predisposed to this pattern of dermatitis.[87] Clinically, lichen simplex is characterized by a plaque of scaly skin with a marked pattern of lichenification. Areas frequently affected include the lower portions of the legs, posterior neck, scalp, forearms, perianal skin, scrotum, and vulva. Treatment includes administration of oral antipruritic agents such as hydroxyzine, especially at bedtime, hydration of the skin, and application of a corticosteroid ointment. In some patients, the use of topical corticosteroids under occlusion, the use of preparations containing tar, and the intralesional injection of corticosteroids may be necessary to achieve relief.

HAND AND FOOT ECZEMA

The etiology of an eczematous eruption on the hands or feet may be difficult to determine and in many cases may be multifactorial. Possible causes of hand and foot eczema are listed in Table 5–13. One must consider scabies and tinea as possible causes of hand and foot eczema and examine appropriate skin scrapings. Acute tinea pedis, particularly vesicular tinea pedis, may be accompanied by a "sympathetic" eruption ("id" reaction) on the hands without the fungus being found there. Therefore, tinea pedis must be ruled out, even when both hands and feet are involved. We have not listed nummular eczema, dyshidrotic eczema, or lichen simplex as causes of hand and foot eczema because we consider them to represent reaction patterns rather than causes.

TOPICAL THERAPY

The objectives of topical therapy for an eczematous dermatitis include relief of itching, gentle cleansing and debridement, and restoration of proper hydration. These may be accomplished by the application of topical medications, usually corticosteroids. The ultimate goal is a comfortable patient in whom the cutaneous barrier has been restored.

A localized acute or subacute dermatitis with vesiculation and exudation is best treated with wet compresses. Several layers of soft cloth may be dipped in tap water and wrapped around the involved skin after the excess moisture

TABLE 5–13 POSSIBLE CAUSES OF HAND AND FOOT ECZEMA

Cause	Common Sites
Atopic dermatitis	Hands and feet
Irritant contact dermatitis	Hands and feet
Allergic contact dermatitis	Hands and feet
Tinea	Feet
Tinea pedis with "id" reaction	Hands and feet
Scabies	Hands
Photodermatitis (polymorphic light eruption, photoallergic drug eruption)	Hands (dorsal surface)

has been squeezed out. The compress is moistened again and reapplied at intervals of 15 to 30 minutes. In most instances, tap water is preferable to Burow's solution, saline solution, or potassium permanganate solution, since it is readily available and does not require mixing. The uniform moistness of wet compresses and their cooling effect will give significant relief of itching. Wet compresses also cleanse and hydrate the cutaneous surface. Topical corticosteroid creams may be applied either under the wet compresses or during the intervals between the application of compresses.

A chronic dermatitis, characterized by scaling and fissuring, should be treated with a combination of hydration and lubrication. Hydration is achieved by soaking the involved area in water for 15 to 20 minutes. While the surface is still moist, a thin film of lubricant should be applied in the form of a bath oil or lubricating lotion or a thicker, greasier preparation, such as petrolatum or Aquaphor. The lubricant may also act as the base for a corticosteroid ointment. Hydration usually relieves itching and gently cleanses the surface, while moistening the stratum corneum. Lubrication helps to maintain hydration by retarding evaporation from the surface, and in the case of a corticosteroid ointment, by delivering anti-inflammatory medication. A chronic dermatitis may also be treated by the application of a corticosteroid preparation under an occlusive covering, such as Saran Wrap. Such therapy is cumbersome and obviously unsuitable for large areas of dermatitis. In most cases, we first attempt hydration and application of a corticosteroid ointment without occlusion.

For the extremely uncomfortable patient with a widespread eczematous eruption, the technique of wet dressings may provide significant benefit. This procedure may be performed at home if the patient has proper assistance, but is best performed by trained personnel in the hospital. Wet dressings (Table 5–14) usually relieve itching within 24 hours, remove scales, exudates, and crusts, and maintain hydration of the stratum corneum. When applied under the wet dressings to hydrated skin, a low potency topical corticosteroid cream, such as fluocinolone 0.01 per cent, is very effective. The technique of wet dressings is especially suited to the highly symptomatic patient with extensive atopic dermatitis.

TABLE 5–14 TECHNIQUE OF WET DRESSINGS

Apply a thin film of a low potency corticosteroid cream to the skin.

Moisten absorbent gauze (or soft cloth) in warm tap water and squeeze out the excess water.

Apply the wet dressing to the skin.

Cover the wet dressings with dry flannel or towels pinned in place.

Remove the dressings and repeat the procedure every four to six hours. Do not allow the dressings to dry.

Change the materials used for the dressings every 24 hours or more often if needed.

Place a portable heater at the bedside if the patient finds the dressings too cooling.

REFERENCES

1. Mihm, M. C., Jr., Soter, N. A., Dvorak, H. F., et al.: The structure of normal skin and the morphology of atopic eczema. J. Invest. Dermatol., 67:305, 1976.
2. Coca, A. F., and Cooke, R. A.: On the classification of the phenomena of hypersensitiveness. J. Immunol., 6:63, 1923.
3. Hill, L. W., and Sulzberger, M. B.: Evolution of atopic dermatitis. Arch. Dermatol., 32:451, 1935.
4. Rostenberg, A., and Solomon, L. M.: Infantile eczema and systemic disease. Arch. Dermatol., 98:41, 1968.
5. Hellerstrom, S., and Lidman, H.: Studies of Besnier's prurigo (atopic dermatitis). Acta Derm. Venereol., 36:11, 1956.
6. Rajka, G.: Prurigo Besnier (atopic dermatitis) with special reference to the role of allergic factors. I. The influence of atopic hereditary factors. Acta Derm. Venereol., 40:285, 1960.
7. Baer, R. L.: Atopic Dermatitis. Philadelphia, J. B. Lippincott, 1955.
8. Haynal, A., and Schnyder, U. U.: Funfunddreseissig auslesefrei Zwillinge mit asthma bronchiale und neurodermitis. Archiv. Vererbungsforsung, 35:455, 1960.
9. Rajka, G.: Atopic Dermatitis. Philadelphia, W. B. Saunders, 1975.
10. Möller, H.: Atopic winter feet in children. Acta Derm. Venereol., 52:401, 1972.
11. Ofuji, S., and Uehara, M.: Follicular eruptions of atopic dermatitis. Arch. Dermatol., 107:54, 1973.
12. Wells, R. S., and Kerr, C. I.: Clinical features of autosomal dominant and sex-linked ichthyosis in English population. Br. Med. J., 1:947, 1966.
13. Ingram, J. T.: Besnier's prurigo: An ectodermal defect. Br. J. Dermatol., 67:43, 1955.
14. Watkins, D.: Pityriasis alba, a form of atopic dermatitis. Arch. Dermatol., 83:915, 1961.
15. Sulzberger, M. B., and Herrmann, F.: The Clinical Significance of Disturbances of Sweat. Springfield, Ill., Charles C Thomas, 1954.
16. Whitfield, A.: On the white reaction (white line) in dermatology. Br. J. Dermatol., 50:71, 1938.
17. Ramsay, C.: Vascular changes accompanying white dermographism and delayed blanch in atopic dermatitis. Br. J. Dermatol., 81:37, 1969.
18. Lobitz, W. C., Jr., and Campbell, C. J.: Physiologic studies in atopic dermatitis (disseminated neurodermitis). I. The local cutaneous response to intradermally injected acetylcholine and epinephrine. Arch. Dermat., 67:575, 1953.
19. Eyster, W. H., Jr., Roth, G. M., and Kierland, R. R.: Studies on the peripheral vascular physiology of patients with atopic dermatitis. J. Invest. Dermatol., 18:37, 1952.
20. West, J. R., Kierland, R. R., and Liton, E. M.: Atopic dermatitis and hypnosis. Arch. Dermatol., 84:579, 1961.
21. Naylor, P. F. D.: The reaction to friction of patients with flexural eczema. Br. J. Dermatol., 67:385, 1955.
22. Rajka, G.: Prurigo Besnier (atopic dermatitis) with special reference to the role of allergic factors. I. The evaluation of skin reactions. Acta Derm. Venereol., 48:186, 1968.
23. Cronin, E., Bandmann, H. J., Calnan, C. D., et al.: Contact dermatitis in the atopic. Acta Derm. Venereol., 50:183, 1970.
24. Jones, H. E., Lewis, C., and McMarlin, S. L.: Allergic contact sensitivity in atopic dermatitis. Arch. Dermatol., 107:217, 1973.
25. Kempe, C. H.: Studies on smallpox and complications of smallpox vaccination. Pediatrics, 26:176, 1960.
26. Copeman, P. W. M., and Wallace, H. J.: Eczema vaccinatum. Br. Med. J., 2:906, 1964.
27. Wheeler, C. E., and Abele, D. C.: Eczema herpeticum: Primary and recurrent. Arch. Dermatol., 93:162, 1966.
28. Mailman, C. J., Miranda, J. L., and Spock, A.: Recurrent eczema herpeticum. Arch. Dermatol., 89:815, 1964.
29. Monif, G. R. G., Brunell, P. A., and Hsiung, G. D.: Visceral involvement by herpes simplex virus in eczema herpeticum. Am. J. Dis. Child., 116:321, 1968.
30. Leyden, J. L., Marples, R. R., and Kligman, A. M.: *Staphylococcus aureus* in the lesions of atopic dermatitis. Br. J. Dermatol., 90:525, 1974.
31. Buckley, R. H., Wray, B. B., and Belmaker, E. Z.: Extreme hyperimmunoglobulinemia E and undue susceptibility to infections. Pediatrics, 49:59, 1972.
32. Hanifin, J. M.: Personal communication, 1976.
33. Clark, R. A., Root, R. F., Kimball, H. R., et al.: Defective neutrophil chemotaxis in a child with recurrent infection. Ann. Intern. Med., 78:595, 1973.
34. Hill, H. R., Quie, P. G., et al.: Raised serum-IgE levels and defective neutrophil chemotaxis in three children with eczema and recurrent bacterial infections. Lancet, 1:183, 1974.
35. Hill, H. R., Ochs, H. D., and Quie, P. G.: Defect in neutrophil granulocyte chemotaxis in Job's syndrome of recurrent "cold" staphylococcal abscesses. Lancet, 2:617, 1974.
36. Jones, H. E., Reinhardt, J. E., and Rinaldi, M. G.: Immunologic susceptibility to chronic dermatophytoses. Arch. Dermatol., 110:213, 1974.

37. Lobitz, W. C., Jr., Honeyman, J. R., and Winkler, N. W.: Suppressed cell-mediated immunity in two adults with atopic dermatitis. Br. J. Dermatol., 86:317, 1972.
38. Longemore, L.: Atopic dermatitis and keratoconus. Aust. J. Dermatol., 11:139, 1970.
39. Nicolis, G. D., and Helwig, E. B.: Exfoliative dermatitis. Arch. Dermatol., 108:788, 1973.
40. Ishizaka, K., and Ishizaka, T.: Biological function of gamma E antibodies and mechanisms of reaginic hypersensitivity. Clin. Exp. Immunol., 6:25, 1970.
41. Stanworth, D. R.: Immunochemical mechanisms of immediate type hypersensitivity reactions. Clin. Exp. Immunol., 6:1, 1970.
42. Cormane, R. H., Husz, S., and Hamerlinck, F.: Immunoglobulin and complement-bearing lymphocytes in allergic contact dermatitis and atopic dermatitis (eczema). Br. J. Dermatol., 90:597, 1974.
43. Ogawa, M., Berger, P. A., McIntyre, O. R., et al.: Immunoglobulin E in atopic dermatitis. Arch. Dermatol., 103:575, 1971.
44. Clendenning, W. E., Clark, W. E., Ogawa, M., and Ishizaka, K.: Serum IgE studies in atopic dermatitis. J. Invest. Dermatol., 61:233, 1973.
45. Stone, S. P., Muller, S. A., and Gleich, G. J.: Immunoglobulin E levels in atopic dermatitis. Arch. Dermatol., 108:806, 1973.
46. Gurevitch, A. W., Heiner, D. C., and Reisner, R.: IgE in atopic dermatitis and other common dermatoses. Arch. Dermatol., 107:12, 1973.
47. Johnson, E. E., Irons, J. S., Patterson, R., and Roberts, M.: Serum IgE concentration in atopic dermatitis. J. Allergy Clin. Immunol., 54:94, 1974.
48. Jones, H. E., Inouye, J. C., McGerity, J. L., and Lewis, C. W.: Atopic disease and serum immunoglobulin E. Br. J. Dermatol., 92:17, 1975.
49. Kumar, L., Newcomb, R. W., and Hornbrook, M.: A year-round study of serum IgE levels in asthmatic children. J. Allergy Clin. Immunol., 48:305, 1971.
50. Johansson, S. G. O., and Juhlin, L.: Immunoglobulin E. in "healed" atopic dermatitis, and after treatment with corticosteroids and azathioprine. Br. J. Dermatol., 82:10, 1970.
51. Cohen, S. G., Sapp, T., and Reese, D.: Homocytotrophic antibody function in the mouse. J. Allergy Clin. Immunol., 54:263, 1974.
52. Okumura, K., and Tada, T.: Regulation of homocytotropic antibody formation in the rat. III. Effect of thymectomy and splenectomy. J. Immunol., 106:1025, 1971.
53. Ishizaka, K., and Kishimoto, T.: Regulation of antibody response in vitro. II. Formation of rabbit reaginic antibody. J. Immunol., 109:65, 1973.
54. Geha, R. S., Colten, H. R., and Schneeberger, E.: Cooperation between thymus-derived and bone marrow-derived lymphocytes in the antibody response to ragweed antigen E in vitro. J. Clin. Invest., 56:386, 1973.
55. Kikkawa, Y., Kamimura, K., Hamajima, T., et al.: Thymic alymphoplasia with hyper-IgE-globulinemia. Pediatrics, 51:690, 1973.
56. McGready, S. J., and Buckley, R. H.: Depression of cell-mediated immunity in atopic eczema. J. Allergy Clin. Immunol., 56:393, 1975.
57. Palacios, J., Fuller, E. W., and Blaylock, W. K.: Immunological capabilities of patients with atopic dermatitis. J. Invest. Dermatol., 47:484, 1966.
58. Fjelde, A., and Kopecka, B.: Cell transformation and mitogenic effects in blood leukocyte cultures of atopic dermatitis patients. Acta Derm. Venereol., 47:168, 1967.
59. Rogge, J. L., and Hanifin, J. M.: Depressed leukocyte chemotaxis and lymphocyte transformation in severe atopic dermatitis. Clin. Res., 24:97A, 1976.
60. Luckasen, J. R., Sabab, A., Goltz, R. W., and Kersey, J. H.: T and B lymphocytes in atopic eczema. Arch. Dermatol., 110:375, 1974.
61. Taylor, B., Norman, A. P., Orgel, H. A., et al.: Transient IgA deficiency and pathogenesis of infantile atopy. Lancet, 2:111, 1973.
62. Kaufman, H. S., and Hobbs, J. R.: Immunoglobulin deficiencies in an atopic population. Lancet, 2:1061, 1970.
63. Michaelsson, G.: Decreased phagocytic capacity of the neutrophil leukocytes in patients with atopic dermatitis. Acta Derm. Venereol., 53:279, 1973.
64. Dahl, M. V., Matula, G., Leonards, R., and Tuffanelli, D. L.: Incontinentia pigmenti and defective neutrophil chemotaxis. Arch. Dermatol., 111:1603, 1975.
65. Szentivanyi, A.: The beta adrenergic theory of the atopic abnormality in bronchial asthma. J. Allergy, 42:203, 1968.
66. Carr, R. H., Busse, W. W., and Reed, C. E.: Failure of catecholamines to inhibit epidermal mitosis in vitro. J. Allergy Clin. Immunol., 51:255, 1973.
67. Reed, C. E., Busse, W. W., and Lee, T. P.: Adrenergic mechanisms and the adenyl cyclase system in atopic dermatitis. J. Invest. Dermatol., 67:333, 1976.
68. Sulzberger, M. B.: Atopic dermatitis. In Fitzpatrick, T. H. (ed.): Dermatology in General Medicine. Part 3. New York, McGraw-Hill, 1971.
69. Sedlis, E.: Conference on infantile eczema. Some controlled observations with topical therapy. J. Pediatr., 66:(Suppl.) 255, 1965.
70. Fischer, R. W.: Comparison of antipruritic agents administered orally. JAMA, 203:418, 1968.

71. Cook, T. J., MacQueen, D. M., Wittig, H. J., et al.: Degree and duration of skin test suppression and side effects with antihistamines. J. Allergy Clin. Immunol., *51*:71, 1973.
72. Blank, I. H.: Factors which influence the water content of the stratum corneum. J. Invest. Dermatol., *18*:433, 1952.
73. Frey, J. R., and Wenk, P.: Experimental studies on the pathogenesis of contact eczema in the guinea pig. Int. Arch. Allergy Appl. Immunol., *11*:81, 1957.
74. Turk, J. L.: Delayed Hypersensitivity. New York, John Wiley, 1967.
75. Miller, A. E., and Lewis, W. R.: Studies on the contact sensitization of man with simple chemicals I. J. Invest. Dermatol., *61*:261, 1973.
76. Najarian, J. S., and Feldman, J. D.: Passive transfer of contact sensitivity by tritiated thymidine-labeled lymphoid cells. J. Exp. Med., *117*:775, 1963.
77. Landsteiner, K., and Chase, M. W.: Experiments on transfer of cutaneous sensitivity to simple chemicals. Proc. Soc. Exp. Biol. Med., *49*:688, 1942.
78. North American Contact Dermatitis Group: The frequency of contact sensitivity in North America 1972–74. Contact Dermat., *1*:277, 1975.
79. Fisher, A.: Contact Dermatitis. Philadelphia, Lea & Febiger, 1973.
80. Uehara, M., Takahashi, C., and Ofuji, S.: Pustular patch test reactions in atopic dermatitis. Arch. Dermatol., *111*:1154, 1975.
81. Christensen, O. B., and Möller, H.: External and internal exposure to the antigen in the hand eczema of nickel allergy. Contact Dermat., *1*:136, 1975.
82. Hellgren, L., and Mobacken, H.: Nummular eczema—clinical and statistical data. Acta Derm. Venereol., *49*:189, 1969.
83. Shelley, W. B.: Dyshidrosis (pompholyx). Arch. Dermatol., *68*:314, 1953.
84. Ingram, J. T.: The seborrheic diathesis. Arch. Dermatol., *76*:157, 1957.
85. Editorial: Seborrheic dermatitis. Br. Med. J., *1*:436, 1973.
86. Strauss, J. S., and Pochi, P. E.: The human sebaceous gland. Its regulation by steroidal hormones and its use as an end organ for assaying androgenicity in vivo. Recent Prog. Horm. Res., *19*:385, 1963.
87. Singh, G.: Atopy in lichen simplex (neurodermatitis circumscripta). Br. J. Dermatol., *89*:625, 1973.

6

PHOTODERMATOSES

GUINTER KAHN, M.D.

INTRODUCTION

Sensitivity to light may result from many different causes. The classification of abnormal light reactions in children has been impeded by the rarity of many of the conditions, which are largely unstudied and infrequently reported. In addition, children with certain inherited photoeruptions, such as xeroderma pigmentosum and ataxia-telangiectasia, often do not survive into adult life, making the study of these diseases still more difficult.

Pediatric and adolescent photoeruptions should be considered separately from light sensitivity problems that occur in adult life, since there tend to be significant differences in etiology. In some conditions, photosensitivity becomes much less severe after puberty. In others, such as systemic and topical drug photosensitivity, adults are affected much more frequently than children. In both children and adults, photosensitivity may be a secondary symptom associated with underlying problems of inheritance, cancer, immunology, and growth.

Light-induced diseases found in young children and adolescents are classified in this chapter, and new information is presented that may be helpful in making difficult diagnoses. The general and specific management of each condition is included, together with suggestions on how the physician may evaluate photodermatoses in the office.

Knowing the distribution of the sun's energy on the earth's surface helps us understand the reactions of skin to light. Ultraviolet light (UVL) is emitted by the sun in a continuous spectrum. Wavelengths of less than 290 nanometers (nm) are absorbed by ozone in the atmosphere. Less than 1 per cent of all solar radiation reaching the surface of the earth lies in the ultraviolet spectrum of 290 to 400 nm. About 0.2 per cent of this radiation is from wavelengths of 290 to 320 nm (ultraviolet B or UVB), which readily produce erythema or sunburn. More than 99 per cent of solar radiation consists of visible, infrared and longer, wavelengths.

Other factors that influence the amount of solar radiation reaching the skin are season, latitude, environmental pollution, and time of day. The sunburn-inducing UVB spectrum of sunlight increases during the warm seasons, in clear unpolluted atmospheres, at latitudes nearest the equator, and during the hours of 9 A.M. to 4 P.M.[1] It is useful to know that diseases such as systemic lupus erythematosus, skin carcinoma, and xeroderma pigmentosum are induced primarily by UVB because, as a preventive measure, one can avoid direct sunlight during the hours of greatest intensity or remain behind window glass, which blocks and absorbs UVB rays. The importance of latitude in the incidence of skin carcinoma is evident, since the frequency of cutaneous carcinoma doubles with every increase in latitude of 10 degrees as one approaches the equator.[2] Ten degrees latitude spans about the distance between the northern and southern United States.[3]

The rate at which solar radiation can inflict damage is influenced by both the hereditary characteristics of the skin and the amount of pigment (melanin) in the epidermis. The ability to neutralize damaging photochemical reactions enzymatically is inherited. People of Celtic ancestry develop skin carcinoma earlier and more frequently than other blond- or red-haired groups living in similar environments. Nevertheless, all light-complexioned people are susceptible to photic damage because their skin fails to filter detrimental radiation. The ability to repair UVL-damaged DNA is another important factor. A decrease in DNA repair occurs in xeroderma pigmentosum (XDP), an inherited disorder in which exposure to sun leads to the development of skin cancer in early childhood (see further on).

PHOTOSENSITIVITY

The general term used to describe the adverse effects of light on the skin is photosensitivity. Photosensitivity is divided into two subtypes, phototoxicity and photoallergy. Phototoxicity is common and will occur in any person overexposed to the wavelengths of light that cause sunburn. Phototoxicity is exaggerated by the presence in the skin of phototoxins, such as coal tar, psoralens, or chlorpromazine. Erythema and edema appear a few hours after the first exposure and peak several hours later. Photoallergy is uncommon and depends on molecular alteration and the formation of haptens by the appropriate wavelengths of light energy. Light-induced antigens interact with T cells to produce cell-mediated hypersensitivity. Photoallergy is characterized by an induction (incubation) period of about ten days. Thereafter, small amounts of light may produce widespread eruptions, which develop about one day after subsequent exposure. Solar urticaria represents an immediate (type I, IgE-mediated) type of hypersensitivity reaction which occurs minutes after exposure to the appropriate wavelengths of light. A review of photosensitivity has been done by Epstein.[4]

Eruptions of the skin in children caused by sensitivity to light are not rare. Some of these disorders are acquired, while others are inherited. In this chapter, we shall discuss the photodermatoses of childhood and adolescence. These include: basal cell nevus syndrome (BCNS), xeroderma pigmentosum (XDP), polymorphous light eruption (PLME), Hartnup disease, Rothmund-Thomson syndrome (poikiloderma congenitale), Bloom's syndrome, ataxia-telangiectasia (AT), Cockayne's syndrome, pellagra, congenital erythropoietic porphyria (EP), erythropoietic protoporphyria (EPP), acquired porphyria cutanea tarda (PCT), systemic and topical photosensitization, solar urticaria, and lupus erythematosus (LE).

BASAL CELL NEVUS SYNDROME (Nevoid Basal Cell Carcinoma)

Basal cell carcinomas *usually* occur in the sun-exposed skin of middle-aged, light-complexioned, outdoor-loving individuals. However, in patients with basal cell nevus syndrome (BCNS), skin tumors in the form of basal cell carcinomas appear as early as the second year of life. The most florid eruption appears during the second decade, whether the skin has been exposed to sunlight or not (see Plate I-C), since UVL plays only a partnership role in the carcinogenic feature of this symptom complex. Patients with BCNS also manifest multiple congenital abnormalities of the osseous, endocrine, and central nervous systems.

BCNS is inherited as an autosomal dominant trait with variable expressivity. The requisite for diagnosis is the presence of numerous basal cell carcinomas. These most commonly appear on the face and chest at puberty.[5] In addition, skin abnormalities frequently include cysts, milia, and lipomas[6] as well as the pits on the palms and soles that are a distinctive finding.

Skeletal abnormalities are found chiefly in the mandible, ribs, metacarpals, vertebrae, and skull. Bossing of the skull gives it a pagetoid appearance. Sometimes the nasal root is broadened and the pupils are widely separated (dystopia canthorum). Ocular and neural anomalies are also common. The falx cerebri and dura may contain calcifications. A variety of tumors may occur in this syndrome, including cysts and glial tumors of the brain, leiomyomas of the esophagus, uterus, and mesentery, adrenal cortical adenomas, ovarian fibromas, and medulloblastomas. Cysts in the mandible are another common occurrence. Overall, UVL plays a minor role in the pathogenesis of BCNS.

XERODERMA PIGMENTOSUM*

Xeroderma pigmentosum (XDP) is an autosomal recessive disease that occurs about once in every 250,000 births. The clinical manifestations are found predominantly on sun-exposed areas of the skin and eyes,[7] although some patients have short stature and neurological abnormalities. Approximately 50 per cent of affected individuals develop an acute sensitivity to sunlight in early infancy. All patients develop freckles, usually before two years of age and subsequently exhibit signs of severe sun damage, such as dryness, scaling, hypopigmentation, telangiectasia, atrophy, and actinic keratoses. Basal cell carcinomas, squamous cell carcinomas, and malignant melanomas of the skin and eyes occur with alarming frequency. Without treatment,

---

*The section on xeroderma pigmentosum was written by Kenneth H. Kraemer, M.D., Research Associate, National Institutes of Health, Bethesda, Maryland.

victims of xeroderma pigmentosum usually die at an early age from the spread of these neoplasms.

In 1968, Cleaver reported that cultured skin fibroblasts from patients with XDP had a markedly diminished ability to repair DNA molecules damaged by ultraviolet light.[8] Under normal circumstances, when UVL causes the induction of thymine disorders (covalent bonds between adjacent thymines on a DNA strand), these are removed by an excision and repair system. An enzymatic system excises the abnormal dimers as well as some adjacent nucleotides and fills the resulting gap by replicating a portion of the opposing strand of DNA (repair replication).

The reduced ability to perform DNA excision and repair in various XDP cell types has been demonstrated by other investigators using several different techniques. Epstein and his colleagues[9] demonstrated reduced, UV-induced, unscheduled DNA synthesis (UDS) — an autoradiographic measure of excision repair — in vivo in epidermal cells and in the dermal fibroblasts of patients with XDP. Robbins and his associates (1974)[7] found that XDP lymphocytes repair DNA more slowly than normal but continue their repair process for a longer time. The XDP lymphocytes ultimately incorporate as much tritiated thymidine (a measure of excision repair) as normal lymphocytes after UV irradiation. Thus, the DNA repair defect in XDP appears to be a reduced rate of repair. Also, different patients have different rates of DNA repair.

Binuclear cells, formed by fusing fibroblasts from certain pairs of XDP patients, have been found to exhibit normal ultraviolet-induced DNA repair,[10] which implies that each of the fused fibroblasts had a different DNA repair defect. Since each fibroblast supplied what the other lacked, it was said to complement the other. Thus, each fibroblast represented a different complementation group. When fused, pairs of XDP fibroblasts with the same DNA repair defect still demonstrated reduced UDS and thus were categorized in the same complementation group. Subsequent fusion studies have shown that at least five complementation groups are represented in XDP fibroblasts.[11] This implies that there are at least five different DNA excision repair defects associated with the disease. Each complementation group has been found to have a characteristic rate of UDS.[11] Restoration of UDS in all five groups also has been demonstrated in vitro by treating XDP fibroblasts with a purified bacteriophage endonuclease and inactivated Sendai virus.[12]

XDP cells with defective DNA repair are more sensitive than normal cells to killing by UVL, as measured by colony-forming ability in tissue culture. In addition, XDP cells are more sensitive than normal cells to killing by carcinogens, such as 4-nitroquinoline-1-oxide, benzanthracene oxide, and N-acetoxy-2-acetylaminofluorene.[7] Cell survival after treatment with these agents apparently is related to a normal and functioning DNA repair system.

Several XDP "variant" patients have been described who have the classic features of XDP but have normal DNA excision and repair function. Fibroblasts from these patients are more sensitive to destruction by UVL than normal fibroblasts are.[13] Studies of fibroblasts from three of these variant patients have demonstrated a defect in another DNA repair system — postreplication repair.[14]

Endogenous or exogenous chemicals, unidentified at present, may cause damage to central nervous system neurons (which do not divide) and result in the progressive mental deterioration seen in some XDP patients.[7]

DIAGNOSIS AND TREATMENT

An early diagnosis of XDP is made possible by measuring UV-induced UDS in cultured skin fibroblasts. This has been accomplished in patients as young as five months of age. Similarly, prenatal diagnosis of XDP has been made, using cultured cells obtained by amniocentesis. This procedure has been followed in cases of families with an affected child who has XDP with diminished UDS.[15]

The goal of therapy in XDP is to minimize morbidity and mortality from neoplasms. The patient and his family must be taught the dangers of UV light and how to minimize UVL exposure. We advise the following: severely limiting outdoor exposure during daylight hours; wearing long hair styles and protective clothing, including glasses; and regularly applying a sunscreen (such as titanium dioxide compound or para-aminobenzoic acid in an alcohol base) to exposed skin. We teach the patients to examine themselves closely and frequently and advise regular visits to a physician in order to detect and treat neoplastic lesions as they arise. Cutaneous neoplasms in patients with XDP may be treated by the usual modalities, such as excision, electrodesiccation and curettage, and irradiation. Fluorouracil applied topically is also a useful treatment for premalignant lesions.[16]

POLYMORPHOUS LIGHT ERUPTION (PMLE)

There are two types of polymorphous light eruptions. An hereditary, autosomal dominant form occurs in American Indian tribes living in a geographic area from Mid-Canada to South America.[17] However, it is not found in Eskimos or in Indians of the Pacific Northwest. About 70 per cent of affected patients develop an eruption by the age of ten, which usually begins on the face as an acute eczematous process. Thereafter, other exposed areas may become involved, especially the lower lip, external ears, and dorsal surfaces of the hands. Typically, papules and crusts develop on an erythematous base. Vesicles and bullae are uncommon lesions. After puberty, the disease tends to abate, and the lesions become circumscribed plaques (Fig. 6–1). Scarring follows trauma and infection. The lesions recur each spring as the intensity of the sun's UVB emission increases. PMLE in American Indians differs from PMLE described in other populations throughout the world in its hereditary pattern, onset, and inciting UVL spectrum wavelengths.

In the second form of PMLE a familial predisposition is absent, and the onset of symptoms occurs in late adolescence or early adulthood. In nonfamilial PMLE, both urticaria and blisters may occur, although one type of lesion generally predominates. European and American studies of nonfamilial PMLE indicate that UVB, long-wavelength UVL (UVA), and visible light all can cause the eruption in some patients.[18] The global distribution of PMLE is erratic, as it is in the United States. It is not related to latitude, since PMLE is almost unknown in India, Japan, and Florida. Thus, the second form of PLME is polymorphous in its clinical presentation, geographical and demographical distribution, activating light wavelength, age of onset, microscopic appearance, and therapy.

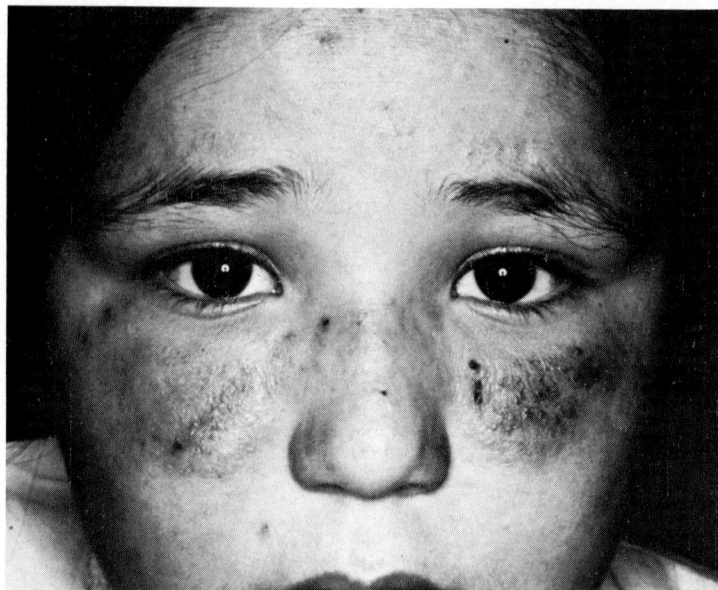

FIGURE 6–1 Circumscribed plaques on the face of an adolescent girl with polymorphous light eruption.

The only feature all patients with PMLE have in common is an abnormal reaction to sun exposure. No biochemical, allergic, metabolic, or endocrine abnormalities have been found in affected individuals. Haxthausen incorporated summer prurigo and the hydroas into a single classification.[19] Since the patients he described were identical clinically to those with PMLE and also exhibited no abnormalities in laboratory tests, they probably suffered from PMLE. Before making the diagnosis of PMLE, one should exclude, by appropriate laboratory tests, the presence of porphyria and its variants, lupus erythematosus, photoallergic and phototoxic dermatoses, solar urticaria, actinic reticuloid, lymphocytic infiltrates, and insect bite infiltrates.

A standard photo test technique is used to provoke a lesion that suggests the diagnosis of PMLE. This consists of exposing an uninvolved (normal skin) forearm to 3 to 5 minimal erythema-producing doses of UVB every 24 to 72 hours, up to five times on successive sessions. In 32 of 37 patients, Epstein was able to reproduce the lesions of PMLE 3 to 14 days after such UVL exposure.[20]

PMLE occurs even in blacks, whose skin has a high melanin content which acts as an excellent sun shield. Therefore, it follows that topical sun protectants provide inadequate screening in severe cases of sensitivity. Orally administered chloroquine and hydroxychloroquine sulfate tablets may be partially effective in decreasing sensitivity to sunlight. Periodic ophthalmological consultations to avert chloroquine retinopathy are mandatory when such drugs are prescribed. Systemic steroids help to alleviate the process, but the biological consequences of the necessary dose and the length of therapy are often prohibitive. Mild reactions may be controlled by applying generous amounts of 5 to 10 per cent para-aminobenzoic acid in alcohol to affected areas in the morning and applying a strong steroid ointment in the evening. Beta-carotene given orally in doses of 90 to 180 mg/day[21, 22] has been shown to be helpful in some patients.

HARTNUP DISEASE

The signs and symptoms of Hartnup disease are similar to those of pellagra, which results from a deficiency of nicotinamide (NA). Hartnup disease is an autosomal recessive aminoaciduria in which symptoms become milder after puberty.

Between the ages of three and nine, the eruption appears as red, rough, eczematous areas on surfaces exposed to light, heat, friction, or pressure. The sites most often involved are the face, dorsa of the hands, wrists, elbows, knees, and inframammary and perineal folds. Lesions are sharply demarcated, red, and scaly (Fig. 6–2). The gastrointestinal tract may be abnormal along its entire length, glossitis and diarrhea being the most common symptoms. Tryptophan transport in the jejunum and proximal kidney tubules is impaired. The symptoms of Hartnup disease may be the result of tryptophan shunting.[23]

Since it is believed that the symptoms of Hartnup disease are due to a lack of nicotinamide (NA), one should be able to correlate this lack with the particular pathological characteristics of Hartnup disease. Man can synthesize NA from tryptophan in the presence of B vitamins, but tryptophan deficiency may occur in alcoholics, food faddists, and victims of starvation. Tryptophan deficiency also results from rapid NA metabolism in febrile and thyrotoxic states as well as in pregnancy. Pellagroid changes are also found in the carcinoid syndrome, since tryptophan is transformed excessively into 5-hydroxytryptamine (serotonin). Isonicotinic acid hydrazide, a drug commonly used to treat tuberculosis, competes metabolically with NA and under some circumstances may induce pellagra. Pellagra thus may be secondary to diet, drugs, the carcinoid syndrome, or Hartnup disease.

In Hartnup disease, central nervous system symptoms may begin as irri-

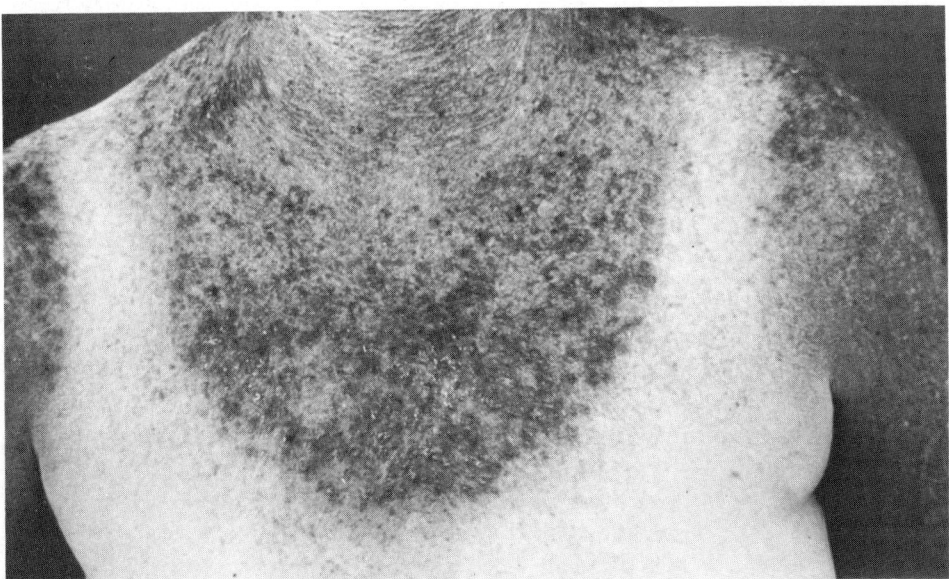

FIGURE 6–2 Pellagrinous skin lesion, sharply demarcated and scaly, may be induced by diet, drugs, carcinoid syndrome, or Hartnup disease.

tability and end as paralysis and insanity. These symptoms and signs may resemble those of pellagra, but mental retardation and cerebellar ataxia almost always are prominent features of Hartnup disease. Affected subjects also have reduced stature, the average height of Hartnup adults being about 4 inches less than their normal growth curves would indicate.

Because wavelengths of light that induce pellagrous skin symptoms are unknown, photo testing with specific wavelengths is not practical. However, exposure to midday sun does induce the lesions. Hartnup syndrome can best be indentified by studying urinary and fecal amino acids under controlled conditions.

Hydroxykynureninuria and congenital tryptophanuria are even more rare but may mimic Hartnup disease. The symptoms and eruptions are similar but begin at an earlier age and are caused by enzymatic defects occurring at different points in the metabolic pathway of tryptophan.[24]

BLOOM'S SYNDROME

This rare autosomal recessive disorder is characterized by light-induced telangiectatic erythema and stunted growth. Photosensitivity begins in the first weeks of life, manifested by lesions on the face and upper extremities that resemble those of systemic lupus erythematosus. Infants with Bloom's syndrome are small at birth, unlike endocrinopathic dwarfs whose size at birth is normal. Children with Bloom's syndrome grow to a greater height than true dwarfs, but remain shorter and appear more wizened than normal children. Their endocrine function and intelligence appear to be normal. Bloom's syndrome occurs primarily in Jewish children (50 per cent) and predominantly in Jewish male children (80 per cent). The specific wavelengths of light causing the erythema are unknown.

Affected individuals often develop malignant tumors early in life. Four of the first five patients identified developed one or more malignancies (leukemia in three cases, tongue carcinoma in one). Among 50 patients who survived infancy, eight developed various kinds of tumors, while another three who reached the age of 30 developed tumors of the gastrointestinal tract.[25] Extensive chromosomal breakage appears to contribute to such tumor formation, with increased abnormal chromosome configurations found in the bone marrow, peripheral blood, and skin. Quadriradial figures are most common. Chromosome number and karyotype are usually normal. Normal skin fibroblasts grown in culture show occasional aberrations (1 to 2 per cent) in appearance, but in Bloom's syndrome up to 15 per cent of these cells have such abnormalities.

Patients with Bloom's syndrome often develop serious and sometimes fatal gastrointestinal and respiratory tract bacterial infections early in life. The advent of antibiotics may have increased the survival of these patients, and perhaps for this reason the entity has been recognized only in recent years. Defects in both humoral and cellular immune function may account for the infections. Immunoglobulin synthesis is decreased in response to pokeweed mitogen (PWM) and cell-mediated immunity is diminished, as measured by one-way mixed lymphocyte culture. Immunological abnormalities of Bloom's syndrome are therefore diffuse, involving both B cell and T cell function.[26] The biological relationships that link immunological impairment, chromosomal abnormalities, UV hypersensitivity, and cancer formation remain to be clarified.

COCKAYNE'S SYNDROME

This syndrome is rarer than Bloom's syndrome and is characterized by dwarfism, light sensitivity, telangiectasia, and a 4 to 1 male-female preponderance.

Cockayne's syndrome seems to be recessively inherited and is most frequently seen in people of British lineage. The syndrome begins in the second year of life and develops progressively. Thinning of the subcutaneous fat causes a birdlike facies, and long extremities, vertebral abnormalities, and progressive ataxia add to the birdlike and aged habitus. Other abnormalities include optic degeneration, deafness, mental retardation, and thickened skull bones.[27] Biochemical studies of the blood and urine have yielded normal results, as have endocrine and chromosomal studies.

The skin of patients with Cockayne's syndrome becomes atrophic and develops striae, and scalp and body hair are sparse. Patients usually die from atheromatous vascular disease before the age of 30. Unlike progeria, plasma lipids are found to be normal in Cockayne's syndrome.[28]

ATAXIA-TELANGIECTASIA (AT)

This autosomal recessive condition is characterized by vascular abnormalities of the cerebellum and skin. Ataxia becomes apparent when the affected child attempts to walk. Drooling and peculiar eye movements also occur in the first years of life, but during this time there are no seizures, indications of mental retardation, or speech defects. Telangiectasia appears on sun-exposed skin and conjunctivae between the ages of three and six and remains permanently. At puberty, speech becomes dysarthric, intelligence deteriorates, and growth is retarded. The skin becomes tight, as in scleroderma, and a red, scaly dermatitis resembling seborrheic dermatitis appears. Hypopigmentation and café au lait spots are also occasionally found.

Varying immunodeficiencies are found in this syndrome. Low serum levels of IgA with or without low serum IgE occur in about 60 per cent of patients. Hypoplasia of the thymus and the germinal centers of lymph nodes has also been described. Prolonged survival of homologous skin grafts and a lack of response to common antigen skin tests have also been noted. Elevated levels of alpha-feto protein, which inhibits antibody production and lymphocyte stimulation by T cell mitogens, may contribute to the immunodeficiency.[29, 30] Impaired immunological defenses also may be responsible for the repeated sinopulmonary infections that start to afflict children between four and six years of age. Other infections are not common. Infections plus pulmonary fibrosis often lead to death by adolescence, although survival up to age 40 has been reported. The relationship of the scleroderma-like skin to the fibrotic lungs has not been studied, to our knowledge.

Ataxia-telangiectasia is a chromosomal breakage syndrome, in which the cells show abnormal fragility and chromosomal instability when exposed to x-ray, although not to UV.[31] Since tissues with chromosomal abnormalities are predisposed to malignant change, it is not surprising that patients with AT have an incidence of lymphoreticular malignancy of about 10 per cent. The relatives of such patients also have a five times greater than average risk of dying from malignancy.[32] Management of this disorder consists of early detection of malignancy by performing periodic white blood cell counts and lymph node biopsies, along with control of infection.

ROTHMUND-THOMSON SYNDROME (Poikiloderma Congenitale)

This autosomal recessive syndrome begins at three to six months of age and is fully expressed after three to seven years. Atrophy, telangiectasia, and hypo- and hyperpigmentation develop following the onset of erythema on the face and extremities (Plate I–D). About one third of patients develop a variety of cataracts, approximately two thirds develop bony defects, and the majority have sparse hair and defective nails. The disease varies in severity from patient to patient. The sine qua non of the syndrome is the presence of reticulated atrophy that simulates chronic radiodermatitis. As in radiodermatitis, carcinomatous changes develop in some adults.[33] Results of chromosomal and other laboratory studies are normal.[34]

DISEASES OF THE PIGMENTARY SYSTEM

Diseases in which sun damage is secondary to impaired pigmentation include albinism, vitiligo, and phenylketonuria. The primary defect in these disorders is inadequate melanin production. Phototoxicity (sunburn) occurs from excessive exposure to UVB. Vitiligo is discussed further in Chapter 18.

PORPHYRIA

All of the porphyrias indicate a defect in porphyrin synthesis, and many are inherited. Those types that are associated with photosensitivity, especially those that occur in childhood, will be discussed in detail.

PORPHYRIA CUTANEA TARDA (PCT)

This disease is very rare in children, with only three cases reported in children under 15 years of age.[35] Two of these cases were induced by excessive iron storage. PCT induced by chemicals (acquired or drug-induced porphyria) is discussed in this section.

VARIEGATE (MIXED) PORPHYRIA

This disease, transmitted by an autosomal dominant trait, represents a combination of acute intermittent porphyria* and PCT. Symptoms occur only after puberty.

---

*Acute intermittent porphyria (AIP) is not manifest before puberty and appears to have no cutaneous features.

HEREDITARY COPROPORPHYRIA

In this rare form of variegate porphyria, only four of 20 patients described experienced photosensitivity.[36]

ACQUIRED (DRUG-INDUCED OR TOXIC) PORPHYRIA

Acquired PCT may be induced in apparently normal individuals by excessive iron intake or by ingestion of chlorinated insecticides. An outbreak of toxic porphyria occurred in Turkey after the fungicide hexachlorobenzene (used on wheat crops) was introduced. The resulting syndrome occurred more severely and more frequently in children than in adults.[37] The prominence of focal hyperpigmentation and hirsutism in these patients gave rise to the term "monkey children," even though bullous skin lesions, hepatomegaly, and arthritic changes were found in half of them. After the ingestion of hexachlorobenzene ended, most patients remained symptomatic and continued to excrete porphyrins for more than two years.[38] The acquired form of porphyria is clinically indistinguishable from PCT except that hyperpigmentation and hypertrichosis are more prominent in the former, whereas bullous and erosive skin lesions are more common in the latter.

Gamma benzene hexachloride (lindane) is generally used to treat scabies in children and adults. The topical application of lindane in scabies has not induced PCT, although Harber states that it is capable of doing so.[39] Since gamma benzene hexachloride and hexachlorobenzene are not related chemically, this finding is unrelated to cases of PCT induced by the ingestion of insecticides.

The diagnosis of PCT is made by examining the urine under a Wood's light to detect pink-orange fluorescence and is supported by a biopsy specimen containing a subepidermal non-inflammatory bulla. The diagnosis is confirmed by finding large amounts of uroporphyrins (Types I and III) in a 24-hour urine specimen.

After the offending chemical has been removed, acquired porphyria should be treated by phlebotomy, which may be performed weekly until hemoglobin levels approach 11 gm/100 ml. The mechanism of improvement is unknown. Hypertrichosis and hyperpigmentation are more resistant to treatment than are erosive or bullous lesions.

ERYTHROPOIETIC PORPHYRIAS

The erythropoietic porphyrias begin in early childhood and manifest themselves as persistent photosensitivity. There are two types: erythropoietic porphyria (EP) or Günther's disease and erythropoietic protoporphyria (EPP).

Erythropoietic Porphyria (EP). EP becomes manifest shortly after birth when diapers are stained pink by red urine, which is saturated with uroporphyrin I (UP). Uroporphyrin I is a photosensitizer that circulates in the blood to the skin, where visible light (400 to 410 nm and 500 to 600 nm) photoreacts with it to cause severe redness and bullae. Since visible light is present throughout the day and penetrates window glass, the process is unremitting. The exposed body parts, including the face and hands, become ulcerated, infected, fibrotic, gnarled, and mutilated. Deposition of UP in teeth and nails discolors them a dirty brown and causes them to fluoresce an orange-red color upon exposure to UVL. The legendary werewolves of the Middle Ages are reputed to have had EP, which explains their nocturnal habits, mutilated hirsute facies and hands, and discolored nails and teeth.[40]

Fewer than 100 patients with this autosomal recessive condition have been reported. Ninety per cent of them have had severe hemolytic anemia and splenomegaly, necessitating splenectomy. (The spleen apparently traps the fragile, UP-laden red blood cells.) Death often occurs in childhood from anemia and secondary infection. Postmortem examinations have revealed that almost every organ in the body contained red fluorescence.

The diagnosis is made by demonstrating large quantities of UP I in the urine of patients with this unique clinical presentation. Treatment is difficult and not always effective, although remissions have been reported after splenectomy and beta-carotene therapy.[41]

Erythropoietic Protoporphyria. EPP is an autosomal dominant disease that usually develops between the ages of two and 10 years. Burning pain and edematous erythema occur 5 to 30 minutes after exposure to sunlight, even through window glass. Eventually scars form, especially on the nose, ears, borders of the lips, and dorsum of the hand (Fig. 6-3). Excess protoporphyrin (PP), a photosensitizer, is present in large amounts in red blood cells,* serum, feces, and skin.

Since its description in 1961, several hundred cases of EPP have been recognized. A few patients have developed cholecystitis, gallstones, and liver failure, presumably from the accumulation of protoporphyrins in biliary

---

*Excess RBC coproporphyrins have been described in a variant form of this disease, erythropoietic coproporphyria.

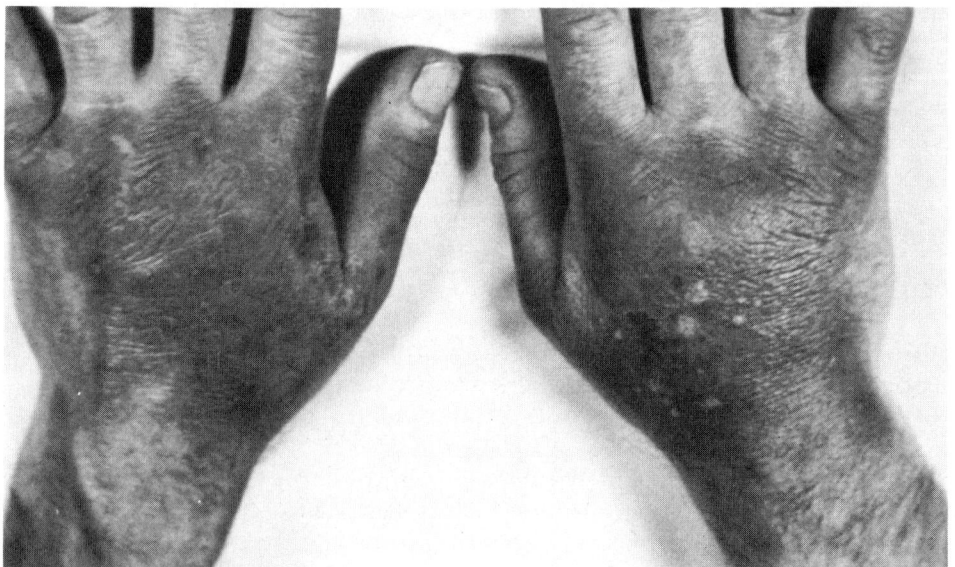

FIGURE 6-3 Dorsa of the hands acutely thickened after sun exposure in a patient with erythropoietic protoporphyria.

canaliculi. One study has suggested that the liver also contributes to protoporphyrin production.[42] If this theory proves to be true, EPP represents the only porphyric disease with biochemical defects of both hepatic and erythropoietic cells.

The diagnosis of EPP is aided by fluorescent microscopic examination of red blood cells. Sections of skin contain dense amorphous material around the papillary and other superficial dermal blood vessels. Photosensitized vessels of the upper dermis appear to exude a foamy material that gives rise to perivascular hyalinization.[43] Direct immunofluorescent study of microscopic sections of involved skin reveals heavy deposits of IgG around these vessels. A rapid screening test for free erythrocyte porphyrin (FEP) is available from Columbia University.*[44] It uses a few drops of blood from a finger stab collected on filter paper. FEP is found to be elevated in cases of EPP, iron deficiency, and lead intoxication. The urine of EPP patients contains no abnormal porphyrins, in contrast to that of EP and PCT patients.

Beta-carotene (Solatene) effectively reduces EPP symptoms without affecting protoporphyrin levels. Patients take 1 to 10 capsules (30 to 300 mg) in divided doses with meals. Individual dosage is titrated to provide adequate photoprotection. Serum levels of 400 to 800 mcg per 100 ml may be achieved in four to six weeks and should provide maximal protection against the noxious effects of UV light. Unfortunately, the skin becomes carotenemic, most visible as orange staining of the palms and soles. Stools may be orange and loosely formed. Vitamin A levels do not rise above normal. All but five of 135 patients using beta-carotene were able to spend more time exposed to sunlight without experiencing adverse effects.[45] No side effects other than orange skin tone and loose stools were noted following six years' administration of the drug. The mechanism of protection has not been established, but the most prevalent theory credits the quenching of free radical energy formed in the skin.

SOLAR URTICARIA

Solar urticaria is a rare disease of unknown etiology. It does not appear to be inherited, and it may begin at any time in life, including early childhood. In the approximately 100 patients who have been studied, UVL and visible light were found to cause erythema and urticarial wheals on the skin from 2 to 30 minutes after exposure. The itching, burning, erythema, and urticaria receded in one to four hours. It is difficult to categorize these patients, since individual variation exists in the activating light spectrum, the severity of symptoms, the ability to overcome the condition, the response to therapy, and the ability of the phenomenon to be passively transferred to normal individuals.[46] Passive transfer tests are positive mainly in patients sensitive to UVB.[47] It appears that the IgE serum factor is passively transferred and that light causes the release of an antigenic factor. Histamine is not the mediator of the inflammatory response in these patients.[48]

Light-induced urticaria also may be caused by porphyria, by photodynamic reactions with coal tar derivatives, by sulfonamides (and other drugs),

---

*Columbia University Medical Center, 161 Fort Washington Ave., New York, N.Y.10032.

and by lupus erythematosus. The diagnosis is made by excluding drug photosensitization, systemic lupus erythematosus, and porphyria. It includes photo testing for immediate (2 to 30 minutes) wheal formation (Plate I–E) and studying urine and red blood cells for the presence of abnormal porphyrins. Vesicular responses in children with solar urticaria probably represent some of the cases of "hydroa" often described in the older literature.

The major therapeutic approach is to help the patient avoid sunlight. Window glass and sunscreens may provide some protection, depending on the provocative wavelengths. Some patients respond to antihistamines, others to chloroquine, but so far none have been found to benefit from beta-carotene. Ramsey successfully induced tolerance to sunlight by hourly exposure to artificial and natural photic radiation.[49] After the action spectrum for whealing was determined, this treatment resulted in the elimination of the urticaria in eight patients.

LUPUS ERYTHEMATOSUS

Both the systemic form (SLE) and the more localized discoid form (DLE) of lupus erythematosus may occur in childhood and adolescence, although both forms are uncommon. DLE is particularly rare in children, with fewer than ten cases under the age of 12 reported from the Mayo Clinic. In both DLE and SLE, the symptoms, prognosis, and treatment are similar for both children and adults.[50] Sun exposure causes lesions on the skin in only about 30 per cent of such patients. Sun-sensitive patients respond to shielding from the activating wavelengths (UVB).[51] Children with a disease resembling or identical to LE have recently been described in families associated with deficiencies in complement cascade; including C1r, C1s, C2, C4, and C5. C2 is the deficiency most frequently encountered. Virtually all the patients with an LE-like disease are photosensitive[52] but most do not have complement at their epidermal-dermal junction or elevated antinuclear antibody (ANA) titers.

The range of symptoms of C2 deficiency varies from no disease to severe generalized LE with pyogenic infections. Of 38 homozygous C2-deficient patients described in the literature, 14 had LE, with approximately equal distribution between SLE and DLE. The relationship between C2 deficiency and LE is probably not fortuitous, as 18 of 19 patients typed for histocompatibility locus belong to HL-A types 10 and B18.[53]

These complement deficiencies are managed today by treating the related diseases, such as SLE, DLE, and pyoderma. In one report, a patient with normal humoral and cellular immunity and an LE-related syndrome improved after levamisole hydrochloride therapy.[54] Complement levels remain unchanged in spite of clinical exacerbations or remissions. A more complete review of the LE-related complement deficiency syndromes has been done by Jordan and Provost.[55]

It is evident that familial complement defects should be sought in children who have unexplained photosensitivity. Determination of the total hemolytic complement (CH50) titers is the best *screening* test for this disorder because it detects all of the deficiencies associated with a lupus-like illness. Complement defects may be missed if only C3 or total complement levels are determined. HL-A typing is also useful.

SYSTEMIC AND TOPICAL PHOTOSENSITIVITY ERUPTIONS

A survey of 200 photosensitized patients in Malaysia indicated that 6 per cent of the subjects were under 10 years of age and 11 per cent were between the ages of 10 and 20, with the youngest child being one and one-half years of age.[56] Patients were not classified by cause (systemic or topical), and the etiology of the majority of photoeruptions was not identified. Some known causes of photosensitivity reactions are discussed in the following section.

SYSTEMIC PHOTOSENSITIZATION

Drug-induced photoeruptions occur infrequently in children, since most common photosensitizing drugs are rarely given to children. Among these photosensitizing drugs are chlorpromazine, psoralens, and the sulfonamides (including sulfonylurea derivatives, which serve as anti-diabetic agents, and thiazide diuretics), and demeclocycline hydrochloride. Most of these drugs, except for the sulfonamide derivatives, induce phototoxic reactions, so that any child receiving a large enough dose plus adequate exposure to sunlight can develop a light-induced reaction. Psoralens have been used chiefly in the treatment of vitiligo and psoriasis. Although the instructions in the package insert in the *Physicians' Desk Reference* recommend that psoralens not be given to children under 12, data to substantiate the need for this precaution are not included. Psoralens have been administered for more than 25 years to children throughout the world, and although cataract and skin tumor formation have been reported in mice treated with psoralens, they have not been reported in children.[57, 58]

In contrast to phototoxic reactions, other drug eruptions are photoallergic, resulting from the interaction of light plus a chemical that produces a cell-mediated immune reaction. Sulfonamide derivatives, such as thiazide diuretics and sulfonylurea antidiabetic agents, are the chief causes of photoallergic reactions in adults, but children seldom receive these drugs. Photoallergy in children is rarely caused by griseofulvin.

TOPICAL PHOTOSENSITIZATION

Although coal tar and its dye derivatives are time-honored topical agents prescribed for children, it is difficult to find reports of childhood photosensitization resulting from the use of these products. Most of the available reports concern adults who contacted these substances in an industrial setting. Perhaps the mild phototoxic effect they may confer on atopic, psoriatic, or infected skin is expected as part of the therapeutic response.[59]

Photoeruptions induced by contact with plants are classified as phytophotodermatitis. They are caused primarily by certain perfumed products in or on a plant containing psoralens. Psoralen (furocoumarin) is a transient, capricious metabolite found in wild and cultivated grasses, fruits, and flowers. It is especially abundant after a rainy growing season in limes, carrots, celery, figs, and bergamot extracts. The skin that has had prior exposure to these substances and is then exposed to UVA (320 to 400 nm) develops redness and blisters conforming to the pattern of contact with the plant. Hyperpigmentation then follows at the same sites after about five days and may persist for months.

Halogenated salicylanilides, found as antibacterial and antifungal agents in soaps, creams, and cleansers, have caused photocontact dermatitis.[60] Since 1974, they are no longer ingredients in products used in interstate commerce in the United States. Strangely, salicylanilde photosensitivity never did seem to affect children or teenagers. Similarly, it was never possible to photosensitize guinea pigs in the first week of life to salicylanilides.

Topical photosensitization is an expected part of the treatment when psoralens are used to treat vitiligo or psoriasis. Unwanted systemic and topical photosensitization is treated by avoiding the offending agent. Since the spectrum of light that induces these eruptions includes both UVA and UVB, the responsible UVL may penetrate window glass and non-opaque sunscreens. Affected persons must avoid the photosensitizer and sunlight.

MISCELLANEOUS DISEASES AGGRAVATED BY SUNLIGHT

Numerous dermatoses are aggravated by sunlight, which causes erythema and acts as a form of trauma that may incite new eruptions. Examples include psoriasis (10 per cent of patients are light-sensitive), atopic dermatitis (16 per cent of patients are worse during the summer), lichen planus, granuloma annulare (rare), and herpes simplex. Neither the mechanisms nor the wavelengths of light aggravating these conditions is known. A similar lack of knowledge prevails in familial diseases in which UVL may play an inciting role. These include a familial benign chronic pemphigus (Hailey-Hailey disease) and keratosis follicularis (Darier's disease).

Lichen planus tropicus (actinicus) occurs on the exposed skin of children more often than adults. Light, heat, and poor nutrition may be responsible for the eruption, according to studies made in the Middle East.[62]

Pemphigus foliaceus, which occurs in children, is also aggravated by UVL. The distribution of lesions supports the clinical impression that sun exposure elicits this disease.

PHOTOPROTECTION

Various types of topical and oral therapy indicated for specific photodermatoses have been discussed throughout this chapter. In addition, there are some general treatment principles that should be followed by anyone who is going to be exposed to sunlight.

Prevention of sun damage is the best treatment and may be accomplished in the following manner: Avoid exposure to sunlight that causes erythema (9 A.M. to 4 P.M.); wear protective clothing such as wide-brimmed hats and long-sleeved shirts; let the hair grow long; wear lipstick or a lip protectant; apply protective sun barrier materials (sunscreens) prior to beginning sun exposure.

PABA (para-aminobenzoic acid) and its esters provide adequate protection against normal sun exposure and are effective in preventing photodermatoses. However, they are not effective protection for conditions provoked by UV wavelengths longer than 320 nm, such as the porphyrias, chemically-induced photosensitization, and some solar urticaria. Patients with these conditions need to apply opaque substances that physically block out light, such as heavy makeup or sunscreens containing zinc oxide or titanium dioxide. These patients are photosensitive throughout the daylight hours and are susceptible even to light that passes through window glass or through thin, porous clothing.

Adherence to these guidelines in younger years will prevent chronic sun damage and skin cancer in later years, since damage from ultraviolet light is cumulative. Physicians must impress upon their patients the value of good "solar hygiene."

OFFICE MANAGEMENT

The office management of pediatric photodermatoses may be conveniently divided into history-taking, physical examination, and use of laboratory tests. Each of these is discussed in detail, with salient comments included about important findings.

HISTORY

1. What is the age at onset? What amount of light is needed to produce the rash? How long after exposure does the rash appear? How long does the rash last?

Note: Most metabolic abnormalities start between two and ten years of age, but EP may begin earlier. EPP and solar urticaria may begin within an hour after exposure; other conditions may take several days before becoming manifest. Sunburn may subside within hours, but the redness of most photodermatoses persists for days. (Solar urticaria is the exception and usually lasts only about an hour.)

2. Does the condition show a seasonal occurrence?

Note: PMLE often begins in the late spring in northern latitudes.

3. What are the effects of artificial light and light passing through window glass or clothing?

Note: Photoeruptions produced through glass or clothing or brought on by exposure to white fluorescent light are indicative of UVA (long wavelength) sensitivity, i.e., porphyria and chemical photoreactions. (Fluorescent white bulbs give off 365 nm light in small amounts.)

4. Are symptoms of itching or burning present?

Note: EPP may cause burning or paresthesias.

5. Is the patient using any drugs or topical materials?

Note: Demethylchlortetracycline and coal tar are the most common offenders in children. Psoralens in flora and in perfumes must be considered.

6. Does the patient have a past history of tumors, mental retardation, unstable gait, intolerance to foods, arthropathies, or liver or gallstone problems?

Note: Methods used to rule out inherited and metabolic photoeruptions have been discussed earlier in this chapter.

7. Is there a family history of skin tumors, consanguinity, light sensitivity, skin problems, or inherited diseases?

PHYSICAL EXAMINATION

1. Parts of the body affected abnormally by sunlight include the face, ears, neck, V of chest, outer arms, and dorsal hands. Areas free of rash are under the chin and behind the ears, the palms, and those parts of the body covered by clothing.

Note: When the latter regions are involved, it indicates a severe or altered photosensitivity eruption or non-photodermatitis.

2. What is the appearance of the rash? Is there redness only or raised redness (urticaria), blisters, papules, or plaques?

Note: EPP and solar urticaria may have raised redness, and PMLE may show several types of lesions. Photoeruptions are better characterized by their distribution than by the type of lesion present.

LABORATORY EQUIPMENT AND PROCEDURES

1. A Wood's light (medium pressure mercury bulb) with filter (range UVA) is used in screening urine for EP and PCT. A Wood's light without filter (range UVA, UVB, and UVC) is used for the following: minimal erythema dose (MED) determination, wavelength screening via window glass (long UVA versus others), photo patch and phototoxin testing, and diagnostic disease reproduction.

The unfiltered bulb gives off about three MED's on the back of a light-complexioned person when held at 10 cm for five minutes. Window glass should be placed in the path of one half of the beam, allowing only light of wavelengths greater than 320 nm (i.e., UVA) to pass through. Any redness under the area covered by window glass is abnormal (except that which may occur temporarily if heat is not conducted away). Light through window glass is also used for photo patch testing to determine the cause of or to rule out photoallergy.[63] The reproduction of PMLE and LE by adequate doses of UVB from the Wood's light has been mentioned earlier. This lamp costs about $150. It must be turned on ten minutes before using. The bulb gives off heat that can easily be conducted away by an ordinary fan.

2. Urinalysis is done to detect the orange-pink fluorescence of EP and PCT (under Wood's light) and aminoaciduria of the Hartnup syndrome.

3. Blood tests (fingerstick screening test) are used to diagnose EPP (see pages 134–135).

4. Skin biopsy and immunofluorescence are aids to the diagnosis of PMLE, LE, PCT, and EPP, especially since only PMLE specimens do not fluoresce. They are also used to rule out severe sunburn, photoallergy, atopic dermatitis, and insect bite reactions.

In summary, the office management of suspected pediatric photodermatoses should include taking a thorough light-oriented history and physical examination, performing a skin biopsy and photo tests with an adequate light source, and ordering appropriate screening tests on urine, skin, and blood.

REFERENCES

1. Daniels, F., Jr.: Physical factors in sun exposure. Arch. Dermatol., *85*:358, 1962.
2. Urbach, F., Epstein, J. H., and Forbes, P. D.: Ultraviolet carcinogenesis. *In*: Fitzpatrick, T. B. (ed.): Sunlight and Man. Tokyo, University of Tokyo Press, 1974.
3. Willis, I.: Photosensitivity. Int. Dermatol., *14*:326, 1975.
4. Epstein, J. H.: Photodermatoses. *In* Malkinson, F. D., and Pearson, R. W. (eds.): Yearbook of Dermatology. Chicago, Year Book Medical Publishers, 1971.
5. Berlin, N. I., Van Scott, E. J., Clendenning, W. E., et al.: Basal cell nevus syndrome. Ann. Intern. Med., *64*:403, 1966.
6. Clendenning, W. E., Block, J. E., and Radde, I.: Basal cell nevus syndrome. Arch. Dermatol., *90*:38, 1964.
7. Robbins, J. H., Kraemer, K. H., Lutzner, M. A. et al.: Xeroderma pigmentosum—an inherited disease with sun sensitivity, multiple cutaneous neoplasms, and abnormal DNA repair. Ann. Intern. Med., *80*:221, 1974.
8. Cleaver, J. E.: Defective repair replication of DNA in xeroderma pigmentosum. Nature, *218*:652, 1968.
9. Epstein, J. H., Fukuyama, K., Reed, W. B., et al.: Defect in DNA synthesis in skin of patients with xeroderma pigmentosum demonstrated in vivo. Science, *168*:1477, 1970.
10. Deweerd-Kastelein, E. A., Keijzer, W., and Boorsma, D.: Genetic heterogeneity of xeroderma pigmentosum demonstrated by somatic cell hybridization. Nature, *238*:80, 1972.
11. Kraemer, K. H., Coon, H. G., Petinga, R. A., et al.: Genetic heterogeneity in xeroderma pigmentosum: Complementation groups and their relationship to DNA repair rates. Proc. Natl. Acad. Sci. USA, *72*:59, 1975.
12. Tanaka, K., Sekiguchi, M., and Okada, Y.: Restoration of ultraviolet-induced unscheduled DNA synthesis of xeroderma pigmentosum cells by the concomitant treatment with bacteriophage T4, endonuclease V and HVJ (Sendai virus). Proc. Natl. Acad. Sci. USA, *72*:4071, 1975.
13. Maher, V., Ouellette, L. M., Mittlestate, M., and McCormick, J. J.: Synergistic effect of caffeine on the cytotoxicity of ultraviolet irradiation and of hydrocarbon epoxides in strains of xeroderma pigmentosum. Nature, *258*:760, 1975.
14. Lehmann, A. R., Kirk-Bell, S., Arlett, C. F., et al.: Xeroderma pigmentosum cells with normal levels of excision repair have a defect in DNA synthesis after UV-irradiation. Proc. Natl. Aca. Sci. USA, *72*:219, 1975.
15. Ramsay, C. A., Coltart, T. M., Blunt, S., et al.: Prenatal diagnosis of xeroderma pigmentosum—report of the first successful case. Lancet, *2*:1109, 1974.
16. Kraemer, K. H., and Robbins, J. H.: Xeroderma pigmentosum. *In*: Maddin, S. (ed.): Current Dermatologic Management, St. Louis, C. V. Mosby, 1975, pp. 316–318.
17. Birt, A. R., and Davis, R. A.: Hereditary polymorphic light eruption of American Indians. Int. J. Dermatol., *14*:105, 1975.
18. Magnus, I. A.: Action spectra of various photodermatoses. *In*: Fitzpatrick, T. B. (ed.): Sunlight and Man. Tokyo, University of Tokyo Press, 1974.
19. Haxthausen, H.: Hudsygdomme fremkaldt af Lyset. V. Pios. Boghandel, Povl Branner, Kopenhagen, 1919.
20. Epstein, J. H.: Polymorphous light eruptions; phototest technique studies. Arch. Dermatol., *85*:502, 1962.
21. Swanbeck, G., and Wennersten, G.: Treatment of polymorphous light eruptions with beta-carotene. Acta Derma. Venereol., *52*:462, 1972.
22. Nordlund, J. J., Klaus, S. N., Mathews-Roth, M. M., and Pathak, M. A.: New therapy for polymorphous light eruption. Arch. Dermatol., *108*:710, 1973.
23. Halvorsen, K., and Halvorsen, S.: Hartnup disease. J. Pediatr., *31*:29, 1963.
24. Efron, M. L., and Gallagher, W. F.: Hartnup disease. *In*: Fitzpatrick, T. B., et al. (eds.): Dermatology in General Medicine. New York, McGraw-Hill, 1971.
25. German, J.: Genes which increase chromosomal instability in somatic cells and predispose to cancer. *In*: Steinberg, A. G., and Bearn, A. G., (eds.): Progress in Medical Genetics. New York, Grune & Stratton, 1972.
26. Hutteroth, T. H., Litwin, S. D., and German, J.: Abnormal immune responses of Bloom's syndrome by lymphocytes in vitro. J. Clin. Invest., *56*:1, 1975.
27. Srivastava, R. N., Gupta, P. C., Mayekav, G., and Roy, S.: Cockayne's syndrome in two sisters. Acta Paediatr. Scand., *63*:461, 1974.
28. Macdonald, E. B., Fitch, K. D., and Lewis, I. C.: Cockayne's syndrome. Pediatrics, *25*:997, 1960.

29. Waldman, T. A., and McIntire, K. R.: Serum alpha-feto protein levels in patients with ataxia telangiectasia. Lancet, 2:1112, 1972.
30. Murgita, R. A., and Tomasi, T. B., Jr.: Suppression of the immune response by alpha-feto protein on the primary and secondary antibody response. J. Exp. Med., 141(2): 269, 1975.
31. Taylor, A. M. R., Harnden, D. G., Arlett, C. F., et al.: Ataxia telangiectasia: A human mutation with abnormal radiation sensitivity. Nature, 258:427, 1975.
32. Swift, M.: Genetic syndromes and predisposition to malignant neoplasms. Int. J. Dermatol., 14:733, 1975.
33. Silver, H. K.: Rothmund-Thomson syndrome: An oculocutaneous disorder. Am. J. Dis. Child., 111:182, 1966.
34. Kristensen, J. K.: Poikiloderma congenitiale—an early case of Rothmund-Thomson syndrome. Acta Derma. Venerol., 55:316, 1975.
35. Kansky, A.: Porphyria cutanea tarda in a two year old girl. Br. J. Dermatol., 90:213, 1974.
36. Hunter, J. A. A., Khan, S. A., Hope, E., et al.: Hereditary coproporphyria. Br. J. Dermatol., 84:301, 1971.
37. Cam, C., and Nigogoysan, G.: Acquired toxic porphyria cutanea tarda due to hexachlorobenzene. JAMA, 183:88, 1963.
38. Chisholm, J. J.: Inborn errors of metabolism. In: Vaughan, V. C., and McKay, R. J. (eds.): Nelson Textbook of Pediatrics. 10th ed., Philadelphia, W. B. Saunders, 1975, p. 469.
39. Harber, L. C., and Bickers, D. R.: The porphyrias. In Malkinson, F., et al. (eds.): Yearbook of Dermatology. Chicago, Year Book Medical Publishers, 1975, pp. 9–49.
40. Levere, R. D., and Kappas, A.: The porphyric diseases of man. Hosp. Pract., 5:61, 1970.
41. Seip, M., Thume, P. O., and Eriksen, L.: Treatment of photosensitivity in congenital erythropoietic porphyria with beta-carotene. Acta Derm. Venereol., 54:239, 1974.
42. Scholnick, P., Marver, H. S., and Schmid, R.: Erythropoietic protoporphyria: Evidence for multiple sites of excess protoporphyrin formation. J. Clin. Invest., 50:203, 1971.
43. Konrad, K., Honigsman, H., Gschnait, F., and Wolff, K.: Mouse model for protoporphyria II. Cellular and subcellular events with photosensitivity flare of the skin. J. Invest. Dermatol., 65:300, 1975.
44. Poh-Fitzpatrick, M. B., Piomelli, S., Young, P., et al.: Rapid quantitative assay for erythrocyte porphyrins. Arch. Dermatol., 110:225, 1974.
45. Mathews-Roth, M. M.: For the super light-sensitive: Carotene. Med. World News, 19:90, 1976.
46. Ive, H., Lloyd, J., and Magnus, I. A.: Action spectra in idiopathic solar urticaria. A study of 17 cases with a monochromator. Br. J. Dermatol., 77:229, 1965.
47. Harber, L. C., Holloway, R. M., Wheatley, V. R., and Baer, R.: Immunologic and biophysical studies in solar urticaria. J. Invest. Dermatol., 41:439, 1963.
48. Sams, W. M., Jr.: Solar urticaria: Studies of the active serum factor. J. Allergy Clin. Immunol., 45:295, 1970.
49. Ramsay, C. A.: The treatment of solar urticaria by inducing tolerance to artificial or solar radiation. Proc. 4th American Society of Photobiology Program. Denver, 1976, p. 110.
50. Hanson, V., and Kornreich, H.: Systemic rheumatic disorders ("collagen disease") in childhood: Lupus erythematosus, anaphylactoid purpura, dermatomytosis, and scleroderma. I. Bull. Rheum. Dis., 17.435, 1967.
51. Freeman, R. G., Knox, J. M., and Owens, D. W.: Cutaneous lesions of lupus erythematosus induced by monochromatic light. Arch. Dermatol., 100:677, 1969.
52. Kohler, P.: Inherited complement deficiencies and systemic lupus erythematosus: An immunologic puzzle. Ann. Intern. Med., 82:420, 1975.
53. Agnello, V. S.: C_2, HLA roles in systemic lupus erythematosus. Skin and Allergy News, 7:59, 1976.
54. Levy, S. B.: Deficiency in the second component of complement and lupus erythematosus. Reported at the American Academy of Dermatology, Chicago, 1976.
55. Jordan, R. E., and Provost, T.: In: Malkinson, F. D., and Pearson, R. W. (eds.): Yearbook of Dermatology. Chicago, Year Book Medical Publishers, 1976, p. 9.
56. Nagreh, D. S.: Photodermatitis—study of the condition in Kuantan, Malaysia. Contact Dermat., 1:27, 1975.
57. Cloud, T. M., Hakim, R. E., and Griffin, A. C.: Photosensitization of the eye with methoxsalen: II, Chronic effects. Arch. Ophthalmol., 66:689, 1961.
58. Griffin, A. C., Hakim, R. E., and Knox, J.: The wavelength effect upon erythemal and carcinogenic response in psoralen treated mice. J. Invest. Dermatol., 31:289, 1958.
59. Epstein, E.: Contact dermatitis in children. Pediatr. Clin. North Am., 18:839, 1971.
60. Calnan, C. D., Harman, R. R. M., and Wells, G. C.: Photodermatitis from soaps. Br. Med. J., 73:1266, 1961.
61. Alani, M. D.: Studies on the induction of allergic photodermatitis in newborn guinea pigs. Acta Allergol., 27:50, 1972.
62. Zawahry, M.: Lichen planus tropicus. Dermatologica, 4:251, 1965.
63. Magnus, I. A.: Clinical Aspects of Dermatological Photobiology. Philadelphia, J. B. Lippincott, 1975.

PSORIASIS IN ADOLESCENCE

E. DORINDA LOEFFEL, M.D.

INTRODUCTION

To date, there has been little attempt to differentiate psoriasis in adolescence from psoriasis in other age groups. Psoriasis in teenagers is usually mentioned only as a statistic in studies of childhood psoriasis (up to 16 years of age) or adult psoriasis (over 19 years of age), with emphasis on the age of onset.

With increasing medical awareness of the unique physical changes and special emotional needs that develop during adolescence,[1,2] it seems appropriate to consider psoriasis in teenagers from a separate viewpoint, searching for characteristics that set it apart from psoriasis in other age groups. An attempt to understand the psychiatric implications of the disease for teenagers is particularly important, so that physicians can anticipate crises precipitated by psoriasis and perhaps help prevent them.

Many of the ideas in this chapter have come directly from teenage patients, who often seem relieved to discuss their special problems and also seem surprised that somebody is willing to listen. Gaining the confidence of a teenager with psoriasis through concerned attention is often a key step toward developing a plan of treatment whose success depends on the willing cooperation of the patient.

PREVALENCE

Psoriasis in adolescence is not a skin problem commonly encountered by the dermatologist or pediatrician, although most physicians care for at least a few such patients. Adolescent patients with psoriasis generally are widely scattered, so that there are few accumulated data available. The true prevalence of teenage psoriasis is unknown, although several studies[3-8] suggest that over one third of all patients with psoriasis first develop symptoms before or during adolescence. The prevalence of psoriasis in the general population has been estimated to be 1 to 3 per cent in several countries,[3, 4, 9–11] with between two and eight million people affected in the United States alone.[12] The recently completed National Health Survey found the prevalence of psoriasis among 50,000 randomly selected people between one and 74 years of age to be 0.55 per cent.[13] If this figure is extrapolated to the entire population (approximately 220 million), about 1.2 million people have psoriasis, of whom at least 400,000 experienced it as teenagers.

AGE OF ONSET

Several studies of psoriatic patients suggest that the peak time of onset of the disease occurs before the age of 20. A 1975 study in Great Britain found that the peak age of onset was between five and nine in girls and between 15 and 20 in boys, with an overall peak age of onset (regardless of sex) between 15 and 20.[3] In the same study of 419 patients with psoriasis, 34.8 per cent of males and 39.4 per cent of females developed the disease before the age of 20. A 1954 British study showed similar findings, with psoriasis beginning before the age of 20 in 34.5 per cent of males and 40.9 per cent of females.[5] In Scandinavia, approximately 45 per cent of all patients with psoriasis experience onset of the disease before the age of 16.[6] In the Faroe Islands, 70.5 per cent of males and 74.9 per cent of females with psoriasis had developed it before the age of 20, with a median age of onset of 12 years in females and 13 years in males.[4] In the United States, estimates of onset before age 20 vary from 31.8 per cent of 464 consecutive psoriasis patients[7] to 35 per cent of 5600 psoriatic patients responding to a questionnaire.[8] From 9 to 10 per cent of psoriasis cases in the United States apparently begin in the age group under 10 years.[7, 8] In Japan, one study of psoriasis patients revealed that 19 per cent of patients developed the disease between 10 and 19 years of age.[14]

During childhood and early adolescence, psoriasis is seen more frequently in girls than in boys and also appears to start earlier in girls. Approximately twice as many girls (180 patients) as boys (88 patients) developed the disease before age 16 in one United States study of 268 childhood cases.[15] Similar findings were noted in Denmark, with 64 per cent of 245 children under age 16 being female in one study,[6] and 68 of 100 children being female in another.[16] In the group of 245 Danish childhood cases, the average age of onset was 7.8 years for girls and 8.5 years for boys.[6] In Great Britain, 60.5 per cent of 157 patients who developed psoriasis before age 20 were female.[3]

INHERITANCE

There is little doubt that psoriasis is an inherited disease, although it often appears capriciously among family members. In the Faroe Islands, where all family members could be examined directly, a familial incidence of 91 per cent was found.[17] Other studies have found lower but significant percentages of positive family histories of psoriasis, generally in the range of 34 per cent[18] to 36 per cent.[19] The onset of psoriasis at an early age is likely to be associated with recognized familial tendencies.[18] A positive history of psoriasis among relatives of children and adolescents with psoriasis has been found in 40 to 48 per cent of those studied in Great Britain,[18] 52 per cent in the United States,[15] and 59 per cent in Denmark.[6]

If neither parent has the disease, approximately 2.45 per cent[7] to 7.5 per cent[20] of the patient's siblings will have psoriasis. However, if one parent has psoriasis, the percentage of affected siblings increases to between 9 and 15 per cent.[7, 20] If both parents have psoriasis, approximately 50 per cent of the siblings of an affected offspring will also develop the disease.[20] If one parent has psoriasis, the offspring who develops psoriasis will almost always manifest it by the age of 30.[3]

A strong genetic influence has also been demonstrated in twins, who are considered to be an "affected twin pair" if either or both have psoriasis. In one study of 41 affected pairs of monozygotic twins, each twin of 30 pairs developed psoriasis at an early age.[21] In 13 of these 30 affected pairs, psoriasis occurred in each twin before the age of 10 years.[21] Another study reported finding psoriasis in both twins in 13 out of 21 affected pairs of monozygous twins.[22]

It has been postulated that the inheritance of psoriasis is multifactorial, needing a combination of genetic and environmental factors to induce it.[20, 23] Statistical analysis of family history data from 698 psoriatic patients is more consistent with multifactorial inheritance than with any simple mode of inheritance, such as autosomal dominant or recessive patterns.[20, 23] There is also an association between psoriasis and the inheritance of certain HL-A histocompatibility antigens, particularly Bw17, B13, B27, and Bw37.[24]

PRECIPITATING FACTORS

Many environmental stimuli seem to precipitate psoriatic lesions, including drug eruptions, emotional crises, and surgical procedures with resulting cutaneous scars. In children and teenagers, two factors appear to be of major importance: systemic infections and localized trauma to the skin.

The most common infection to precipitate psoriasis is streptococcal pharyngitis, which usually precedes a flare of psoriasis by two to three weeks. The resulting psoriasis is usually of the guttate type (Plate I–A), with hundreds of tiny lesions appearing suddenly over the trunk and extremities.[25] In one Danish study of children with psoriasis, 38 out of 245 children had the initial onset of psoriasis after a sore throat, while 113 out of 245 children had subsequent aggravation of psoriasis following pharyngitis.[6] An elevated antistreptolysin O (ASO) titer of over 200 Todd units was present in 60 per cent of the children in the same study.

Another Danish study revealed that 38 of 100 children initially developed psoriasis after sore throats, and 58 had serological evidence of preceding beta-hemolytic streptococcal infection.[16] A study in Sweden reported that 64 per cent of 65 patients with guttate psoriasis had sore throats preceding the psoriasis flares, and that 65 per cent had elevated ASO titers.[26] In a retrospective study of 5600 patients, Farber and Nall[8] found that sore throats reportedly precipitated the onset of psoriasis in 17 per cent of children who developed the disease before age 10 and in 32 per cent of children who developed it between the ages of 10 and 19. Another study in the United States found elevated ASO titers in 17 out of 20 patients with acute psoriasis, in contrast to only one patient in 50 with chronic plaque-type psoriasis.[26]

TABLE 7-1 PRECIPITATING CAUSES OF PSORIASIS LESIONS IN ADOLESCENTS

Precipitating Cause	Injury to Skin
ATHLETICS	Abrasions, lacerations, scratches Wear and tear injuries (rope burn, karate chop) Abrasions caused by rubbing of athletic uniform or equipment (football pads, catcher's mask, bathing suit, tennis racquet, saddle) Sunburn Insect bite Poison ivy (oak) dermatitis
COSMETIC PRACTICES	Nicking and perifollicular lesions caused by shaving, especially legs and underarms, and eyebrow plucking Infection caused by ear piercing Damage to hair caused by hot comb straightening, sleeping on curlers, and use of irritating sprays and dyes Contact allergy from perfumes, soaps, cosmetics, aftershave lotion
HOBBIES	Chemical irritation from exposure to solvents (painting, photography) Abrasion caused by rubbing of tools (gardening, carpentry, sewing, hunting)
WORK	Chemical irritation (housework, hairdressing) Abrasion caused by rubbing of tools and equipment (farming, construction)
STUDY HABITS	Pressure and abrasion from writing, typing, leaning on elbows
NERVOUS HABITS	Abrasion and infection from biting nails, rubbing skin
CLOTHING AND JEWELRY	Pressure and constriction of shoes (heel, toe, Achilles tendon), girdle, wristwatch, eyeglasses, belt, bra
MEDICAL PROCEDURES	Surgical scars (elective and cosmetic surgery should be avoided, especially on the face) Reaction to allergy test (scratch and intradermal) Reaction to smallpox vaccination Reaction to liquid nitrogen treatment Rubbing of plaster cast
OTHER CONDITIONS THAT TRAUMATIZE THE SKIN	Sunburn Insect bites Contact dermatitis Generalized drug eruption Herpes simplex Herpes zoster Acne Pityriasis rosea Furuncles Tinea pedis Tinea cruris Perianal candidiasis

It has been postulated that a streptococcal toxin may be deposited in dermal capillaries, causing damage to both vessels and overlying skin.[27] A similar mechanism could also be postulated for other infections that precipitate flares of psoriasis, including scarlet fever, chickenpox, measles, sinusitis, and infected dentition. If these infections do indeed act as endogenous stimuli that traumatize the skin, they could induce subsequent psoriatic lesions through a mechanism known as the Koebner phenomenon.[16] This refers to the ability of a traumatic stimulus applied to clinically normal skin to cause the formation of a psoriasis lesion in the damaged area (Plate II–B). It has been shown that both dermal and epidermal injury are necessary to induce a Koebner response.[28, 29] Although external physical trauma is most commonly associated with this response, the role of endogenous trauma also needs to be considered. In addition to streptococcal toxin, bacteremia, and viremia (Plate II–B), perhaps other circulating substances, such as drugs or hormones, could induce a Koebner response.[30] Conceivably, two factors that commonly cause psoriasis to flare—stress and the withdrawal of systemic steroids or other immunosuppressive drugs—somehow induce a Koebner response.

External trauma to the skin usually induces lesions of psoriasis in injured areas 10 to 14 days following trauma,[29] with a range of seven to 29 days.[30] Although this phenomenon probably occurs eventually in most cases, many patients fail to recognize it until the association is pointed out. In a questionnaire study, only 11 per cent of 1537 patients with psoriasis seemed aware of the role of trauma.[19] Various other studies have found higher degrees of awareness, reaching 40, 47, 52, and 76 per cent of patients sampled.[8, 10, 15, 31]

Many types of external trauma have been implicated as causes of the Koebner phenomenon, most of which produce well-demarcated lesions of psoriasis localized to small areas. Many of these apply particularly to teenagers and can be conveniently grouped according to typical adolescent activities. A list of common causes of Koebner responses is found in Table 7–1, and several are illustrated in Plate II–B to E.

SIGNS OF PSORIASIS

Certain areas of the body are especially prone to develop psoriatic lesions and should be routinely checked during a skin examination. These areas include the scalp, ears, forehead, eyebrows, trunk, elbows, knees, nails, gluteal crease, and genitalia (Plate III–A, B, D, and E and Plate IV–A). The patient may be unaware of some of the lesions, especially in the nails and gluteal cleft. Unsuspected lesions that have not been altered by previous treatment may be extremely helpful in establishing the diagnosis.

In children and adolescents, psoriasis is often first noticed in the scalp, where it may be mistaken for seborrheic dermatitis or tinea capitis (Plate VIII–D). In one study, the scalp was involved in 82 per cent of children with psoriasis.[6] Lesions varied from well-demarcated erythematous plaques with thick silvery scale to generalized erythema with thick adherent scale resembling a cap. The scale of psoriasis is non-greasy (in contrast to seborrheic dermatitis) and reappears in profusion within 24 hours after shampooing the hair. When the scalp is involved, thick scale often accumulates behind the ears and may also be present inside the ears, where it forms thick waxy plugs that may itch or interfere with hearing.

Scalp lesions frequently involve the frontal hairline and may extend downward onto the upper forehead. Patients with such lesions often wear a hairstyle that effectively covers the upper part of the face. In general, children and adolescents have much more facial involvement than do adults. Nyfors[6] found facial lesions in 43 per cent of affected children. Lesions may involve the eyebrows and nasolabial folds, as in seborrheic dermatitis, or may occur in a perioral distribution. At times, the entire forehead may be involved. Sunburn may induce lesions over the entire face or in a butterfly distribution over the cheeks and nose. The pressure of glasses rubbing on the nose, temples, or posterior auricular folds may also induce lesions. Facial lesions are among the most distressing to teenagers, interfering with their self-image and greatly diminishing their self-confidence. Lesions on the face cannot be hidden, although girls can sometimes cover them with makeup. Any type of lesion remaining on the face may lead to dissatisfaction with treatment, even if other psoriatic lesions have cleared.

Certain areas of the body tend to develop the thick, scaly, irregularly-shaped plaques commonly associated with psoriasis, although in children and teenagers the plaques tend to be thinner, softer, and less permanent than in adults.[15] In addition to the scalp, the elbows and knees are typical locations of psoriatic plaques. On the chest and back, plaques sometimes become confluent, forming geographic patterns resembling a map (Plate III–C). On the trunk and elsewhere, the plaques are often strikingly symmetrical. The thickest plaques are frequently located on the lower legs, especially over the shins.

The trunk is the area most commonly involved in the typical guttate flare of psoriasis (Plates II–A and III–C), in which hundreds of tiny lesions may erupt suddenly. These lesions are usually ovoid, thin, and only slightly scaly, are 2 mm to 1 cm in diameter, and are scattered evenly over the trunk and proximal extremities. The face is sometimes involved, but the palms, soles, and distal extremities are usually spared. As discussed earlier, a guttate flare is frequently associated with a streptococcal throat infection. Some clinicians believe that guttate lesions are the most common type of psoriasis lesions seen in childhood.[32] In the two Danish studies, 44 per cent and 34 per cent of children with psoriasis had developed guttate lesions.[6,16] It is estimated that psoriasis begins as a guttate explosion in 14 to 17 per cent of all patients.[23] Guttate flares tend to continue throughout the teenage years and into early adulthood but decrease with age. This presentation of psoriasis must be differentiated particularly from pityriasis rosea, secondary syphilis, and maculopapular generalized drug eruption.

Lesions similar to guttate psoriasis but centered around hair follicles are seen fairly commonly in children and teenagers, although they are rare in adults.[32] Such *follicular psoriasis* is sometimes localized to the anterior tibial and olecranon areas, where it occurs as patches of horny spikes.[32] In teenage girls, the follicular localization on the legs is probably the result of trauma to the hair follicles caused by shaving. Follicular psoriasis may also be more generalized, at times resembling pityriasis rubra pilaris[32] or widespread guttate psoriasis.

Psoriasis may occur primarily on the palms and soles, sparing most other body areas (Plate IV–B). These lesions are usually symmetrical and often involve only part of the palm or sole. They must be distinguished from contact dermatitis, atopic eczema, and dermatophyte infection. At times, the lesions of the palms and soles become very thick and develop deep, painful, linear fissures. Occasionally, such lesions may contain many large sterile pustules, although this is uncommon in children and teenagers. Psoriasis lesions on the palms and soles sometimes develop as a Koebner response to various activities. Holding a tennis racquet, baseball bat, or hammer may induce lesions on the palms and fingers, and the rubbing of boots or shoes during strenuous activity may cause lesions on the feet.

A clue to the diagnosis of psoriasis on the hands and feet may come from examination of the nails, which undergo characteristic changes in up to 50 per cent of patients.[33-35] These changes include tiny pits or indentations in the nail plate, thickening of the nail plate with hyperkeratotic crumbly debris beneath the nail, and onycholysis of the nail plate as it becomes separated from the nail bed. This permits air to enter underneath the nail plate and results in white opaque discoloration of the distal edge of the nail (Plate IV–A). The frequency of nail changes in teenagers has not been reported but presumably lies between the 14 per cent occurrence reported in children[6] and the 50 per cent estimated for adults.[8, 33-34]

Psoriasis in the genital area occurs in children and teenagers, although its frequency is difficult to determine. The Stanford questionnaire study found that 49 per cent of males and 33 per cent of females reported genital involvement, and 44 per cent of the entire group reported perianal involvement at some time during the course of the disease.[8] The perianal and gluteal cleft areas and the umbilicus tend to be untreated by the patient and should always be examined when the diagnosis of psoriasis is in doubt (Plate IV–C). Lesions in these areas are likely to be moist, macerated, and fissured.[36] In infants, this probably represents a Koebner response to irritation of the skin produced by urine, diapers, and fecal material.[37] Occasionally, involvement of the genital area may persist through childhood and into adolescence. In girls, such psoriasis tends to be found in the mons pubis, labia majora, and inguinal folds. Irritation of the labia due to vaginal moniliasis with itchy discharge may induce a Koebner response, as may the pressure of a girdle, garter belt, or underpants with elastic leg bands. In boys, psoriasis lesions in the genital area tend to be localized to the penis, inguinal folds, and perianal area. Teenage males may develop lesions from the rubbing of athletic supporters or condoms. Genital lesions become particularly embarrassing to both sexes when they become sexually active.

SYMPTOMS OF PSORIASIS

The symptoms of psoriasis generally fall into the categories of itching, pain, and emotional stress.

Itching. Many patients with psoriasis never experience itching or have it only mildly and occasionally, while others suffer from severe intermittent or constant itching. The pruritus that occurs in psoriasis is frequently worse at night (as it is in many skin diseases) and may interfere with sleep. Sweating precipitated by active exercise, hot baths, electric blankets, and sunbathing may trigger itching. Some patients experience severe pruritus after the application of tar-containing medications, which may rule out their use.

Pain. Pain occurring with psoriasis usually results from the development of fissures, infection, or arthritis.

FISSURES. Fissures are deep linear cracks that develop in thick plaques of psoriasis exposed to the stress of movement, such as extension or flexion of the hand or digit. They occur most commonly on the hands and feet, particularly on the fingers, palms, soles, heels, and plantar base of the toes. The fissures extend into the dermis, involving many nerve fibers, and are consequently very sensitive to trauma. They often cause complete disability, interfering with walking and preventing working with the hands. A few people also develop painful fissures in thick plaques located on the trunk and thighs.

SUPERFICIAL INFECTION. Pain associated with psoriatic lesions may also result from infection of plaques with *Staphylococcus aureus* (Plate IV–D). Approximately 50 per cent of patients with psoriasis are carriers of *Staphylococcus aureus*, with organisms much more numerous on psoriatic plaques than on normal skin.[38] Psoriatic lesions may become heavily colonized by *Staphylococcus aureus* without signs of clinical infection.[39, 40] At times, however, the infected plaques develop clinical signs of infection, including suppuration and crusts.[38] Such impetiginized lesions become covered by thick or thin yellow crusts overlaying moist red surfaces. These lesions are usually tender and are frequently surrounded by erythema and edema. If the infected lesions are on the legs, pitting edema may develop on the feet.

ARTHRITIS. Pain associated with psoriasis may also result from coexisting arthritis (Plate V–A), since approximately 8 per cent of patients with psoriasis suffer from an associated erosive arthritis.[41] Although children and teenagers seldom develop psoriatic arthropathy,[6, 42] they occasionally have asymmetrical involvement of a few scattered joints, particularly the terminal interphalangeal joints of the fingers and toes. Severe psoriasis of the fingers and toes with marked nail involvement is associated with erythematous, painful, sausage-like swelling of the digits.[43] In teenagers, the sacroiliac joint is seldom affected by arthritis, in contrast to adults with psoriatic arthritis. Arthritis beginning during the teenage years may continue to worsen, leading occasionally to marked crippling and disability in young adulthood. Psoriatic arthritis should be suspected in seronegative patients who lack rheumatoid nodules but have erosive arthritis of the terminal interphalangeal (TIP) joints and asymmetrical involvement of other joints, including metatarsophalangeal joints and the sacroiliac joint.[43] The determination of the HL-A histocompatibility antigens may be a helpful diagnostic test, as HL-A B27 is strongly associated with psoriatic arthritis, ankylosing spondylitis, Reiter's disease, and postinfectious reactive arthritis.[44]

Emotional Stress. In many teenagers, the most serious symptoms connected with psoriasis are emotional. Emotional strain is commonly expressed as embarrassment, pent-up hostility with depression, and worry about the future.

EMBARRASSMENT. Like most patients with psoriasis, teenagers become very concerned about their appearance. They worry especially about what their friends think of their "ugly skin" and fear social ostracism within their peer group. They are extremely embarrassed by their skin and go to great lengths to hide the disease with clothing and makeup. The inability to go swimming in a public place or to participate in certain athletic activities that would reveal their skin frequently causes them great unhappiness. Adolescents are also embarrassed by the excessive scale that forms on their skin, including severe dandruff on the scalp, which leads to teasing by their peers. Fear of leaving a trail of scale often rules out the common teenage activity of spending the night at a friend's house, as the patient does not want to leave embarrassing scale in the bed or on the floor.

HOSTILITY WITH DEPRESSION. Embarrassment often merges with hostility when the teenager is faced with the common questions, "What is the matter with your skin?" and "Is it catching?" Patients usually answer with something about a "skin allergy," not liking to mention the term "psoriasis," which usually engenders further questions and explanations. Teenagers deeply resent these questions and may become very hostile toward the people who ask them, particularly if they are curious casual acquaintances or complete strangers. In addition, they may experience a gnawing irritation brought on by anger at their own skin,[45] which is in a "constant state of disgrace," as one teenager put it. This underlying tension seems to be continuously present when skin lesions are visible or threatening to erupt, and it may lead to serious depression. Well-meaning parents and friends who suggest new types of treatment unconsciously add to feelings of anger and depression. Sometimes, a teenager will completely withdraw from social relationships with friends and family, spending most of his time alone. Alcohol or drugs may become a substitute for friendship. The teenager may refuse to apply any type of treatment, saying "What's the use, since the psoriasis will come right back." This attitude is particularly upsetting to parents, who may unconsciously nag the teenager about applying treatment. In some cases, psoriasis probably serves to magnify pre-existing poor relationships with parents and friends, becoming the "root of all evil" in the patient's mind.

WORRY ABOUT THE FUTURE. In the later years of adolescence, teenagers begin to worry about how their future will be affected by psoriasis, especially if the disease is severe and cosmetically disfiguring. They doubt that anyone will hire them, and they may even lack the self-confidence to seek a job. They also worry about marriage, concluding that they are far too ugly to be sexually desirable. Certain lesions of psoriasis, such as thickened fingernails or severe dandruff, may become focal points that damage the teenager's self-image. Unfortunately, the high premium put on good looks during adolescence fosters the fear of physical imperfection and may keep a shy teenager with psoriasis from ever attempting any social relationships. Later, this same fear may stifle physical intimacy, with the patient's being unwilling to shock a potential sexual partner with the sight of florid psoriasis. Even if these physical and emotional barriers are successfully bridged, the worry about having children who are affected by psoriasis may replace them. Many teenagers worry about passing the disease to their children, and some conclude that they either should not marry or else should never have children.

Fortunately, many teenagers cope with psoriasis without apparent difficulty, accepting it as a necessary evil that must be tolerated. Many of them may have only mild psoriasis, while others with more severe disease are probably well adjusted and secure both at home and at school and receive constant reassurance that "beauty is more than skin deep."

DIAGNOSIS

Prior to beginning treatment, the diagnosis of psoriasis should be documented by photographs showing typical skin lesions (Plate V–B, a and b) or by a skin biopsy showing typical histopathological development. Treatment rapidly alters the appearance of psoriatic plaques, which become flat, less red, and non-scaly. Histologically, skin lesions also change rapidly with treatment, particularly if topical steroid preparations are used.

A skin biopsy specimen can be obtained easily with a 3 mm punch, which causes a small round wound that should be closed with a stitch to promote healing. The characteristic histopathological changes in psoriasis include: acanthosis, elongation of the rete ridges (Plate V–C), layered parakeratosis (nuclei retained in the thickened stratum corneum), thinning of the granular layer, clubbing of the dermal papillae, and mild inflammatory cell infiltrate in the dermis.

The diagnosis needs to be documented for future reference by other physicians, who may have to treat the patient when the skin lesions are atypical of psoriasis. The diagnosis of psoriasis may be very difficult to make, particularly if the presenting lesions are intertriginous, palmoplantar, or pustular, or if they resemble a generalized erythroderma.

PROGNOSIS

Psoriasis is a chronic disease whose exacerbations and remissions are often unpredictable. The Stanford questionnaire survey of adults with psoriasis found that remissions of the disease occur in approximately 39 per cent of patients.[8] In contrast, another study of patients under the age of 16 found that psoriasis was persistent in only 71 of 245 patients (29 per cent).[6] In general, the course of psoriasis tends to be more severe and persistent when it begins in childhood than when it begins later in life.[4, 15, 18, 23]

The effects of psoriasis on major life decisions, such as education, occupation, and marriage, are difficult to determine and probably not fully recognized by most patients. In Sweden, a study to determine the influence of psoriasis on socioeconomic factors revealed that older adults who had developed psoriasis before age 20 had had significantly fewer marriages.[46] Psoriasis as a factor in divorce was cited by 18 per cent of men and 7 per cent of women interviewed.[46] In general, the onset of psoriasis before age 20 did not affect either the level of education or the choice of employment. Education was believed to have been significantly influenced by psoriasis in 11 per cent of males and 16 per cent of females, while choice of vocation was affected in 19 per cent of males and 14 per cent of females. Psoriasis was felt to have a detrimental effect on work in 11 per cent of males and 8 per cent of females, and work was felt to adversely affect psoriasis in 19 per cent of males and 14 per cent of females. Psoriasis led to a change of occupation in 16 per cent of males and 9 per cent of females. Overall, the questioning of psoriatic patients of all ages led to the conclusion that psoriasis influenced education, vocation, and present occupation in 30 per cent of males and 20 per cent of females.[46]

TREATMENT

The treatment suggested to a teenage patient will necessarily depend on the type and extent of psoriasis and on the evaluation of possible precipitating factors. Other considerations that will influence the choice of treatment include: emotional state of the patient, cooperation of the parents, travel time required to obtain treatment, availability of inpatient and outpatient facilities for intensive care, season of the year in climates where the amount of natural sunlight varies greatly, and cosmetic acceptability of certain therapeutic agents.

Each treatment plan should be tailored as much as possible to the convenience of the individual and should allow for the continuation of normal daily activities at school. The patient should be encouraged to participate in the development of a treatment plan that is both practical and cosmetically acceptable. For instance, the teenager may express a preference for ointments (which keep the skin greasy) or for creams in vanishing bases (which are readily absorbed into the skin). The teenager should be put in charge of carrying out his own treatment to encourage cooperation and to eliminate potential friction with oversolicitous parents.

The first step in the treatment of adolescent psoriasis should be evaluation of possible precipitating factors. If guttate psoriasis is present, a search should be made for evidence of beta-hemolytic streptococcal infection. Laboratory studies should include a throat culture, ASO titer, and urinalysis. If a streptococcal infection is present, it should be treated with penicillin or erythromycin. If the adolescent has a history of recurrent "strep throat," the antibiotic should be given in the presence of a guttate flare of psoriasis, even if no current strep infection exists. If recurrent crops of guttate lesions are associated with recurrent streptococcal sore throats and enlarged tonsils, a tonsillectomy should be considered.[47] A retrospective study in Denmark showed that 71 per cent of 74 patients (ages four to 33) with refractory psoriasis experienced marked improvement in their skin condition following tonsillectomy.[47] A similar study in Russia found improvement in 51 of 57 patients with chronic tonsillitis and psoriasis following tonsillectomy.[48]

In addition to throat infections, other sources of infection and possible causes of lesions should be sought. In adolescent boys, fungal infections of the feet and groin should be watched for, along with various lesions induced by athletic activity. Although adolescent girls may also develop lesions from such sports as tennis and horseback riding, their psoriatic lesions are often induced by cosmetic practices. Shaving the legs results in trauma to hair follicle orifices and may induce perifollicular psoriasis lesions, while accidentally nicking the skin with the razor may cause psoriatic lesions in the injured areas. Lesions induced by pressure from jewelry, elastic undergarments, and uncomfortable shoes are also common in adolescent girls. Table 7–1 may be helpful in identifying other sources of a Koebner phenomenon.

Emotional trauma that may precipitate psoriatic lesions should also be discussed with the patient alone and with his parents. Events immediately preceding the development of lesions should be examined, along with major crises and emotional upsets that occurred prior to other episodes of psoriatic exacerbation. It is possible that emotional trauma generated at home can be reduced or eliminated by the physician's meeting with the whole family in order to educate them about the disease and to permit them to express their attitude toward it. Family members need to realize that the disease is chronic, inherited, and not contagious and that it is sometimes magnified by emotional stress. Parents should recognize the adverse effects of continually nagging the adolescent about carrying out treatments. They should also realize the therapeutic benefits of maintaining a harmonious atmosphere at home and of encouraging the adolescent to live a normal life. The family should be advised also that the treatment of psoriasis should not be allowed to dominate family life or disrupt family schedules.

An attempt to anticipate and prevent social and emotional crises at school is also worthwhile. The nature of psoriasis should be explained to teachers, so that students won't be subjected to embarrassing questions or told to "go home and wash with lye soap."* Certain rules may have to be relaxed, such as requirements for taking swimming or basketball, which would unduly expose large areas of skin. Participating in group showers also should not be required, as exposure of the entire skin could prove very humiliating to the adolescent. The negative reaction of classmates and their parents to the disease should also be anticipated. The fear that psoriasis is contagious may cause the patient to be shunned in social situations and force his exclusion from certain group activities.

The pharmacological treatment of psoriasis may be conveniently divided into three approaches: topical, intralesional, and systemic.

TOPICAL TREATMENT

Topical treatment should always be tried first, as it is the safest and one of the most effective methods of treating psoriasis. Unfortunately, it may be both messy and time-consuming, making it at best a nuisance or at worst unacceptable to the patient. Since it does little good to prescribe a therapeutically sound topical program that the patient rejects, every effort should be made to keep medications cosmetically acceptable and to design a program that is simple to carry out and realistic in its time requirements. Before any topical treatment program is declared a failure, the degree of compliance with therapy should be determined, and the patient should be given a two to three week trial of intensive topical treatment under medical supervision in a hospital. If the disease still remains resistant to topical therapy, evaluation for systemic therapy may be undertaken.

Convincing a teenager to try a topical treatment is often the first obstacle to overcome, particularly if he has used topical salves in the past. Like many older patients, the adolescent with psoriasis may quickly become disillusioned with medical care and openly hostile toward any treatment resembling previously prescribed medications. Like other psoriatic patients, the adolescent begins to make the rounds of physicians, searching for a quick and easy "cure," eventually exhausting the resourcefulness of everyone concerned. Such a patient becomes depressed by the chronicity of the disease and frequently grasps at any new treatment promoted in the press, even if it calls for extensive travel or expense. Understandably, the teenager with psoriasis wants a permanent cure for the disease and has difficulty grasping the concept that not all skin disease is curable. It is sometimes helpful to compare the chronicity of psoriasis with that of heart disease or diabetes mellitus in order to demonstrate that successful control is possible, even though no cure is available. Once the teenager understands this, it becomes easier to "sell" a topical program designed to eliminate unsightly lesions and uncomfortable symptoms. Giving

---

*A quotation from a teenage patient.

the patient the hope of looking normal again is extremely important. The physician's enthusiasm will greatly influence the teenager's motivation to carry out a prescribed treatment. Teenagers should never be told, "You are stuck with your psoriasis and had better learn to live with it," since this will quickly discourage them from trying any type of therapy.

Topical treatment should initially include the combined use of tar preparations, topical steroids, and ultraviolet light. While each of these may be effective alone under some circumstances, their combined use greatly increases the likelihood of bringing about a rapid remission of the disease. Any treatment of psoriasis will generally be most successful during the summer months, when exposure to strong natural sunlight has a beneficial effect in most psoriatic cases. If natural sunlight is consistently available, daily exposure between the hours of 10 A.M. and 2 P.M. is recommended, beginning with an exposure time of about 20 minutes for persons of medium pigmentation. Care must be taken to avoid sunburn, which could precipitate new psoriatic lesions in burned areas. The exposure time can usually be increased by about five minutes daily, with the aim of inducing only slight erythema on the skin. Some patients with psoriasis plan periodic vacations to sunny climates for therapeutic sunbathing. This might be considered for teenagers during the Christmas or Easter school vacation, although sunbathing on a public beach may pose psychological problems if the psoriasis is very noticeable.

ULTRAVIOLET LIGHT THERAPY

If natural sunlight is unreliable, a substitute source of ultraviolet light should be found. Small portable sunlamps promoted for home use are not suitable because only a small area of skin can be exposed at any one time. It is too impractical, unreliable, time-consuming, and dangerous* to keep shifting a small light from place to place in order to irradiate all involved areas.

Artificial sunlight exposure can be provided best in a walk-in ultraviolet light booth containing eight or more four-foot-long UVB sunlamp bulbs. A "light box" with 14 bulbs allows an initial safe exposure time of one minute in Caucasians, two minutes in Orientals and Latins, and three minutes in blacks. The treatment time can then be increased by one-minute increments with each successive treatment until the desired point of minimal erythema is reached. Treatment may be given every day or two to three times a week. In a booth with 14 bulbs, the maximum exposure tolerated without burning is usually 10 to 15 minutes for Caucasians and 15 to 25 minutes for blacks.

UVB light sources are also available in many health clubs. UVB light booths are available commercially and may be purchased for home use, although these booths are not standardized and pose some hazards. Plans are available for constructing a home light box, using an empty closet lined with aluminum foil and containing eight bulbs.[49]

During any ultraviolet light therapy, special sunglasses or goggles must be worn to prevent eye damage. Signs reminding the patient to wear these glasses

---

*Dangerous because overlapping areas receive double doses of UV light. Also, these lights are not standardized and change in potency with time.

should be posted outside and inside all ultraviolet light booths. A record of light exposure treatment should also be kept to guard against excessive exposure time, with resulting sunburn. The patient should be warned not to apply perfume, cologne, or aftershave lotion before ultraviolet light exposure, as these substances may contain photosensitizers that can induce severe sunburn.

Tar Preparations

Prior to ultraviolet light exposure, a thin layer of tar should be applied to the skin.[50] This is most easily accomplished by taking a bath containing two capfuls of Zetar emulsion (30 per cent coal tar) or Balnetar (2.5 per cent coal tar), which leave a barely visible coating of tar on the skin. Additional tar should be applied to the skin at bedtime, preferably in the form of a cream or ointment. The traditional preparation of 5 per cent crude coal tar in petrolatum is effective but extremely messy. It may not be practical for home use, since greasy tar will stick to everything the patient touches. A similar problem arises with the use of a coal tar derivative, anthralin (dithranol 0.1, 0.2, or 0.4 per cent) in paste form, which crumbles and falls off the skin, staining bedclothes and carpets. Seville[51] claims to have ameliorated this problem by substituting a stiff ointment for the paste. Another disadvantage of anthralin paste is its irritant potential for normal skin, so that it must be applied only to psoriatic plaques, which is very time-consuming. The advantages of anthralin paste are that it causes rapid flattening of thick psoriatic plaques, and few patients fail to respond.[52]

A more cosmetically acceptable tar-derived preparation is LCD (liquor carbonis detergens), commonly applied in 5 to 10 per cent concentrations in cold cream. Although this cream has a mild tar odor, it rubs into the skin fairly well and does not permanently stain clothing or bedding. Any tar preparation that is used overnight should be washed off in the morning in a bath containing small amounts of liquid tar. If the patient's skin tends to dry out with daily bathing, a bath oil such as Alpha-Keri (which has many of the ingredients contained in Balnetar) may be added to the water.

Topical Steroids

For daytime use, a topical steroid cream or ointment applied once or twice daily to affected skin is helpful.[53] Application should be delayed until after ultraviolet light exposure so as not to interfere with the interaction of tar and light. Patients with dry skin often prefer a steroid ointment that provides long-lasting lubrication, especially in winter. Other patients prefer steroid in a vanishing cream base, which is absorbed into the skin without leaving a greasy film to rub off onto clothing or books.

The choice of a steroid preparation should be governed by both the cost and potency of the compound. Several reasonably economical products are available in half-pound or one-pound jars, including hydrocortisone 1.0 per cent, triamcinolone acetonide 0.025 per cent or 0.1 per cent (Kenalog, Aristocort), and fluocinolone acetonide 0.01 per cent (Synalar). The long-term use of more potent topical steroid preparations, particularly under plastic wrap occlusion, should be discouraged because of possible systemic absorption[53] and localized cutaneous atrophy.[54] In particular, the very potent topical steroids such as betamethasone 17-valerate (Valisone), fluocinonide (Lidex), and "HP" (high potency) forms of triamcinolone acetonide and fluocinolone acetonide should not be used on the face, where unsightly skin atrophy with marked telangiectasia may develop. If such changes are seen in a patient with psoriatic lesions on the face, hydrocortisone cream should be substituted for the potent compounds to permit the skin to recover from the steroid-induced atrophy.

The advisability of using topical steroids for treatment of psoriasis has been questioned by Seville,[55] since he found the relapse time to be shorter in those patients treated with topical steroids. His study, conducted in 1968, involved hospitalized patients treated with either combinations of topical steroids and dithranol paste or with dithranol paste alone. Patients treated with the combination of topical steroid and dithranol experienced a return of psoriasis lesions within a mean time of 5.3 weeks following discharge from the hospital, in contrast to a mean relapse time of 27.9 weeks in patients treated with dithranol alone, a statistically significant difference. It was postulated that systemic absorption of steroids had occurred with transient pituitary-adrenal suppression, which caused a rebound of psoriasis when the steroids were removed.

Therapy for Lesions of Scalp and Nails

Psoriatic lesions of the scalp and nails require special types of treatment, since they do not respond well to the therapies described. Most scalp lesions clear with daily tar shampoos, followed by twice daily application of a steroid lotion such as Synalar solution or Valisone lotion. Persistent lesions may also be treated by overnight application of either anthralin (0.4 per cent) scalp pomade or 10 per cent LCD in Nivea oil. Thick scale on the scalp may be loosened prior to shampooing by massaging mineral oil into the scalp and covering it with a hot moist towel for 15 minutes. Scalp lesions often readily respond to treatment, although cessation of treatment may lead to rapid recurrence of scaling. In contrast, nail lesions of psoriasis are a major therapeutic challenge, although sometimes they regress spontaneously during remission of psoriatic lesions.

If nail lesions persist and cause a cosmetic problem to the patient, long-term treatment with topical 1 per cent 5-fluorouracil cream or solution may be undertaken, with twice daily application around the nails.[56] If this fails, injections of small amounts of triamcinolone into the proximal nail folds once monthly may be successful,[57] but it is a painful form of treatment.

INTRALESIONAL THERAPY

The injection of triamcinolone into psoriatic plaques is also helpful when plaques have remained resistant to topical therapy and are present on uncovered parts of the body. Specifically, triamcinolone acetonide 2 to 4 mg/cc may be injected into a plaque with a #27 needle or dermojet. This procedure may be repeated if necessary at monthly intervals. More frequent injections augment the risk of skin atrophy and adrenal suppression. Although corticosteroids can be used with reasonable safety in topical application and intralesional injection, they have too many undesirable effects when they are given systemically. Psoriasis often improves initially with either intramuscular or oral steroids but gradually becomes refractory to the dosage schedule and requires higher and higher doses for control. Many patients in the past have developed the Cushing syndrome from this treatment, with unfortunate complications of obesity, muscle wasting, diabetes mellitus, and osteoporosis.[53] When systemic corticosteroids are removed from the treatment program, severe generalized psoriasis frequently develops, requiring long periods of hospitalization.

SYSTEMIC THERAPY

Systemic therapy of any type is rarely warranted in the treatment of teenagers with psoriasis. The immediate benefits of such effective systemic agents as the antimetabolites must be weighed against the potential long-term health risks that accompany their use. However, if psoriasis is refractory to topical treatment and has caused physical, emotional, or economic disability, the use of systemic agents should be seriously considered. An adolescence made unhappy by skin disease may permanently destroy self-confidence and scar a personality for life. Every effort should be made to enhance the teenager's self-image at a time when great emphasis is placed on physical appearance.[1] The parents of a teenager with psoriasis are often desperate for help and more than willing to have their child try any treatment that offers help. Too often, physicians shy away from effective systemic agents for fear of potential toxicity to the patient and concomitant medico-legal problems. However, one survey showed that a significant majority of dermatologists would use methotrexate, a systemic medication, if they had psoriasis.[58] Long-term risks must be weighed not only against the appearance of the eruption but also against loss of self-confidence, possibly resulting in severe depression and potential suicide.

The most dependable and most rapidly acting drug available for the treatment of psoriasis is methotrexate, which has now been used for almost 20 years. Methotrexate is a folic acid antagonist that acts to reduce the amount of DNA produced by epidermal cells.[58] The drug effectively inhibits DNA synthesis in rapidly dividing cells in the basal layer of the epidermis. In psoriasis, these cells have a cycle approximately 12 times faster than normal (every 37.5 hours instead of the normal 457 hours).[59] Since the psoriatic cell cycle is approximately 37 hours, and methotrexate inhibits DNA synthesis for a minimum of 12 hours, three doses of methotrexate given 12 hours apart will theoretically affect an entire population of psoriatic basal cells.[60] This principle provides the basis for the weekly dosage schedule of methotrexate most commonly used.

Therapy is started with one tablet (2.5 mg). Methotrexate is next administered the same day of the following week, when two tablets are taken 12 hours apart. The third week, one tablet is given three times over a 36-hour period. The number of tablets is increased at the rate of two or three per week to a maximum of three to four tablets every 12 hours for three doses. This schedule allows a prolonged rest period for the recovery of non-psoriatic dividing cells that might have been affected by the drug. It also decreases the side effects that may result from taking larger doses of methotrexate with shorter rest periods. These include bone marrow suppression, mouth ulcerations, and liver damage. Undesirable and sometimes serious side effects found with the 36-hour administration schedule are nausea, weakness, and stomach irritation. These complications may necessitate discontinuing this form of therapy.

The long-term effects of methotrexate remain uncertain, particularly those related to liver toxicity.[61] Prior to initiating methotrexate treatment, a thorough laboratory evaluation should be made of the patient's renal, hepatic, and hematological systems. A liver biopsy is also recommended, particularly if the patient drinks significant amounts of alcohol or has any history of liver problems.[12] During methotrexate therapy, the patient's white blood count should be checked at least once monthly, and a complete blood count and liver and kidney function tests should be repeated every three to four months. Once a complete remission of psoriasis has been obtained, the drug should be stopped. The patient should be made to understand that methotrexate may not be taken continuously over many years because of its potential toxicity and that *it is contraindicated in pregnancy.**

Another antimetabolite drug, hydroxyurea, is also useful and perhaps safer in treating psoriasis, even in the presence of liver damage.[63-65] Hydroxyurea, which is commonly used to treat chronic myelogenous leukemia, selectively inhibits DNA synthesis by interrupting the cell cycle at the same phase as methotrexate. The dose of hydroxyurea is 0.5 g twice daily. The maximum response to hydroxyurea is usually seen after eight weeks, and the drug should be discontinued after 12 weeks for a rest period of at least three to four weeks. A second course of hydroxyurea may then produce a maximum response in about three weeks.

The most frequent systemic effect of hydroxyurea is macrocytosis, although reversible marrow suppression, with depressed white blood cells, hemoglobin, and platelets, also occurs. Complete blood counts with platelet counts should be performed approximately every two weeks to guard against significant marrow depression. Other side effects include lassitude, vertigo, mouth ulcers, nasal, rectal, and vaginal bleeding, and a flu-like syndrome.[64] In addition to blood counts, laboratory tests should include monthly evaluation of liver and kidney functions. The drug should be withheld if the white blood count drops below 4000 per cu mm, indicating the presence of bone marrow depression. The lowest possible effective dose of hydroxyurea should be used as maintenance. The drug should be stopped if the skin clears completely.

The administration of antimetabolite drugs in teenage psoriasis is controversial, and their use should not be encouraged or prolonged. However, they may provide a helpful temporary crutch during times of serious emotional trouble. In rare cases, they become absolutely vital for controlling severe psoriasis. The antimetabolites generally represent the "ace in the hole" treatment that succeeds when all other forms of treatment fail. However, they should be treated with respect.

SUPPORTIVE THERAPY

A final part of the treatment of adolescent psoriasis is the physician's active interest in the patient's problems. The patient should be encouraged to

---

*Patients should be advised that this drug may cause fetal deformity.

ventilate anxiety. Certain topics tend to cause great concern, including strained relationships with parents, emotional and social problems resulting from psoriasis (such as fear of sexual activity and pregnancy), and vocational plans that might be influenced by psoriasis. The physician should particularly watch for signs of depression related to the skin disease. If great unhappiness develops, consideration should be given to group therapy sessions for teenagers with psoriasis.

In summary, the following steps should be included in treatment of teenage psoriasis:

1. Evaluate possible precipitating causes, including throat infections, emotional trauma, and sources of physical trauma to the skin.

2. Anticipate and attempt to prevent emotional crises at home and school by educating the teenager's family and teachers about psoriasis.

3. Encourage the teenager to participate in the development of a treatment plan that is realistic in terms of time, convenience, and ease of administration.

4. Begin treatment with topical application of cosmetically acceptable tar preparations followed by ultraviolet light exposure. Daily tar shampoos should be included as well as topical steroid preparations for the skin and scalp. Consider hospitalization to carry out this treatment under supervision, particularly if the disease is widespread and the patient is greatly discouraged or depressed.

5. If topical therapy fails, consider the use of systemic drugs for short periods to tide the teenager over emotional crises.

6. Encourage the teenager to talk about personal problems related to psoriasis, and give friendly guidance whenever possible.

REFERENCES

1. Delano, J. G.: Psychiatric implications of the teenager's problems. JAMA, *184*:125, 1963.
2. Blotcky, M. J.: Adolescence—When isn't it "just a phase?" JAMA, *237*:2232, 1977.
3. Holgate, M. C.: The age-of-onset of psoriasis and the relationship to parental psoriasis. Br. J. Dermatol., *92*:443, 1975.
4. Lomholt, G.: Psoriasis: Prevalence, Spontaneous Course, and Genetics: A Census Study on the Prevalence of Skin Diseases in the Faroe Islands. Copenhagen, GAD, 1963.
5. Ingram, J. T.: The significance and management of psoriasis. Br. Med. J., *2*:823, 1954.
6. Nyfors, A., and Lemholt, K.: Psoriasis in children—A short review and a survey of 245 cases. Br. J. Dermatol., *92*:437, 1975.
7. Steinberg, A. G., Becker, S. W., Fitzpatrick, T. B., and Kierland, R. R.: A genetic and statistical study of psoriasis. Am. J. Hum. Genet., *3*:267, 1951.
8. Farber, E. M., and Nall, M. L.: The natural history of psoriasis in 5600 patients. Dermatologica, *148*:1, 1974.
9. Ingram, J. T.: The uniqueness of psoriasis. Lancet, *1*:121, 1964.
10. Hellgran, L.: Psoriasis: The Prevalence in Sex, Age, and Occupational Groups in Total Populations in Sweden: Morphology, Inheritance and Association with Other Skin and Rheumatic Diseases. Stockholm, Almquist and Wiksell, 1967.
11. Farber, E. M., and Peterson, J. B.: Variations in the natural history of psoriasis. Calif. Med., *95*:6, 1961.
12. Whedon, G. D.: Introduction to psoriasis. *In*: Farber, E. M., and Cox, A. J. (eds.): Proceedings of the International Conference on Psoriasis. Stanford, Stanford University Press, 1971, pp. 1–2.
13. Johnson, M-L. T.: Prevalence of Dermatological Disease Among Persons 1–74 Years of Age: United States Advance Data from Vital and Health Statistics of the National Center for Health Statistics. No. 4. Washington, D.C., U.S. Dept. of Health, Education and Welfare, 1977.
14. Yasuda, T., Ishikawa, E., and Mori, S.: Psoriasis in the Japanese. *In*: Farber, E. M., and Cox, A. J. (eds.): Proceedings of the International Conference on Psoriasis. Stanford, Stanford University Press, 1971, pp. 25–34.

15. Farber, E. M., and Carlsen, R. A.: Psoriasis in childhood. Calif. Med., *105*:415, 1966.
16. Asboe-Hansen, G.: Psoriasis in childhood. *In*: Farber, E. M., and Cox, A. J. (eds.): Proceedings of the International Conference on Psoriasis. Stanford, Stanford University Press, 1971, pp. 53–59.
17. Lomholt, G.: Environment and genetics in psoriasis. *In*: Farber, E. M., and Cox, A. J. (eds.): Proceedings of the International Conference on Psoriasis. Stanford, Stanford University Press, 1971, pp. 21–24.
18. Church, R.: The prospect of psoriasis. Br. J. Dermatol., *70*:139, 1958.
19. Farber, E. M., Bright, R. D., and Nall, M. L.: Psoriasis: A questionnaire survey of 2144 patients. Arch. Dermatol., *98*:248, 1968.
20. Watson, W., Cann, H. M., Farber, E. M., and Nall, M. L.: The genetics of psoriasis. Arch. Dermatol., *105*:197, 1972.
21. Farber, E. M., Nall, M. L., and Watson, W.: Natural history of psoriasis in 61 twin pairs. Arch. Dermatol., *109*:207, 1974.
22. Haro, A. S.: Psoriasis in twins. Ann. Med. Intern. Fenn., *44*:225, 1955.
23. Watson, W., and Farber, E. M.: Psoriasis in childhood. Pediatr. Clin. North Am., *18*:875, 1971.
24. Karvonen, J., Tiilikainen, A., and Lassus, A.: HL-A antigens in psoriasis. A family study. Ann. Clin. Res., *8*:298, 1976.
25. Maeyens, E., Jr., and Tindall, J. P.: Psoriasis guttata associated with B-hemolytic streptococci. Cutis, *9*:481, 1972.
26. Norrlind, R.: Psoriasis following infections with hemolytic streptococci. Acta Derm. Venereol., *30*:64, 1950.
27. Whyte, H. J., and Baughman, R. D.: Acute guttate psoriasis and streptococcal infection. Arch. Dermatol., *89*:350, 1964.
28. Farber, E. M., Roth, R. J., Ascheim, E., et al.: Role of trauma in isomorphic response in psoriasis. Arch. Dermatol., *91*:246, 1965.
29. Shelley, W. B., and Arthur, R. P.: Biochemical and physiological clues to the nature of psoriasis. Arch. Dermatol., *78*:14, 1958.
30. Holzmann, H., Krapp, R., Hoede, N., and Morsches, B.: Exogenous and endogenous provocation of psoriasis—A contributor to the Koebner phenomenon. Arch. Dermatol. Forsch., *249*:1, 1974.
31. Braun-Falco, O., Burg, G., and Farber, E. M.: Psoriasis: Eine Fragebogenstudie Bei 536 Patienten. Munch. Med. Wochenschr., *114*:1, 1972.
32. Michelson, H. E.: The unusual in psoriasis. Arch. Dermatol., *78*:9, 1958.
33. Crawford, G. M.: Psoriasis of the nails. Arch. Dermatol. Syph., *38*:583, 1938.
34. Zaias, N: Psoriasis of the nail—A clinical-pathologic study. Arch. Dermatol., *99*:567, 1969.
35. Lewin, K., DeWit, S., and Ferrington, R. A.: Nail involvement in psoriasis: A clinicopathological study. *In*: Farber, E. M., and Cox, A. J. (eds.): Proceedings of the International Conference on Psoriasis. Stanford, Stanford University Press, 1971, pp. 111–123.
36. Laouenan, P.: Psoriasis inversus. *In*: Sidi, E., Zagula-Mally, Z. W., and Hincky, M. (eds.): Psoriasis. Springfield, Ill., Charles C Thomas, 1968, p. 34.
37. Andersen, S. L. C., and Thomsen, K.: Psoriasiform napkin dermatitis. Br. J. Dermatol., *84*:316, 1971.
38. Marples, R. R., Heaton, C. L., and Kligman, A. M.: *Staphylococcus aureus* in psoriasis. Arch. Dermatol., *107*:568, 1973.
39. Selwyn, S., and Chalmers, D.: Dispersal of bacteria from skin lesions: A hospital hazard. Br. J. Dermatol., *77*:349, 1965.
40. Noble, W. C., and Savin, J. A.: Carriage of *Staphylococcus aureus* in psoriasis. Br. Med. J., *1*:417, 1968.
41. Wright, V.: Psoriasis and arthritis. Br. J. Dermatol., *69*:1, 1957.
42. Bellaiche, A.: Psoriasis and arthritis. *In*: Sidi, E., Zagula-Mally, Z. W., and Hincky, M. (eds.): Psoriasis. Springfield, Ill., Charles C Thomas, 1968, p. 99.
43. Baker, H., Golding, D. N., and Thompson, M.: Atypical polyarthritis in psoriatic families. Br. Med. J., *2*:348, 1963.
44. Isomaki, H., Koota, K., Martio, J., et al.: HL-A 27 and arthritis. Ann. Clin. Res., *7*:138, 1975.
45. Graham, D. T.: The relation of psoriasis to attitude and to vascular reactions of the human skin. J. Invest. Dermatol., *22*:379, 1954.
46. Molin, L.: Psoriasis. Acta Derm. Venereol., *53*(72):1, 1973.
47. Nyfors, A., Rasmussen, P. A., Lemholt, K., and Eriksen, B.: Improvement of refractory psoriasis vulgaris after tonsillectomy. Dermatologica, *151*:216, 1975.
48. Lukovsky, L. A., Nesterenko, G. B., Tytar, G. M., and Bashmakov, G. V.: The immediate and remote results of tonsillectomy in patients with chronic tonsillitis and psoriasis. Vestn. Otorinolaringol., *32*:23, 1970.
49. Zimmerman, M. C.: Ultraviolet light therapy. Arch. Dermatol., *78*:646, 1958.
50. Grupper, C.: The chemistry, pharmacology, and use of tar in the treatment of psoriasis. *In*:

Farber, E. M., and Cox, A. J. (eds.): Proceedings of the International Conference on Psoriasis. Stanford, Stanford University Press, 1971, pp. 347–356.
51. Seville, R. H.: Simplified dithranol treatment for psoriasis. Br. J. Dermatol., 93:205, 1975.
52. Harris, D. R., and Ferrington, R. A.: The chemistry, pharmacology, and use of anthralin in the treatment of psoriasis. In: Farber, E. M., and Cox, A. J. (eds.): Proceedings of the International Conference on Psoriasis. Stanford, Stanford University Press, 1971, pp. 357–365.
53. Stoughton, R. B.: Corticosteroids in psoriasis. In: Farber, E. M., and Cox, A. J. (eds.): Proceedings of the International Conference on Psoriasis. Stanford, Stanford University Press, 1971, pp. 367–375.
54. Jones, E. W.: Steroid atrophy—A histologic appraisal. Dermatologica, 152(1):107, 1976.
55. Seville, R. H.: Relapse rate of psoriasis worsened by adding steroids to a dithranol regime. Br. J. Dermatol., 95:643–646, 1976.
56. Fredriksson, T.: Topically applied fluorouracil in the treatment of psoriatic nails. Arch. Dermatol., 110:735, 1974.
57. Abell, E.: Treatment of psoriatic nail dystrophy. Br. J. Dermatol., 86:79, 1972.
58. Rees, R. B., Bennet, J. H., and Maibach, H. I.: Methotrexate for psoriasis. Arch. Dermatol., 95:2, 1967.
59. Weinstein, G. D., and Frost, P.: Abnormal cell proliferation in psoriasis. J. Invest. Dermatol., 50:254, 1968.
60. Weinstein, G. D., and Frost, P.: Methotrexate for psoriasis—A new therapeutic schedule. Arch. Dermatol., 103:33, 1971.
61. Weinstein, G. D., Roenigk, H., Maibach. H., et al.: Cooperative study: Psoriasis-liver-methotrexate interactions. Arch. Dermatol., 108:36, 1973.
62. Roenigk, H. R., Jr., Maibach, H. I., and Weinstein, G. D.: Use of methotrexate in psoriasis. Arch. Dermatol., 105:363, 1972.
63. Leavell, U. W., Jr., and Yarbro, J. W.: Hydroxyurea: A new treatment for psoriasis. Arch. Dermatol., 102:144, 1970.
64. Rosten, M.: Hydroxyurea: A new antimetabolite in the treatment of psoriasis. Br. J. Dermatol., 85:177, 1971.
65. Moschella, S. L., and Greenwald, M. A.: Psoriasis with hydroxyurea—An 18 month study of 60 patients. Arch. Dermatol., 107:363, 1973.

PYOGENIC INFECTIONS

PRUDENCE B. STEWARDSON-KRIEGER, M.D.
AND NANCY B. ESTERLY, M.D.

NORMAL CUTANEOUS FLORA

The appropriate interpretation of cultures obtained from cutaneous surfaces requires a knowledge of the normal flora of skin. Because skin is continuously in contact with microbes in the environment, it is often difficult to differentiate pathogenic organisms from those that are resident or commonly transient. Since the cutaneous factors that favor or inhibit the growth of diverse organisms vary with age, the clinician who treats both infants and adolescents is better equipped to interpret laboratory microbial data if he is familiar with the age-related differences of skin flora.

Most of the cutaneous microbial population resides in the superficial stratum corneum and in the upper portion of the hair follicle.[1] Areas of the skin surface with relatively high moisture content, such as the axillae, groin, and toe webs, support substantially greater numbers of organisms than other body areas.[2] The concentration on the skin of free fatty acids produced by the action of cutaneous bacteria on sebaceous gland lipids is a major determinant of microbial selection, increased concentrations being associated with greater inhibition of certain classes of bacteria.[3,4] The skin of the adolescent has less eccrine gland activity and water content and greater sebaceous and apocrine gland activity than that of the preadolescent child. Normal adult skin flora is not established until puberty, when the types (varieties) of host organisms become more limited than in childhood.[5,6]

The normal cutaneous flora is predominantly gram-positive. In most individuals, the skin harbors both aerobic and anaerobic species of *Corynebacterium*, known as diphtheroids. Members of this genus are the most common microbial residents of human skin.[7] These pleomorphic rods, found primarily within the follicular canal, can be cultured from many body regions.[8] Corynebacteria play an important role in the ecology of the cutaneous surface, as some species are capable of hydrolyzing sebum triglycerides to free fatty acids,[3] which inhibit the growth of other species of bacteria. The increased sebaceous gland activity that occurs at puberty allows these organisms to attain their greatest numbers during adolescence, when skin conditions are most favorable for their growth.[5] The diphtheroids are antigenically related to both mycobacteria and *Nocardia*,[9] and some *Corynebacterium* infections were formerly attributed to one of these other bacterial groups. In most instances, diphtheroids are non-pathogenic, but they can become opportunistic pathogens in the debilitated host and are causally related to several specific skin diseases.

The other most common microbial skin residents belong to the family *Micrococcaceae*, which includes the genera *Staphylococcus* and *Micrococcus*.[10] After puberty, the majority of skin staphylococci are *Staphylococcus epidermidis* (formerly *S. albus*), which are found predominantly in the upper part of the hair follicle.[8] They are most frequently recovered from the face, the axillae, and the groin.[11] Together with the diphtheroids, they probably play an important role in the development of axillary odor.[12] Although usually non-pathogenic, they are frequently implicated in infections associated with surgically placed prosthetic devices.[13]

The micrococci and *Staphylococcus saprophyticus* (formerly *Micrococcus* groups M1 through M4) are common non-pathogenic skin commensals in both children and adults. *Staphylococcus saprophyticus* may occasionally cause cystitis, particularly in adolescent girls and young women.[14] Coagulase-positive staphylococci, or *Staphylococcus aureus*, are not considered members of the normal cutaneous flora of glabrous skin in adults but are frequent transients acquired from carriage sites such as the anterior nares and perineum.[2, 15] Although nasal carriage is extremely common in infancy, carriage rates decline with age and range from 10 to 40 per cent after puberty.[16] However, carriage rates are higher among hospital personnel, hospitalized patients, and patients with skin disorders.[17]

Beta-hemolytic streptococci are not usually considered normal skin flora, although epidemiological studies of geographic areas where streptococcal pyoderma is endemic indicate that there may be exceptions.[18, 19] Eczematous skin conditions may predispose to beta-hemolytic streptococcal skin carriage.[20] Alpha-hemolytic streptococci constitute the principal aerobic flora of the mouth,[21] and they are often cultured from the faces and hands of older children and adults.[19] Infants frequently carry alpha-hemolytic streptococci over their entire integument, probably because of lower concentrations of surface free fatty acid, but such wide cutaneous distribution is uncommon in older children and adolescents.[15] Both beta- and alpha-hemolytic streptococci are causative agents of several specific skin infections.

Two additional genera of gram-positive bacteria, *Clostridium* and *Bacillus*, are isolated frequently enough from skin lesions to require brief mention.[22] The *Bacillus* species, particularly *Bacillus subtilis*, are prevalent saprophytes in the environment and may be part of the resident skin flora in childhood.[15] However, they are only frequent transients after puberty. The anaerobic clostridia are also widespread in nature, and although often transient on intact skin, are not part of the normal skin flora. They are responsible for some serious cutaneous infections, especially in postsurgical and burn patients,[22] but their colonization of the wounds of such patients is not necessarily evidence of infection.

Most gram-negative enteric bacilli are seldom resident on normal adolescent or adult skin, although they are frequently recovered from the skin of young infants.[23] This is probably because of the low humidity of healthy adult skin and the higher moisture content of the infant's cutaneous surface.[24] *Proteus* species, however, can be recovered from the nasal mucosa and toe webs, particularly after puberty.[23] Organisms of the non-enteric genus *Acinetobacter* are common residents of the axillae, groin, and toe webs in childhood and adulthood,[23] but these bacteria are rarely pathogenic in normal persons. Conditions that continuously expose the skin to excessive moisture cause increased carriage of gram-negative enteric organisms and may predispose to cutaneous infection with these agents.[23, 24] Dermatophyte infections have also been shown to be associated with an increase in the bacterial colonization of the skin.[25]

Only a few fungal species are considered residents of normal human skin.[2] Most adolescents and adults carry *Pityrosporum* species, but only *Pityrosporum orbiculare* is known to be potentially pathogenic. Several *Candida* species, including *Candida albicans*, are frequently isolated from skin continually exposed to moisture, although this finding is much less common in older children and adolescents than in infants.[26] Dermatophyte species, the most common causes of fungal skin infection, are most frequently found in areas where the stratum corneum is thick, such as the soles of the feet.[2, 26] Their presence is not necessarily indicative of disease.[26] Dermatophytic colonization of the feet is relatively rare before adolescence but is very common among post-adolescent males.[26]

Since a number of the microbial species designated as normal resident flora or frequent transients are also common agents of skin infection, cultural data are often less important in the diagnosis of cutaneous disorders than careful evaluation of the epidemiological and clinical characteristics of the skin lesions. However, when the clinician has a basic understanding of normal cutaneous ecology, microbial cultures can be helpful adjuncts in the assessment of primary and secondary microbial skin disease.

PYOGENIC SKIN INFECTIONS

Pyogenic (pus-forming) skin infections, collectively referred to as the pyodermas and excluding the granulomatous and fungal-like bacterial skin diseases, occur very frequently prior to puberty. The adolescent more closely resembles the adult than the child in his susceptibility to pyoderma, and the common pyodermas of childhood are seen much less often in the post-pubescent age group. Although they are not strictly pyodermas, infections of the subcutaneous tissues, namely cellulitis and fasciitis, will be discussed because of their common etiological relationships to pyogenic skin diseases.

The two most frequent causes of pyoderma are Group A beta-hemolytic streptococci, or *Streptococcus pyogenes*, and *Staphylococcus aureus*. The lesions caused by these agents can often be distinguished on clinical grounds. Less commonly, cutaneous and subcutaneous infections are caused by clostridia and the gram-negative bacilli, including *Pseudomonas*. *Corynebacterium* skin infections will be discussed with the fungal diseases, because they are not pyogenic and because they more closely resemble the mycoses histopathologically.

INFECTIONS PREDOMINANTLY CAUSED BY STREPTOCOCCI

The streptococci are classified both by their ability to hemolyze red blood cells in vitro (alpha, beta, or gamma hemolysis) and by their immunological reaction with group-specific rabbit antisera (Groups A through T).[27] Most human infections are caused by Group A beta-hemolytic aerobic streptococci, but alpha- and non-hemolytic streptococci, microaerophilic streptococci, and several non-Group A beta-hemolytic streptococci are potentially pathogenic.[28] In laboratory cultures, these organisms grow in chains, but in spreading infected lesions, single and diplococcal forms frequently occur.[27]

IMPETIGO CONTAGIOSA

Impetigo contagiosa is a very common, acute, superficial pyoderma characterized by discrete and coalescent lesions that begin as subcorneal vesicles, quickly become pustular, and soon rupture, leaving thick, yellowish-brown crusts. These lesions usually heal without scarring (Fig. 8–1). The infection is primarily caused by Group A beta-hemolytic streptococci, although the etiological role of staphylococci in non-bullous impetigo is often debated.[29] Group B beta-hemolytic streptococcus has been reported to cause the disease in infants.[30] The peak incidence is in the preschool and grammar school population, but reported series include many teenagers as well.[31-33] In one study, the infection rate declined more sharply with age among females than among males.[34] It has been observed frequently in young servicemen stationed in the tropics[35] and is more common during the summer months, in warm, moist climates, and under crowded conditions.[36] Lesions show a predilection for the forearms and especially the lower parts of the legs and are less often located on the face than are the lesions of staphylococcal bullous impetigo.[31]

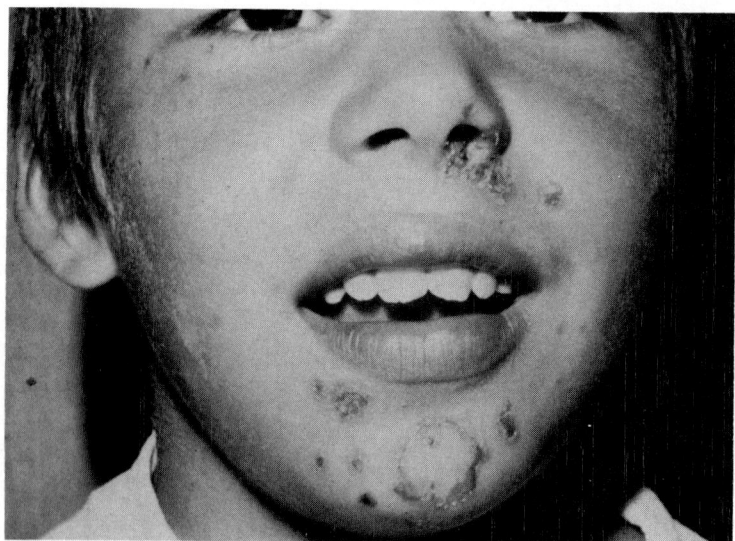

FIGURE 8–1 Crusted lesions of streptococcal impetigo on the face of a 12-year-old boy.

Infection is thought to occur when a minor break in the epidermis, such as a mosquito bite, permits the inoculation of organisms acquired by intimate contact with an individual who has actively infected lesions.[37] Specific pyoderma strains may be present on normal skin for days to weeks before the onset of clinical lesions.[38] Streptococci are probably not transmitted from the respiratory tract to the skin, but rather the reverse.[39] Although mild lymphadenopathy is usually present in patients with impetigo, systemic reactions are rare. The course of the disease is often chronic, with individual lesions persisting for more than a week and overall infection continuing for months, primarily because of autoinoculation by scratching.

Acute rheumatic fever does not occur as a sequela of streptococcal skin infection, but acute nephritis occurs in up to 15 per cent of patients with impetigo after a latent period of approximately three weeks.[40] However, this complication is distinctly uncommon after six years of age, unlike post-pharyngitis nephritis, which has a somewhat older peak incidence age.[40] Although post-pyoderma nephritis most often follows streptococcal impetigo, it may be caused by other types of streptococcal skin and subcutaneous infections. A limited number of antigenic or M types of Group A streptococci are associated with impetigo, and only a few of these are nephritogenic, in particular Types 2, 49, and 53 through 63.[37, 41] The small number of strains involved probably explains the rarity of recurrent attacks of post-pyoderma nephritis. Although nephritis has not been observed to follow skin infection with non-Group A streptococci, it has been reported in association with Group C pharyngitis.[42] There is a theoretical possibility that streptococcal Groups C and G may precede post–infectious nephritis because they are antigenically similar to Group A streptococci,[28] produce similar extracellular enzymes, and can cause identical soft tissue infections.

Laboratory findings. Fresh vesicles and pustules are more likely to yield pure cultures of streptococci than older crusted lesions, which are often contaminated or superinfected with *Staphylococcus aureus*. Gram-stained smears of unruptured lesions contain polymorphonuclear leukocytes mixed with epithelial debris and occasional coccal forms. Smears of older lesions frequently contain secondarily acquired staphylococci and may be misleading diagnostically. Leukocytosis may or may not occur but is not a prominent feature. In uncomplicated streptococcal impetigo, the antistreptolysin O titer does not usually rise significantly, whereas the anti-deoxyribonuclease B titer often is markedly elevated, and the antihyaluronidase titer is moderately elevated.[43–45] Peak antibody response to the streptococcal extracellular enzymes usually occurs from 20 to 40 days after the onset of disease. In view of the variability of post-streptococcal infection antibody responses, which are dependent on both the streptococcal strain and the site of infection,[44] a multiple antibody hemagglutination technique (Streptozyme) that screens five major streptococcal antibodies has been developed and is now generally available.[46]

Differential diagnosis. The differentiation between primary streptococcal and primary staphylococcal impetigo has been repeatedly discussed in the literature, and the unique features of each have been reiterated.[29] Impetigo contagiosa can be confused with varicella zoster viral infections, herpes simplex lesions, allergic contact dermatitis, and occasionally with dermatophyte skin infections. The epidemiology and distribution of lesions are sufficiently different in each of these disorders to distinguish them from impetigo.

Treatment. Local care traditionally includes the gentle soaking of lesions several times daily in tepid water to remove crusts, plus daily bathing with an antibacterial soap. However, recent animal experiments have suggested that removal of crusts does not contribute to healing and that scrubbing with antibacterial soap may be harmful.[47] Cleansing may be followed by the application of an antibacterial salve, but the efficacy of topical antibiotic therapy alone has not been established.[47-49] Appropriate hygienic precautions should be observed to prevent both autoinoculation and the spread of organisms to other persons. Systemic therapy either with a single intramuscular injection of benzathine penicillin G or with a 10-day course of oral phenoxymethyl penicillin should be prescribed. Infrequently, a patient may require therapy for a more prolonged period. Occasionally, significant secondary infection with staphylococci may require the use of a semisynthetic penicillin, preferably oral cloxacillin or dicloxacillin. Erythromycin, cephalexin, and clindamycin are active against streptococci and penicillinase-producing staphylococci and are effective alternatives for the penicillin-allergic individual.[50] However, the occasional serious gastrointestinal side effects of clindamycin require that it be prescribed with caution for the patient with only minor infection. Unfortunately, it has not been convincingly demonstrated that antibiotic therapy prevents post-pyoderma nephritis.[48, 51]

ECTHYMA

Ecthyma refers to a skin lesion or lesions that resemble impetigo in onset and appearance but evolve more slowly to the crusted stage and extend deeper into the dermis to form a purulent ulcer with elevated margins. Healing is slow and often accompanied by scarring. Lesions most commonly occur on or below the knees in debilitated persons. The causative agent is usually Group A beta-hemolytic streptococcus.

Treatment is similar to that for impetigo contagiosa, with the addition of cleansing the lesions with hydrogen peroxide two or three times daily.

ERYSIPELAS

Erysipelas is an uncommon, rapidly spreading epidermal and subepidermal infection, usually caused by Group A beta-hemolytic streptococci.[52] *Streptococcus* Group C[53] and *Streptococcus pneumoniae*[54] also may infrequently cause erysipelas. The lesion is bright red, indurated, tender, and hot, with a raised and sharply-defined irregular border. It is generally singular and does not demonstrate central clearing. Lymphadenopathy and lymphangitis are frequent, and formation of microabscesses and bullae in the tissues is common as the lesion progresses (Fig. 8–2). Erysipelas may occur on any part of the body, but the lesion has a predilection for the face and lower portions of the legs. Patients of any age may acquire this infection, but debilitated individuals and the very young and very old are more often affected. The disease is rare in the normal adolescent.

As with impetigo, infection is probably acquired when minor or major trauma to the skin permits the inoculation of organisms into the superficial

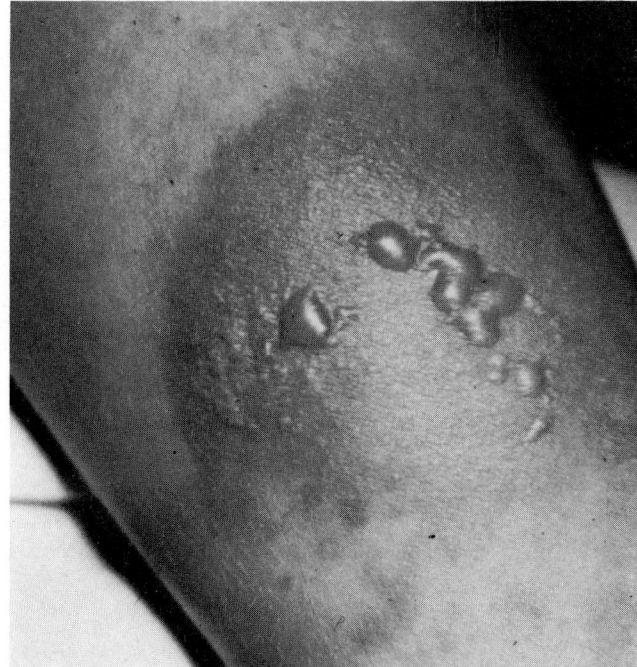

FIGURE 8–2 Erysipelas of the leg, demonstrating a well-defined margin and superficial blisters.

dermis, but this disease is not particularly contagious in contrast to impetigo.[52] It was once a common postoperative complication, prior to the introduction of strict aseptic surgical technique. The disease has an abrupt onset heralded by chills, fever, vomiting, headache, and arthralgia. It may recur repeatedly at the same body site, and subsequent attacks may be milder than the initial episode. Permanent tissue damage and lymphedema may result from such repeated attacks.

Laboratory findings. Pure cultures of the etiological agent may be obtained by injecting a small amount of sterile, preservative-free saline into the advancing border of the lesion with a small-gauge needle and aspirating the injected material. Careful microscopic examination of a Gram-stained smear of this aspirate may reveal the causative organisms. Patients with erysipelas usually sustain a marked leukocytosis with a predominance of polymorphonuclear leukocytes and immature granulocytes. One or more blood cultures should be obtained before antibiotic therapy is initiated.

Differential diagnosis. Erysipelas is differentiated from deeper or subcutaneous forms of cellulitis by the sharply demarcated border of the lesion. Erysipelas may simulate streptococcal necrotizing cellulitis and necrotizing fasciitis, but the differentiation between the three syndromes is unclear, and they may represent part of a streptococcal cellulitis spectrum.[55] Erysipelas occasionally may be confused with the cutaneous manifestations of acute dermatomyositis or systemic lupus erythematosus. This confusion is most likely to arise when erysipelas occurs in a mid-facial butterfly distribution. The history, physical examination of the patient, and laboratory data relevant to connective tissue disease (see Chapter 16) as well as the lack of response to antibiotic therapy should serve to differentiate these connective tissue diseases from erysipelas. Uncommonly, contact dermatitis, which most often is not accompanied by fever and other systemic symptoms, may be initially confused with erysipelas. A severe reaction to insect bites occasionally may resemble erysipelas.

Treatment. The patient with erysipelas often is severely ill and should be hospitalized. Antipyretics and fluid therapy are often required. Parenteral administration of penicillin, initially with aqueous penicillin G every four hours, should be undertaken promptly. When the patient's condition improves, therapy may be completed with 10 days of either intramuscular administration of procaine penicillin G or oral administration of phenoxymethyl penicillin. The local application of cool compresses and the elevation of an affected extremity are important adjuncts of antibiotic therapy.

CELLULITIS

Cellulitis refers to infection of the subcutaneous tissues, most often caused by Group A beta-hemolytic streptococci but sometimes secondary to infection with *Staphylococcus aureus*.[56] While *Hemophilus influenzae* Type b is an important problem in the pediatric patient less than six years of age, it is rarely a cause of cellulitis in the adolescent and adult.[57] In periorbital and orbital cellulitis secondary to paranasal sinus infection, *Streptococcus pneumoniae* may be the offending agent.

Cellulitis is characterized by a diffuse, edematous area of erythema that is warm and tender to palpation. The infection is usually subacute, but the patient may be febrile and moderately ill. The adolescent generally manifests a less pronounced systemic reaction than the young child or infant. The potential for severe septic or metastatic complications exists if the cellulitis is left untreated,[56] but many minor localized infections probably resolve without medical attention.

The infection frequently follows a break in the skin caused by trauma or an insect bite, but the wound may not always be detectable. Cellulitis may complicate one of the superficial pyodermas, such as impetigo or furunculosis, and is a frequent component of wound infection.[56] The presence of lymphangitis and lymphadenopathy is indicative of streptococcal causation. Staphylococcal infections are generally more purulent and localized than is streptococcal disease, which tends to exhibit more rapid spread at the periphery of each lesion. A clear differentiation between these two most common etiologies cannot be made clinically at the onset of infection. Cellulitis is not limited to a particular age group.

Laboratory findings. The laboratory evaluation of cellulitis should follow that outlined for erysipelas. A white blood cell count will frequently but not invariably reveal a leukocytosis with a shift to the left, depending on the extent and severity of the lesion. At least two blood samples should be cultured from any patient with systemic manifestations. One should avoid a needle aspiration of bone or joint spaces through infected skin or subcutaneous tissue because such procedures may lead to osteomyelitis or septic arthritis.

Differential diagnosis. When cellulitis involves an extremity and no wound is apparent, the localized tenderness and systemic symptoms may cause the physician to consider the possibility of osteomyelitis or septic arthritis. However, edema and erythema of the overlying skin and subcutaneous tissues are not hallmarks of bone and joint infections. In septic arthritis, the entire circumference of the limb is often enlarged, whereas cellulitis is not often circumferential. In septic arthritis, joint movement is excruciatingly painful, whereas cellulitis does not seriously restrict joint mobility. The patient with osteomyelitis may often refuse to bear weight on the involved extremity, whereas the patient with cellulitis often arrives in the physician's office limping. Uncommonly, cellulitis may be confused with early photodermatitis, with lupus erythematosus and dermatomyositis, or with angioneurotic edema. A carefully taken history and additional clinical features of these diseases (see Chapters 16 and 18) should serve to differentiate them from cellulitis.

Treatment. Local measures should include the application of moderate heat and the elevation of an affected extremity. In minor streptococcal infections, oral phenoxymethyl penicillin may be prescribed, but severe disease requires the use of parenterally administered penicillin, as prescribed for erysipelas. For lesions without systemic manifestations, in which the etiological agent is unknown or suspected to be staphylococcus, either oral cloxacillin or dicloxacillin may be prescribed. For more severe disease of unknown or staphylococcal origin, a semisynthetic penicillin such as oxacillin administered parenterally is preferred. Erythromycin is an acceptable alternative for minor infection in the penicillin-allergic patient but should not be used in the patient with severe staphylococcal disease. Clindamycin is recommended as an effective alternative for the treatment of serious staphylococcal disease.[58]

BLISTERING DISTAL DACTYLITIS

Blistering distal dactylitis is a unique beta-hemolytic streptococcal infection of the fingertips, characterized by a superficial blister filled with a thin purulent exudate (Fig. 8–3).[59] It is not accompanied by signs of systemic illness and is easily treated by incision and drainage, and penicillin administered orally. Four of the thirteen patients described by Hays were aged 10 years or older.[59] The infection probably occurs more frequently than is currently recognized.

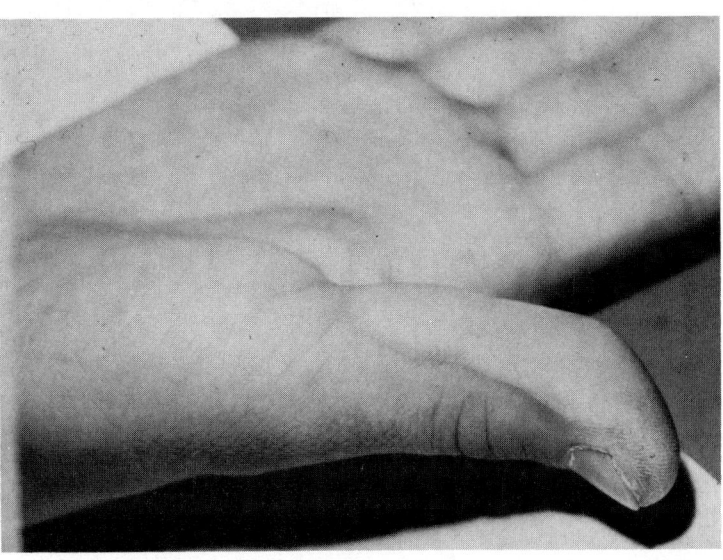

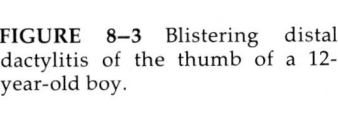

FIGURE 8–3 Blistering distal dactylitis of the thumb of a 12-year-old boy.

INFECTIONS PREDOMINANTLY CAUSED BY STAPHYLOCOCCI

The most important genera of the family Micrococcaceae are *Staphylococcus* and *Micrococcus*. The genus *Staphylococcus* includes the species *Staphylococcus aureus, Staphylococcus epidermidis,* and *Staphylococcus saprophyticus,* of which only *Staphylococcus aureus* is commonly associated with human infections. Coagulase production is a useful indicator of potential pathogenicity, since *Staphylococcus aureus* produces coagulase and all other Micrococcaceae do not. *Staphylococcus aureus* is further divided into four groups by bacteriophage typing, with a large number of phage types in each group. Although superficial infections can be caused by any of the phage groups, phage Group II organisms have been implicated in several specific primary staphylococcal skin diseases.[60] Since coagulase-negative *Staphylococcus epidermidis* is one of the dominant flora of the normal skin, it is frequently present in cultures and smears obtained from cutaneous surfaces. However, it is only rarely pathogenic and is not known to be responsible for cutaneous infection. *Staphylococcus saprophyticus* (formerly *Micrococcus* subgroups M1 through M4) is also resident on human skin but is not thought to be an agent of skin disease.

With the exception of the staphylococcal scalded skin syndromes,[61] which are not true pyodermas, cutaneous staphylococcal skin disease is not confined to a particular age group.[62] However, certain common localized infections, such as those of the bearded region in men, are unique to the post-adolescent age groups.

BULLOUS IMPETIGO AND TOXIC EPIDERMAL NECROLYSIS

The etiology of impetigo has been the subject of frequent debate, but it is now generally agreed that at least two distinct clinical forms occur: impetigo contagiosa, caused primarily by *Streptococcus pyogenes*, and bullous impetigo, caused by *Staphylococcus aureus*.[40] The latter is characterized by the appearance of large, localized, intraepidermal bullae that persist for longer periods than the transient vesicles of streptococcal impetigo and subsequently rupture spontaneously to form very thin crusts (Fig. 8–4). Bullous impetigo is considered by some investigators to be one of the forms of the staphylococcal scalded skin syndrome,[61] but it differs from the other forms in that generalized exfoliation does not occur and the Nikolsky sign is negative. This group of diseases has been shown to be caused by an epidermolytic toxin produced by some strains of phage Group II staphylococci[63] and rarely by certain phage Group I staphylococci.[64] The etiological agent is present in and isolated from cutaneous lesions only in the localized, impetiginous form. In staphylococcal scarlatina and generalized exfoliative disease, the staphylococcal infection occurs at other body sites such as the ears, eyes, or nose, and the toxin is believed to be circulating.[65]

Although scalded skin syndrome is common in infants and young children under the age of 10, it was formerly believed that adolescents and adults were resistant. However, the disease has been demonstrated in a number of adults,[66, 67] most of whom have been immunodeficient or debilitated. Experiments

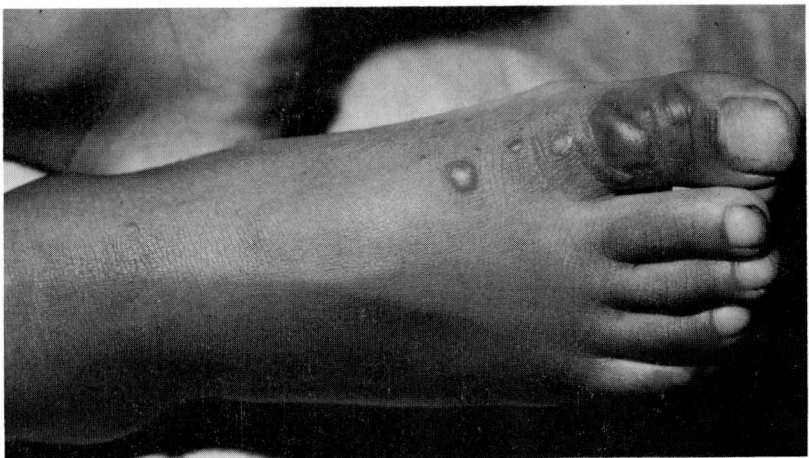

FIGURE 8-4 Grouped lesions of bullous impetigo on the dorsum of the foot and great toe.

performed with human volunteers have shown that adults are susceptible to the purified staphylococcal toxin when it is injected intracutaneously.[68] Most patients with uncomplicated bullous impetigo are otherwise well and without systemic symptoms,[61] but some cases have occurred as a complication of overwhelming staphylococcal infection.[66]

Laboratory findings. The fluid contents of an unruptured bulla will reveal the presence of phage Group II staphylococci, most frequently Type 71.[61] A punch biopsy specimen will show the plane of cleavage to be intraepidermal and subgranular, with minimal inflammatory infiltration of the underlying dermis. In patients with uncomplicated disease, the blood culture is almost never positive, but blood cultures should be obtained from any patient with systemic symptoms.[66]

Differential diagnosis. The non-localized, more severe forms of the scalded skin syndrome must be differentiated from drug-induced toxic epidermal necrolysis, which is more common in patients over 10 years of age than the similar disease caused by staphylococci. Histologically, the drug-induced disease shows a subepidermal cleavage plane and is accompanied by intracellular edema of the epidermal tissues as well as basal cell degeneration.[69] Erythema multiforme, which has many features similar to drug-induced toxic epidermal necrolysis, may also cause diagnostic confusion. The lesions of localized scalded skin syndrome or bullous impetigo may mimic the non-infectious bullous diseases, such as pemphigus and bullous pemphigoid, both of which occur mainly in middle-aged and elderly persons. These diseases are distinguished by distinctly different histological features and by characteristic immunofluorescent staining patterns.

Treatment. Oral therapy with a penicillinase-resistant penicillin should be instituted and continued for at least five to seven days or until the lesions resolve. Cephalexin and erythromycin are acceptable substitutes in the penicillin-allergic patient. The ruptured lesions should be gently cleansed until healing takes place, which ordinarily should be no longer than a week.

FOLLICULITIS

Infection of a hair follicle is a common occurrence and is most often caused by *Staphylococcus aureus*, although streptococci, gram-negative bacilli, and even *Pityrosporum* species can be etiological agents.[70, 71] Folliculitis usually remains superficial and is then termed Bockhart's impetigo or ostia folliculitis. It is characterized by the presence of tiny, white-to-yellow pustules at the openings of the pilosebaceous canals (Fig. 8–5). Commonly infected sites include the scalp, extremities, and perioral and perinasal regions of the face. Lesions occur most frequently in persons with poor hygiene or on skin sites occluded by dressings or oils. The infection occasionally leads to considerable inflammation of the surrounding tissues. The use of prolonged antibiotic therapy for acne vulgaris has resulted in an increased incidence of antibiotic-resistant, gram-negative folliculitis in the adolescent and young adult age group.[70]

Therapy should include enhanced personal cleanliness and the use of a mild antibacterial soap. Local antibiotic ointments may be used, but systemic drugs are unnecessary in uncomplicated cases. If the folliculitis is secondary to prolonged systemic antibiotic therapy, cessation of therapy is indicated. It should be superseded by the institution of antibiotics based on bacterial culture and sensitivity data. The application of a benzoyl peroxide preparation is frequently helpful in instances of chronic low-grade folliculitis.

SYCOSIS VULGARIS

Sycosis vulgaris or sycosis barbae, a deep folliculitis of the bearded region of men, is precipitated and exacerbated by shaving. Nasal carriers of staphylo-

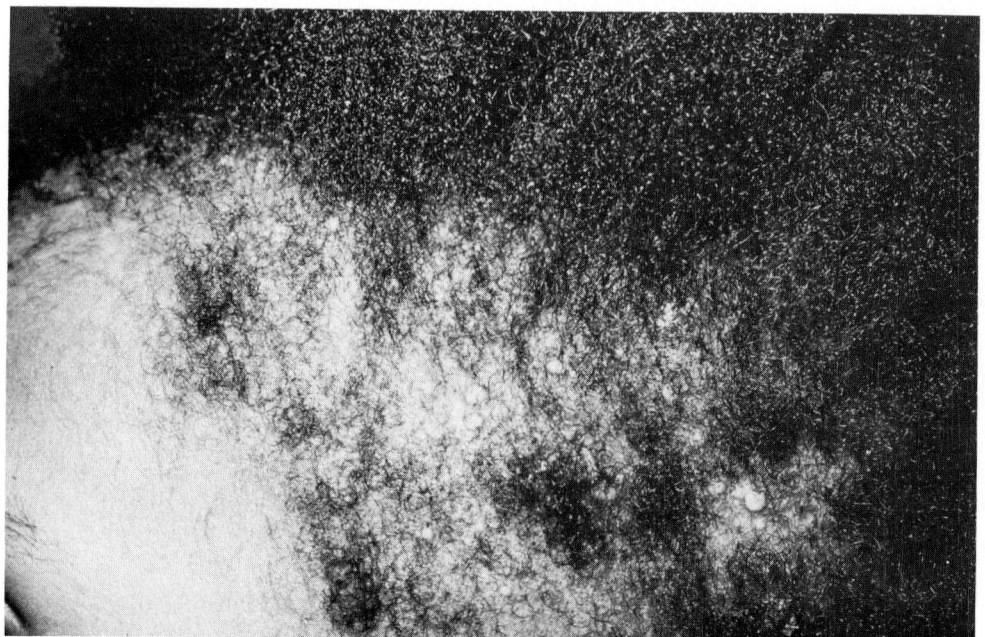

FIGURE 8–5 Tiny pustules of staphylococcal folliculitis on the anterior scalp.

cocci may be more susceptible to this infection, which tends to be recurrent. Inflammation and induration of the surrounding skin can become quite severe. Phage Group II, Type 71 staphylococci have been associated with sycosis vulgaris.[72]

Differential diagnosis. This entity may be confused with pseudofolliculitis of the beard, a non-infectious condition in men with very curly hair that is caused by the reentry or ingrowth of short, curved hairs after shaving. Pseudofolliculitis has also been reported in curly-haired women who pluck rather than shave their legs.[73] Bacterial folliculitis must also be differentiated from tinea barbae.

Treatment. The condition may be resistant to treatment. Therapy should consist of the application of warm compresses with a mild antibacterial solution several times a day, followed by the application of an antibacterial ointment. Infected hairs should be epilated with a small forceps, and the frequency of shaving should be reduced. The use of fresh, alcohol-cleaned razor blades or electric razor heads is indicated. If the condition is particularly severe or recurrent, systemic therapy with an appropriate antistaphylococcal agent may be of benefit.

Furunculosis and Carbunculosis

Superficial folliculitis may persist and worsen to form a perifollicular staphylococcal abscess, referred to as a furuncle or boil. Such lesions are very common[74] and progress from localized erythema and induration to central necrosis and suppuration, subsequently discharging their contents onto the skin surface. They tend to become chronic and recurrent and favor such locations as the gluteal region, the axillae, and the posterior aspect of the neck. When a lesion is composed of several confluent furuncles with multiple drainage points, it is termed a carbuncle. These larger abscesses are most common in the thick skin at the back of the neck in older and debilitated persons. Some patients with chronic furunculosis or carbunculosis can be shown to have diabetes or an underlying immunodeficiency,[75] but many repeatedly afflicted individuals have no demonstrable impairment of host defenses.

Laboratory findings. Although staphylococci are responsible for the vast majority of cutaneous abscesses, the occasional implication of other bacteria or fungal species makes the Gram stain and culture of lesions important procedures. Although the patient with a common furuncle does not usually have systemic symptoms, carbunculosis may be accompanied by fever, leukocytosis, and bacteremia. Any patient with systemic symptoms should have a complete blood count and at least two blood cultures drawn prior to the institution of antibiotic therapy. Bacterial sensitivities of staphylococcal species should be obtained, since these organisms are capable of resistance to numerous antibiotics.[76]

Differential diagnosis. Furunculosis is often confused with hidradenitis suppurativa, which is a chronic infection of the apocrine sweat glands, usually of the axillae, groin, and perineum. Since the latter condition frequently requires surgical intervention and perhaps prolonged antibiotic therapy, its differentiation from common furunculosis is important.

Treatment. Initial management of acute furunculosis consists of the frequent application of hot, moist compresses to speed localization and spontaneous drainage. Larger lesions may require a small incision or repeated needle aspiration to aid drainage, but such procedures are contraindicated until the lesion is well-localized and obviously fluctuant. Incision of facial or nasal lesions entails the risk of direct spread of infection to the cavernous sinus. Systemic antibiotics are indicated for large or multiple lesions, lesions located on the face, and lesions in patients with fever or other systemic symptoms. Because of the increasing prevalence of penicillinase-producing staphylococci, penicillin is no longer acceptable for the initiation of antistaphylococcal therapy. One of the penicillinase-resistant penicillins, such as cloxacillin administered orally or oxacillin parenterally, should be prescribed instead.[76] The cephalosporin antibiotics may be considered in the penicillin-allergic patient, but a small percentage of such patients also exhibit allergic reactions to cephalosporins. In such cases, clindamycin and vancomycin are third-choice alternatives but should be reserved for use in serious infections. Erythromycin is preferred for mild, acute staphylococcal infection in the penicillin-allergic patient but is not recommended for serious or recurrent disease because it may promote the emergence of resistant organisms.[77] When it is employed, antibiotic therapy should be continued until the lesions heal.

The treatment of chronic and recurrent furunculosis is often difficult. Improved personal hygiene may be of some benefit. It should include a daily bath with an antibacterial soap and frequent hand washing to prevent autoinoculation with organisms from nasal and perineal carriage sites. A unique form of therapy that has received some attention is the deliberate colonization of chronic furunculosis patients with a strain of *Staphylococcus aureus* of low pathogenicity. This method is referred to as bacterial interference treatment and has been shown to be effective in a number of instances.[78]

INFECTIONS PREDOMINANTLY CAUSED BY MICROAEROPHILIC AND ANAEROBIC BACTERIA

Microaerophilic and anaerobic skin and subcutaneous infections most often affect tissues injured by trauma or surgical procedures. The classification of these syndromes in the literature is very confusing, but several entities can be regarded as unique. While usually secondary infections of injured tissues, these infections may resemble several of the primary bacterial soft tissue diseases such as erysipelas, and the original wound may not always be obvious. Since the therapy of these infections frequently includes surgical intervention, it is important to differentiate them from non-surgical soft tissue infections.[55]

ERYSIPELOID

Erysipeloid[80] is a cutaneous infection that is generally regarded as an occupational disease, since it is found almost exclusively in fishermen, butchers, kitchen workers, and others who handle raw meat, poultry, and fish.

The causative organism, *Erysipelothrix insidiosa* (formerly *E. rhusiopathiae*), is a gram-positive, non-encapsulated, non-spore-forming rod that can be recovered from dead animal matter.

Localized erysipeloid infections present as a violaceous, non-suppurative cellulitis, usually on the hands or wrists. Erythema and edema begin approximately two to seven days after traumatic inoculation of the organism. The lesion is elevated, with a sharply defined, irregular border, and may display central clearing and arcuate and polycyclic margins. Vesicles may occur on occasion. The lesions are migratory, with involution of some areas and expansion of others. Swelling of the tissues may restrict movement of the fingers, but lymphangitis and lymphadenitis are not associated. Pain and itching are usual symptoms.

A more generalized form of erysipeloid, with fever, arthralgia, and a widespread skin eruption, may occur infrequently. An initial lesion is present at the site of inoculation on the hand, and gradual enlargement takes place over a period of months. Lesions may occur remote from the site of inoculation until a large portion of the body surface becomes involved. The lesions have sharply marginated, gyrate or festooned borders and may persist for weeks to months. A rare form of erysipeloid, with systemic endocarditis, purpura, joint involvement, and a characteristic hemorrhagic necrosis of the ears, also has been described.[81]

Laboratory findings. The organism can be recovered from a saline aspirate of a skin lesion but is most reliably obtained from a full-thickness skin biopsy of the active advancing margin. Since the organisms are located deep in the dermis, superficial cultures are unrewarding unless the lesions are extremely inflamed. The organism grows on routine non-selective media and forms long filaments and chains.

Differential diagnosis. The lesions may be confused with those of erysipelas. However, erysipelas lesions are solitary, do not demonstrate central clearing, and are usually found on the legs or face. Other types of cellulitis also have to be considered in the differential diagnosis. The diffuse type of erysipeloid must be distinguished from erythema multiforme.

Treatment. Penicillin is the drug of choice for this disease and should be administered in doses of 1.2 to 3 million units per day, depending on the severity and extent of the disease. For localized disease, 1.2 million units of benzathine penicillin G are usually adequate. The organism is also sensitive to tetracycline, erythromycin, and chloramphenicol, any of which may be used for treatment of the penicillin-sensitive individual.

CLOSTRIDIAL CELLULITIS

Anaerobic, necrotizing cellulitis produced by one of the anaerobic, gram-negative bacilli of the genus *Clostridium* is usually accompanied by cutaneous crepitation secondary to gas formation in the tissues.[55] The lesion is characterized by the presence of thin, superficial blebs that contain a foul-smelling, hemorrhagic fluid, plus soft tissue edema that may extend some distance from the wound. The infection is generally accompanied by moderate local pain and systemic toxicity, but the patient does not become as critically ill as the patient with clostridial myonecrosis (gas gangrene). Gram stain of drainage material is frequently positive for the offending agent, but since wound contamination with these organisms is common, their presence alone is not necessarily indicative of invasive disease. While clostridial cellulitis is not as severe an infection as myonecrosis, therapy should include immediate wide excision and drainage of tissue in addition to the prompt administration of penicillin G parenterally.[79] Antitoxin therapy is not necessary.

NON-CLOSTRIDIAL GAS-FORMING CELLULITIS

A number of organisms, including gram-negative enteric bacilli, *Bacteroides* species, and anaerobic streptococci, are capable of causing an infection that resembles clostridial cellulitis.[55, 82] These infections are not usually accompanied by the systemic toxicity and intense local pain that are associated with clostridial infections.[55] Surgical excision of tissues is not necessary, and therapy should consist of local wound care plus the administration of appropriate antibiotics.

HEMOLYTIC STREPTOCOCCUS GANGRENE

Necrotizing streptococcal cellulitis, or hemolytic streptococcus gangrene, is an infrequent infection of the dermis and subcutaneous tissues that has an appearance similar to erysipelas. It is accompanied by vascular thrombosis, ischemia, and cutaneous gangrene.[83] Like most streptococcal soft tissue infections, it generally follows skin trauma or surgery. The acute onset of this infection is accompanied by moderate to severe systemic symptoms. Initially, the lesions resemble erysipelas but fail to respond to antibiotic therapy and instead become markedly edematous, brownish in hue, and devitalized, with large blebs forming in the relatively hypoesthetic skin. The lesion should be considered a surgical emergency, requiring immediate wide incision and drainage.[83] Parenteral aqueous penicillin G administration and fluid therapy should be instituted without delay.

Hemolytic streptococcus gangrene must be differentiated from erysipelas and necrotizing fasciitis. Clostridial cellulitis is differentiated by the presence of more intense wound pain and gas formation in the tissues.

NECROTIZING FASCIITIS

Necrotizing fasciitis is similar to and may be accompanied by hemolytic streptococcus gangrene but involves the deeper or fascial layers of the subcutaneous tissues.[84] Group A hemolytic streptococci are the bacteria most frequently isolated from these lesions, but hemolytic staphylococci[85] and several gram-negative organisms have been implicated as well. It has been suggested that the disease is caused by the synergistic effects of two or more organisms.[55] Necrotizing fasciitis secondary to anaerobic gram-negative bacteria is usually not confined to the subcutaneous tissue but involves the underlying muscle as well.[86]

Infection usually follows trauma or surgery, with an acute onset accompanied by severe systemic symptoms and intravascular hemolysis. The lesion is initially characterized by local hypoesthesia and mild discoloration and edema of the overlying skin, which is easily dissected from the underlying muscle.[55] If therapy is delayed, necrotizing cellulitis and cutaneous gangrene frequently follow.

As with hemolytic streptococcus gangrene, emergency surgical intervention, consisting of wide incision and drainage, is indicated. Initial antibiotic therapy should include the intravenous administration of a penicillinase-resistant penicillin plus an aminoglycoside, pending the results of bacterial cultures.[55] Appropriate supportive measures, including electrolyte and blood transfusion therapy, may be of vital importance.

PROGRESSIVE BACTERIAL SYNERGISTIC GANGRENE

Meleney's progressive bacterial synergistic gangrene is an uncommon late postoperative surgical complication characterized by the development of swelling, tenderness, and erythema in the skin surrounding a surgical wound.[55] It is most frequently seen in neglected or debilitated patients. The cutaneous changes are accompanied by systemic toxicity and wound pain. The lesion progresses to an area of central necrosis that subsequently ulcerates and is surrounded by a purple border of induration. Bacteriological data indicate that the entity is the result of the synergistic combination of a microaerophilic gamma streptococcus with either *Staphylococcus aureus* or a gram-negative bacillus.[82] Appropriate therapy includes both surgical debridement and excision of necrotic tissue and administration of broad-spectrum antibiotics.[55]

MELENEY'S ULCER

The term "Meleney's ulcer" usually refers to a chronic, undermining, ulcerative lesion or lesions caused by microaerophilic streptococci.[87] Since Meleney also described progressive bacterial synergistic gangrene and hemolytic streptococcus gangrene,[88] the association of his name with these syndromes may cause confusion. Meleney's ulcers occur following trauma or surgical procedures after a period of some days or even weeks and are characterized by the appearance of deep subcutaneous erosions that connect with similar secondary lesions via subcutaneous tracts. The infection persists for months and is not accompanied by systemic symptoms. Therapy consists of surgical debridement in addition to appropriate antibiotics. Some cases of what has been called Meleney's ulcer in the past were probably examples of pyoderma gangrenosum (see Chapter 18).

INFECTIONS CAUSED BY PSEUDOMONAS

The gram-negative non-fermenting bacillus *Pseudomonas aeruginosa* can be responsible for a variety of cutaneous infections. This organism demonstrates tropism for vascular endothelium, and several types of skin lesions may accompany *Pseudomonas* septicemia, including localized areas of necrotizing cellulitis, erythematous nodules, hemorrhagic vesicles, and the painless necrotic ulcers referred to as ecthyma gangrenosum.[89] These lesions occur in critically ill, debilitated patients and almost always herald a fatal outcome.

Acute otitis externa is a painful infection of the external auditory canal in which *Pseudomonas aeruginosa* is the most frequently isolated bacterial agent.[90] The condition occurs predominantly in older children and is common among persons who swim frequently. Local treatment with Burow's solution and topical antibiotic drops is usually effective. Chronic otitis externa is frequently the result of seborrheic dermatitis.

The green nail syndrome refers to an exquisitely tender paronychia and onychia, often accompanied by a greenish-blue discoloration of the nail bed.[91] A similar greenish discoloration of the nail is sometimes seen in candidal onychia, which is a more chronic, but relatively painless condition. *Pseudomonas* nail infection occurs most frequently in persons who spend long periods of time with their hands immersed in water. The infection tends to resist treatment but sometimes responds to drying of the infected area plus topical antibiotic therapy. Often the nail must be removed in order to achieve access to the affected nail matrix and bed.

Pseudomonas toe web infection occurs in persons whose feet are continually exposed to moisture, because of either occlusive footgear or chronic immersion.[92] In addition to scaling and maceration, the involved skin may exhibit a faint greenish tinge. As with *Pseudomonas* paronychia, the infection responds to drying and topical antibiotic therapy.

REFERENCES

1. Montes, L. F., and Wilborn, W. H.: Location of bacterial skin flora. Br. J. Dermatol., 81(1):23, 1969.
2. Marples, M. J.: The normal microbial flora of the skin. In: Skinner, F. A., and Carr, J. G. (eds.): The Normal Microbial Flora of Man. New York, Academic Press, 1974, pp. 7–12.
3. Pukvel, S. M., Reisner, R. M., and Sakamoto, M.: Analysis of lipid composition of isolated human sebaceous gland homogenates after incubation with cutaneous bacteria. Thin layer chromatography. J. Invest. Dermatol., 64:406, 1975.
4. Ricketts, C. R., Squire, J. R., and Topley, E.: Human skin lipids with particular reference to the self-sterilizing power of the skin. Clin. Sci. Mol. Med., 10:89, 1951.
5. Noble, W. C., and Somerville, D. A.: Microbiology of Human Skin. Philadelphia, W. B. Saunders, 1974, pp. 284–301.
6. Woodroffee, R. C. S., and Shaw, D. A.: Natural control and ecology of microbial populations on skin and hair. In: Skinner, F. A., and Carr, J. G. (eds.): The Normal Microbial Flora of Man. New York, Academic Press, 1974, pp. 13–34.
7. Noble, W. C., and Somerville, D. A.: Microbiology of Human Skin. Philadelphia, W. B. Saunders, 1974, pp. 79–99.
8. Imamura, S.: The localization and distribution of gram-positive cocci in normal skin and in acne lesions. J. Invest. Dermatol., 65:244, 1975.
9. Davis, B. D., Dulbecco, R., Eisen, H. N., et al.: Microbiology. New York, Harper & Row, 1973, pp. 681–706.
10. Baird-Parker, A. C.: The basis of the present classification of staphylococci and micrococci. Ann. N.Y. Acad. Sci., 236:7, 1974.
11. Noble, W. C.: Skin carriage of the Micrococcaceae. J. Clin. Pathol., 22:249, 1969.
12. Shehadek, N. H., and Kligman, A. M.: The bacteria responsible for axillary odor. J. Invest. Dermatol., 41:3, 1963.
13. Holt, R. J.: The pathogenic role of coagulase-negative staphylococci. Br. J. Dermatol., 86(8):42, 1972.
14. Maskell, R.: Importance of coagulase-negative staphylococci as pathogens in the urinary tract. Lancet, 1:1155, 1974.

15. Ehrenkranz, N. J.: Transmission of *Staphylococcus aureus* in man: Epidemiologic and experimental studies. *In:* Maibach, H. I., and Hildrick-Smith, G. (eds.): Skin Bacteria and Their Role in Infection. New York, McGraw-Hill, 1965, pp. 201–215.
16. Williams, R. E. O.: Healthy carriage of *Staphylococcus aureus*. Its prevalence and importance. Bacteriol. Rev., *27*:56, 1963.
17. Noble, W. C., Williams, R. E. O., Jevons, M. P., and Shooter, R. A.: Some aspects of nasal carriage of staphylococci. J. Clin. Pathol., *17*:79, 1964.
18. Dajani, A. S., Ferrieri, P., and Wannamaker, L.: Endemic superficial pyoderma in children. Arch. Dermatol., *108*:517, 1973.
19. Noble, W. C., and Somerville, D. A.: Microbiology of Human Skin. Philadelphia, W. B. Saunders, 1974, pp. 160–171.
20. Noble, W. C.: An epidemic of streptococcal infection in a skin hospital. Br. J. Dermatol., *81*:259, 1969.
21. Hardie, J. M., and Bowden, G. H.: The normal microbial flora of the mouth. *In:* Skinner, F. A., and Carr, J. G. (eds.): The Normal Microbial Flora of Man. New York, Academic Press, 1974, pp. 47–83.
22. Noble, W. C., and Somerville, D. A.: Microbiology of Human Skin. Philadelphia, W. B. Saunders, 1973, pp.192–195.
23. Noble, W. C., and Somerville, D. A.: Microbiology of Human Skin. Philadelphia, W. B. Saunders, 1974, pp.172–184.
24. McBride, M. E., Duncan, W. C., and Knox, J. M.: Physiological and environmental control of gram-negative bacteria on skin. Br. J. Dermatol., *93*:191, 1975.
25. Bibel, D. J., and LeBrun, J. R.: Effect of experimental dermatophyte infection on cutaneous flora. J. Invest. Dermatol., *64*:119, 1975.
26. Noble, W. C., and Somerville, D. A.: Microbiology of Human Skin. Philadelphia, W. B. Saunders, 1974, pp. 206–224.
27. Davis, B. D., Dulbecco, R., Sisen, H. N., et al.: Microbiology. New York, Harper & Row, 1973, pp.707–726.
28. Duma, R. J., Weinberg, A. N., Medrek, T. F., and Kunz, L. J.: Streptococcal infections. Medicine, *48*(2):87, 1969.
29. Dajani, A. S., Ferrieri, P., and Wannamaker, L. W.: Natural history of impetigo. II. Etiologic agents and bacterial interactions. J. Clin. Invest., *51*:2863, 1972.
30. Belgaumkar, T.: Impetigo neonatorum congenita due to group B beta-hemolytic streptococcus infections. J. Pediatr., *86*:982, 1975.
31. Dillon, H. C.: Impetigo contagiosa: Suppurative and non-suppurative complications. I. Clinical, bacteriologic, and epidemiologic characteristics of impetigo. Am. J. Dis. Child., *115*:530, 1968.
32. Freeman, R.: Streptococcal infection in a large general hospital. J. Clin. Pathol., *24*:300, 1971.
33. Glezen, W. P., deWalt, J. L., Lindsay, R. L., and Dillon, H. C.: Epidermic pyoderma caused by nephritogenic streptococci in college athletes. Lancet, *1*:301, 1972.
34. Bassett, D. C. J.: Streptococcal pyoderma and acute nephritis in Trinidad. Br. J. Dermatol., *86*(8):55, 1972.
35. Allen, A. M., Taplin, D., and Twigg, L.: Cutaneous streptococcal infections in Vietnam. Arch. Dermatol., *104*:271, 1971.
36. Taplin, D., Lansdell, L., Allen, A. M., et al.: Prevalence of streptococcal pyoderma in relation to climate and hygiene. Lancet, *1*:7802, 1973.
37. Dillon, H. C.: Streptococcal infections of the skin and their complications: Impetigo and nephritis. *In:* Wannamaker, L. W., and Matsen, J. M. (eds.): Streptococci and Streptococcal Diseases: Recognition, Understanding, and Management. New York, Academic Press, 1972, pp. 571–587.
38. Dudding, B. A., Burnett, J. W., Chapman, S. S., and Wannamaker, L. W.: The role of normal skin in the spread of streptococcal pyoderma. J. Hyg., *68*:19, 1970.
39. Ferrieri, P., Dajani, S. S., Wannamaker, L. W., and Chapman, S. S.: Natural history of impetigo. I. Site of sequence of acquisition and familial patterns of spread of cutaneous streptococci. J. Clin. Invest., *51*:2851, 1972.
40. Wannamaker, L. W.: Differences between streptococcal infections of the throat and of the skin. N. Engl. J. Med., *282*:23, 1970.
41. Fox, E. N.: M proteins of group A streptococci. Bacteriol. Rev., *38*:57, 1974.
42. Duca, E., Teodorivici, G., Radu, C., et al.: A new nephritogenic streptococcus. J. Hyg., *67*:691, 1969.
43. Potter, E. V., Moran, A. F., Poon-King, T., and Earle, D. P.: Characteristics of beta-hemolytic streptococci associated with acute glomerulonephritis in Trinidad, West Indies. J. Lab. Clin. Med., *71*:126, 1968.
44. Kaplan, E., Anthony, B., Chapman, S., et al.: The influence of the site of infection on the immune response to group A streptococci. J. Clin. Invest., *49*:1405, 1970.
45. Bisno, A. L., Nelson, K. E., Waytz, P., and Brunt, J.: Factors influencing serum antibody responses in streptococcal pyoderma. J. Lab. Clin. Med., *81*:410, 1973.

46. Klein, G. C., and Jones, W. L.: Comparison of the Streptozyme test with the antistreptolysin O, antideoxyribonuclease B and antihyaluronidase tests. Appl. Microbiol., *21*:257, 1971.
47. Dajani, S. S., Hill, P. L., and Wannamaker, L. W.: Experimental infection of skin in the hamster simulating human impetigo. II. Assessment of various therapeutic regimens. Pediatrics, *48*:83, 1971.
48. Dillon, H. C.: The treatment of streptococcal skin infections. J. Pediatr., *76*:676, 1970.
49. Esterly, N. B., and Markowitz, M.: The treatment of pyoderma in children. JAMA, *214*:1862, 1970.
50. Dillon, H. C., and Derrick, C. W.: Clinical experience with clindamycin hydrochloride. I. Treatment of streptococcal and mixed streptococcal-staphylococcal skin infections. Pediatrics, *55*:205, 1975.
51. Dajani, A. S., Ferrieri, P., and Wannamaker, L.: Endemic superficial pyoderma in children. Arch. Dermatol., *108*:517, 1973.
52. Wilson, G. S., and Miles, A.: Topley and Wilson's Principles of Bacteriology, Virology, and Immunity. Baltimore, Williams & Wilkins, 1975, pp. 1908–1947.
53. Birkhaug, K. E.: Studies on the biology of the *Streptococcus erysipelatis*. Johns Hopkins Med. J., *36*:248, 1925.
54. Milstein, P., and Gleckman, R.: Pneumococcic erysipelas: A unique case in an adult. Am. J. Med., *59*:293, 1975.
55. Baxter, C. R.: Surgical management of soft tissue infections. Surg. Clin. North Am., *52*:1483, 1972.
56. Shulman, J. A., and Nahmias, A. J.: Staphylococcal infections: Clinical aspects. *In:* Cohen, J. O. (ed.): The Staphylococci. New York, John Wiley & Sons, 1972.
57. Rasmussen, J. E.: *Hemophilus influenzae* cellulitis: Case presentation and review of the literature. Br. J. Dermatol., *88*:547, 1973.
58. Abramowicz, M. (ed.): The Medical Letter on Drugs and Therapeutics. New Rochelle, N.Y., The Medical Letter, Inc., 1976.
59. Hays, G. C., and Mullard, J. E.: Blistering distal dactylitis: A clinically recognizable streptococcal infection. Pediatrics, *56*:129, 1975.
60. Ehrenkranz, N. J.: Transmission of *Staphylococcus aureus* in man—Epidemiologic and experimental studies. *In:* Maibach, H. I., and Hildrick-Smith, G. (eds.): Skin Bacteria and Their Role in Infection. New York, McGraw-Hill, 1965.
61. Melish, M. E., and Glasgow, L. A.: Staphylococcal scalded skin syndrome: The expanded clinical syndrome. J. Pediatr., *78*:958, 1971.
62. Kay, C. R.: Sepsis in the home. Br. Med. J., *1*:1048, 1962.
63. Melish, M. E., Glasgow, L. A., and Turner, M. D.: The staphylococcal scalded skin syndrome: Isolation and partial characterization of the exfoliative toxin. J. Infect. Dis., *125*:129, 1972.
64. Kondo, I., Sakurai, S., and Sarai, Y.: New type of exfolatin obtained from staphylococcal strains belonging to phage groups other than group II, isolated from patients with impetigo and Ritter's disease. Infect. Immun., *10*:851, 1974.
65. Dajani, S. S.: The scalded skin syndrome: Relation to phage group II staphylococci. J. Infect. Dis., *125*:548, 1972.
66. Epstein, E. H., Flynn, P., and Davis, R. S.: Adult toxic epidermal necrolysis with fatal staphylococcal septicemia. JAMA, *229*:425, 1974.
67. Elias, P. M., and Levy, S. W.: Bullous impetigo: Occurrence of localized scalded skin syndrome in an adult. Arch. Dermatol., *112*:856, 1976.
68. Elias, P. M., Fritsch, P., Tappliner, G., et al.: Experimental staphylococcal toxic epidermal necrolysis (TEN) in adult humans. J. Lab. Clin. Med., *84*:414, 1974.
69. Peck, G. L., Herzig, G. P., and Elias, P. M.: Toxic epidermal necrolysis in a patient with graft-versus-host reaction. Arch. Dermatol., *105*:561, 1972.
70. Leyden, J. J., Marples, R. R., Mills, O. H., and Kligman, A. M.: Gram-negative folliculitis: Complication of antibiotic therapy. Br. J. Dermatol., *88*:533, 1973.
71. Potter, B. S., Burgoon, C. F., and Johnson, W. C.: *Pityrosporum* folliculitis: Report of seven cases and review of pityrosporum organism relative to cutaneous disease. Arch. Dermatol., *107*:388, 1973.
72. Spittelhouse, K. E.: Phage-types of *Staphylococcus pyogenes* isolated from impetigo and sycosis barbae. Lancet, *2*:378, 1955.
73. Dilaimy, M.: Pseudofolliculitis of the legs. Arch. Dermatol., *112*:507, 1976.
74. Gould, J. C., and Cruikshank, J. D.: Staphylococcal infection in general practice. Lancet, *2*:1157, 1957.
75. Louria, D. B.: Factors predisposing to clinical infections of the skin. *In:* Maibach, H. I., and Hildick-Smith, G. (eds.): Skin Bacteria and Their Role in Infection. New York, McGraw-Hill, 1965, pp.75–84.
76. Wise, R. I.: Modern management of severe staphylococcal disease. Medicine, *52*:295, 1973.
77. Pestka, S., Vince, R., LeMahieu, R., et al: Induction of erythromycin resistance in *Staphylococcus aureus* by erythromycin derivatives. Antimicrob. Agents Chemother., *9*:128, 1976.

78. Strauss, W. G., Maibach, H. I., and Shinefield, H. R.: Bacterial interference treatment of recurrent furunculosis. JAMA, *208*:861, 1969.
79. Weinstein, L., and Barza, M. A.: Gas gangrene. N. Engl. J. Med., *289*:1129, 1973.
80. Nelson, E.: Five hundred cases of erysipeloid. Rocky Mt. Med. J., *52* 40, 1955.
81. Klauder, J. V.: *Erysipelothrix rhusiopathiae* infection in swine and in human beings. Arch. Dermatol., *50*:151, 1944.
82. Gorbach, S. L., and Bartlett, J. G.: Anaerobic infections. N. Engl. J. Med., *290*:1177, 1237, 1289, 1974.
83. Strasberg, S. M., and Silver, M. S.: Hemolytic streptococcus gangrene. An uncommon but frequently fatal infection in the antibiotic era. Am. J. Surg., *115*:763, 1968.
84. Rea, W. J., and Wyrick, W. J.: Necrotizing fasciitis. Ann. Surg., *175*:957, 1970.
85. McCloskey, R. V.: Scarlet fever and necrotizing fasciitis caused by coagulase-positive hemolytic *Staphylococcus aureus*, phage type 85. Ann. Intern. Med., *78*:85, 1973.
86. Stone, H. H., and Martin, J. D.: Synergistic necrotizing cellulitis. Ann. Surg., *175*:202, 1972.
87. Meleney, F. L.: Clinical Aspects and Treatment of Surgical Infections. Philadelphia, W. B. Saunders, 1949.
88. Meleney, F. L.: A differential diagnosis between certain types of infectious gangrene of the skin with particular reference to hemolytic streptococcus gangrene and bacterial synergistic gangrene. Surg. Gynecol. Obstet., *56*:847, 1933.
89. Forkner, C. E., Frei, E., Edgcomb, J. H., and Utz, J. P.: *Pseudomonas* septicemia. Am. J. Med., *25*:877, 1958.
90. McKelvie, M., and McKelvie, P.: Some aetiological factors in otitis externa. Br. J. Dermatol., *78*:227, 1966.
91. Goldman, L., and Fox, H.: Greenish pigmentation of nail plates from *Bacillus pyocyaneous* infection. Arch. Dermatol., *49*:136, 1944.
92. Taplin, D., Zaias, N., and Rebell, G.: Skin infections in a military population. Dev. Ind. Microbiol., *8*:3, 1969.

9 | VIRAL INFECTIONS

ROSALYN WEINTRAUB, M.D.

INTRODUCTION

Adolescents are subject to the same viral infections of the skin that occur at other ages. Some viral infections, such as verruca vulgaris, may have a greater frequency during adolescence; others, such as molluscum contagiosum and herpes simplex, become more prevalent with sexual maturity. By puberty, the majority of the population either has been vaccinated against or has been infected with most of the childhood viral exanthems. Because these have always been of clinical interest, new exanthems and atypical presentations of older ones continue to be described.

Since the late 1960's, there has been significant advancement in the rapid laboratory diagnosis of viral infections. Isolation and identification of some viral agents, such as herpes simplex virus (HSV), may be obtained in two to three days; rubella and other viruses may take from three to four weeks to isolate.[1] New studies using fluorescent antibody techniques, gel diffusion, and electron microscopy have expedited the diagnosis of viral infections. With the introduction of phosphotungstic acid for rapid negative staining, some viruses contained in crusts and vesicles can be identified in minutes by electron microscopy.[2]

Viruses are strict intracellular parasites. The virion contains a core of one nucleic acid, either RNA or DNA, and a protein outer coat or capsid, which is the antigenic part of the virus. Viruses lack ribosomes and therefore depend on the use of the host cells' enzyme systems. They reproduce by inducing the host cell to synthesize new viral material. Viruses blend with the metabolic material of the host cell and in some conditions may be undetectable until some stimulus causes the cell to produce new viral particles. Viral infection is often detected histologically by the presence of inclusion bodies in the nucleus or cytoplasm of the cell.

Viral infections of the skin may vary in their morphological appearance. Lesions may be erythematous macules or papules, vesicles, pustules, or occasionally urticarial. Viral infections can also induce epidermal cells to proliferate, causing the characteristic tumors of molluscum contagiosum, warts, and milker's nodule. These infections are confined completely to the epidermis. Other viruses, after an initial incubation and proliferation in the skin, may disseminate to other organs.

Vaccines have been important in the prevention of many viral diseases, such as polio, measles, mumps, rubella, and smallpox. However, the management of viral diseases has been limited to symptomatic therapy, since few chemotherapeutic agents are capable of killing viruses without injuring the host.[3] Host defenses against viral infections include (1) humoral antibodies produced in response to antigenic stimulation by viruses, (2) local antibodies (IgA) produced in the mucous secretions of the gastrointestinal, respiratory, and urinary tracts, which can prevent infection at the point of entry of the virus, and (3) serum antibodies that protect against systemic invasion by the virus. In addition, interferon, a non-antibody polypeptide produced by viral-infected cells, makes cells of the same species resistant to infection by other viruses.

Besides vaccines, interferon, and interferon inducers, antiviral therapy also includes chemotherapy and more recently, phototherapy. The characteristic resistance of viral infections to treatment with antibiotics may be related to the viruses' use of the host enzyme systems to reproduce. Any attempt to interfere with these systems has disastrous effects on the host.

Although the intracellular location of the virus makes it particularly resistant to antibiotics, several new antiviral drugs may be effective. Amantadine hydrochloride, useful in influenza A_2, interferes with entry of the virus into the host cell. 5-Iodo-2'-deoxyuridine inhibits the enzymes necessary for synthesis of nucleic acid precursors and also competes with nucleotides for incorporation into nucleic acid. This drug has been effective in herpes simplex infections of the eye. Cytosine arabinoside (Ara-C), a nucleoside analogue, is effective against DNA core viruses and has been used in herpes zoster and cytomegalic inclusion disease. These agents are quite toxic, for by interfering with viral replication they also interfere with synthesis of host cell DNA. Rifampicin inhibits poxvirus and adenovirus in vitro and because of its low toxicity was thought to be a very promising drug. Unfortunately, its lack of toxicity is associated with a lack of antiviral activity. Methisazone has been remarkably effective in the treatment of smallpox. By preventing the formation of complete viral particles, it inhibits late protein synthesis. Viral components are produced but are not assembled into complete viruses. In tissue culture, methiasazone has a broad spectrum of activity, but it has been used primarily for the prevention of smallpox.[4, 5]

Interferons are proteins endogenously produced by cells in response to viral infection. Interferons disrupt the combination of viral messenger RNA and cellular ribosomes, thereby preventing the synthesis of viral proteins. One substance, poly I:C, a synthetic double-stranded RNA, is now under study as a compound to induce interferon production. Although there is active interest in the treatment of viral infections, specific antiviral agents are still under investigation.

HERPES SIMPLEX VIRUS (HSV)

Infections with herpes simplex viruses are probably the most common viral infections of humans. The layman usually refers to these infections as fever blisters or cold sores. These viruses have a universal distribution, and almost all adults have been infected at some time. Dowdle and Nahmias[6] showed that the causative agent, herpesvirus hominis (a DNA-containing virus), is differentiated into antigenic Types I and II, each having individual biological and morphological properties. They can be differentiated by their cytopathic effect and plaque size on tissue culture: Type II produces larger pocks on egg chorioallantoic membranes (Fig. 9-1). The DNA is chemically distinct in each type, and each shows a marked difference in pattern of skin infection, depending on age of host, venereal exposure, and site of infection.[7] HSV Type I occurs more often in non-genital infections. The greatest initial incidence is during childhood; antibody to Type I often is evident by two to five years of age. In older patients, HSV Type I may be isolated from the face and upper trunk.[3, 8]

Neonatal herpes is usually caused by Type II virus. Since HSV-II is spread venereally, it is more common in sexually active adolescents and adults and may be transmitted to the neonate at birth. Antibodies to HSV-II increase at puberty.

The relationship of HSV Type II to cervical cancer has been of concern. The oncogenic potential of other herpesviruses is well known, and recent clinical investigations have implicated HSV as a cause of cervical dysplasia and carcinoma.[9] Rapp has shown that HSV can transform hamster embryo fibroblasts into neoplastic cells.[10] The incidence of cancer of the cervix is much higher in females with antibodies of HSV-II than it is in matched controls. Antigens produced by HSV in cell culture are related to antigens derived from cervical carcinomas. Although HSV may be related to cervical carcinoma, only a small fraction of females with HSV-II infection develop cancer. Therefore, other factors must be important.[3, 11]

Disseminated herpes simplex infection involves the initial entry of the virus, followed by primary viremia. In the next (progressive) stage, the virus disappears from the blood but multiplies in the cells of infected organs. This is followed by a third "florid" stage, with a secondary viremia and the seeding of multiple organ systems. In the final stage, or recovery, the virus clears from the blood and diminishing amounts of virus are found in the involved viscera. In

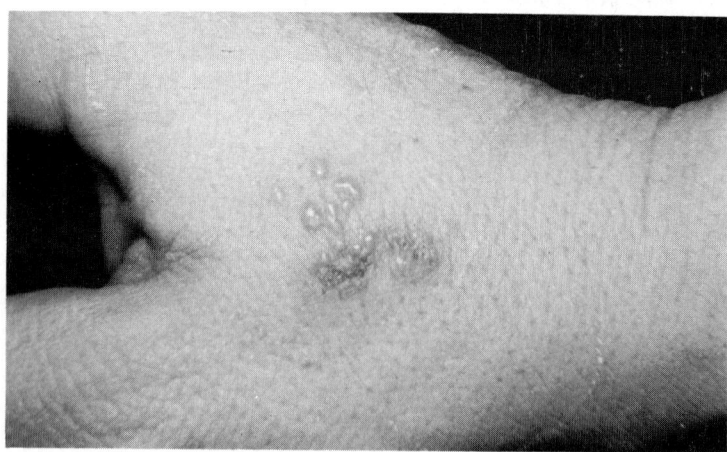

FIGURE 9-1 Herpes simplex. (Courtesy of Dr. Adnan S. Dajani.)

the dissemination of virus from the respiratory or genital tract to neural tissue, mature virions may be distributed along peripheral nerves by streaming through the axoplasm or by cell-to-cell transmission within the Schwann sheath surrounding the nerve. This may explain the occasional zosteriform presentation of HSV.[12] HSV has also been found in cadavers in both the sacral and the trigeminal ganglia.

PRIMARY HERPES SIMPLEX

Infections with HSV are classified as primary, recurrent, and chronic. Primary infection denotes the first exposure to HSV-I or HSV-II. Since most primary infections with HSV are subclinical or unapparent, they are characterized only by the development of antibodies to the virus. When it is clinically manifest, the primary infection tends to be more severe than recurrent infections with the same virus type.[13] There is also a spectrum of severity of the primary infection, ranging from subclinical infection (50 per cent) to severe involvement of all organs of the body. The incubation period is from two to 20 days.[11] Neutralizing antibodies develop in one to four weeks; IgM antibodies develop in the first two weeks, followed by IgA and IgG antibodies. Herpes simplex is rare before four months of age, as passively transferred maternal antibodies protect most infants from infection. However, the incidence of primary infection rises after one year of age and becomes frequent thereafter.

The most common primary clinical presentation of HSV Type I infection is gingivostomatitis, characterized by a sudden high fever. Vesicles develop in the oral cavity and soon become eroded and ulcerated. The gingivae are swollen, drooling is constant, and marked cervical lymphadenopathy appears. This painful condition usually persists for 10 days to two weeks. Although gingivostomatitis occurs predominantly in children, young adults may be affected as well.

Keratoconjunctivitis also may occur as a primary herpetic infection. It is characterized by edema, erythema, vesicles, and erosions of the conjunctiva and cornea. Marked pain and photophobia are present; occasionally blindness may result. Although it is usually caused by HSV-I, keratoconjunctivitis in newborn infants may be caused by a Type II infection.

Primary cutaneous inoculation herpes simplex is a less common presentation of HSV. It results from the implantation of the virus in traumatized skin. In wrestlers, it has been called herpes gladiatorum. Dentists, hygienists, and anesthesiologists are subject to a herpetic whitlow or paronychia from contact with infected saliva. This primary infection may be accompanied by systemic symptoms.[14] Often these paronychias are mistaken for pyogenic infections.[15] Herpetic paronychia may also occur by autoinoculation from nailbiting in patients with herpetic stomatitis.[16]

Primary herpes may cause a meningoencephalitis clinically indistinguishable from that caused by other viral agents. Diagnosis is difficult in that the patient may present with only an antecedent rhinitis or pharyngitis without skin lesions. Biopsy of brain tissue may be the only method of establishing a definitive diagnosis. The mortality rate has been high with all therapeutic efforts.

Primary vulvovaginitis or balanitis is usually caused by HSV Type II. Vesicles rapidly become eroded, and marked edema of the genitalia may be present, along with associated regional adenopathy, fever, and constitutional symptoms. Herpes cervicitis may be associated with vulvovaginitis or may occur independently. HSV is found more frequently in the cervical area than in the external genitalia and may be discovered in routine Papanicolaou cervical smears in asymptomatic patients.[17] In males, the primary HSV infection may cause a urethritis accompanied by severe dysuria and regional adenopathy but without any visible skin findings.

Genital herpes occurs frequently in teenagers. One half of the females with genital herpes and one quarter of the males are in this age group. There is also a significant association with other venereal diseases. Infrequently, genital lesions occur in children. Aside from the clinical and psychological problems related to genital herpes, females with herpes simplex infections during pregnancy develop more severe primary herpes, perhaps because of the relative immunosuppression at this time.[11] Transmission of the virus to the infant may occur early in gestation, accounting for a higher incidence of abortion and premature births. It may also occur at delivery, when the infant may be infected transplacentally or by direct contact with the virus in the birth canal.[17]

NEONATAL HERPES INFECTION

Neonatal herpes is caused predominantly by HSV Type II. It varies from a relatively mild disorder limited to the skin to a severe, often fatal, systemic infection.[11] Several cases of herpes simplex presenting with grouped vesicles in a zosteriform distribution have been observed in newborn infants.[18] Often the clinical manifestations of fever, cyanosis, and hepatosplenomegaly must be differentiated from other viral infections of newborns, such as rubella and cytomegalovirus, which present as a TORCH syndrome (*T*oxoplasma, *O*ther, *R*ubella, *C*ytomegalovirus, and *H*erpes simplex virus). The lungs, liver, adrenal glands, central nervous system, gastrointestinal tract, and occasionally the skin and mucous membrane may be involved. Whether neonatal herpes can be prevented by Cesarean section in females with genital herpes who are close to term is now being determined. Approximately 50 per cent of infants delivered vaginally become infected, and of these, half are severely damaged or die of herpetic infection. Amniocentesis performed close to the time of delivery in a mother with genital herpes may be helpful. If HSV is found in the amniotic fluid, vaginal delivery is contraindicated.[19]

Primary infection with rapid systemic dissemination occurs in immunologically impaired patients and in those receiving immunosuppressant drugs such as azathioprine or corticosteroids. Severely malnourished patients may present initially with herpetic gingivostomatitis and rapidly progress to hepatitis with dissemination of the HSV infection. Almost 35 per cent of patients with renal transplants develop herpes simplex infections.

KAPOSI'S VARICELLIFORM ERUPTION

Kaposi's varicelliform eruption is a severe infection of the skin with HSV, vaccinia virus, or varicella in a patient with an underlying skin disorder. This is most common with atopic dermatitis, but association with Darier's disease and severe thermal burns also has been reported. The physician must examine the margins of burns for the presence of vesicles. Kaposi's varicelliform eruption has a predilection for infants and children, but patients of any age may be affected. Clinically, there is a sudden development of umbilicated, varicelliform lesions in the area of the skin most involved in the dermatosis. There is marked malaise, toxicity, fever up to 105°F (40.8°C), edema of the involved skin, and marked lymphadenopathy. The peak of the illness usually occurs within 10 days, but the entire course may last up to four weeks. Because of the decline in smallpox immunization, HSV is the major cause of Kaposi's varicelliform eruption today. The two viruses can be differentiated by a Tzanck smear. HSV produces intranuclear inclusions and multinucleated giant cells, while vaccinia virus produces cytoplasmic inclusions. Occasionally, Kaposi's varicelliform eruption becomes a recurrent infection in susceptible individuals.

RECURRENT HERPES SIMPLEX

Recurrent herpes simplex infections are seen in patients previously infected with HSV and are thought to be caused by reactivation of a latent or quiescent infection.[20] It has also been shown that infectious virus can reinfect an individual who has a high titer of herpes-neutralizing antibodies.[21] Injecting vaccines to increase serum antibodies therefore would seem an irrational therapy for recurrent herpes. These patients have a high level of neutralizing antibodies present at the onset of the recurrent infection, and there is little fluctuation of the antibody level during the illness. After peripheral infection, the herpes virus remains in some form in the regional nerve ganglia.[12] Many clinicians believe that recurrent HSV originates from these ganglia and spreads distally to the skin. HSV Type II has been recovered from the sacral ganglia and Type I from the trigeminal ganglion. The recurrent disease tends to be more benign than the primary; it is self-limiting and the lesions usually heal within two weeks.

The precipitating cause of recurrent herpes may be any stress or emotional upset, sunlight, fever, onset of menses, gastrointestinal disorder, dental extraction, or exposure to cold, to note a few causes. The onset is heralded by burning or itching at the site of involvement, followed within a few hours to days by the appearance of small (2 to 3 mm) vesicles grouped on an erythematous base. These vesicles, which rapidly become purulent and crusted, heal in one to two weeks. The most common sites of involvement are the lips, perioral area, and face, followed by the anogenital area, buttocks, and thighs. A recurrent herpes simplex virus infection may affect the eye, producing a severe keratitis or keratoiritis. However, corneal transplants have been fairly successful once the infection has cleared. It is known that some patients may develop a recurrent encephalitis or a recurrent Kaposi's varicelliform eruption.

HSV also may precipitate recurrent erythema multiforme.[22] This has been associated with HSV-I, but recently two cases with HSV-II infections were reported. One unusual case followed a herpes-related cervicitis and was characterized by the persistence of large crusted plaques from which virus was recovered. A second case, which followed HSV Type II recurrent herpes progenitalis, showed no evidence of virus in the lesions of erythema multiforme. Rarely, a severe type of neuralgia accompanies some recurrent HSV infections. This unusual variant seems to be more recalcitrant to therapy.

CHRONIC HERPES SIMPLEX

A chronic cutaneous form of HSV infection has been seen only in patients with impaired immunity and in those receiving immunosuppressive drugs. These individuals may develop chronic destructive skin lesions without dissemination of the infection.[23] Low antibody titers are found. The lesions may be single or multiple ulcers with hemorrhagic crusting, and the borders may have characteristic vesicles. They are resistant to therapy.[24]

Diagnosis of HSV by tissue culture of the virus can often be made in one to two days. Once the virus is isolated, serological tests can differentiate Type I from Type II. Rising antibody titers distinguish primary infections from recurrent ones. More rapid diagnosis of infections is possible with the use of fluorescent antibody techniques.

TREATMENT

Treatment of herpes simplex virus infection is primarily symptomatic, as no specific therapy is yet available. Many drugs have been tested and found either ineffective or occasionally harmful. In the early stages, vesicles are opened, and alcohol, ether, chloroform, or liquid nitrogen is applied. In recurrent infections, ways of eliminating precipitating factors, such as sunlight exposure or emotional stress, are considered first. Iododeoxyuridine has been beneficial in the treatment of herpetic keratitis but has not been too effective in herpes labialis and herpes progenitalis. Although it was initially reported to promote rapid healing in these sites, no controlled studies exist to document its efficacy. Iododeoxyuridine has also been used in HSV-related encephalitis, but the results to date are difficult to interpret.[21] Photoinactivation of HSV after the application of supravital dyes (proflavine and neutral red), followed by exposure to light, caused inactivation of the virus in vitro. However, the resulting defective viral particles caused cell cultures to lose contact inhibition, and the question of potential oncogenicity has arisen. Furthermore, there is reason to doubt the efficacy of this treatment in vivo. Drugs in investigational use in herpes simplex virus infections include adenine arabinoside (Ara-A), cytosine arabinoside (Ara-C), 5-iodo-2'-deoxyuridine, trifluorothymidine, and phosphonoacetic acid.[25] All of these agents interfere with the DNA metabolism of cells, and thus all may be extremely toxic.[4, 21] Vaccines also are currently being studied. They have been used in recurrent HSV infection, even though the host already has high antibody levels. Again, there is concern about the use of HSV vaccine because of its possible oncogenicity. Immunogens containing no viral DNA would be a more acceptable treatment if they could be shown to be effective. There is no information on the use of steroids in HSV infections. Their use in the eye is contraindicated without concurrent administration of antiviral drugs.

VARICELLA-ZOSTER INFECTIONS

It is interesting to compare HSV with the varicella-zoster virus (V-Z), since both these herpesviruses cause a distinctive primary infection that is often followed by a reactivation of the endogenous virus after a variable latent period. In both conditions, the virus has been recovered from regional nerve ganglia.

Varicella (chickenpox) and herpes zoster are caused by the same virus and a morphological distinction cannot be made by tissue culture, electron microscopy, fluorescent antibody studies, or complement fixation tests. Studies have indicated that susceptible children inoculated with vesicle fluid from patients with herpes zoster contracted typical varicella, while those with a previous history of varicella did not develop any lesions. Furthermore, patients with herpes zoster produce only IgG complement-fixing antibody (usually a secondary or anamnestic response), while patients with varicella produce IgM complement-fixing antibody initially, followed by the production of IgG antibody. Sera from patients recovering from herpes zoster have a much higher antibody titer than sera from convalescing varicella patients. Because herpes zoster is caused by a reactivation of endogenous virus, its incidence in childhood is low. It has been reported rarely in infants whose mothers had varicella during pregnancy. Its incidence increases with age.[26]

VARICELLA

Varicella is a highly contagious, acute, exanthematous disease, caused by herpesvirus varicellae. Its communicability is such that 90 per cent of the population of the western world has been infected by the time they reach adulthood. There is a peak incidence between the ages of two and eight years. Although it may occur in all seasons, varicella is more frequent in the winter and spring in temperate climates. The transmission of the virus by the respiratory tract seems to occur early in the disease, as it is difficult to recover virus from the nasopharynx; however, the virus is easily recovered from the characteristic vesicles.

CLINICAL SIGNS

Clinically, varicella has an incubation period of 10 to 20 days. A 24-hour prodrome of fever, headache, and malaise may occur; the fever and eruption appear simultaneously. A transient scarlatiniform or morbilliform exanthem is seen on the trunk, face, and scalp (Fig. 9–2). These macules quickly become papules developing a unilocular small vesicle, in the center which results in the characteristic "dewdrop on a rose" appearance. This vesicle rapidly becomes turbid and slightly unbilicated. The lesion dries and is rendered non-infective with crusting. These vesicles erupt in three to five crops over a period of two to four days, so that lesions characteristic of every stage of development are present. Eventually, all lesions become crusted and if they are not secondarily infected heal in two to three weeks without scarring.

The exanthem appears abruptly first on the trunk, face, and scalp. Lesions

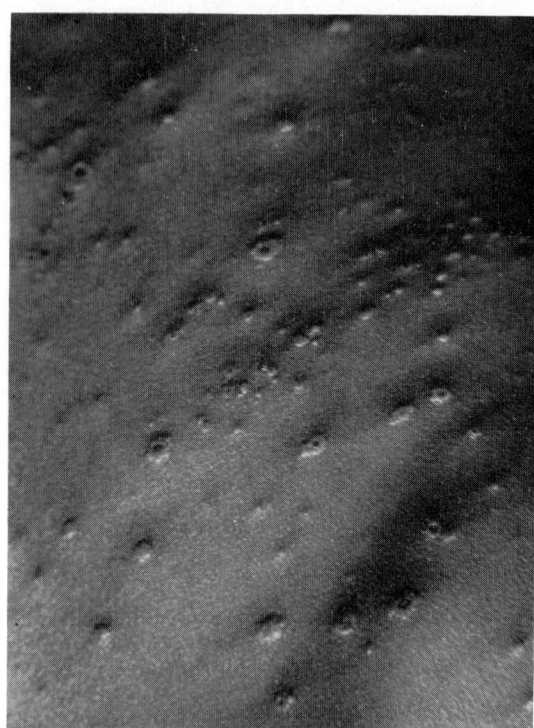

FIGURE 9–2 Chickenpox.

are most concentrated at these sites. The axillae and proximal portions of the extremities, thighs, and upper arms are more extensively involved; the distal palms and soles are usually spared. Mucous membranes are characteristically involved, and ulcers may be present on the palate and anterior tonsillar pillars, conjunctiva, vulva, pharynx, and even larynx. Systemic symptoms of fever, headache and malaise may last as long as active lesions appear but in general such systemic symptoms are mild in children. Pruritus is often the most severe symptom, and the resulting scratching may lead to secondary bacterial infection of the lesions. Other complications of varicella include thrombocytopenic purpura, mild encephalitis, and keratitis. Occasionally, unusual lesions are observed, such as polycyclic bullae resulting from the coalescence of vesicles. Hemorrhagic blisters with petechiae are likely to occur in immunologically weakened patients. Patients receiving chemotherapy for malignancy, those with renal transplants or autoimmune diseases, as well as those taking steroids may develop hemorrhagic varicella, an often fatal variant of the disease. Lowering the dose of steroids in these patients is contraindicated.

When varicella occurs in older adolescents and adults, the systemic symptoms tend to be more severe and the exanthem more profuse than in children. Adults also develop viral pneumonia as a complication of varicella more frequently than children do. If varicella occurs during pregnancy, the fetus may be unaffected, infected in utero, or infected at the time of delivery. Infection that takes place early in gestation may be manifested after birth by cicatrizing lesions of the extremities and by neuromuscular disorders. Congenital infections may also present at birth or shortly thereafter as typical varicella. More common is neonatal varicella with onset 10 to 28 days after birth.

This condition varies from a benign infection to a severe, often fatal, disorder.

The diagnosis of varicella is usually made clinically. The differentiation from variola is important but may be difficult in some cases of modified smallpox. Electron microscopic studies of vesicle contents can rapidly distinguish herpesvirus from poxvirus. A Tzanck smear may help if the intranuclear inclusions of the herpesvirus can be differentiated from the intracytoplasmic inclusions of the poxvirus. A characteristic rise in varicella-zoster antibody titer will also aid in the differential diagnosis.

Treatment

The treatment of varicella is symptomatic, and usually includes hygienic measures, aspirin for fever and pruritus, drying lotions, and soothing baths. Zoster-immune globulin, prepared from the plasma of patients recovering from herpes zoster, will prevent varicella if it is administered within 72 hours of the initial exposure. High-risk children (those with defective cell-mediated immunity, malignancies, or leukemia, and those receiving steroids or antimetabolites) are not protected as successfully, but the disease, if it occurs, is much milder. Zoster-immune globulin (ZIG) is not useful once the eruption has appeared. In newborn infants whose mothers have varicella at delivery, ZIG may prevent infection.[27]

HERPES ZOSTER

Herpes zoster is an acute vesicobullous eruption in a dermatomal distribution caused by reactivation of an endogenous, latent, varicella-zoster virus. It is thought that after an initial varicella infection, the varicella-zoster virus remains dormant in cells of the dorsal root ganglia or cranial nerve ganglia. The mechanisms that activate the virus are not known, although cold, trauma, x-irradiation, and altered immunity are considered important. Once activated, the varicella-zoster virus propagates along the affected sensory or cranial nerve to the skin, where infection causes the typical intraepidermal vesicles, which are identical to the vesicles of varicella. Pathologically, axon degeneration and demyelinization of posterior horn cells, and to a lesser degree anterior horn cells, occur. This may account for the occasional paresis associated with herpes zoster.

Clinical Signs

The incubation period after the initial varicella infection is unknown. The outstanding prodromal symptom is pain of variable severity in a dermatomal distribution, occurring one to 10 days before the vesicular eruption. The pain is described as dull, sharp, burning, or lancinating. Occasionally, the pain and the eruption occur simultaneously. The lesions resemble those of varicella but more often tend to appear in groups, concentrated at the proximal portion of the sensory or cranial nerve distribution (Fig. 9–3). The grouping is almost always unilateral along one or occasionally

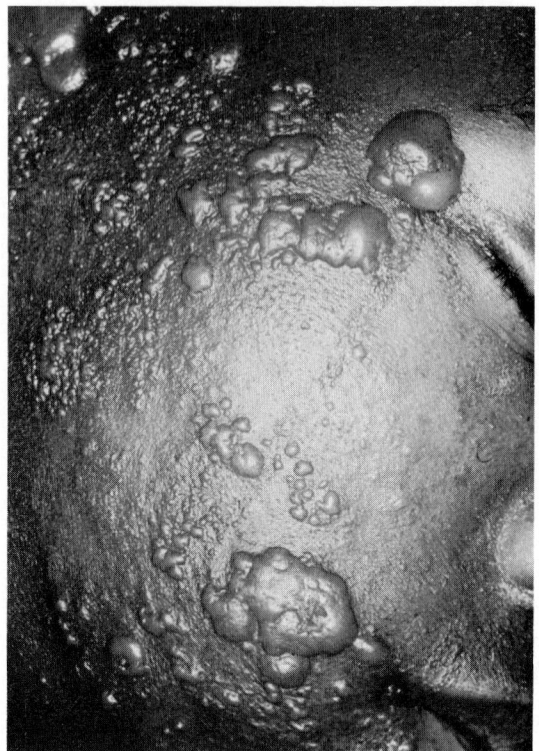
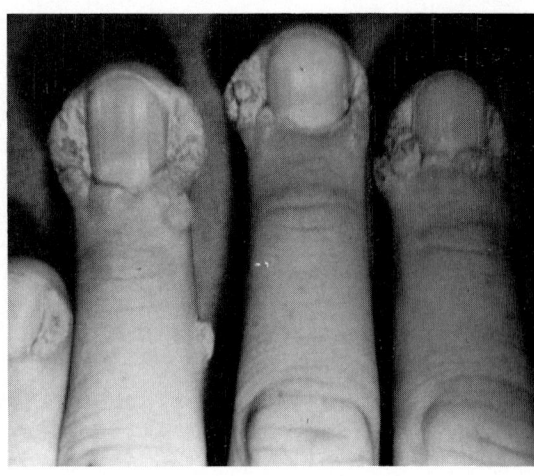

FIGURE 9-3 *A,* Herpes zoster. *B,* Verrucae vulgaris of the fingers.

two dermatomes. The evolution of the lesions from vesicles on an erythematous base to pustules and then to crusted lesions concludes with healing in two to two-and-half weeks. Lymphadenopathy, fever, and chills may also be present. Unlike varicella, scarring is common in herpes zoster. A few scattered vesicles may appear on other parts of the body, suggesting that a viremia has occurred. Immunosuppressed patients may develop a generalized herpes zoster infection that is indistinguishable from varicella.

In herpes zoster, the most common site of sensory nerve involvement is the skin innervated by thoracic ganglia (D_2), followed by the lumbosacral ganglia (L_2). The fifth and seventh cranial nerves are most frequently involved. Specific syndromes are associated with varicella-zoster infection of the various sensory and cranial ganglia.

Fifty per cent of cases with involvement of the ophthalmic division of the trigeminal nerve will have ocular complications. Vesicles on the side and tip of the nose indicate involvement of the nasociliary branch of the trigeminal nerve. Since this nerve gives rise to the ciliary nerve, which innervates the iris, ciliary body, and cornea, infection may lead to conjunctivitis, keratitis, corneal scarring, or panophthalmitis. If the ciliary ganglion is involved, a temporary or permanent Argyll Robertson pupillary reaction may be observed.

Zoster of the geniculate ganglion causes the Ramsay Hunt syndrome of tinnitus, deafness, vertigo, and sometimes deep facial pain simulating a dental abscess. Painful vesicles may appear on the uvula, palate, anterior tongue, auricle, and postauricular areas. The muscles of facial expression may be paralyzed, simulating a Bell's palsy.

Involvement of the glossopharyngeal ganglion causes pain in the ear and pharynx and produces vesicles in these areas. Vagal nerve involvement may cause cardiac and epigastric distress and paralysis of the larynx. Involvement of the phrenic nerve may cause hemidiaphragmatic paralysis. Thus, patients with herpes zoster of the neck should have a chest x-ray examination to check for this complication. With thoracic herpes zoster, pleural friction rubs are often present. Lumbosacral involvement may present initially as renal colic, and urinary retention may be a problem.[26]

The clinical diagnosis of herpes zoster is not difficult, although occasionally herpes simplex may occur in a zosteriform distribution. Although the viruses are indistinguishable on Tzanck smear, differential diagnosis may be made serologically or by isolating the virus.

Post-herpetic neuralgia is a severe problem but is extremely unusual in people under fifty. Approximately 4 per cent of patients with herpes zoster develop a generalized infection. Patients with defects of cell-mediated immunity, as in Hodgkin's disease, lymphomas, and chronic lymphatic leukemia, are more susceptible to herpes zoster than those with humoral defects, as in multiple myeloma.

TREATMENT

A study of treatment with steroids in early herpes zoster found that no dissemination occurred. Steroids were not found to be hazardous in a large series of patients with both Hodgkin's disease and herpes zoster.[29] The stage of Hodgkin's disease was a more critical determinant of dissemination of herpes zoster than was any treatment given the patients.

Treatment of herpes zoster is usually symptomatic, as the disorder is self-limited. Aspirin, analgesics, drying lotions, application of ethyl chloride, and flexible collodion painted on hyperesthetic areas have been useful. In patients over 60, high doses of steroids early in the course of the disease may reduce the incidence of post-herpetic neuralgia. Unfortunately, there have been reports of generalized herpes following the administration of systemic steroids in elderly patients, and some physicians feel that encephalitis may be precipitated when cranial nerves are involved. Individuals who develop herpes zoster in the course of steroid therapy are not at any greater risk of complications or of disseminated zoster than the general population. It is recommended that they be maintained on their medication throughout the illness. Recurrent herpes zoster is extremely rare and more likely to be recurrent herpes simplex in a zosteriform distribution.

WARTS

Warts are probably the most common viral infection of the skin and mucous membranes. Although they may vary in structure or clinical appearance, depending upon location, they are all caused by the same human papovavirus. Warts are primarily an infection of childhood and young adulthood. The viral etiology of verrucae has been known since 1907, when Cufio first transmitted the lesion by means of a cell-free ultrafiltrate. Ultrafiltrates of infected tissue cultures have produced verrucae in recipients,[30] and the virus has been successfully cultured.[31] Inoculation of material from one type of wart can give rise to other morphological varieties of verrucae. Autoinoculation is common; a single lesion is frequently surrounded by satellite lesions, and new lesions may occur on opposing skin surfaces.

Human papovavirus is one of the papillomaviruses, a subgroup of the papovaviruses. (Papova is an acronym for papilloma, polyoma, and vacuolating.) These are all oncogenic DNA viruses. Electromicroscopic studies have identified the virus as a spherical particle, 52μ in diameter, which is located next to the nucleus of the cell.[32] In verrucae, large vacuolated cells in the stratum spinosum have basophilic inclusions in their nuclei. Actually, two types of intranuclear inclusions have been reported. The basophilic inclusions appear to be aggregated viral particles, while the eosinophilic inclusions contain no viral elements and are seen both in the nuclei and cytoplasm of cells.[33] They seem to be composed of keratotic-like material and are probably a degeneration product related to abnormal keratinization.[34-36]

Fluorescent antibody techniques have shown localization of the wart antigen to the nuclei of cells in the stratum granulosum and lower portion of the stratum corneum.[37] Circulating wart virus antibodies have also been detected. With active infection, IgM is present; IgG occurs with increased frequency when the wart has been present over one year.[38] The longer the duration of the warts or the greater the number of lesions, the lower the serum antibody levels found.[39] When patients with regressing or non-regressing warts were compared, it was found that warts were rejected by patients with IgG antibodies, and cell-mediated immunity increased at resolution. Unfortunately, this immunity is short-lived, usually of no more than three months' duration.[38, 40]

The relationship between the human papovavirus and the epithelial cell is of interest. Two types of infection are noted in papovaviruses; (1) replicative, in which the virus reproduces itself and releases virions to infect adjacent cells, and (2) transformational, in which the viral genome is integrated into the germinative cells, causing heritable changes that are passed on to all progeny.[41] Studies of enzyme systems in humans seem to favor the latter type. In heterozygote females with two types of isoenzymes (a and b) in their skin, the warts produced had only one isoenzyme, either a or b. The wart was therefore believed to be a clone of cells arising from a single transformed keratinocyte.

Epidermodysplasia verruciformis is a rare familial disorder in which an eruption of flat warts appears during childhood and persists to undergo malignant degeneration. This disorder, shown to be caused by human papovavirus, causes verrucae when the virus is transmitted.[42]

Massing and Epstein's studies showed an incidence of warts of 7 to 10 per cent in the general population, with a much higher incidence in institutionalized patients. New lesions are more likely to occur in individuals who are already infected. Age is an important factor, with warts being less common in infancy and early childhood. The incidence increases during the school years with the peak at age 12 to 16, then decreases to age 20. After this, there is a general decline in the incidence of warts. In early childhood, the sexes appear to be equally affected. After age six, warts are more common in females.[44]

Because of a long incubation period, the transmission of warts has been difficult to study. However, warts are spread directly by contact with wart-infected tissue or indirectly by contact with virus-contaminated objects. Autoinoculation is very common.[36] Communal bathrooms, gymnasiums, tattooing, and sharing of contaminated materials, such as combs, have been associated with epidemics of warts.

With the exception of the feet, warts usually occur on areas that are unprotected by clothing. The virus enters the skin directly in minor abrasions, as seen in the rapid spread of flat warts in the bearded area. Pathologically, all verrucae are characterized by hyperplasia, hyperkeratosis, and acanthosis. There is hyperplasia of all layers of the epidermis. Vacuolated cells may be present in the stratum malpighii and granular layers. The basal layer is intact, but mitotic figures may extend for several layers. The intrapapillary papillae are elongated and contain blood vessels that extend into the wart, causing bleeding when the wart is trimmed. This may be helpful in differentiating warts from clavus (corns).

CLINICAL APPEARANCE

The clinical appearance of warts depends on their location. They vary primarily in degree of epithelial proliferation and keratinization.

Common Wart. Verruca vulgaris, or common wart, may be single or multiple, occurring anywhere but most frequently on the hands. These warts are sharply circumscribed firm papules, with a rough keratotic surface, usually 1 to 5 mm in diameter. Occasionally, a large mass of warts is produced by the confluence of individual papules.[45]

Flat Wart. Verruca plana juvenilis, or flat wart, is a discrete, slightly elevated, flat papule. It is commonly seen on the face, the dorsa of the hands, and the anterior tibial surfaces. These warts are frequently multiple, and often hundreds are present. Epidermodysplasia verruciformis, a generalized eruption of flat warts, has potential for malignant transformation into Bowen's carcinoma.

Digitate Wart. Digitate or filiform warts project as fingerlike or threadlike structures. They occur on the face and neck of young adults and may be confused with acrochordon or epidermal nevi.

Plantar Warts. Plantar warts occur on the plantar surface of the foot and occasionally on the palms. They do not extend above the surface of the surrounding skin. Plantar warts are covered by a hyperkeratotic material that resembles ordinary callus, but when they are pared, small bleeding points are visible. Most plantar warts occur beneath the heel or in the metatarsal area. They may be single or multiple and occasionally form a lesion composed of closely grouped small warts, called a mosaic wart. These are more resistant to therapy. Pain on pressure can be severe with plantar warts.

Condylomata Acuminata. Condylomata acuminata present a special problem. An exuberant, moist, polypoid growth occurs in the intertriginous spaces of the genitalia and the perianal region. These warts become fungating masses, which are often secondarily infected, at times involving the mucous membranes of the anus, vulva, and penis. Large cauliflower masses may develop, particularly during pregnancy, which often resolve spontaneously after delivery. Studies have shown that these genital warts have a venereal transmission.[46] Serological studies in one laboratory suggest that the genital wart virus may differ from the common wart virus in its antigenic structure.[47]

Laryngeal Papillomas. Laryngeal papillomas may occur at any age but can be a serious problem in early infancy. These papillomas are seen in a high percentage of infants whose mothers had genital warts at the time of delivery.[48] Laryngeal papillomas have been shown to contain human papovavirus like virions under the electron microscope.[49] As with other verrucae, spontaneous regression may occur, but recurrences after surgical removal are common.[43, 50]

TREATMENT

Just as warts vary in clinical manifestations, they also vary greatly in natural history. They may persist relatively unchanged for several years or may suddenly develop multiple satellite lesions. Some warts disappear spontaneously after several months or years (their average duration is two-and-one-half years).[32, 44, 51] Many therapists feel that some home remedies, including stump water and lard, have been as successful as some of the widely used therapeutic agents prescribed by physicians. Because of the high rate of spontaneous cure, any therapy that causes significant scarring, especially on an area such as the plantar surface of the foot, should be avoided.[52, 53] Therapy has been primarily destructive, but more recently immunotherapy and chemotherapy have been used.[32] Electrodesiccation, curettage, and cryosurgery are the methods most frequently employed. Surgical excision may be followed by pain and scarring, however, and recurrences are common on or near the scar. X-ray therapy is seldom used today.

Application of liquid nitrogen is the therapy of choice and is less likely to damage the dermis. However, when liquid nitrogen is used, the clinician must avoid freezing the digital vessels and nerves at the sides of fingers. Damage to the nail matrix can cause permanent nail dystrophy if the therapy is too intensive.

Chemocauterants used in treating warts include 0.7 per cent cantharidin[65] in flexible collodion,[54] 40 per cent salicylic acid plasters, and a preparation of 10 per cent salicylic acid and 10 per cent lactic acid in flexible collodion. Other chemicals, such as trichloroacetic acid, phenol, and nitric acid have also been used.

Exfoliative lotions, such as retinoic acid (Retin-A) have been helpful in treating flat warts. Podophyllin (20 per cent) in tincture of benzoin is used for condylomata acuminata. This solution is painted on, allowed to dry, and removed in four to six hours. The treatment is repeated weekly. One must be sure the patient is not pregnant, as podophyllin is absorbed systemically and may be very toxic.[56] Condylomata may also be excised or electrodesiccated, but care must be taken to avoid possible orificial stricture.

More recently, immunotherapy with dinitrochlorobenzene (DNCB),[36] smallpox vaccines and autologous wart vaccines, has come into use. Patients were first sensitized to DNCB. After DNCB was applied topically, a cell-mediated immune response resulted in destruction of the wart. However, the potential complications of smallpox vaccination and autologous vaccines make them unacceptable at this time. The use of transfer factor and chemotherapy with 5-fluorouracil and bleomycin is also currently being studied.[26] Warts may recur in spite of therapy. Patients with renal transplants, those receiving immunosuppressive medication, and those with depressed cellular immunity, as in Hodgkin's disease or lymphomas, present management problems because of their resistance to therapy.

MOLLUSCUM CONTAGIOSUM

Molluscum contagiosum was first described by Bateman over 150 years ago. Juliusberg established the causative agent as a filterable virus. This mildly contagious disease, which affects only the skin and conjunctivae, is characterized by the appearance of pearly, flesh-colored, firm, umbilicated papules 2 to 5 mm in diameter (Fig. 9–4). A central punctum develops in the umbilicated area from which a curdlike material can be expressed. These lesions occur on all parts of the body, singly or in clusters. They are more common on the face, breasts, genitalia, and inner surfaces of the thigh, less common on the conjunctival or mucosal surfaces, and extremely rare on the palms and soles.[57]

The disease is seen most frequently in children and young adults. Its distribution is worldwide, and it may occur sporadically or in small epidemics in schools and institutions. An incidence of one to 12 per 1000 has been observed in patients attending a dermatology clinic.[58] While a history of

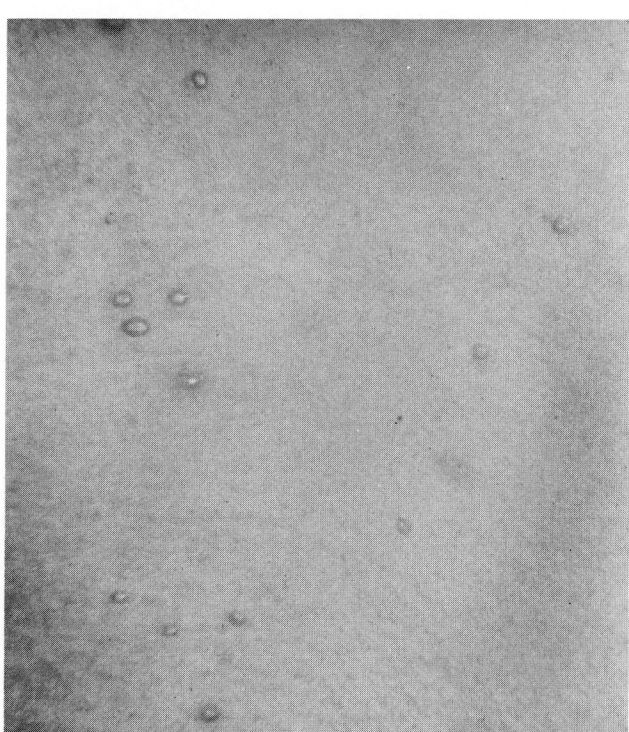

FIGURE 9–4 Molluscum contagiosum.

physical contact is rare in the common sporadic case, molluscum contagiosum is spread by close physical contact. It is often transmitted in swimming pools, Turkish baths, gymnasiums, and overcrowded living quarters. It can result from surgical procedures and tattooing. In adolescents and adults, molluscum contagiosum may be venereally transmitted; lesions occur frequently in the pubic area.[59, 60] Once infection has occurred, the disease is usually spread by autoinoculation caused by scratching.

In its size, shape, structure, and characteristic inclusion bodies, the molluscum contagiosum virus belongs to the poxviruses, the largest of all the vertebrate viruses.[58, 61] Identification of molluscum or Henderson-Patterson bodies, epidermal cells stuffed with elementary bodies of the virus, is easily made. Although the molluscum contagiosum virus has not been isolated and propagated in tissue cultures, it does affect tissue cells, which undergo cytopathic changes. An abortive infection in these cells has been produced, and transfer has been possible in human volunteers.[62, 63]

The viral antigen is not very potent. Until the agar gel diffusion technique showed humoral antibodies in 40 per cent of patients, only low titer complement-fixing antibodies had been demonstrated. The fluorescent antibody technique has shown the presence of humoral antibodies (89 per cent positive) and also localized antibodies on molluscum bodies.[55, 64] Patients infected with molluscum contagiosum virus have circulating antibodies with a very low titer, which disappears rapidly with healing of the lesions. In fluorescent antibody studies, antigen was not obvious until the intracytoplasmic inclusions had formed.[65]

PATHOGENESIS

Pathologically, hypertrophied epidermis extends into the dermis without breaking the limiting basement membrane. Proliferation is mainly confined to the basal layer, with the cell hypertrophy accompanied by rapid renewal time (three days versus a normal six days). Viral replication, characterized by the presence of Henderson-Patterson inclusion bodies, is not seen below the lower cells of the stratum spinosum.[58, 66] These inclusion bodies, consisting of mature and immature virus and cell debris, increase in size as the infected cells migrate to the stratum granulosum. After finally filling the host cells and pushing aside the nucleus, the characteristic mature hyalinized intracytoplasmic inclusion body, or molluscum body, is formed.[66, 67] Uninfected epidermal cells are interspersed among infected cells. Epstein, in thymidine studies, showed two populations of cells in each lesion. These included (1) infected cells that moved rapidly (nine to 15 days) and lost contact inhibition, and (2) uninfected cells that moved slowly (nine to 30 days).[68]

CLINICAL FINDINGS

The lesions develop by inoculation after an incubation period of two to eight weeks. In most cases, the diagnosis is established by typical umbilicated papules, but several unusual pictures have been described. Solitary lesions, especially large ones occurring on the face and scalp, may resemble furuncles, basal cell epitheliomas, keratoacanthomas, verruca vulgaris, or angiofibromas.[69] An eyelid lesion may simulate a sebaceous cyst or chalazion and may be associated with conjunctivitis. A miliary type of molluscum contagiosum, first described by Whitfield, consists of numerous, small, pruritic papules, suggesting seborrheic dermatitis. Plaques of 50 to 100 individual lesions, described as agminated, occurred in two cases of molluscum contagiosum, with involvement of the penis, pubis, and inner thigh.[70]

Although this infection is generally considered non-inflammatory, an inflammatory reaction may occur when the papules become disrupted and the contents are discharged into the dermis. A granulomatous reaction, resembling that seen in acne vulgaris or a ruptured sebaceous cyst, has been described. A molluscum dermatitis may develop with up to 10 cm of acute dermatitis surrounding the molluscum contagiosum papule. The dermatitis clears after the molluscum papule is removed.[71] This dermatitis may represent a delayed hypersensitivity reaction to a molluscum contagiosum virus antigen.[72] Widespread eruptive molluscum contagiosum also has been observed in patients with atopic dermatitis.[73] It has been postulated that these patients are more susceptible to viral infections than the general population.[74] Molluscum contagiosum has also caused extensive eruptions in immunosuppressed patients.

TREATMENT

Although the lesions of molluscum contagiosum often persist for months or years, most resolve spontaneously or as a result of an inflammatory response that develops after trauma or bacterial infection. Since the lesions are benign and usually resolve, any method of treatment that is potentially scarring should be avoided. Some of the commonly used therapies include: (1) spraying with ethyl chloride, followed by curettage, (2) electrodesiccation under local anesthesia, (3) application of cantharidin 0.9 per cent in flexible collodion, (4) cryosurgical freezing of lesions and, (5) administration of local cauterizing chemicals, such as phenol and trichloroacetic acid.

EXANTHEMATOUS DISEASES

Many systemic viral illnesses are accompanied by eruptions on the skin called exanthems. These may be macules, papules, pustules, vesicles, or petechiae, and often the virus may be isolated from the particular lesion. The clinical characteristics of the classic exanthems are fully described in any pediatric text. These disorders for the most part are encountered in childhood, and by adolescence either they have occurred or the child has been immunized against them. We are concerned with atypical presentations of well-known disorders and with some of the newer exanthems (Table 9–1).

TABLE 9–1   CLINICAL FINDINGS IN NEWER EXANTHEMS

	Skin	Mouth	Virus
COXSACKIE			
Herpangina	—none	—ulcers with hyperemic borders —vesicles: uvula, palate, anterior pillars, posterior pharynx	Coxsackie A9,2,4,5
Hand, foot, mouth	—papulovesicles distal extremities first, proximal borders: fingers, dorsa and ulnar border of hands —maculopapular lesions: buttocks	—herpangina	Coxsackie A16,5,10
A. Aseptic meningitis	—maculopapules and vesicles may resemble varicella but without pustules	—none	Coxsackie A9
B. Aseptic meningitis	—maculopapular and morbilliform, central distribution	—none	Coxsackie A4
C. Aseptic meningitis	—morbilliform exanthem, central distribution —fever disappears with onset	—none	Coxsackie B1,3,4,5
ECHO			
	—maculopapular exanthem occasionally vesicular —may have petechiae	—punched out ulcers: tonsillar pillars —gray-white papules simulate Koplik's	ECHO 9,4,6,14,18
Boston exanthem	—maculopapular (central distribution) —exanthem appears with defervescence	—punched out ulcers: soft palate and tonsillar pillars	ECHO 16,1,2,3,5 7,11,19

RUBEOLA

Rubeola (measles) is a highly contagious endemic myxovirus infection with an incubation period of two weeks. After a prodrome of fever, conjunctivitis, cough, and the presence of an enanthem (Koplik's spots), the exanthem appears. Starting as an erythematous, discrete, macular eruption in the scalp and spreading to the chest, these discrete macules become confluent and raised, presenting the characteristic rubelliform picture. After two to three days, a brownish discoloration is noted, and a fine scale may be present. The exanthem of measles is thought to be a delayed hypersensitivity response to measles antigen; normal cell-mediated immunity is necessary for the development of the eruption. Patients with severe defects in cell-mediated immunity are unable to get rid of the virus, suffer severe complications such as pneumonia, and do not develop the exanthem. However, in the absence of competent humoral immunity, e.g., agammaglobulinemia, there is no such problem. Interestingly, a depression of cell-mediated immunity occurs during the natural disease, as evidenced by anergic response to tuberculin. There is also a leukopenia that may be associated with defects in neutrophil chemotaxis.

During the early years of measles immunization, inactivated killed measles virus vaccine was used. It was given in three monthly doses and only occasionally followed by administration of live attenuated vaccine, as recommended in 1974 by the American Academy of Pediatrics. Some of the immunized children developed a severe illness with an unusual exanthem after being exposed to wild measles virus. Atypical reactions were also reported in children reimmunized with live vaccine. These were usually severe local reactions at the site of injection, similar to the Arthus reaction.

After immunization the illness associated with wild virus infection, atypical measles, is characterized by high fever, headache, myalgia, and cough. This is followed by a maculopapular exanthem involving first the distal portions of the extremities and the palms and soles (which are often edematous) and then extending to the trunk. Occasionally, the lesions are vesicular, urticarial, or purpuric (Fig. 9–5A, B, and C). A severe pneumonia, pleural effusion, and hilar adenopathy may be present. This serious illness, lasting one to two weeks, is thought to be caused by the accumulation of wild virus on mucosal surfaces. There the virus encounters circulating antibody, and the combination results in immune complex disease in the lung. Because of the severity of this illness, it is recommended that children who received only killed vaccine be reimmunized with live attenuated vaccine.

RUBELLA

Rubella is a viral exanthem often encountered in adolescents and young adults. In children it is a very mild, self-limited disorder. However, many children escape infection only to develop a more severe disease as young adults. Before the 1964 epidemic, 20 to 30 per cent of young adults had been shown to have no antibodies to rubella. A high incidence of infection in this age group was found in military camps and institutions.

Although the initial illness is often subclinical or very mild in children,

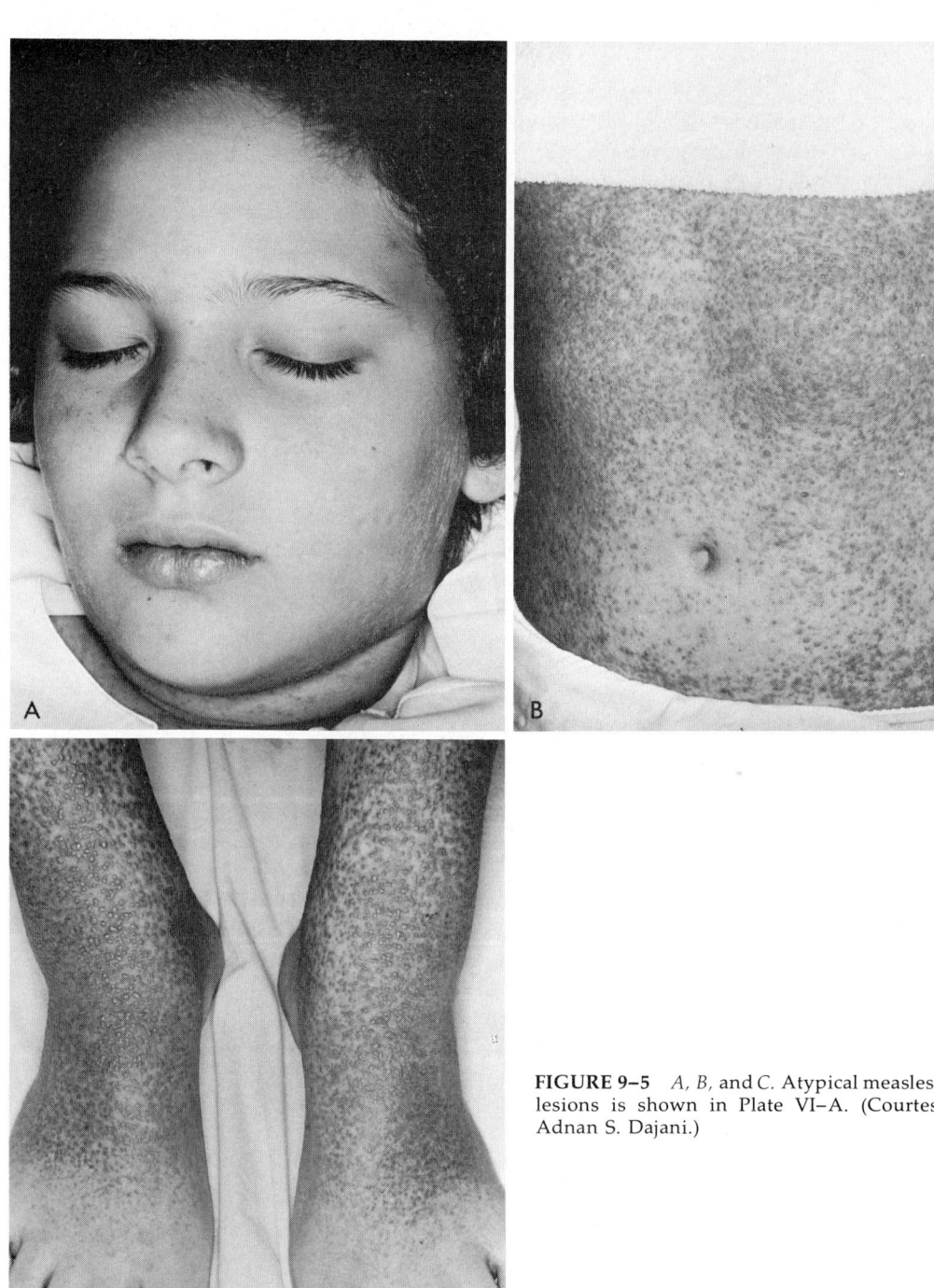

FIGURE 9–5 *A, B,* and *C.* Atypical measles. Color of lesions is shown in Plate VI–A. (Courtesy of Dr. Adnan S. Dajani.)

adults may have a four to five day prodrome of fever, malaise, headache, and respiratory symptoms. The exanthem occurring in 25 per cent of cases may vary from a faint blush to the more usual rash, starting with a macular eruption on the face that rapidly spreads to the trunk and extremities and clears in three days. An enanthem of petechiae on the soft palate may be present, and adenopathy may be prominent.

In adult or post-pubertal females, polyarthritis and polyarthralgia may occur. These conditions may persist for several weeks and may be associated with transient positive latex fixation tests for rheumatoid factor. Arthritis is less likely to occur in males and is uncommon in children.

The consequences for the infant whose mother developed rubella during early pregnancy are severe. A live attenuated vaccine has been developed, although antibody titers are not as high as after natural infection. With vaccination, a mild rash and lymphadenopathy may occur, but the most frequent complaint is arthralgia, which is usually mild and transient. A full-blown arthritis with pain, tenderness, swelling, effusion, and carpal tunnel syndrome has been reported. Because vaccination during pregnancy is contraindicated, hemagglutination-inhibition antibody tests should be performed when rubella is suspected in pregnant women.

ENTEROVIRUS INFECTION

The enteroviruses are the leading cause of some of the "newer" exanthems. Although they occur more commonly in children, they occasionally infect adults. Both epidemics and sporadic occurrences are common. In temperate climates, there is an increased incidence during late summer and fall. Virus has been recovered from the throat and respiratory tract for one to two weeks and from the stool for up to months after the infection.

Clinical expressions of these disorders are protean. In general, they cause fever, malaise, nausea, vomiting, diarrhea, hepatitis, pharyngitis, upper respiratory infections, pleurodynia, pneumonia, myocarditis, nephritis, orchitis, stomatitis, parotitis, meningitis, and encephalitis. As far as dermatological findings are concerned, the exanthems produced by the enteroviruses are not specific, as in measles or rubella, and one agent may cause various eruptions in the course of the same epidemic. Thus, maculopapular, vesicular, petechial, and urticarial lesions may all be seen. These exanthems and some enanthems occur more frequently in small children, and at adolescence the incidence of exanthems markedly declines.[75]

The most distinctive of the newer exanthems is hand, foot, and mouth syndrome caused primarily by Coxsackie A16 viral infection and occasionally by Coxsackie viruses A5 and A10. This infection occurs in late summer and fall. It spreads rapidly among children, and the disease may be transmitted to the parents of infected children. After an incubation period of four to six days and a prodrome of fever and malaise, an enanthem of vesicles and ulcers occurs on the palate, uvula, and tonsillar pillars in 90 per cent of cases. This infection is easily confused with aphthous stomatitis. In two thirds of patients, an exanthem appears on the hands and feet, first as maculopapules, later as grey vesicles on a slightly erythematous base. The lateral sides and dorsum are usually more involved than the palms and soles. Occasionally, a maculopapular eruption appears on the buttocks of children. This disorder frequently has been misdiagnosed as insect bites, poison ivy or an "id" reaction.[76]

Coxsackie A4, a common cause of aseptic meningitis, often presents with a non-specific maculopapular eruption, but an unusual symptom complex with vesicular lesions simulating chickenpox has also been observed. Another frequent cause of aseptic meningitis, ECHO 9 virus is frequently seen in children and in 50 per cent of cases is associated with an exanthem. It is usually maculopapular, but petechial eruptions are also seen. Occasionally, punched-out ulcers occur on the soft palate.

Boston exanthem, an uncommon infection, is caused by ECHO 16 and other viruses. After an incubation period of three to eight days, fever, anorexia, sore throat with punched out ulcerative lesions on the soft palate, and cervical lymphadenopathy occur. The fever disappears with the onset of the rubelliform exanthem, which extends to palms and soles and lasts from one to five days.

Coxsackie B5 has been associated primarily with aseptic meningitis and pleurodynia but may be implicated in paralytic disease, orchitis, hepatitis, neonatal encephalitis, and myocarditis. The exanthem is usually maculopapular, but petechial and urticarial lesions have been described; these exanthems occur at the time of defervescence.

SUMMARY

In summary, viral infections of the skin that occur at adolescence include those typical of childhood and those associated with sexual maturity. Herpes simplex Type II, molluscum contagiosum, and venereal warts, diseases that have shown a marked increase, are in the latter group. Certain diseases, such as rubella, herpes simplex, varicella, and condylomata acuminata, which may lead to laryngeal papillomas, are particularly important because of their effects on the newborn infant.

The epidemiological pattern of viral infections changes, and new viruses gain prominence while others fade in importance as causes of disease. Because of this, we can expect new viral entities and changes in earlier ones.

REFERENCES

1. Artenstein, M.S., and Demis, J.J.: Recent advances in the diagnosis and treatment of viral diseases of the skin. N. Engl. J. Med., *270*:1101, 1964.
2. Blank, H., Davis, C., and Collins, C.: Electron microscopy for the diagnosis of cutaneous viral infections. Br. J. Dermatol., *83*:69, 1970.
3. Blank, H.: Herpes simplex: From vesicles to cancer. J. Dermatol., *2*:53, 1975.
4. Alford, C. Z., Jr., and Whitley, R. J.: Treatment of infections due to herpes virus in humans: A critical review of the state of the art. J. Infect. Dis., *133*:101, 1976.
5. Fitzpatrick, T. B., Arndt, K. A., Clark, W. H. Jr., et al.: Dermatology in General Medicine. New York, McGraw-Hill, 1971.
6. Dowdle, W., Nahmias, A., Harwell, R., and Pauls, F.: Association of antigenic type of herpes virus hominis to site of viral recovery. J. Immunol., *99*:974, 1967.
7. Josey, W. E., Nahmias, A. J., and Naib, Z. M.: The epidemiology of type II (genital) herpes simplex virus infection. Obstet. Gynecol. Surv., *24*:295, 1972.
8. Blank, H., and Haines, H.: Viral diseases of the skin, 1975: A 25-year perspective. J. Invest. Dermatol., *67*:169, 1976.

9. Nahmias, A. J., Naib, Z. M., and Josey, W. E.: Epidermological studies relating genital herpetic infections to cervical carcinoma. Cancer Res., 34:1111, 1974.
10. Rapp, F., and Duff, R.: Oncogenic conversion of normal cells by activated herpes simplex viruses. Cancer, 34:1353, 1974.
11. Nahmias, A. J., and Roizman, B.: Infection with herpes simplex viruses I and II. N. Engl. J. Med., 289:667, 719, 781, 1973.
12. Stevens, J. G., and Cook, M. L.: Latent herpes simplex in ganglia of mice. Science, 173:843, 1971.
13. Nahmias, A. J., Josey, W. E., Naib, Z. M., et al.: Perinatal rise associated with maternal genital herpes simplex virus infection. Am. J. Obstet. Gynecol., 110:825, 1971.
14. Friedrich, E. R., Cole, W., and Middelkamp, J. N.: Herpes simplex: Clinical aspects and electron microscopic findings. Am. J. Obstet. Gynecol., 104:758, 1969.
15. Rosato, F. E., Rosato, E. F., and Plotkin, S. A.: Herpetic paronychia, an occupational hazard of medical personnel. N. Engl. J. Med., 382:804, 1970.
16. Muller, S. A., and Herrmann, E. C.: Association of stomatitis and paronychias due to herpes simplex. Arch. Dermatol., 101:396, 1970.
17. Amstey, M. S.: Genital herpes virus infection. Clin. Obstet. Gynecol., 18:89, 1975.
18. Music, S. I., Fine, E. M., and Togo, Y.: Zoster-like disease in the newborn due to herpes simplex virus. N. Engl. J. Med., 284:24, 1971.
19. Nahmias, A. J.: Herpes simplex infections. South. Med. J., 68:1191, 1975.
20. Docherty, J. L., and Chapan, M.: The latent herpes simplex virus. Bacteriol. Rev., 38:337, 1974.
21. Ashton, H., Frank, E., and Stevenson, C. J.: Herpes simplex virus infections and idoxuridine. Br. J. Dermatol., 84:496, 1971.
22. Shelley, W. B.: Herpes simplex virus as a cause of erythema multiforme. JAMA, 201:3, 1967.
23. Muller, S. A., Herrmann, E. C., Jr., and Winkelmann, R. K.: Herpes simplex infections in hematologic malignancies. Am. J. Med., 62:102, 1971.
24. Logan, W. S., Tindall, J. P., and Elson, M. L.: Chronic cutaneous herpes simplex. Arch. Dermatol., 103:606, 1971.
25. Adams, H. G., Benson, E. A., Alexander, E. R., et al.: Genital herpetic infection in men and women: Clinical course and effect of topical application of adenine arabinoside. J. Infect. Dis., 133:151, 1976.
26. Burgoon, C. F., Jr., Burgoon, J. S., and Baldridge, G. D.: The natural history of herpes zoster. JAMA, 164:265, 1957.
27. Brunell, P. A., and Gershon, A. A.: Passive immunization against varicella-zoster infections and other modes of therapy. J. Infect. Dis., 127:415, 1973.
28. Caleb, M. H., and South, M. A.: Measles and the immune system. Cutis, 18:755, 1976.
29. Eaglestein, W. H., Katz, R., and Brown, J. A.: The effects of early corticosteroid therapy on the skin eruption and pain of herpes zoster. JAMA, 211:1681, 1970.
30. Mendelson, C. G., and Kligman, A. M.: Isolation of wart virus in tissue culture. Arch. Dermatol., 83:559, 1960.
31. Eisinger, M., Kucarova, O., Sarkar, N. H., et al.: Propagation of human wart virus in tissue culture. Nature, 256:432, 1975.
32. Pass, F.: Warts, biology and current therapy. Minn. Med., 57:844, 1974.
33. Oriel, J. D., and Almeida, J. D.: Demonstration of virus particles in human genital warts. Br. J. Vener. Dis., 46:37, 1970.
34. Almeida, J. D., Howatson, A. F., and Williams, M. G.: Electron microscope study of human warts; sites of virus production and nature of the inclusion bodies. J. Invest. Dermatol., 38:337, 1962.
35. Cornelius, C. E., Witkowski, J. A., and Wood, M. G.: Viral verruca, human papovavirus infection. Arch. Dermatol., 98:377, 1968.
36. Russo, L., Russo, A., and Russo, V.: Immunotherapy of warts. Lancet, 1:921, 1975.
37. Noyes, W. F.: Verrucae: Virus structure, localization of antigens, and comparison with the Shope papilloma. Cancer Res., 28 321, 1968.
38. Morison, W.: In vitro assay of cell-mediated immunity to human wart antigen. Br. J. Dermatol., 90:531, 1974.
39. Pyrhönen, S., and Penttinen, K.: Wart-virus antibodies and the prognosis of wart disease. Lancet, 2:1330, 1972.
40. Matthews, R. S., and Shirodarea, P. V.: Study of regressing warts by immunofluorescence. Lancet, 1:684, 1973.
41. Niimura, M., Pass, F., Wooley, R., and Sourer, C. A.: Primary tissue culture of human wart derived epidermal cells (keratinocytes). J. Natl. Cancer Inst., 54:563, 1975.
42. Jablonska, S., Dabrowski, J., and Jakubowicz, K.: Epidermodysplasia verruciformis as a model in studies on the role of papovaviruses in oncogenesis. Cancer Res., 32:583, 1972.
43. Curtis, W. W., and Aklin, R. J.: Immunotherapy of condyloma acuminata. JAMA, 225:994, 1973.

44. Massing, A. M., and Epstein, W. L.: Natural history of warts. Arch. Dermatol., *87*:306, 1963.
45. Gold, S.: The enigma of viral warts. Practitioner, *211*:265, 1973.
46. Oriel, J. D.: Natural history of genital warts. Br. J. Vener. Dis., *47*:1, 1971.
47. Almeida, J. D., and Goffe, A. P.: Wart viruses. Br. J. Dermatol., *83*:698, 1970.
48. Cook, T. A., Brunschwig, J. P., Butel, J. S., et al.: Laryngeal papilloma: Etiologic and therapeutic considerations. Ann. Otol. Rhinol. Laryngol., *82*:649, 1973.
49. Boyle, W. F., Riggs, J. L., Oshiro, L. S., and Lennette, E. H.: Electron microscopic identification of papovavirus in laryngeal papilloma. Laryngoscope, *83*:1102, 1973.
50. Cook, T. A., Cohn, A. M., Brunschwig, J. P., et al.: Wart viruses and laryngeal papillomas. Lancet, *1*:732, 1973.
51. Tagami, H., Ogino, A., Takigawa, M., et al.: Regression of placid warts following spontaneous inflammation — A histopathological study. Br. J. Dermatol., *90*:147, 1974.
52. Clarke, G. H. V.: The charming of warts. J. Invest. Dermatol., *45*:15, 1965.
53. Barr, A., and Coles, R. B.: Warts on the hands — A statistical survey. Trans. St. Johns Hosp. Dermatol. Soc., *55*:69, 1969.
54. Einbinder, J., Parshley, M. S., Walzer, R., and Sanders, S.: The effect of cantharidin on epithelial cells in tissue culture. J. Invest Dermatol., *52*:291, 1969.
55. Epstein, W. L., Senecal, I., Kransnobrod, H., and Massing, A. M.: Viral antigens in human epidermal tumors: Localizations of an antigen to molluscum contagiosum. J. Invest. Dermatol., *40*:51, 1963.
56. Ridley, C. M.: Toxicity of podophyllum. Lancet, *3*:698, 1972.
57. Wenner, H. A.: Virus diseases associated with cutaneous eruptions. Prog. Med. Virol., *16*:269, 1973.
58. Postlethwarte, R.: Molluscum contagiosum — A review. Arch. Environ. Health, *21*:432, 1970.
59. Lynch, P. J., and Minkin, W.: Molluscum contagiosum of the adult. Arch. Dermatol., *98*:141, 1968.
60. Jacobs, P. H.: Molluscum contagiosum. Aerospace Med., *41*(10):1196, 1970.
61. Pirie, G. D., Bishop, P. M., Burke, D. C., and Postlethwarte, R.: Some properties of purified molluscum contagiosum virus. J. Gen. Virol., *13*:311, 1971.
62. Chang, T., and Weinstein, L.: Cytopathic agents isolated from lesions of molluscum contagiosum. J. Invest. Dermatol., *37*:433, 1961.
63. Barbanti-Brodano, G., Mannini-Palenzona, A., Varioli, O., et al.: Abortive infection and transformation of human embryonic fibroblasts by molluscum contagiosum virus. J. Gen. Virol., *24*:237, 1974.
64. Raskin, J.: Molluscum contagiosum, tissue culture and serologic study. Arch. Dermatol., *87*:552, 1963.
65. Epstein, W. L., and Kligman, A. M.: Treatment of warts with cantharadin. Arch. Dermatol., *77*:508, 1958.
66. Sutton, J. S., and Burnett, J. W.: Ultrastructural changes in dermal and epidermal cells of skin infected with molluscum contagiosum virus. J. Ultrastruct. Res., *26*:177, 1969.
67. Middelkamp, J., and Munger, B. L.: The ultrastructure and histogenesis of molluscum contagiosum. J. Pediatr., *64*:888, 1964.
68. Epstein, W. L., and Fukugaina, K.: Maturation of molluscum contagiosum virus in vivo: Quantitative electron microscopic autoradiography. J. Invest. Dermatol., *60*:73, 1973.
69. Kaye, J. W.: Problems in therapy of molluscum contagiosum. Arch. Dermatool., *94*:454, 1968.
70. Mehregan, A. H.: Molluscum contagiosum. Arch. Dermatol., *84*:175, 1961.
71. Henao, M., and Freeman, R. G.: Inflammatory molluscum contagiosum. Arch. Dermatol., *90*:479, 1964.
72. Kipping, H. F.: Molluscum dermatitis. Arch. Dermatol., *103*:106, 1971.
73. Solomon, L. M., and Telner, P.: Eruptive molluscum contagiosum in atopic dermatitis. Can. Med. Assoc.J., *95*:978, 1966.
74. Block, S. H.: Eczema and molluscum contagiosum. JAMA, *223*:195, 1973.
75. Horstmann, D. M.: Viral exanthems and enanthems. Pediatrics, *41*:867, 1968.
76. Miller, G. D., and Tindall, J. P.: Hand-foot-and-mouth disease. JAMA, *203*:827, 1968.

GENERAL REFERENCES

Demis, D. J., Dobson, R. H., and McQuire, J.: Clinical Dermatology. New York, Harper & Row, 1976.
Domonkos, A. N.: Andrews' Diseases of the Skin. 6th ed. Philadelphia, W. B. Saunders, 1975.
Moschella, S. L., Pillsbury, D. M., and Hurley, H. J.: Dermatology. Philadelphia, W. B. Saunders, 1975.
Rook, A., Wilkinson, D. S., and Ebling, R. J. G.: Textbook of Dermatology. Philadelphia, F. A. Davis, 1968.

SCABIES AND PEDICULOSIS

10

MILTON ORKIN, M.D.

SCABIES

Epidemics of scabies occur in 30-year cycles. Although the cyclical nature of these epidemics is not well understood, immunological factors, especially delayed hypersensitivity, probably play a significant role.[1] Each scabies epidemic usually lasts about 15 years,[2] with a 15-year gap between the end of one epidemic and the beginning of the next. The current worldwide epidemic began in most countries in 1964,[3] and should abate by about 1980. In both urban and rural areas of the United States, scabies has become increasingly prevalent in the last few years.[4]

Scabies frequently affects children and adolescents. Adopted children from foreign countries, especially South Korea and Vietnam, have a high incidence of scabies, which may become manifest after their arrival in the United States.[4]

CLASSIC SCABIES

Classic scabies has been seen less frequently in the current epidemic, compared with past ones.[4,6] The distribution of the eruption is a helpful diagnostic sign. The hands are often the first area to manifest cutaneous changes. The lesions, which are frequently eczematous, occur mainly on the finger webs and the sides of the digits. The flexor surfaces of the wrists are commonly involved, as are the extensor surfaces of the elbows (lesions may be nodular but more commonly are dry and eczematous) and the anterior axillary folds. The lesions are typically symmetrical. The female breast often has eczematous lesions, and papular lesions may be present on the abdomen, particularly around the umbilicus. Penile involvement is characteristic (Fig. 10–1). Another

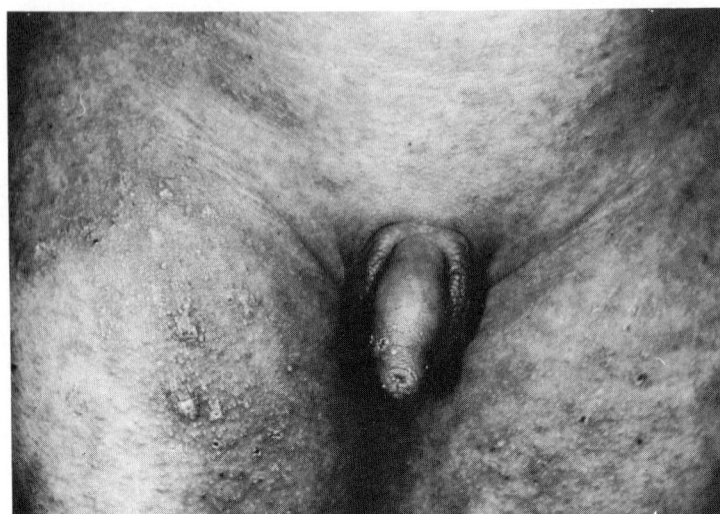

FIGURE 10–1 Scabies. Papular and eczematous eruption on abdomen, penis, and thighs. (Courtesy of Ervin Epstein, Sr., M.D.)

site with a predilection for lesions is the crease in the lower buttocks at the junction of the upper thigh.[5] Scabies is caused by the mite *Sarcoptes scabiei.*

The pathognomonic run, or burrow, consists of a short, wavy, dirty-looking line; it is seen much less frequently in the current epidemic. Small erythematous papules, which are often excoriated, are present on most parts of the body. Secondary eczematization and infection may overshadow the more typical features. Itching is characteristically nocturnal.

SPECIAL FORMS OF SCABIES

In forms other than classic scabies the infestation may be more difficult to diagnose. Scabies in hygienically clean individuals is common, signs and symptoms are minimal, and burrows are difficult to find. Scabies in infants may suggest other conditions because of extensive eczematous changes, and atypical distribution involving the head, neck, palms, and soles. Nodular scabies, animal-transmitted scabies, Norwegian scabies, scabies "incognito," and scabies associated with syphilis are other variant forms.

PRINCIPLES OF MANAGEMENT[5]

1. Establish the diagnosis. The diagnosis should be made with certainty, preferably by identifying the mite—in direct skin scrapings (Fig. 10–2) or at times by cutaneous biopsy—prior to instituting therapy. If the mite cannot be demonstrated, the suggestive signs and symptoms should be reviewed; the more numerous the features of scabies, the greater the likelihood that the diagnosis is correct.

2. Select an appropriate scabicide. This includes consideration of risk to benefit ratio. A decision about risk to benefit ratio must take into account the efficacy of the agent. Unfortunately, there has been only limited interest in

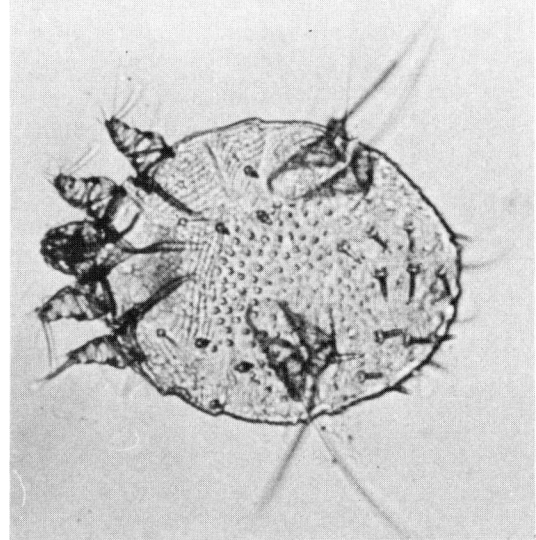

FIGURE 10-2 Scabies. Scrapings taken directly from the skin show the adult mite.

comparative, controlled efficacy trials of scabicides since the second World War.

3. Limit the quantity of medication ordered. Patients tend to apply topical preparations more often and for longer periods (sometimes weeks or months) than the physician has prescribed. The exact amount of the preparation required for appropriate treatment should be estimated and ordered. Approximately 30 gm (1 ounce) of a topical preparation is required to cover the trunk and extremities of an average adult adequately; proportionately less is needed for children and infants. If, for example, there are three adult equivalents (two parents and two small children) to be treated, and the medicament is to be applied for one night, the prescription should be written for a total of 90 gm (30 gm per application for three adult equivalents for one night). "No refill" should be specified in the prescription. An irritant dermatitis may result from too frequent use of a scabicide. If the patient mistakes this dermatitis for persistent scabies, a cyclical use of the scabicide may ensue. Systemic absorption of the active therapeutic agent is also a matter for concern.

4. Treat the entire trunk and extremities, not just obvious lesions. The scabicide should be applied thinly but thoroughly from the neck down to cover all areas, with special attention to the hands, feet, and intertriginous areas.

5. The patient should be instructed not to use any local preparations other than those prescribed for the scabies.

6. All members of the patient's household may be treated at the same time as well as sexual partners outside the household. The data in support of this approach are not conclusive, and some physicians prefer to treat only demonstrably infested individuals. Since the incubation period from infestation to manifestation of symptoms may be as long as two months (more typically, less than one month), it is important to recognize the carrier state. The person who has never had scabies may harbor many mites prior to developing pruritus or lesions and may be capable of transmitting the disease dur-

ing this period. This can lead to "ping-pong" chronic reinfestation. Scabies may spread rapidly through a community by means of many such untreated carriers.[6]

Transmission of scabies requires close contact. Generally, it is a family disease and, often, a sexually transmitted disease. Therefore, it is usually unnecessary to treat individuals who are exposed casually, such as office contacts, schoolmates, and visitors. When venereal transmission is suspected, the infested patient should be examined for signs of other venereal disease. Laboratory studies should include a serological test for syphilis and a culture for gonorrhea.

7. At the conclusion of therapy, intimate articles of clothing and bed linen should be machine washed and automatically dried (using the heat cycle in each case), or laundered and ironed, or boiled. It is not necessary to clean outer garments or furniture. The mites survive only briefly away from the human host.

8. The patient should be advised of the natural history of the disease following therapy. It may take several weeks for symptoms and signs to abate after effective treatment, since the hypersensitivity state will not disappear immediately upon destruction of the mites. This is particularly true for atopic individuals, in whom itching and eczematous lesions may persist.

9. Careful explanation and reassurance are vital, since patients frequently react to a diagnosis of scabies with inordinate concern, guilt, and even skepticism.

Some physicians prescribe oral antipruritic agents, such as antihistamines or salicylates, during the course of treatment for scabies. Following the completion of scabicidal therapy a soothing local agent may be applied. Fluorinated topical corticosteroid preparations may potentiate the infestation, and therefore should not be used *prior* to scabicidal therapy.[7]

Systemic antibiotics are seldom required if scabicidal therapy is instituted relatively early in the disease. When there is objective evidence of significant bacterial infection (pyoderma, furunculosis, cellulitis), especially in the immunologically deficient patient, systemic antibiotic therapy is indicated.

Acute glomerulonephritis may supervene in children whose scabietic lesions are also infected with a nephritogenic strain of Streptococcus. This complication has been reported primarily in Trinidad and Africa, specifically among underprivileged patients.[8,9] The possibility of bacterial complication should be considered in any patient with scabies in whom crusting and erythema are prominent. Unfortunately, it has not been shown conclusively that early treatment with systemic antibiotics prevents nephritis.[10] Significant secondary bacterial infection will sometimes cure the scabies, since the mite cannot survive in skin infected by bacteria.[11]

10. The patient with scabies is unlikely to be capable of transmitting the disease 24 hours after treatment with an effective scabicidal agent.

11. Real or apparent treatment failure may be due to noncompliance, reinfestation, irritation from treatment, mite resistance, acarophobia, or a combination of these factors.

Noncompliance with treatment frequently can be documented by taking a careful history. Did the patient follow instructions completely? Were all members of the household and sexual contacts of infested members treated?

The patient or one of his family may be *reinfested* from an outside source. We do not believe this to be a common occurrence.

Chemical irritation may result from too frequent use of a scabicidal agent. It resembles a primary irritant eczematous contact dermatitis. Chemical irritation can be reduced by limiting or controlling the dosage. When chemical irritation occurs, or anxiety prolongs the itching, or an otherwise effectively treated patient is symptomatic because of *hypersensitivity to mite antigen,* the patient often recognizes upon questioning that the quality of the itching is different in character, intensity, or duration from that of the original infestation. However, if the pruritus is the same as that prior to therapy, it may suggest persistent infestation.

True resistance can be proved only by *demonstrating the mites again* in those patients with whom there is reasonable assurance that the medication has been properly applied. Frequently, new lesions develop and old ones fail to heal. Resistance to the most frequently used scabicides has not been proved. Persistent itching is most often due to mite hypersensitivity and is not a sign of resistance. This is a common phenomenon and the patient should be so informed.

Acarophobia (delusion of parasitosis) is not uncommon with or without antecedent scabies or some other cutaneous disease. A diagnosis of acarophobia should not be made until examination has failed to demonstrate actual infestion.[12] Acarophobic patients are firmly convinced their skin is infested. They manifest chronic pruritus (less frequently, other cutaneous symptoms), excoriations and resulting complications, and irritant contact dermatitis from extensive use of chemicals, medicaments, and soap. They often bring scraps of skin and detritus to the physician, believing these to be the parasites. Usually, these patients have significant mental illness and may be referred for psychiatric care, although they frequently resist such suggestions.

12. Some patients may throw off the infestation and undergo spontaneous cure.[11] A hypersensitivity response may play a role in inhibiting reinfestation and thus may participate in the cyclical nature of scabies epidemics.

SPECIFIC AGENTS

Gamma Benzene Hexachloride (GBH, Lindane)

Composition. GBH contains lindane (1 per cent) and inert ingredients (99 per cent).

Advantages. This is the scabicide used most extensively in the United States. The preparation (Gamene) is relatively pleasant and easy to use and is available in cream or lotion form. It is usually an effective treatment.

Most controlled efficacy studies of modern scabicides were done over 20 years ago. Pierce[13] studied 500 patients with scabies in a correctional institution. His evaluation showed that one application of lindane resulted in a slightly superior cure rate and caused few local reactions, compared with one application of other preparations such as crotamiton and benzyl benzoate.

Disadvantages. Irritant contact dermatitis may result from prolonged use of lindane. Feldman and Maibach[14] documented the percutaneous absorption and urinary excretion of lindane. When a tracer of lindane was administered intravenously in humans approximately 25 per cent of the dose appeared in the urine during the subsequent five days. The half-life of urinary excretion of this chemical is approximately 26 hours. Much of the remainder of the lindane was assumed to be excreted in the stool. When lindane in acetone was applied to the forearm, approximately 9 per cent of the 4-mcg/cm^2 application was excreted in the urine over five days. It is probable that percutaneous penetration is greater than 9 per cent because the forearm is one of the least permeable skin sites.[15] The face, cubital fossae, axillae, and scalp permit greater penetration of many chemicals; the scrotum is highly permeable, allowing some chemicals almost total penetration. Assuming that an adult applied 30 gm of 1 per cent lindane, the total applied dose would be 300 mg. If we assume that about 10 per cent will be absorbed, approximately 30 mg will enter the circulation. Because of the slow urinary excretion and the prolonged penetration from the skin, it is possible that significant levels of lindane could accumulate in the blood after repeated applications.

Studies of acute lindane toxicity in animals and cases of poisoning in humans have shown that central nervous system toxicity is a significant factor.[16] Careful studies to determine the presence or absence of subliminal central nervous system toxicity from lindane therapy for scabies have not been performed, nor has such toxicity resulting from topical therapy been proved clinically.

Because of the paucity of clinical studies, it has not been possible to extrapolate data on percutaneous penetration from adults to infants. It has been assumed (but not proved) on the basis of indirect data that percutaneous penetration is greater in infants.[17]

Administration. On the basis of experimental study,[14] the caution advised by Solomon and Esterly,[18] and the lack of toxicological data for the pediatric age group, we prefer not to use lindane in treating infants or young children. We have also modified the frequency and technique of its application in older children and adults and therefore prescribe one application of lindane lotion to be left on for 12 hours and then washed off thoroughly. As with the other scabicides, application is preceded by a soap and water bath, followed by thorough drying. The lotion should be kept away from eyes and mucous membranes. After 12 hours, the medication is thoroughly washed from the skin and is not reapplied. The patient and family members then change to freshly laundered underclothing, pajamas, and bed linens.

Usually a single application of lindane is sufficient treatment. There is theoretical reason for a second application one week later in order to destroy recently hatched larvae and nymphs. These larvae (formed from eggs present at the initial application of the scabicides) may now be susceptible.[19] It is not certain that any of the scabicidal agents is ovicidal. A second application may also be appropriate if there is evidence of treatment failure (instruct the patient again), reinfestation, or resistance. If apparent resistance persists after the second application, a different scabicide may be used.

CROTAMITON

Composition. Crotamiton provides 10 per cent of the synthetic, N-ethyl-o-crotonotoluide in a vanishing cream base (Eurax).

Advantages. Crotamiton is a satisfactory scabicide. We do not know whether it is equally, or more or less, effective than lindane or sulfur ointment.

It has been used as a non-specific antipruritic agent. The itching associated with scabies usually responds rapidly to this medication.

Crotamiton is occasionally irritating. However, it is often irritating if applied to acutely inflamed skin. It should not be used on the eyes or in the oral cavity.

Administration. Crotamiton should be thoroughly massaged into the skin from the neck down, with particular attention to hands, feet, and intertriginous areas. A second application is administered 24 hours later. Clothing and bed linen are changed the next morning, and a cleansing bath is taken 24 to 48 hours after the last application.

Sulfur

Composition. Sulfur preparations must be compounded. They are usually prescribed as precipitated sulfur in concentrations of 5 per cent to 10 per cent in petrolatum. Our preference is for 6 per cent precipitated sulfur in petrolatum. Some prefer to add balsam of Peru (3 per cent) to the sulfur ointment; however, the balsam may cause allergic sensitization.

Advantages. Because this medication has been used safely and effectively for centuries, we prefer it for use with infants and small children.

Disadvantages. The sulfur preparation is messy, stains clothing, and is malodorous; patients may find it less acceptable than the modern scabicides. It may be irritating to the skin, although we have seldom found this to be so when it is used as prescribed. Sulfur should not be used with mercury compounds because of the subsequent formation of hydrogen sulfide which is odoriferous, sometimes irritates the skin, and may form a black deposit on the skin. Despite these drawbacks, the majority of patients treated with sulfur do not complain about its use.

Administration. Sulfur ointment is applied nightly for three nights. The ointment is rubbed into the hands and then applied to the body. Treatment is preceded by a bath. The bath is repeated 24 hours after the last application, at which time all family members should change to freshly laundered underclothing, pajamas, and bed linen. Most patients prefer to take a bath each night before reapplying the sulfur and 24 hours after the final application.

Benzyl Benzoate

Composition. No commercial preparation of benzyl benzoate is available in this country. It may be compounded as an emulsion or lotion in 20 to 35 per cent concentrations. The United States Pharmacopeia (USP) formula is: saponated benzyl benzoate (containing triethanolamine and oleic acid), 275 cc, and water q.s. to make 1000 cc.

Advantages. This preparation is a good scabicide, although it has not been used much in this country since the advent of lindane and crotamiton. It is cosmetically acceptable and does not soil underclothing or bedding. Care should be taken to avoid transferring the solution to the eyes, since it may cause stinging and conjunctivitis.

Disadvantages. Some patients will have increased itching or irritation after the application of this preparation. The male genitalia are especially susceptible to such irritation.

Administration. Benzyl benzoate is applied every night or every other night for a total of three applications.

TREATMENT OF SPECIAL FORMS OF SCABIES

NODULAR SCABIES

About 7 per cent of patients with scabies have a variety of the disease in which reddish-brown, pruritic nodules (Fig. 10–3) develop on parts of the body that are generally covered by clothing (usually the male genitalia, the groin, and the axillary regions). The nodules may simulate lymphoma and histiocytosis X clinically, and lymphoma and arthropod bites histologically. These pruritic nodules are apparently due to an immune reaction to the mite and may persist for up to a year or longer despite scabicidal therapy. The lesions eventually clear spontaneously.[20]

Nodular scabies generally fails to respond to most topical anti-inflammatory agents, including fluorinated corticosteroids applied under occlusive dressings, but may regress with intralesional corticosteroids. Surgical excision is occasionally utilized if intralesional corticoids are ineffective or if the patient is particularly concerned. However, the patient should be advised that scars may result from surgical intervention.

ANIMAL-TRANSMITTED SCABIES

This form of scabies occurs frequently as regional outbreaks in the United States and Canada. The major source of the mite is dogs, whose external ears are frequent sites of involvement. Canine scabies in man differs from human scabies in its greater case of transmission, shorter incubation period, absence of

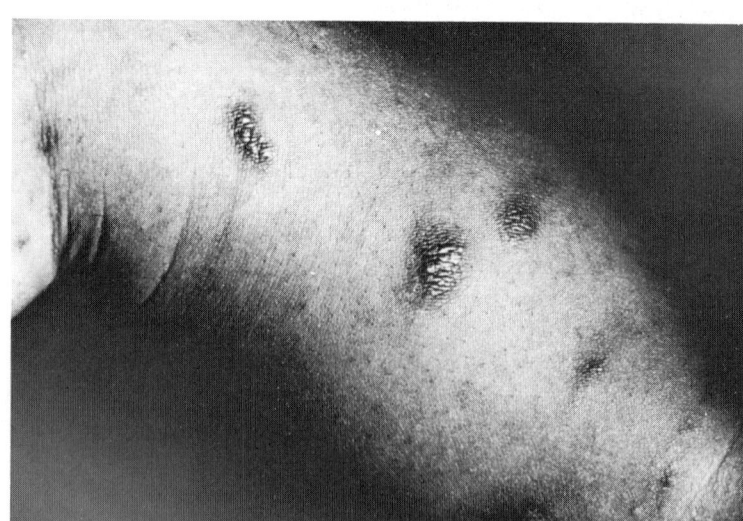

FIGURE 10–3 Nodular scabies.

burrows, distribution, and usual self-limited course (unless the patient is reexposed to the canine source).

It is unnecessary to treat asymptomatic family members or sexual partners outside the household, since the condition usually is not contagious. Symptomatic family members may be treated with supportive measures; however, Smith and Claypoole,[21] among others, believe that treatment with scabicides will shorten the duration of this infestation.

NORWEGIAN (CRUSTED) SCABIES

Norwegian scabies is a rare, highly contagious, exfoliative and crusted dermatitis that causes local epidemics in hospitals and institutions. It has a predilection for the mentally retarded and the physically and immunologically debilitated. Although it usually causes little pruritus, enormous numbers of mites may be found in the exfoliating scales. A therapeutic approach similar to that for common scabies is usually sufficient, although Norwegian scabies responds more slowly and may require the sequential use of lindane, sulfur, and crotamiton. Eradication of the mite may be facilitated by applying keratolytic agents such as 2 per cent salicylic acid cream before applying the scabicide. Other patients and personnel in the institution may require prophylactic treatment. Carslaw and his associates[22] found the immediate environment of patients with Norwegian scabies to be heavily contaminated with mites. They suggested that effective control requires isolation of the afflicted individuals, followed by disinfestation of the individuals and their environment.

PEDICULOSIS

There has been a sharp rise in the frequency of pediculosis capitis and pediculosis pubis in the United States and Western Europe[23] in recent years. The increase is unrelated to socioeconomic levels. One unexplained aspect is the relative immunity of blacks to louse infestation. Pediculosis corporis is seldom seen in the western world today, except in indigent vagabonds and those with poor hygienic habits. Because pediculosis corporis is rare in adolescence, we shall not discuss it in this chapter.

In all three of these obligate parasitic diseases, adult lice are relatively sparsely distributed on the skin. The diagnosis of p. pubis and p. capitis is usually made by identifying the numerous eggs (nits) found on the hair. In p. corporis, adult organisms and nits may be found in the seams of clothing.

PEDICULOSIS PUBIS

Patients with pediculosis pubis are seen more frequently at venereal disease clinics, at student health services, and by family physicians than by dermatologists. Many patients treat themselves, or are treated, with a variety of over-the-counter medications.

Diagnosis. The diagnosis of this pruritic dermatosis is usually made by identifying the eggs. These are attached to the pubic hair shaft by a cement-

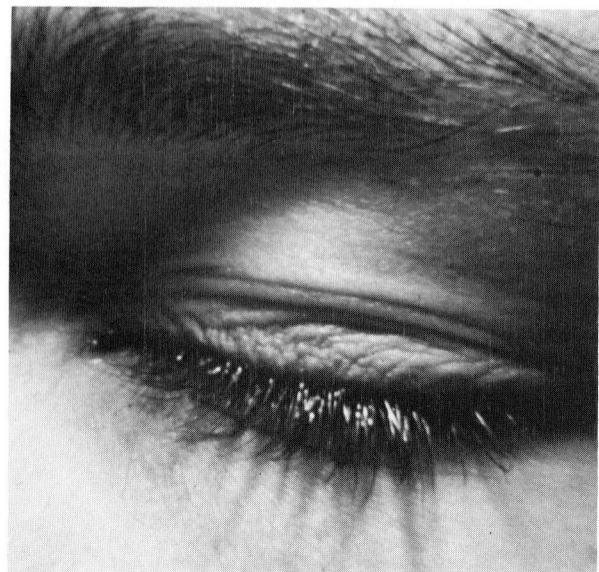

FIGURE 10–4 Phthiriasis palpebrarum (infestation of eyelashes by pubic lice). The nits are found at the base of the cilia.

like substance at a site close to the skin surface. In hairy individuals, the oganisms also may be present on the short hairs of the thighs and trunk and occasionally on the beard and mustache. Involvement of the eyelashes (Fig. 10–4) and the hair on the periphery of the scalp occurs mainly in children. The organism is transmitted to children by close contact with an infested parent or sibling. The diagnosis is confirmed by identifying the nits on plucked hair, using low power light microscopy.

P. pubis is transmitted most often by sexual contact. Like gonorrhea, p. pubis is found more frequently in females aged 15 to 19 than in males of the same age group. After age 20, the frequency is greater in males.[24]

Therapy. Lindane is the most widely used pediculicide. Therapy is preceded by a soap and water bath followed by thorough drying with a towel. A thin layer of lindane lotion* is applied to the infested and adjacent hairy areas, with particular attention to the mons pubis and perianal region. In hairy individuals, therapy should include the thighs, trunk, and axillary regions because involvement at these sites is common. The lotion remains in place for 12 hours and then is washed off thoroughly. Usually one application is sufficient, but a second application one week later may be necessary if viable organisms persist or if new nits appear at the junction of skin and hair. Translucent empty nits (those with no embryo) are signs of inactive infestation and need no further treatment; if there is any doubt, the physician may examine the hairs under a microscope. It is not necessary to shave the area.

The patient's sexual partners should be treated at the same time, although uninfested members of the household need not be. When the eyelashes are involved, yellow oxide of mercury (an old but still effective treatment) may be applied. Anticholinesterase preparations also are effective but may cause ocular symptoms and signs. A simpler method, which we use, is to apply

---

*Some physicians prefer to prescribe lindane shampoo, lathered into affected sites for five minutes and rinsed off thoroughly.

petrolatum thickly to the lashes twice daily for eight days and then to remove the remaining nits with a fine-toothed comb or forceps. If there is scalp involvement, the scalp should be treated concomitantly with lindane shampoo (see therapy of p. capitis).

At the conclusion of treatment, the infested individuals and their sexual partners use clean underclothing, pajamas, sheets, and pillowcases. Infested articles should be machine-washed and automatically dried (using the hot cycle), or boiled, or commercially laundered.

Resistance. P. pubis has shown no resistance to the insecticides.[23] Therapeutic failure is usually due to the patient's noncompliance with instructions, failure to treat sexual contacts, or reinfestation. Pruritus may persist because of irritation caused by the pediculicide (usually from too frequent use), irritation or sensitization to previous medications, or the patient's anxiety. Parasitophobia, with or without preceding pediculosis, is common and is difficult to deal with.

PEDICULOSIS CAPITIS

Persons with head lice are treated more frequently by school nurses, pediatricians, and family physicians than by dermatologists. P. capitis is seen in preschool children of both sexes. In some parts of the country, the frequency decreases in males as children begin to attend school. Teenagers, and occasionally adults, may also be infested. P. capitis is communicated by sharing hats, combs, and brushes, and may be promoted by long hair and elaborate hair styles, particularly those styles that discourage frequent washing and good hygiene. The condition is typically confined to the scalp, particularly the occipital region, and to a lesser degree the postauricular region. Pruritus is a cardinal symptom (although not invariably present); excoriations frequently lead to pyoderma of the scalp and nape, with regional lymphadenopathy.

Diagnosis. The diagnosis is made by identifying the oval nits that are cemented to hairs. In the initial stages of infestation, the nits are attached close to the scalp. Nits are identified by examining plucked hairs under the microscope. One must differentiate nits from seborrheic scales, hair casts, and substances such as hair spray. Nits adhere very tightly to the hair whereas the others may easily be brushed off.

Therapy. Lindane shampoo should be prescribed only in the amount judged necessary for adequate treatment. The patient should be instructed to shampoo the scalp for four minutes (using one tablespoon or less), then to rinse thoroughly, and to dry the hair with a towel. Residual nits may be removed with a fine-toothed comb or forceps. A second shampoo is desirable one week later if viable eggs persist or if new eggs are seen, since the pediculicides are not proved to be ovicidal.[25] Empty nits need not be treated further.

Other children and adults in the household should be examined also, but only those infested should be treated, except for individuals who share a bed with the affected individual.

Following therapy, infested individuals should put on clean clothing. All washable clothing, towels, and bed linens with which they have been in contact should be laundered in hot water. Machine drying with high heat for at least 20 minutes will destroy nits. Clothing that is not washable (e.g., coats, hats, scarves, and sweaters) should be dry cleaned.

Resistance. Resistance of head lice to lindane (and DDT) has been noted in Great Britain,[26] but not in the United States.

SUMMARY

There has been a recent notable increase in scabies and pediculosis pubis and pediculosis capitis. Once the diagnosis is established (preferably by demonstrating the mite or louse), therapy includes consideration of a risk to benefit ratio, explanation of the nature of the infestation to the patient, application of appropriate therapeutic techniques, and follow-up procedures. Resistance of the *Sarcoptes* mite to modern scabicides has been suggested but not proved. Resistance of the head louse and body louse to modern pediculicides has been reported in other countries but not in the United States.

REFERENCES

1. Orkin, M.: Today's scabies, an editorial. Arch. Dermatol., *111*:1431, 1975.
2. Shrank, A. B., and Alexander, S. L.: Scabies: Another epidemic? Br. Med. J., *1*:669, 1967.
3. Orkin, M.: Resurgence of scabies. JAMA, *217*:593, 1971.
4. Orkin, M.: Today's scabies. JAMA, *233*:882, 1975.
4b. Orkin, M., Maibach, H. I., Parish, L. C., and Schwartzman, R. M.: Scabies and Pediculosis. Philadelphia, J. B. Lippincott, 1977.
5. Orkin, M., Epstein, E., and Maibach, H. I.: Treatment of today's scabies and pediculosis. JAMA, *236*:1136, 1976.
6. Mellanby, K.: Scabies. London, E. W. Classey, 1972; Los Angeles, Entomological Reprint Specialists, 1972.
7. Macmillan, A. L.: Unusual features of scabies associated with topical fluorinated steroids. Br. J. Dermatol., *87*:496, 1972.
8. Hersch, C.: Acute glomerulonephritis due to skin disease, with special reference to scabies. S. Afr. Med. J., *41*:29, 1967.
9. Svartman, M., Potter, E. V., Finklea, J. F., et al.: Epidemic scabies and acute glomerulonephritis in Trinidad. Lancet, *1*:249, 1972.
10. Lasch, E. E., Frankel, V., Vardy, P. A., et al.: Epidemic glomerulonephritis in Israel. J. Infect. Dis., *124*:141, 1971.
11. Mellanby, K.: The development of symptoms, parasitic infection and immunity in human scabies. Parasitology, *35*:197, 1944.
12. Wilson, J. W.: Delusions of parasitosis (acarophobia); further observations in clinical practice. Arch. Dermatol., *66*:577, 1952.
13. Pierce, H. E., Jr.: Scabies: Epidemiology and management at correctional institutions. J. Natl. Med. Assoc., *43*:107, 1951.
14. Feldmann, R. J., and Maibach, H. I.: Percutaneous penetration of some pesticides and herbicides in man. Toxicol. Appl. Pharmacol., *28*:126, 1974.
15. Maibach, H. I., Feldmann, R. J., and Milby, T. H.: Regional variation in percutaneous penetration in man. Arch. Environ. Health, *23*:208, 1971.
16. American Medical Association, Council on Pharmacy and Chemistry: Toxic effects of technical benzene hexachloride and its principal isomers. JAMA, *147*:571, 1951.
17. Maibach, H. I., and Fisher, L.: Percutaneous penetration in infants and young children (in preparation).
18. Solomon, L. M., and Esterly, N. B.: Neonatal Dermatology. Philadelphia, W. B. Saunders, 1973, pp. 156–157.
19. Heilesen, B.: Studies on acarus scabiei and scabies. Acta Derm. Venereol. Suppl. XIV, *26*:1, 1946.
20. Konstantinov, D., and Stanoeva, L.: Persistent scabious nodules. Dermatologica, *147*:321, 1973.
21. Smith, E. B., and Claypoole, T. F.: Canine scabies in dogs and in humans. JAMA, *199*:59, 1967.
22. Carslaw, R. W., Dobson, R. M., Hood, A. J. K., et al.: Mites in the environment of cases of Norwegian scabies. Br. J. Dermatol., *92*:333, 1975.

23. Gratz, N. G.: The current status of louse infestations throughout the world. The control of lice and louse-born diseases. Proceedings of the International Symposium on the Control of Lice and Louse-Born Diseases, Pan American Health Organization. Washington, D.C., 1973, p. 23.
24. Fisher, I., and Morton, R. S.: Phthirus pubis infestation. Br. J. Vener. Dis., *46*:326, 1970.
25. Controlling Head Lice. Atlanta, Center for Disease Control, 1975.
26. Maunder, J. W.: Use of malathion in the treatment of lousy children. Community Med., *126*:145, 1971.

11
SYPHILIS

LOUISE E. TAVS, M.D.

SEXUALLY TRANSMITTED DISEASES

Sexually transmitted diseases, particularly gonorrhea and herpes simplex virus Type II infections, have had an explosive increase since the late 1960's. Adolescents are especially at risk from venereal diseases because, although they are sexually active, they are often late in seeking medical attention for venereal infections.[1] During 1975, 999,937 cases of gonorrhea and 80,358 cases of syphilis were reported in the United States. Nationally, 68 per cent of the reported cases of gonorrhea and 44 per cent of the primary and secondary cases of syphilis occurred in persons under 25 years of age. By 1976, the incidence of gonorrhea had risen to 1,007,518.[2] Table 11–1 presents various sexually transmitted diseases and their causative organisms.

ETIOLOGY OF SYPHILIS

Syphilis is a chronic infectious disease caused by *Treponema pallidum*. It is systemic from inception, clinically encompassing a range from asymptomatic latency to protean manifestation. Syphilis is capable of involving almost every organ system of the body and is transmissible to the fetus in utero (Table 11–2). Either early acquired syphilis or late congenital syphilis may be encountered in the adolescent.

In 1905, Schaudinn, assisted by Hoffmann, identified *Treponema pallidum* as the etiological agent of syphilis.[3, 4]

The organism is a slender spirochete of the genus *Treponema*, 6 to 20 μ in length and 0.25 μ in width, with 6 to 14 regular rigid spirals and tapered ends. Its movement in serum is slow and deliberate, but in viscous media and tissue the organism attains greater traction and more rapid propulsion. It moves by rotating on its long axis, which produces a propeller effect with movement forward or backward. Flexion at right angles may occur, with the spirals retaining their taut shape as the organism bends in the middle. *Treponema pal-*

TABLE 11-1 SEXUALLY TRANSMITTED DISEASES

Type	Organism	Disease
Spirochetes	*Treponema pallidum*	Syphilis
Bacteria	*Neisseria gonorrhoeae*	Gonorrhea
	Hemophilus ducreyi	Chancroid
	Calymmatobacterium (Donovania) granulomatis	Granuloma inguinale
	Corynebacterium (Hemophilus) vaginalis	Hemophilus vaginitis
	Chlamydia subgroup A	Lymphogranuloma venereum
Viruses	Herpes simplex virus Types I and II	Herpes simplex genitalis
	Poxvirus	Molluscum contagiosum
	Papovavirus	Condylomata acuminata
Protozoa	*Trichomonas vaginalis*	Trichomoniasis
Fungi	*Candida albicans*	Candidiasis
	Epidermophyton inguinale	Tinea cruris
Parasites	*Sarcoptes scabiei*	Scabies
	Phthirus pubis	Pediculosis pubis
Miscellaneous	*Chlamydia, Escherichia coli,* virus, *Trichomonas, H. vaginalis, Candida,* cocci, *Mycoplasma*	Non-gonococcal urethritis
	Chlamydia, Mycoplasma, allergy, auto-immunity, virus	The Reiter syndrome

TABLE 11-2 CLASSIFICATION OF SYPHILIS

Acquired Syphilis

Primary stage
— Seronegative, darkfield-positive chancre
— Seropositive, darkfield-positive chancre

Secondary stage
— Infectious relapse (mucocutaneous)
— Serological relapse
— Osseous, hepatic, renal relapse, neurorelapse

Early latent stage: No clinical evidence of syphilis except for reactive serological test, including the FTA–ABS test,* and known duration of four years or less.

Late latent stage: No clinical evidence of syphilis except for reactive serological test, including the FTA–ABS test, and known duration of more than four years.

Late stage → Persistent latency

Cardiovascular disorders
Neurosyphilis
Gumma formation (mucocutaneous, osseous, gastric)

Congenital Syphilis
Early congenital stage: Patient is two years of age or less.
Late congenital stage: Patient is over two years of age.

*Fluorescent treponemal antibody–absorption test.

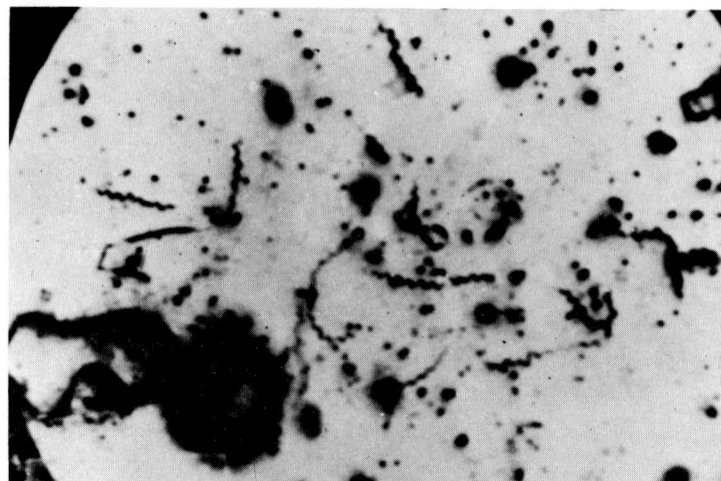

FIGURE 11–1 *Treponema pallidum*.

lidum reproduces by transverse fission, a process that requires 30 to 33 hours to complete (Fig. 11–1).[5]

Electron microscopy demonstrates a central protoplasmic core containing ribosomes, mesosomes, and filamentous nuclear areas. The protoplasm is contained within two membranes: an inner trilaminar cytoplasmic membrane and a delicate outer trilaminar sheath, which is a major osmotic barrier for the cell. Between these two membranes, three to six axial fibrils wind around the central protoplasmic cylinder and act as organs of motility.[6] An outer capsule or protective slimy layer may also be present.

CLINICAL MANIFESTATIONS OF EARLY ACQUIRED SYPHILIS

Although *Treponema pallidum* can penetrate unbroken mucosa, a microscopic abrasion of the tough barrier of the stratum corneum is needed for the organism to penetrate the skin. The incubation period of syphilis ranges from 8 to 90 days, the average being three to four weeks.

The initial syphilitic lesion or chancre appears at the site of penetration by the treponemes. It is usually single and erosive rather than ulcerative, except on glabrous skin. The base is level or slightly depressed. The lesion is clean, with serous or serosanguineous exudate and the color of raw muscle. If it is moist, the erosion may be covered by a delicate pellicle; a crust may form on exposed skin. The margin is sharp (not rolled or undermined), and the base of the lesion is characteristically indurated as a result of edema and dense infiltrate of lymphocytes and plasma cells in the underlying dermis. The induration may be parchment-like and barely palpable or cartilaginous, with a button-like firmness. Or it may be the rubber ball type of induration found in a chancre of the lip or frenum. In about 70 per cent of cases, satellite lymphadenopathy develops one or two weeks after the appearance of the chancre. The satellite bubo of an extragenital chancre tends to be unilateral. In lesions around the genitalia, however, the adenopathy usually is bilateral and involves a chain of

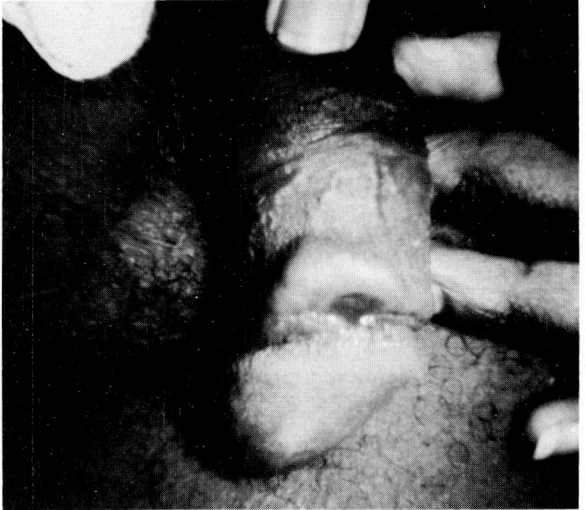

FIGURE 11–2 Chancre at the sulcus coronarius. The erosion is circular with a slightly depressed base and a marked shoulder of induration. Except on glabrous skin, a syphilitic chancre is usually an erosion rather than an ulcer.

nodes. The individual lymph nodes are usually firm, discrete, freely movable under the skin, painless, and give no visible evidence of inflammatory reaction (Figs. 11–2 to 11–6).

Even though a syphilitic chancre is usually painless, pain may occur (1) in a lesion secondarily infected with pyogenic or chancroidal organisms, (2) in a paronychial or felon chancre caused by pressure of the infiltrate underlying the nail, and (3) in a chancre of the tongue containing a central fissure (Table 11–3).

In a series of 584 chancres in the female reported by Davies,[7] the most common sites in order of frequency were the cervix, the lower half of the labia majora, and the fourchette. The vaginal mucosa is rarely the site of a chancre except by extension from the cervix or fourchette. With changing sexual mores, casual, salutatory kissing and fellatio have both become more prevalent. An infectious lesion resulting from these practices, such as a chancre of the lip,

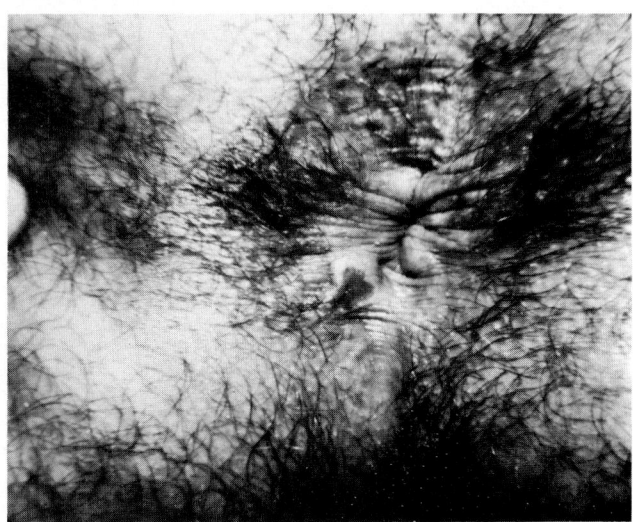

FIGURE 11–3 Fissured type of anal chancre. *Treponema pallidum* organisms were demonstrated on darkfield examination, and the VDRL test was reactive. Occasionally, a diffuse brawny infiltration of all or part of the external or internal anal ring may occur. Multiple fissured chancres also may develop.

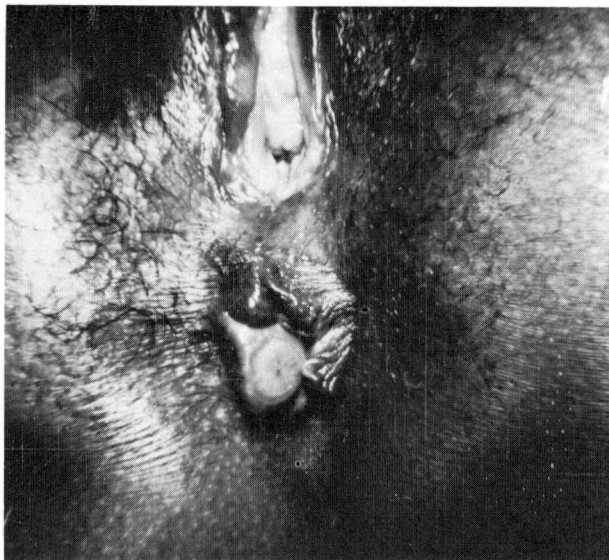

FIGURE 11-4 A typical hunterian chancre of the external ring and adjacent skin of the anus, with marked induration like that of a cartilaginous button, extending slightly beyond the base of the erosion. This patient had a second chancre of the lower third of the labium majorum, the second most common site of chancre in the female.

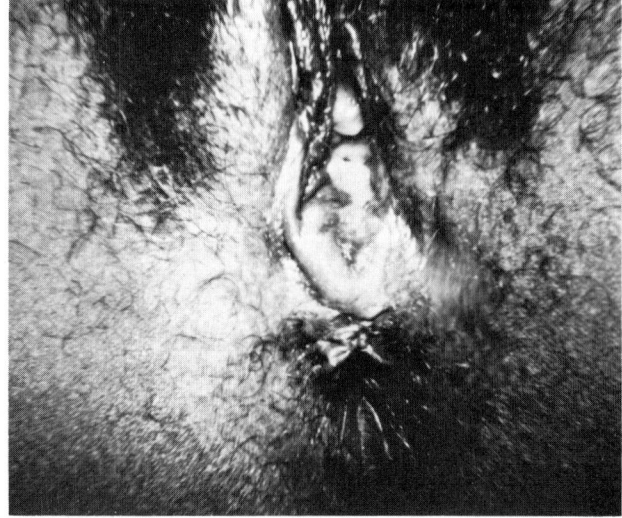

FIGURE 11-5 Chancre of the fourchette. Note the sharply marginated erosion surrounded by a prominent shoulder of induration. This is produced by the infiltration of the underlying round cells and plasma cells. The fourchette is the third most common site of chancre in the female.

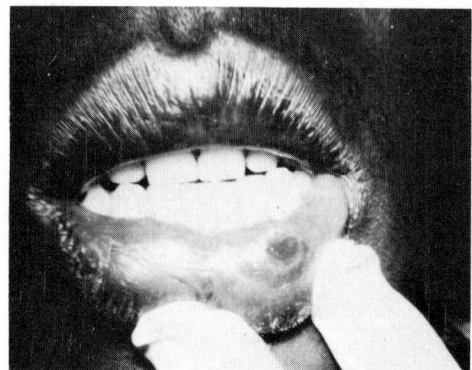

FIGURE 11-6 Syphilitic chancre of the lower lip. Approximately 50 per cent of extragenital chancres occur on the lip. A lesion of the lip that is indurated, slow to develop, and slow to heal, and associated with marked satellite adenopathy often indicates syphilitic chancre or epithelioma. The diagnosis of chancre must have laboratory confirmation, such as a positive darkfield examination, reactive serological test, or occasionally biopsy findings compatible with the diagnosis.

TABLE 11–3 CLINICAL CHARACTERISTICS OF A TYPICAL SYPHILITIC CHANCRE

Relatively long incubation period (8 to 40 days but may be as long as 90 days)
Single (may be multiple)
Painless
Induration present
Erosion rather than ulcer
Sharply defined border
Level or slightly depressed base
Clean base, the color of raw muscle
Serous exudate
Indolent course (2 to 6 weeks)
Regional lymphadenopathy
Healing with atrophic scar, often invisible.

tongue, or tonsil, may be overlooked by the examining physician unless he is alert to the possibility of syphilis.

A chancre may vary from a minute erosion to a large crusted ulcer and may occur on any accessible portion of the body except the hair, teeth, and nails. Depending on its size and the degree of induration, spontaneous healing occurs in two to six weeks, leaving a thin, often imperceptible, atrophic scar.

Since the syphilitic chancre may resemble other lesions that arise from very diverse causes, Table 11–4 presents a differential diagnosis of the syphilitic chancre.

The clinical diagnosis of primary syphilis should be supported by laboratory evidence (such as the identification of *Treponema pallidum* by darkfield microscopy of serum from the lesion or of aspirated lymph node

TABLE 11–4 DIFFERENTIAL DIAGNOSIS OF SYPHILITIC CHANCRE

Genital
Chancroid
Herpes progenitalis
Condylomata acuminata
Carcinoma
Scabies
Trauma
Pyogenic lesion
Sebaceous cyst
Granuloma inguinale
Lymphogranuloma venereum
Fixed drug eruption
Behçet's syndrome

Lip
Herpes simplex
Epithelioma
Pyogenic granuloma
Trauma
Sarcoidosis
Gumma
Blastomycosis
Inoculation tuberculosis

fluid), by immunofluorescent staining of *Treponema pallidum* in serum from the lesion,[8-11] by reactive blood serology, or occasionally by biopsy findings. All serological tests now available are non-reactive during the incubation period.

After the appearance of the chancre, the FTA–ABS test is usually the first to become positive, followed shortly by the RPR* circle card test. Both are usually reactive in primary syphilis within one to two weeks. The VDRL* test becomes reactive soon thereafter; the TPHA* and TPI* tests may be slower to develop positivity.

CLINICAL MANIFESTATIONS OF SECONDARY SYPHILIS

Approximately three to six weeks after the appearance of the chancre (i.e., six weeks to six months after the initial infection has occurred), the secondary stage may become evident. The four cardinal signs of the secondary stage of syphilis are the skin eruption, the mucous patch, condylomata lata, and generalized lymphadenopathy.

CUTANEOUS ERUPTION (Figs. 11–7 to 11–19)

Cutaneous eruption as a sign of secondary stage of syphilis is presented in tabular form (Table 11–5). The other three signs will be discussed in the text.

---

*RPR — Rapid plasma reagin circle card test
VDRL — Venereal disease research laboratory test
TPHA — *Treponema pallidum* hemagglutination test
TPI — *Treponema pallidum* immobilization test

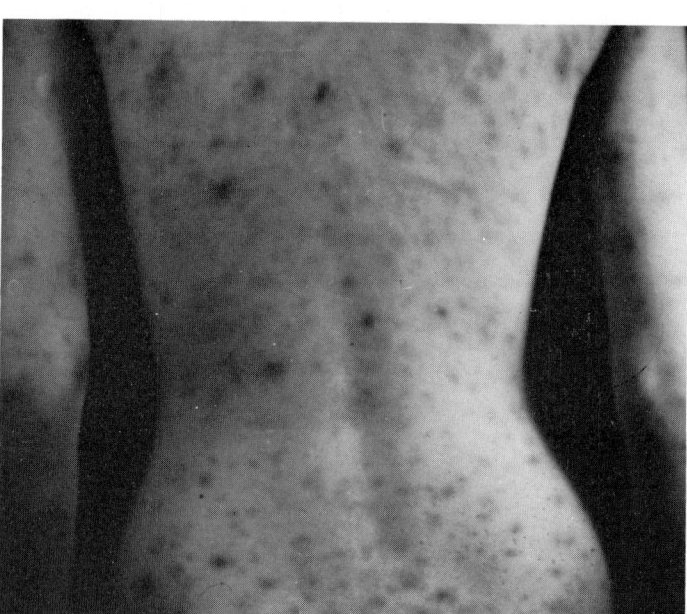

FIGURE 11–7 Maculopapular eruption of secondary syphilis. Associated severe itching usually rules out syphilitic eruption. However, the follicular and psoriasiform secondary syphilids may be mildly pruritic.

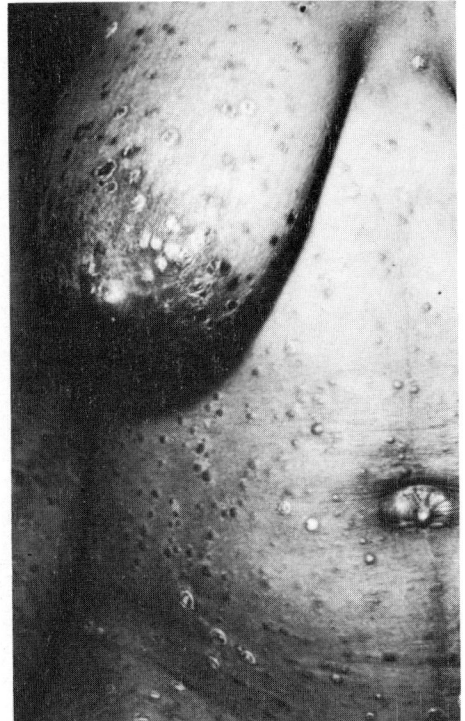

FIGURE 11-8 Papular secondary syphilids. The papules are indurated, flat or rounded, scaling or smooth, of varying size, and coppery red in color. Note the dry, thin, whitish scale that begins in the center of the papule and advances to the periphery to produce a dry collarette of scale.

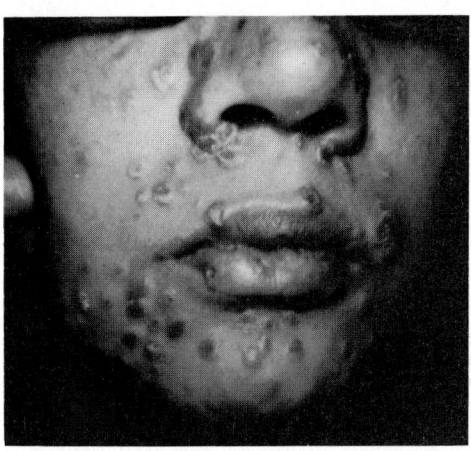

FIGURE 11-9 Papular secondary syphilis. Note the fine, dry collarette of scale on many of the lesions. An involuting papular eruption tends to persist longest in areas of vascular stasis or congestion (such as the rosaceal area of the face) and on the ankles, palms, and soles, provided these areas were included in the original distribution.

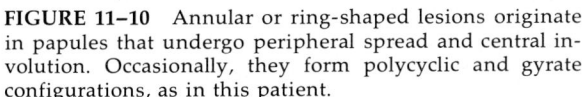

FIGURE 11-10 Annular or ring-shaped lesions originate in papules that undergo peripheral spread and central involution. Occasionally, they form polycyclic and gyrate configurations, as in this patient.

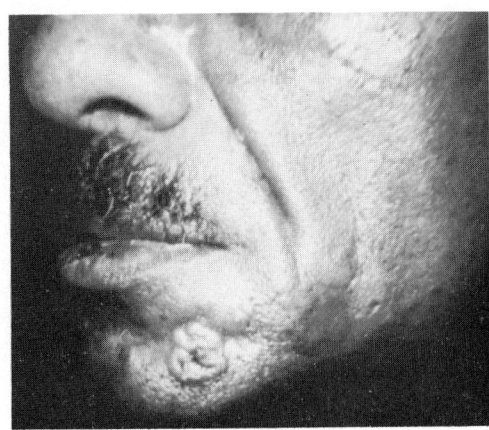

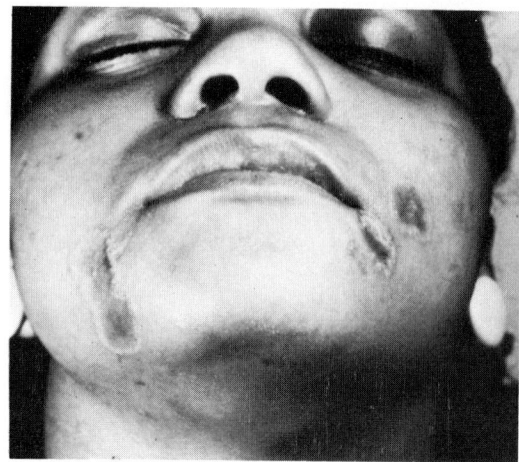

FIGURE 11-11 Annular secondary syphilids. The specimen for darkfield examination should be taken from the raised indurated border. Annular lesions are most commonly seen in blacks and are often a manifestation of infectious relapse. The face, neck, and posterior aspect of the scrotum are common sites for annular lesions.

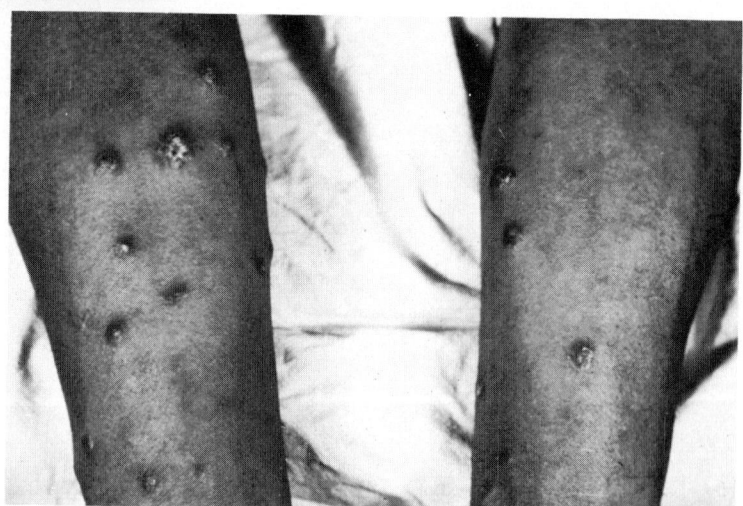

FIGURE 11-12 Nodular secondary syphilids. The lesions are indurated, with a diameter greater than 1 cm. Only a few lesions may be present. They may be flat or rounded and scaling or smooth, and usually are darker in color than papular lesions.

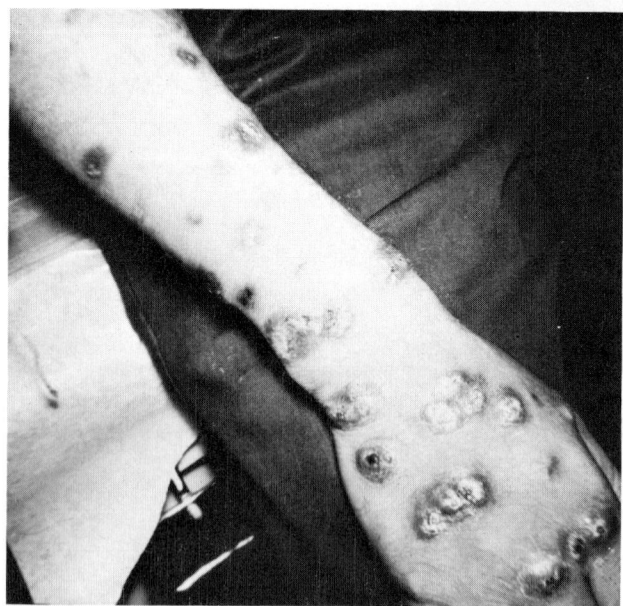

FIGURE 11-13 Pustular secondary syphilid. The surrounding skin is not significantly affected. An inflammatory areola or other sign of infection is rare. Crusts are thick and turtle-backed. They are formed by successive accretions from below, caused by liquefactive necrosis within the lesion. A moist ulcer is present beneath the crust.

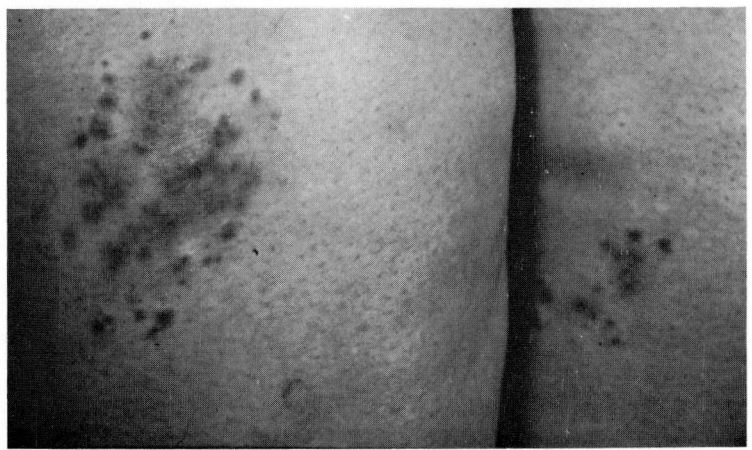

FIGURE 11–14 The corymbose configuration of lesions of secondary syphilis consists of a central large lesion, usually a papule, nodule, or plaque, surrounded by a group of lesser satellites. Cormybose lesions also result from infectious relapse and are distinct evidence of increased severity of the cutaneous reaction.

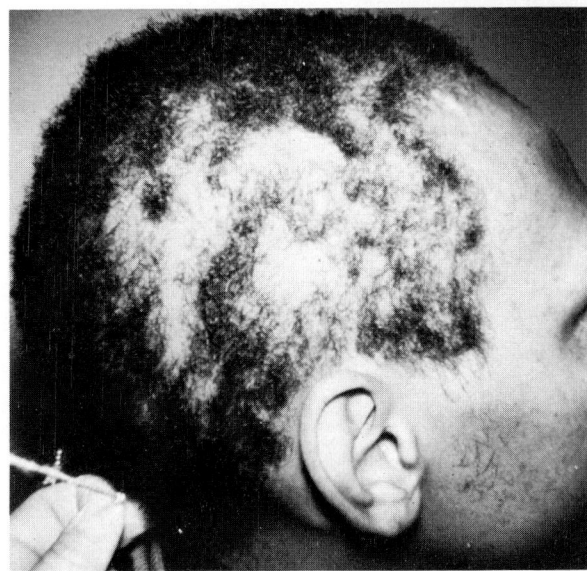

FIGURE 11–15 Typical moth-eaten alopecia of secondary syphilis. The process is better seen at the sides and back of the head where the hair is shorter.

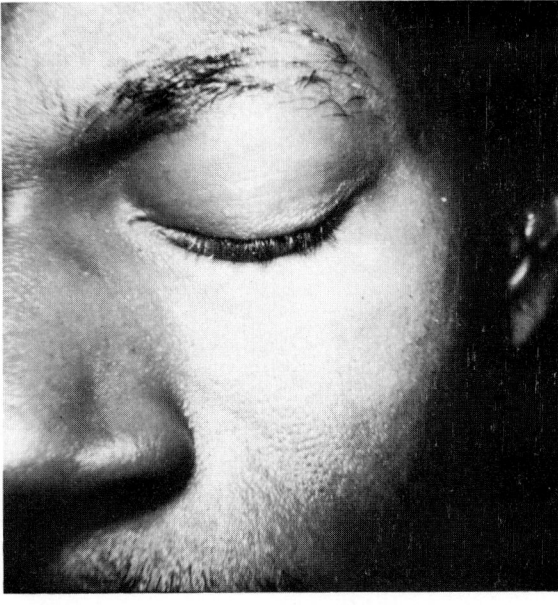

FIGURE 11–16 Hertoghe's sign of moth-eaten hair loss of the lateral half of the eyebrows. This sign may also be seen in some cases of lepromatous leprosy, leukemia, myxedema, acromegaly, and thallium poisoning, and following the use of cytotoxic drugs, such as methotrexate.

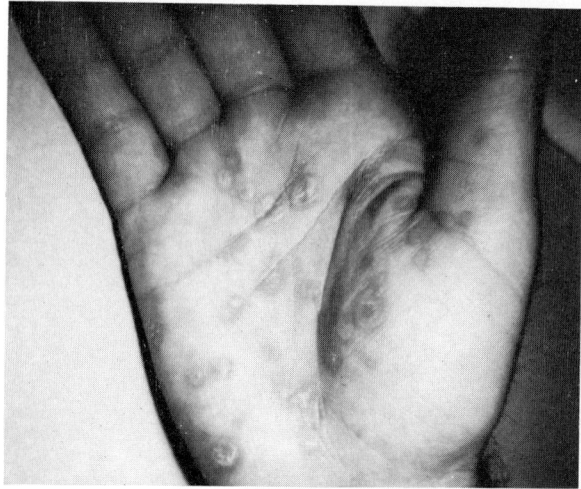

FIGURE 11–17 Maculopapular eruption of the palm. Involvement of palms and soles is usually bilateral. Note the fine, dry collarette of scale on many of the lesions. A papular eruption on the palms or soles with no lesions on the scalp, elbows, or knees, with no patches of dermatitis elsewhere on the body, and with constitutional symptoms, suggests syphilis.

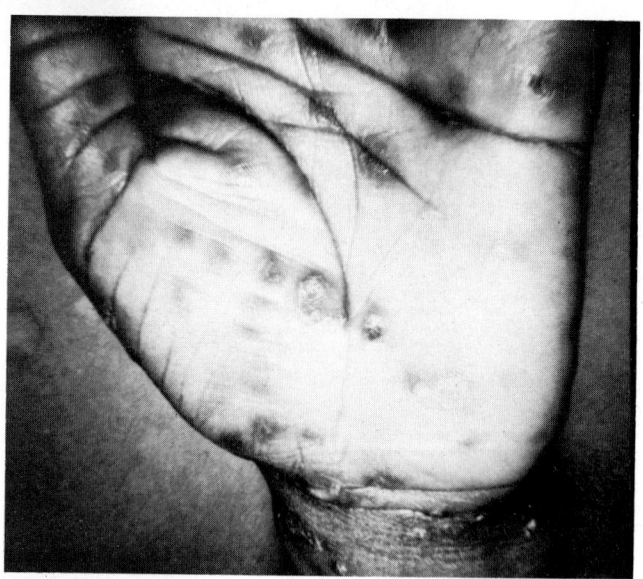

FIGURE 11–18 Secondary syphilids of the palm and wrist. Some papules demonstrate the dry collarette of fine scaling. Several are markedly keratotic and show the characteristic central dell. A keratotic papule with a central dell showing arciform configuration may be a manifestation of a late cutaneous relapse. It is termed "lues cornée" of the palm.

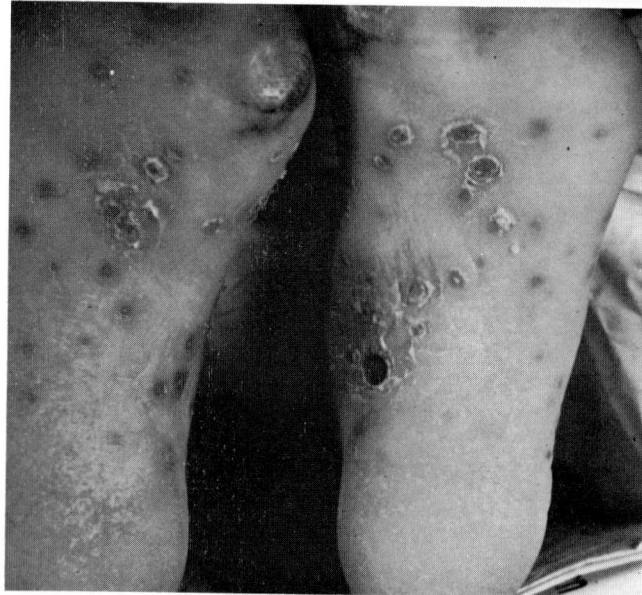

FIGURE 11–19 Papular secondary syphilids of the sole. Although all areas of the sole may be involved to some extent, papular lesions occur predominantly in the longitudinal arch of the foot. Note the fine, dry collarette of scale on many of the lesions.

TABLE 11–5 CUTANEOUS ERUPTION

Type of Lesion	Characteristics
Macular	Pale pink- to rose-colored; no scale; never vesicular; macules remain discrete, not blotchy. Most often seen on abdomen, on thorax below axillae, and over scapulae, rarely seen on face.
Maculopapular	Most common lesion; may be associated with condylomata lata.
Papular	Dull coppery-red color; occurs on face, trunk, extremities, and occasionally on scalp; may be associated with lesions of palms and soles and with mucous patches; frequently shows fine, dry collarette of scale. Condylomata lata often present.
Annular	Most commonly seen on black skin; frequently involves face, neck, and penile and scrotal skin.
Nodular	Lesions are 1 cm in diameter or larger and tend to be few in number.
Pustular	Sterile pustules; adherent brownish crusts overlying an erosion or ulcer; may be associated with chronic alcoholism, malnutrition, or deficient immunological mechanism.
Corymbose configuration	Central large lesion, usually nodular, surrounded by small satellite papules; may be associated with chronic alcoholism or malnutrition, or may represent infectious relapse.
Alopecia	Moth-eaten hair; loss of anagen phase of hair cycle; occurs in about 5 per cent of secondary stage cases; involves hair of scalp and less commonly, hair of beard, vellus hairs of body, and lateral half of eyebrows (Hertoghe's sign). Hair loss is partial, with many small patches but no atrophy; hair regrows.
Palms and soles	Bilateral; may be discrete macules or coppery-red papules, frequently with a fine dry collarette of scale; keratotic lesions may contain a central dell. Lesions of sole are often localized to longitudinal arch.

MUCOUS PATCH (Plate VI–B)

The mucous patch is a papular lesion of the mucosa whose surface has been eroded by moisture and friction. The lesion is slightly raised, round or oval, 5 to 10 mm in diameter, with a central erosion, clean pinkish base, and dull red halo of erythema. There may be a delicate silvery or yellowish pellicle covering the surface. On the tough surface of the tongue, the lesion is usually not eroded but appears as a reddish, flat papule whose surface is devoid of lingual papillae.

The mucous patch is painless and teems with treponemal organisms. It may occur on the tongue surfaces, buccal and labial mucosa, palate and tonsil, cervical and vaginal mucosa, labia minora, penile glans and coronal sulcus, and under the foreskin. Mucous patches have also been demonstrated on the gastric and rectal mucosae.[12–14]

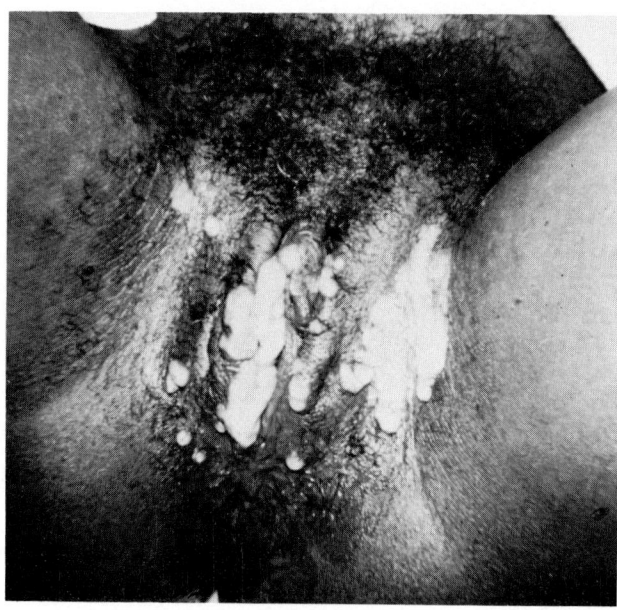

FIGURE 11–20 Condylomata lata of secondary syphilis involving the vulva and groin folds. At sites of moisture and friction, papules may hypertrophy to form button-like plaques with a moist surface and a spongy feel on palpation. The lesions may become confluent to form soft, spongy masses and may be found on the external genitalia, medial thighs, groin folds, and axillae and under pendulous breasts. Condylomata lata are the most infectious lesions encountered in early acquired syphilis.

Condylomata Lata (Fig. 11–20)

Condylomata lata are moist papules that have undergone vegetative hypertrophy at sites of friction and moisture. They appear as round or oval, raised, button-like plaques with a smooth, moist, or spongy surface. They are pinkish-gray in color and often coalesce to form a mass of condylomatous vegetation. These lesions are usually found in the folds of the genitalia, perineum, medial thighs, perianal skin, and in the gluteal cleft. They occur much less frequently under pendulous breasts, in the axillae, on the glans penis, and between the toes. Condylomata lata are the most infectious lesions seen in acquired syphilis. Treponemal counts, performed with special equipment on sera from condylomata lata, have demonstrated a range of 3700 to 246,000 treponemes per cu ml.[15] Experimental evidence indicates that the 50 per cent minimal infective dose for humans is less than 60 *Treponema pallidum* organisms.[16]

Generalized Lymphadenopathy

Generalized involvement of the lymphatic system in secondary syphilis occurs in about 85 per cent of cases. In addition to the inguinal chains, three groups of superficial lymph nodes are frequently affected to such a degree that they can be palpated: the suboccipital, the posterior cervical and postauricular, and the epitrochlear nodes. Occasionally, the deeper lymph nodes of the lateral axillary chain also can be palpated.

CONSTITUTIONAL SYMPTOMS OF SECONDARY SYPHILIS (Fig. 11–21)

About half of patients with secondary syphilis have constitutional symptoms that are usually mild, such as sore throat, low-grade fever, night sweats, rhinitis, and arthralgia.

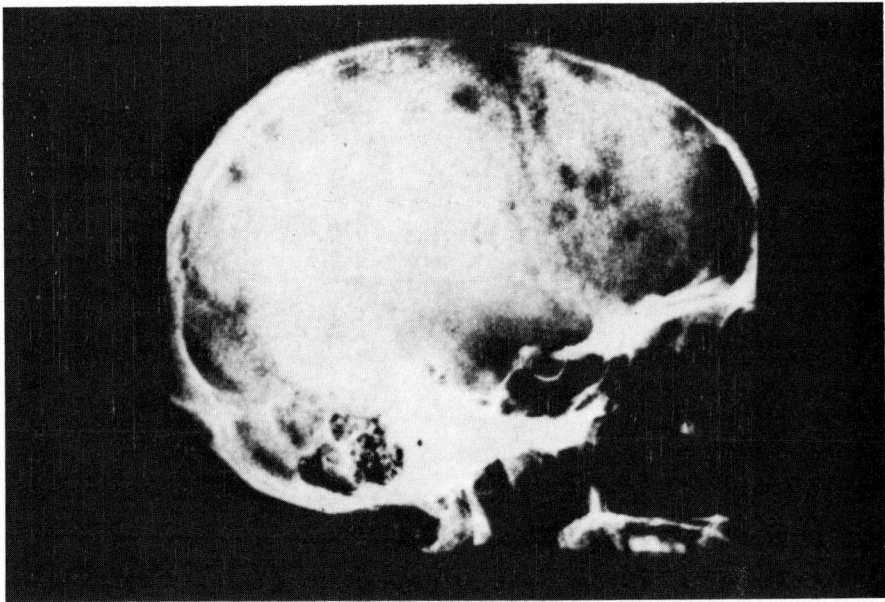

FIGURE 11–21 Localized areas of destructive osteolytic process involving the skull. Cranial spot-like pain may be exactly localized by pressure over the affected area, which may develop during the secondary stage of syphilis or during the subsequent six to 12 months of the infection. Parietal and frontal bones are most commonly affected, although the posterior half of the calvarium may be involved. (*From:* Cabanel, G., Phelip, X., and Gintz, B.: Ostéite cranienne lacunaire de la syphilis secondaire. Presse Med., 79:1755, 1971.)

Headache, a common symptom,[17] may occur as diffuse cephalgia, or as a persistent occipital pain with meningismus, which may be associated with an early syphilitic basilar meningitis. Headache may also occur as spot-like cranial pains resulting from localized syphilitic osteolytic lesions of the skull.[18-21] Localized bone pain caused by periostitis usually involves the tibiae, sternum, skull, and ribs.

On x-ray examination, the osteolytic lesions appear as irregularly circular areas of decreased density and have a moth-eaten appearance. The thinner and more porous bones of the calvarium are the ones most commonly affected. Lesions posterior to the lambdoidal suture are far less common. The inner and outer table or both may be affected. Symptoms of head pain and tenderness often disappear 72 to 96 hours after initiation of antibiotic therapy, but healing may require three to six months.

Differential diagnosis includes pyogenic osteomyelitis, multiple myeloma, tuberculous osteitis, leukemic infiltration, metastatic carcinoma, Hodgkin's disease, eosinophilic granuloma, and hemangioendothelioma.

LIVER INVOLVEMENT

Rather rarely, a hepatitis-associated antigen (HAA)–negative syphilitic hepatitis may develop during the early stages of syphilis, with liver enlargement and tenderness sometimes accompanied by jaundice. Serum alkaline phosphatase levels become elevated out of proportion to the rise in transaminases. Tissue obtained by liver biopsy has shown the pathogenesis of pericholangitis. *Treponema pallidum* has been demonstrated by silver staining techniques and by animal inoculation.[22-24]

KIDNEY INVOLVEMENT

Renal involvement in secondary syphilis has been recognized for at least 150 years. It is most often manifested as a simple mild proteinuria, but occasionally acute syphilitic nephrosis occurs. This is a transient nephrotic syndrome characterized by sudden onset of gross edema, massive proteinuria, hypoproteinemia, frequent oliguria, and hypercholesterolemia. Dramatic recovery has been observed after treatment of the syphilitic infection. Electron microscopy has revealed nodular electron-dense deposits of IgG and complement on the epithelial aspects of the glomerular basement membrane. Fusion of the epithelial foot processes compatible with an immune deposit disease has also been observed.[25-27]

NEURAL INVOLVEMENT

During the first six months to two years of an untreated or inadequately treated infection, early meningovascular neurosyphilis may develop. During the early stages of syphilis, spirochetemia facilitates the passage of treponemes to the central nervous system, where they may escape from meningeal or choroidal vessels, either to float freely in the cerebrospinal fluid or to lodge in the leptomeninges.[28, 29] Since the richest blood supply is at the base of the brain, basilar meningitis, characterized by cranial nerve palsies, headache, and meningismus, may be the outcome. The second, third, seventh, and eighth cranial nerves are most vulnerable; hence ptosis, neuroretinitis, or acute syphilitic auditory neuritis and syphilitic labyrinthitis may result.[30-34] An increased cell count and elevated total protein content of the cerebrospinal fluid are the earliest and most conspicuous signs of meningeal involvement. Subsequently, the non-treponemal antigen tests (e.g., Kolmer-Wassermann complement fixation and VDRL) become reactive. A modified FTA (fluorescent treponemal antibody) test of cerebrospinal fluid is apparently sensitive and specific but is still under evaluation.[35-37]

A clinical diagnosis of secondary syphilis must be supported by laboratory evidence, such as identification of *Treponema pallidum* by darkfield microscopic examination of serum from a lesion, by reactive blood serology, or occasionally by histopathological studies of biopsy material.

RELAPSE IN EARLY SYPHILIS

During the first two years after the spontaneous involution of secondary lesions in untreated syphilis, or after inadequate therapy, the early latent stage may be interrupted by evidence of relapse. This may occur as an infectious relapse of skin or mucosa, with such recurrent secondary symptoms as an annular lesion, a few papules or condylomata lata, oral or genital mucous patches, or lesions of palms and soles. There may be an ocular relapse, such as iritis, or a neurorelapse (i.e., early syphilitic meningitis or meningovascular neurosyphilis). An osseous relapse may be manifested as an area of periostitis or as an osteolytic process. Serological relapse, with an abrupt, marked rise in reagin titer, may precede other forms of relapse.

On the other hand, the latent stage of syphilis may be maintained for years, even for the life of the patient. However, during latency and particularly during the first two years of the infection, showers of treponemes can enter the bloodstream from a focus in the liver or a lymph node; while the organisms are in the blood stream, a pregnant female can infect the fetus in utero.

LABORATORY DIAGNOSIS

The most specific means of diagnosing early syphilis is by direct demonstration of motile *Treponema pallidum* spirochetes in serous exudate from a gently abraded lesion, using darkfield microscopy. Enlarged regional lymph nodes can also be used as a specimen source by aspirating the node and examining the material obtained. Darkfield examination is indicated when lesions of primary, secondary, or infectious relapsing syphilis, or of early congenital syphilis, are present.

Oral lesions present a unique problem. Except for lesions on the lips or the tip of the tongue (sites that can be carefully dried of saliva) darkfield specimens of oral lesions may lead to erroneous interpretation. Saprophytic *Treponema macrodentium* and *T. microdentium,* which are morphologically almost identical to *Treponema pallidum,* hamper the diagnosis of lesions of posterior tongue and tonsil. Elsewhere, saprophytic spirochetes can be identified because they appear more translucent, and their irregular spirals collapse and distort during rapid motion. *T. calligyrum,* sometimes found in the genital area, has rigid regular spirals but is twice as thick as *T. pallidum* and has slightly hooked ends. *Treponema pallidum* has a peculiar brilliance, similar to a tungsten filament. The spirals are rigid and regular, whether at rest or in motion, and the organism drifts unhurriedly with currents in the field. It has been called "the queen of spirochetes."

SEROLOGICAL TESTS

Two main types of tests are used in the serological diagnosis of syphilis:

1. Non-treponemal antigen tests, which measure non-specific antibodies (syphilitic reagins) that are directed against either lipoidal antigens derived from the treponeme itself or a lipoidal antigen that results from interaction of the host tissue and the treponeme.

2. Treponemal antigen tests, which usually employ *T. pallidum* as the antigen to detect specific treponemal antibodies developed in the body.

NON-TREPONEMAL ANTIGEN TESTS

Non-treponemal antigen tests are basically of two types: (a) flocculation tests, and (b) complement fixation tests.

In 1906, Wassermann introduced the complement fixation test for syphilis, using the livers of stillborn congenital syphilitics as antigen. Subsequently, it was shown that other tissues, particularly alcoholic extracts of beef or ox heart, could be used satisfactorily as antigen. In 1931, Kahn introduced a flocculation test that required no complement and could be read macroscopically within a few hours. Modifications of the flocculation test procedure were made by Kline, Hinton, Mazzini, Eagle, and Meinicke. In 1941, Pangborn[38] purified the cardiolipin-lecithin antigen from beef heart. This formed the basis of modern reagin tests, such as the VDRL and RPR flocculation tests and the Kolmer modification of the Wassermann complement fixation test (Table 11–6).

The VDRL and RPR tests are inexpensive, easily performed, and reproducible. If any degree of reactivity is reported, a quantitative test is indicated. The most accurate measure of syphilitic activity is a rising serological reagin titer, and the best measure of response to treatment is a falling titer. Cardiolipin antigen tests may be non-reactive in some cases of early primary syphilis, occasionally in late latent syphilis, and in some manifestations of late syphilis. If an excess of antibody is present, a prozone phenomenon, with inhibition of precipitation, may result. This produces a false negative reaction in the first tube of undiluted serum measured in the flocculation test.[54] However, subsequent dilutions result in reactivity. In some individuals, reagin reactivity is stimulated by other medical conditions, causing a false positive result in a non-treponemal antigen test.

A reactive reagin test is of value for the following reasons:

1. As confirmatory evidence when correlated with the patient's history and clinical evidence of syphilis.

2. As a significant finding when used in conjunction with epidemiological investigations.

3. As a measure of syphilitic activity when a high or rising serological reagin titer is present.

4. As a measure of the adequacy of therapy when the serological reagin titer response after treatment is studied.

5. As a reliable diagnostic tool when a good quantitative reagin test is used to evaluate asymptomatic neonates under investigation for early congenital syphilis.

6. As a particularly specific test in analyzing spinal fluid, since false positive results are extremely rare.[55]

Treponemal Antigen Tests

Treponemal antigen tests, which utilize antigen prepared from virulent *T. pallidum,* measure specific antitreponemal antibody. They are used primarily: (a) to help distinguish between biological false positive reactive and true reactive reagin tests for syphilis, (b) to help establish a correct diagnosis in patients who have clinical evidence of syphilis (particularly late syphilis), but who have non-reactive blood and spinal fluid reagin tests, and (c) to assist in the diagnosis of patients who are suspected epidemiologically of having the disease, but who have non-reactive reagin tests and do not show clinical evidence of syphilis.

Latter cases include the individual with a syphilitic marital partner and the

TABLE 11-6 ANTIBODIES PRODUCED IN SYPHILIS

Antibodies to Lipoidal Antigens (Reagin)

Test	Date First Described	Class of Antibody Detected
Wassermann complement fixation[39]	1906	IgG mainly
Kahn flocculation[40]	1931	IgG, IgM
VDRL flocculation[41]	1946	IgG, IgM
Kolmer-Wassermann[42]	1948	IgG mainly
Rapid plasma reagin flocculation[43]	1957	IgG, IgM
Rapid plasma reagin circle card[44]	1962	IgG, IgM

Antibodies to Treponemal Antigens

ANTIBODIES TO GROUP TREPONEMAL ANTIGENS

Test	Date First Described	Class of Antibody Detected
Reiter protein complement fixation[45, 46]	1957	Non-specific antitreponemal antibodies, IgG mainly

ANTIBODIES TO SPECIFIC ANTI-*T. pallidum* ANTIGENS

Test	Date First Described	Class of Antibody Detected
Treponema pallidum immobilization[47]	1949	IgG mainly
Fluorescent treponemal antibody[48]	1957	IgG, IgM
FTA–Absorption[49]	1964	IgG, IgM
Treponema pallidum hemagglutination[50, 51]	1965	IgG mainly
IgG–FTA–ABS IgM–FTA–ABS[52]	1968	IgG IgM
Micro–*T. pallidum* hemagglutination (MHA–TP)[53]	1970	IgG mainly

non-reactive mother of a congenitally syphilitic child.[55] Once positive, treponemal tests tend to remain reactive for life despite adequate treatment and therefore are not reliable indicators of cure.

False Positive Reactions

False positive reactions to non-treponemal antigen tests result from the production of reagin in response to conditions or infections of non-treponemal origin. Since the replacement of crude antigens with more specific purified cardiolipin-lecithin-cholesterol antigens, the incidence of false positive reactions caused by unrelated disease has shown a marked decrease.

False positive reactions are divided into two groups. The first is acute false positive reactions, which disappear within a ten-month period. These have been associated with such conditions as viral pneumonia, malaria, infectious mononucleosis, infectious hepatitis, lymphogranuloma venereum, chickenpox, and measles, as well as immunization procedures against smallpox, yellow fever, and typhoid.

The second group is chronic false positive reactions, which persist for longer than ten months and often for many years. These reactions may occur with such conditions as collagen diseases (e.g., systemic lupus erythematosus, rheumatoid arthritis, autoimmune hemolytic anemia, and periarteritis nodosa), heroin addiction, lepromatous leprosy, hepatitis, and brucellosis.

There is general agreement that the acute false positive reaction is without serious significance for the patient. However, the chronic false positive reaction is an immunological phenomenon of considerable importance. In addition to the high incidence of autoimmune disease associated with chronic false positive reactivity, the positivity may precede the onset of a collagen disease by many years.[56, 57] A genetic factor also may be involved in the development of the chronic reaction. This may account for the high incidence of raised serum gamma globulin levels, antinuclear factors, rheumatoid factors, and false positive non-treponemal antigen test results in the families of those who show chronic false positive reactions.[58, 59] Biochemical derangements found in the sera of patients with chronic false positive reactions include abnormal values for liver function tests, abnormal immunoglobulins, thyroid antibodies, rheumatoid and lupus erythematosus cell factors, raised erythrocyte sedimentation rate, elevated serum globulin level, anemia, and a high level of circulating anticoagulant. IgM and IgG antibodies are responsible for the false positive reaction. During pregnancy the IgG fraction may cross the placental barrier into the fetal circulation, to disappear a few weeks after birth. No relationship between passively transferred false positive IgG fraction and subsequent development of a chronic false positive test is known.

Non-treponemal antigen tests, such as the VDRL and Wassermann tests, detect antibodies to cardiolipin, which is a complex of diphospholipids found mainly on the mitochondrial inner membrane. Syphilitic reagins may be a type of autoantibody produced by action of the treponemes on body tissues. Autoantibodies found consistently in patients with primary biliary cirrhosis have been described. They react with a lipoprotein component on the mitochondrial inner membrane but are non-reactive with cardiolipin; they also produce 'M' fluorescence with Coon's technique.[60] It has been found that many patients with chronic false positive reactions also showed 'M' fluorescence. The two reactions are considered useful markers of a special immunological abnormality related to connective tissue disease.[61] They may indicate the actual presence of systemic disease or be helpful in identifying those patients who are likely to develop connective tissue disease.

False Positive Reactions to Treponemal Antigen Tests. The FTA–ABS test has proved to be a sensitive, specific test for treponemal antibodies. However, sera from patients with lupus erythematosus may reveal atypical beaded staining of treponemes as well as homogeneous staining like that of syphilitic sera.[62] These reactions are thought to be due to an anti-DNA antibody and can be corrected by treatment of the sera with DNA or nucleoprotein.[63] On rare occasions beaded fluorescence may occur in hepatitis, rheumatoid arthritis, glomerulonephritis, scleroderma, and other autoimmune diseases. Nevertheless, in general it is prudent to approach a confirmed reactive FTA–ABS test as strong evidence of syphilis until proved otherwise.

Although the specificity of the TPHA and MHA (micro-hemagglutination) tests is relatively good, false positive results figure in most published series.[64-66] Therefore, a positive TPHA test in a patient with no clinical evidence or history of syphilis should be verified by the FTA–ABS procedure.

LATE CONGENITAL SYPHILIS

Syphilis is the only important transplacental infection that is both preventable and treatable in utero. Congenital syphilis results when the fetus is infected by the syphilitic organisms of the mother. Since fetal infection does not occur until after organogenesis is complete, it does not lead to congenital malformations. The fetus becomes vulnerable to infection after the 16th week of pregnancy. Treatment of the infected mother prior to that time will almost always prevent infection in the fetus; treatment after this time may cure the disease if infection has taken place. The danger of fetal infection is greatest if the pregnant woman has primary, secondary, or early latent syphilis. It is urged that serological tests be performed at the first prenatal visit, during the third trimester, and at the time of delivery.

Neurosyphilis. Congenital neurosyphilis is a possible consequence of an untreated infection during pregnancy. Congenital neurosyphilis causes mental retardation, meningovascular neurosyphilis with its seizures and hemiplegia, juvenile paresis, and juvenile tabes dorsalis. These manifestations almost always appear before the age of 20.

Early congenital syphilis is comparable to the secondary stage of acquired syphilis, and its manifestations may include skin eruption, rhagades, mucous patches, condylomata lata, snuffles, osteochondritis, periostitis, hepatosplenomegaly, and syphilitic meningitis. Blood serological tests are positive. As an untreated or inadequately treated syphilitic child grows up, the effects of *Treponema pallidum* or its toxins may slowly become apparent with the development of stigmata of late congenital syphilis.

Gummata. Nasopalatine, nasopharyngeal, mucocutaneous, subperiosteal, or hepatic gummata may occasionally develop (Figs. 11–22 and 11–23).

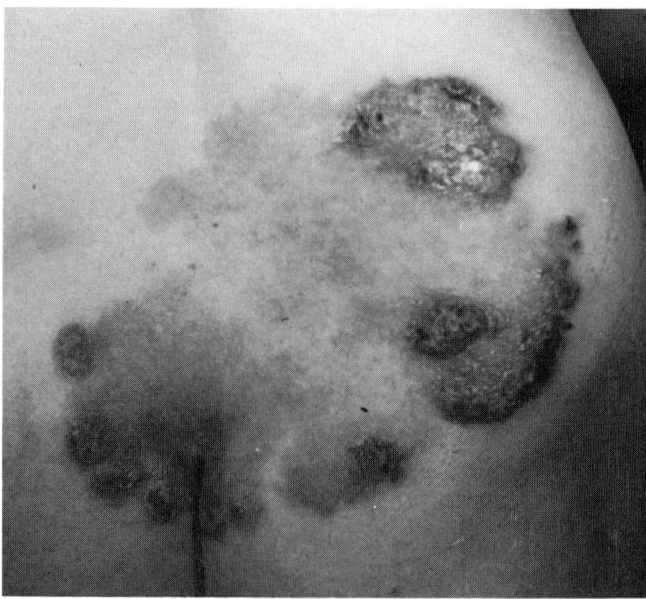

FIGURE 11-22 Nodulo-ulcerative cutaneous late syphilid. This is a classic example of gummatous manifestation of late syphilis, which may occur in late congenital syphilis as well as in late acquired syphilis. It is marked by deep, palpable gummatous infiltration, indolence, and acriform configuration with polycyclic borders. Tissue destruction and replacement occur with or without ulceration. There is a tendency to central or one-sided healing with peripheral extension and persistent hyperpigmentation as healing occurs. The lesion heals with a superficial, atrophic, non-contractile scar. The surrounding skin in the direction of extension is practically normal. (There is no suggestion of metastatic nodule formation beyond the periphery, such as occurs in lupus vulgaris, and no diffuse inflammatory areola, as in a pyogenic process.)

BLOOD SEROLOGICAL REACTIONS IN LATE CONGENITAL SYPHILIS

Treponemal antigen tests (e.g., FTA–ABS) tend to remain reactive for the life of the patient, regardless of antisyphilitic therapy or possible non-reactivity of non-treponemal antigen tests. The reagin tests, although helpful in diagnosing children and adolescents, may spontaneously become non-reactive in patients over 40, or may remain persistently positive despite therapy.

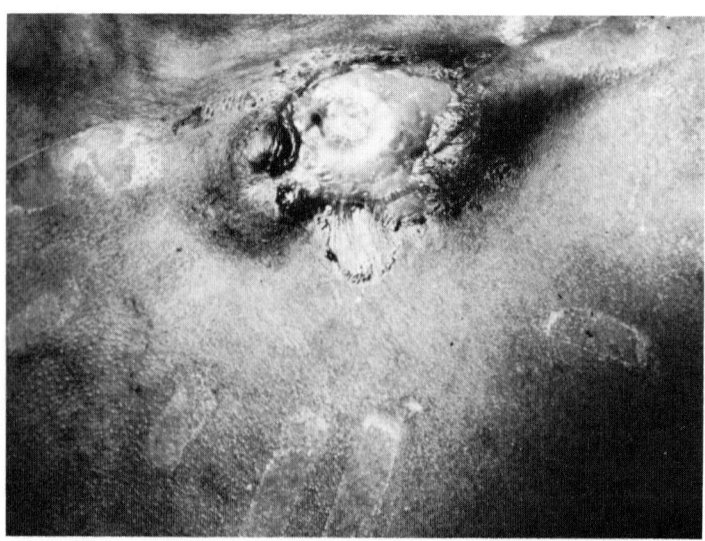

FIGURE 11-23 Gummata of the sternoclavicular joint in an 18-year-old male with late congenital syphilis. There is extension of gummatous osteomyelitis from the sternal end of the clavicle to the sternoclavicular joint as well as extension to the periarticular tissues and overlying skin. Although cranial bone and tibial lesions are more common, gummatous lesions involving the clavicle tend to be more destructive. Bone gummata frequently cause a severe Herxheimer reaction.

PHYSICAL SIGNS OF LATE CONGENITAL SYPHILIS
(Table 11-7)

Facies. The facies of late congenital syphilis is a composite of syphilids and developmental dystrophies. Localized syphilitic periostitis of the frontal eminences of the forehead produces prominent frontal bosses, which were first described by Parrot. Periostitis of the superciliary arches of the frontal bones results in the overhanging brow. When associated with minor degrees of hydrocephalus during infancy, the increased height and thickening of the frontal bones create the appearance of the "Olympian brow," "squarehead," "hot cross bun," or "tower skull." Frontal bossing also may be caused by coexisting rickets.

The saddle bridge deformity of the nose is the end result of the syphilitic rhinitis (snuffles) of the neonatal period. The nasal mucosa becomes eroded, with destruction of underlying bone and cartilage resulting in high perforation of the nasal septum and collapse of the nasal bridge. A gummatous osteitis may also produce perforation of the hard palate or perforation of the nasal septum, with resulting saddle bridge deformity.

Post-Rhagadic Scars. Post-rhagadic scars in linear or retiform arrangement radiate from the lips, chin, cheeks, or perianal skin (Fig. 11–24). They are caused by atrophy of elastic tissue as the deeply fissured lesions found in these areas undergo involution in the infected neonate.

Higouménakis' Sign. The Higouménakis sign, noted after puberty, is the enlargement, usually unilateral, of the medial third of the clavicle.[67-69] The

TABLE 11–7 HALLMARKS OF LATE CONGENITAL SYPHILIS

Major	Secondary	Debatable
Reactive serological test for syphilis	Frontal bosses of Parrot's sign	DuBois' little finger sign
Interstitial keratitis	Higouménakis' sign	High, narrow palatine arch
Hutchinson's incisors	Scaphoid scapulae	Carabelli tubercle
Mulberry (Moon, Fournier) 6 year molars	Dactylitis	Outflung elbow
Eighth nerve deafness	Epiphyseal enlargement	Ulnar deviation of middle finger
Juvenile tabes, paresis	Saddle nose; wideset eyes	
Post-rhagadic scars	Perforation of nasal septum or hard palate	
Saber tibiae	Paroxysmal cold hemoglobinuria	
Clutton's joints (synovitis)		
Choroiditis; primary optic atrophy		
Periostitis; osteitis		
Gummata in nose and throat		

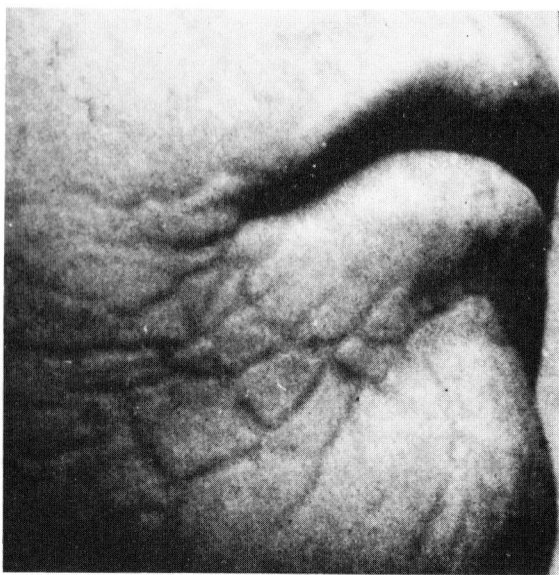

FIGURE 11–24 Post-rhagadic scars of the lip, chin, and cheek. These are linear furrows of the vermilion margin of the lips, which extend into radial or reticular scar-like lesions of the surrounding skin of chin and cheek. They are caused by the loss of elastic tissue in the healing of rhagadic fissures seen in early congenital syphilis. The perianal skin may also be involved.

clavicle begins to ossify before any other bone in the body, developing primary ossification centers in the medial and lateral portions during the fifth to sixth week of fetal life. The secondary ossification center is at the sternal end and does not appear until the 18th to 20th year of life, uniting with the rest of the bone at about the 25th year. *Treponema pallidum,* having a predilection for connective tissue, may remain dormant at the sternal end of the clavicle as well as in certain membranous bones. Syphilitic infection tends to be most evident at sites of active growth. With the development of the ossification center at the sternal end of the clavicle, the syphilitic infection may be reactivated, and osteitis and hyperostosis may result.

Epiphyseal Enlargement. Epiphyseal enlargement resulting in the disproportionate size of joints, is characterized by wide wrists, heavy knees, and outflung elbow. The shortening of the long bones due to epiphyseal changes enhances the appearance of heavy bone structure.

Saber Shin. The saber shin consists of anterior bowing of the tibiae and fusiform enlargement of the middle third of the tibiae. The fibulae may show similar enlargement on x-ray examination; both are a residue of periostitis and chronic syphilitic osteitis.

Scaphoid Scapulae. The scaphoid scapula is a concavity of the vertebral border. The scapula ossifies from seven or more centers, and at birth a large part is osseous. However, the secondary ossification center appears on the vertebral border between the 14th and 20th year of life. Syphilitic reactivation of dormant treponemes, with marked thickening of the vertebral border and adjacent scapular spine caused by periostitis and osteitis, is believed to produce the concavity.

Clutton's Joints (Fig. 11–25). The observation that a chronic, slowly evolving, symmetrical serous synovitis of the knee joints may be a manifestation of congenital syphilis was made by Clutton in 1886.[70] The maximum age of onset is between 8 and 15 years. The involvement is almost always bilateral, with relatively painless, non-tender separation of the joint surfaces due to

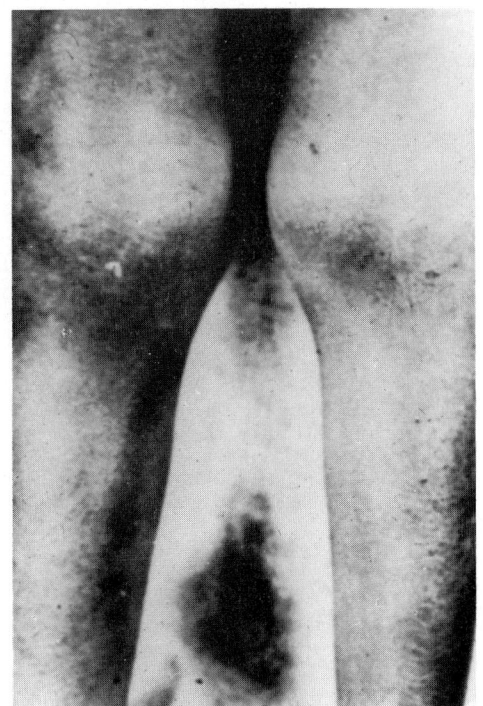

FIGURE 11–25 Clutton's joints. These are bilateral, painless joint effusions producing separation of the joint surfaces, unassociated with bony-joint changes. The knee joints are most commonly involved. Blood serological tests for syphilis are almost uniformly reactive. When the effusion disappears, the joint becomes normal. A stigma of late congenital syphilis, its maximum age of onset is between eight and 15 years.

effusion, but with no x-ray evidence of bone changes. The presence of other stigmata of late congenital syphilis, such as the residue of interstitial keratitis, may aid in the diagnosis. While knee joints are the primary targets, other joints, such as ankles, elbows, or wrists, may be affected. Blood serological tests for syphilis are almost uniformly reactive, as are reagin tests of the joint fluid. Darkfield examination of joint fluid is negative.[71] The synovitis resolves spontaneously after several months, leaving no residual joint damage.[72] There is almost complete absence of response to therapy with either salicylates or antibiotics. However, in these cases, treatment for late congenital syphilis as a general measure is indicated.

Hutchinson's Incisors. This characteristic of late congenital syphilis will be discussed in the following section on abnormalities of the teeth, eyes, and ears.

DISEASES AND ABNORMALITIES OF THE TEETH, EYES, AND EARS IN LATE CONGENITAL SYPHILIS

DENTAL MALFORMATIONS

At birth, the central incisors and first molar teeth of the permanent dentition have reached the stage of morphodifferentiation, while the deciduous teeth are forming enamel and dentin. There is marked cellular activity at the dentino-enamel junction of the permanent teeth, particularly at the apex of the enamel organ.

In the Hutchinson's incisor of late congenital syphilis, the syphilitic

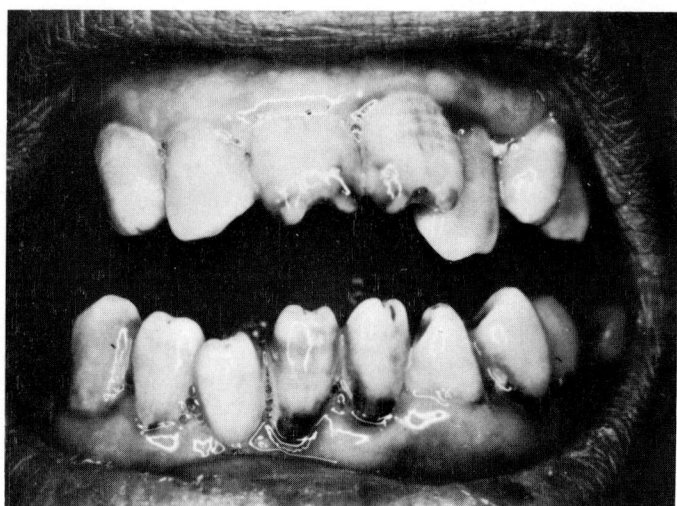

FIGURE 11–26 Hutchinson's incisors of late congenital syphilis. This 48-year-old woman had bilateral corneal residue of interstitial keratitis, complete hearing loss, and typical Hutchinson's incisors. These three signs comprise "Hutchinson's triad" of late congenital syphilis.

infection produces a narrowed and constricted dentino-enamel junction. This distortion determines the basic shape of the tooth, on which normal enamel is laid down about three months after birth.

With the suppressed development of the central dental mamelon, the lateral enamel surfaces of the tooth converge to produce the bulging sides and anterior-posterior thickening of the screwdriver or oat-shaped tooth. With marked hypoplasia at the dentino-enamel junction, one central defect or notch may result, which is covered by fairly normal enamel deposition (Figs. 11–26 and 11–27).[73–76]

Bauer[77] demonstrated that in syphilitic fetuses and neonates, the mesenchymal dental sac and epithelial tooth buds of both deciduous and permanent teeth (particularly those adjacent to the enamel epithelium) harbored a greater number of *Treponema pallidum* organisms than any other tissue of the osseous system. They were evidently conveyed by the dense network of capillaries invading the outer epithelial layer. The periosteum of the jaws also contained treponemes in perivascular tissue. Lymphocytic and plasma cell infiltration and obliterative endarteritis were also evident in the layers of the dental sac adjoining the tooth buds. The tissue reaction was more pronounced in syphilitic neonates than in fetuses, but no disturbances of dentin formation were observed.

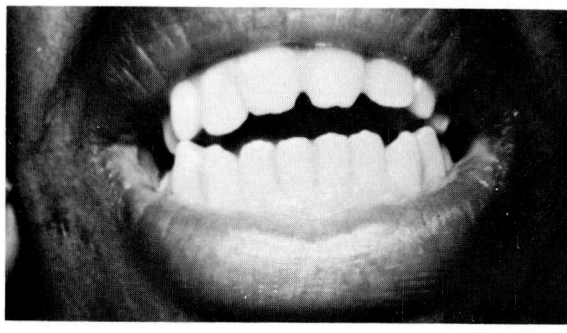

FIGURE 11–27 Hutchinsonian upper central incisor teeth without notching. The diameter of the cutting edge is narrower than the gingival edge, giving a screwdriver shape to the tooth. An anteroposterior thickening produces a barrel shape. Although there is a suggestion of one central notch in each upper central incisor, this is not essential to the diagnosis. The dentino-enamel junction is dwarfed, influencing the shape of the tooth and producing a narrower crown. This should not be confused with enamel hypoplasia, such as may occur in rickets or fluorosis. Traumatic notching occasionally is deceptive.

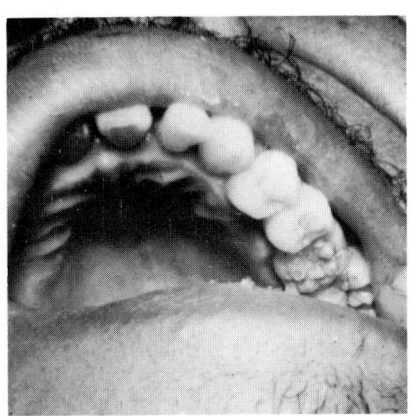

FIGURE 11–28 This is the "mulberry" molar (six year molar of the permanent dentition), also termed "Fournier tooth" and "Moon molar." Note the multiple dwarfed cusps that spring from well within the margin of the narrowed crown and the shoulder of hypertrophied enamel ridge that surrounds the crown.

If treatment for syphilis can be instituted within the first 72 to 80 days of life, the distortion at the dentino-enamel junction of the permanent incisor teeth can be prevented, and when the teeth erupt at age six to seven, they will not show characteristics of the Hutchinsonian incisor.[75, 78] These characteristics are:

1. The cutting edge of the Hutchinson's incisor is narrower than the gingival margin, producing the screwdriver or oat shape.

2. The bulging shoulder of enamel at the sides and back of the crown increases the anterior-posterior diameter, producing a barrel shape.

3. One central notch on the cutting edge of the tooth (not present in all cases).[79]

At birth, the first (six year) molars of the permanent dentition are also at the stage of morphodifferentiation. In the presence of syphilitic infection, there may be constriction of the dentino-enamel junction with resulting narrowed crown surface and a shoulder of enamel bulging out around the sides and back of the crown. From well within the margin of the occlusal surface multiple dwarfed cusps develop that resemble miniature turrets. These malformed teeth are called "mulberry molars" (Fig. 11–28).

There is no correlation between severity of syphilitic infection in the neonatal period and earliest infancy and dental development. These changes should not be confused with actual enamel hypoplasia, which develops at a later time in the growth of the tooth and may be caused by rickets, hypoparathyroidism, or fluorosis. However, enamel hypoplasia may occur in the incisor teeth of the deciduous dentition. A classic Hutchinsonian incisor or mulberry molar may be regarded as pathognomonic of late congenital syphilis. It may affect a single tooth or all of the incisors and first molars.

SYPHILIS OF THE EYE

Histological examination of the eyes of syphilitic fetuses shows treponemes disseminated throughout the organ, including the cornea, sclera, uveal tract, retina, and optic nerve.[80, 81] The high incidence of ocular disease in congenital syphilis therefore is not surprising, but it is remarkable that the eye usually becomes involved relatively late in the disease.

Choroiditis. Choroiditis of congenital syphilis, occurring in about 5 per cent of cases, is probably one of the earliest ocular lesions, although the typical atrophic changes may not be detected until later in life. Involvement of the peripheral choroid results in the characteristic pigmentation of the peripheral fundus, the so-called salt and pepper fundus.[82]

Interstitial Keratitis. Interstitial keratitis is the most common eye lesion of late congenital syphilis. It is usually encountered between the ages of five and 16, although it may appear as early as birth or as late as 30 years of age. According to Duke-Elder,[83] interstitial keratitis is a manifestation of a local antigen-antibody reaction. It may be precipitated either by small-scale treponemal invasion of the antibody-rich cornea and uveal tract or by the release of antigens from organisms elsewhere in the body, which are carried in the blood stream to the sensitized cornea. Intraocular treponemes have been demonstrated in untreated interstitial keratitis.[84, 85]

The active phase of interstitial keratitis usually starts with severe inflammatory symptoms, circumcorneal congestion, lacrimation, photophobia, and pain. There is general clouding of the cornea owing to lymphocytic cellular infiltration. This is followed by vascular invasion of the cornea from the limbus by both superficial and deep ciliary vessels and by secondary necrosis of the corneal lamellae (Fig. 11–29). The superficial vessels may form loops, producing the "salmon patch."

Although all layers of the cornea may be involved to some degree, the major disease occurs in the deeper layers adjacent to Descemet's membrane. Almost invariably synchronous with the infiltration and vascularization of the cornea is the involvement of the iris and anterior uvea. The disease, which is usually bilateral, may persist for several months, after which the infiltrate is absorbed, and the cornea clears steadily from the periphery. The central haziness persists longest, leaving a thin, somewhat mottled scar. The regression of the blood vessels is never complete, persisting throughout life as fine threads or ghost

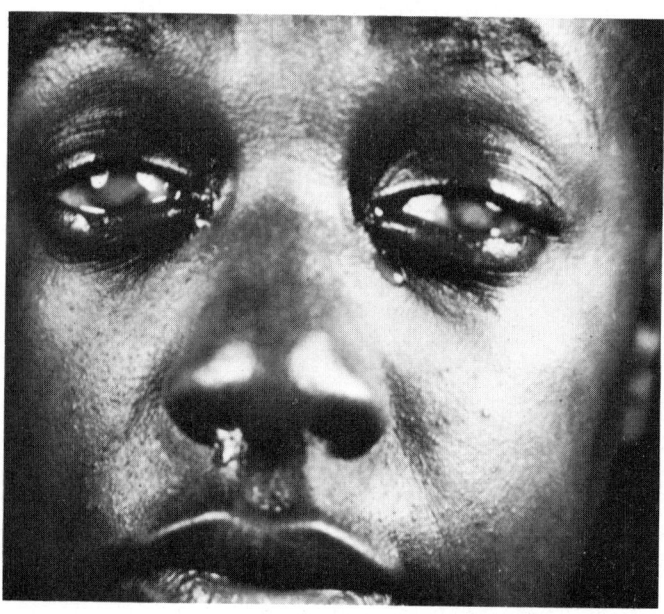

FIGURE 11–29 Interstitial keratitis of late congenital syphilis. This patient demonstrates the bilateral photophobia, bilateral clouding of the cornea, and lacrimation found in this condition. The round cell infiltrate and vascularization involve all layers of the cornea to some degree but particularly involve the substantia propria adjacent to Descemet's membrane. The iris and anterior uvea are usually also involved, increasing pain and lacrimation.

vessels traversing the substantia propria of the cornea. These are easily identifiable under slit-lamp examination.[86]

Recurrences of keratitis have been reported in 9 to 18 per cent of untreated or inadequately treated cases of congenital syphilis, but relapse occurred in only 2 per cent of adequately treated patients.[87] Glaucoma may be a late sequela of interstitial keratitis.

Treatment. Willcox[88] has drawn attention to the scarcity of data on penicillin serum levels when different penicillin preparations are used, when there are variations in dosage and administration, and when probenecid is prescribed.

There are known factors that affect the penetration of antibiotics into the eye. Essentially, the blood-aqueous barrier consists of layers of cells that separate the blood of the capillary vessels within the eye from the intraocular fluids. Lipid-soluble substances traverse the blood-aqueous barrier more freely than do water-soluble substances. Penicillin undergoes ionization in the blood stream and exists almost completely as ions insoluble in lipids. Thus penicillin, which exists in plasma in a water-soluble ionic form, penetrates the blood-aqueous barrier very slowly. In contrast, chloramphenicol, which is more soluble in lipids, travels across the barrier approximately 20 times more rapidly than penicillin G, even though both compounds have similar molecular weights.[89]

The adsorption of a portion of penicillin G on plasma proteins, which are unable to penetrate the blood-aqueous barrier because of their molecular size, means that only the unbound fraction of the antibiotic in the blood stream is available for passage into the eye, although in the presence of uveitis, the barrier may be partially broken down. The efficacy of penicillin G in the treatment of all stages of syphilis is well documented, but clinical evidence shows that ampicillin may be more effective in intraocular syphilitic eye infections.[85, 90]

Cottini and Lazzaro found the concentration of ampicillin needed for the complete immobilization of *Treponema pallidum* was 0.032 mcg/ml.[91] Few venereologists in the United States have reported the use of ampicillin in acquired or congenital syphilis, although it is being used in France. In the treatment of late congenital syphilis with interstitial keratitis, a course of ampicillin following the accepted parenteral dosage of penicillin G may be effective. The topical use of cortisone also is helpful in the control of the inflammatory and exudative phases of corneal involvement (Table 11–8).[92]

Eighth Nerve Deafness

Three main types of hearing loss due to syphilis are encountered in the congenital form of the disease.

Meningo-Neuro-Labyrinthitis. During the first six months to two years of untreated syphilitic infection, a meningovascular or meningoencephalitic neurosyphilis may develop. As a result of the spirochetemia of early congenital syphilis, the organisms are conveyed to the nervous system through the blood stream. Hardy and his associates demonstrated *Treponema pallidum* in the cerebrospinal fluid of seven of 13 neonates with early congenital syphilis.[93] The treponemes may escape from the meningeal or choroidal vessels and either float freely in the cerebrospinal fluid or lodge in the leptomeninges.

TABLE 11-8 TREATMENT OF SYPHILIS

Stage of Disease	Benzathine Penicillin G (PCN–G)	Aqueous Procaine Penicillin G (APPG)	Alternate Antibiotics
Primary syphilis	2.4 million units (1.2 million units in each buttock) IM. Repeat in 1 week. Total: 4.8 million units		500 mg erythromycin or tetracycline every 6 hours (2 gm daily) for 15 days. Total: 30 gm
Secondary syphilis	2.4 million units given IM once weekly for 3 weeks. Total: 7.2 million units		As above
Early latent syphilis	2.4 million units given IM once weekly for 4 weeks. Total: 9.6 million units		2 gm erythromycin or tetracycline daily for 20 days. Total: 40 gm
Late latent syphilis	As above		2 gm erythromycin or tetracycline daily for 30 days Total: 60 gm
Late syphilis: Asymptomatic neurosyphilis Neurovascular Cardiovascular Osseous, visceral, or cutaneous	As above		As above Total: 60 gm
Late syphilis: Symptomatic neurosyphilis (paresis, tabes dorsalis, meningovascular neurosyphilis, primary optic atrophy, eighth nerve deafness)	As above	Alternative: 1,200,000 units APPG IM daily for 2 weeks. Total: 16.8 million units	As above Total: 60 gm
Pregnancy	According to stage of the disease		2 gm erythromycin daily. Total according to stage of the disease
Congenital syphilis: Birth to 4 kg weight	300,000 units IM once weekly for 4 weeks. Total: 1.2 million units	400,000 units/kg body weight divided into 12 injections daily.	
4 to 10 kg weight	600,000 units once weekly for 4 weeks. Total: 2.4 million units		
10 to 30 kg weight	1.2 million units once weekly for 4 weeks. Total: 4.8 million units		
over 30 kg weight (more than 70 lbs)	2.4 million units IM once weekly for 4 weeks. Total: 9.6 million units		

Because the richest blood supply is at the base of the brain, some degree of basilar meningitis (localized or diffuse) is most common. Meningitis is believed to occur in 30 to 50 per cent of infants with prenatal syphilis, an involvement that may be asymptomatic.[94, 95] Cerebrospinal fluid accumulates at the base of the brain in the chiasmatic and pontine cisterna and bathes the emerging cranial nerves. Some of the cerebrospinal fluid escapes from the skull along the first, second, and eighth nerves where the arachnoid membrane blends peripherally with the perineural connective tissue sheaths.

The eighth cranial nerve is particularly vulnerable because the arachnoid space continues for a distance into the bony canal of the acoustic pore before the membrane merges with the perineurium. If treponemes are present in the cerebrospinal fluid of the adjacent cisterna, or if a leptomeningitis becomes more extensive, inflammation of the meningeal sheaths with a syphilitic meningoperineuritis of the eighth cranial nerve may develop. The process may extend concentrically to the acoustic nerve fibers, resulting in a meningoneuritis of the eighth nerve or a meningo-neuro-labyrinthitis.[96, 97]

The predominant histopathological lesion indicates severe degeneration of the organ of Corti, spiral ganglion, and nerve fibers, with round cell infiltration, fibrinous deposit, and hemorrhage in the labyrinth. The resulting hearing loss is usually bilateral. If deafness occurs before speech has been acquired, the child is likely to be a deaf mute.[98] Meningo-neuro-labyrinthitis also may occur as a manifestation of acquired secondary syphilis or as a form of neurorelapse in acquired early syphilis.[31, 97] Since this type of syphilitic deafness is potentially reversible with prompt and adequate treatment, the diagnosis of congenital syphilis in the neonate is of paramount importance.

Sensorineural Hearing Loss of Juvenile Tabes Dorsalis and Juvenile Paresis. In the juvenile form of tabes dorsalis and paresis, a chronic leptomeningitis may extend progressively to the marginal portions of the acoustic nerve and then to the more centrally placed nerve fibers. It causes thinning and degeneration of the nerve fibers, disappearance of axones, breaking up of myelin sheaths, and accumulation of myelin droplets. The cochlear branch of the eighth cranial nerve is particularly vulnerable and the vestibular branch may also be affected.

Deafness almost always occurs before the age of 25, appearing rather suddenly and progressing rapidly over weeks or months. Vestibular symptoms and tinnitus diminish as labyrinthine destruction increases. In our experience, treatment has little effect on this type of hearing loss.

Syphilitic Gummatous Osteomyelitis and Periostitis of the Temporal Bone (Fig. 11–30). In 3[71] to 10 per cent[17, 87] of patients with late congenital syphilis, there is a chronic, low-grade gummatous osteomyelitis and periostitis of the temporal bone. Despite intensive early treatment and healing of early sites of infection, the temporal bone may suddenly become involved in a rapidly progressive disease. Isolation of treponemes that have persisted in the perilymph despite prior antisyphilitic therapy has been reported.[99] Treponemes have also been demonstrated in the endochondral bone of the labyrinthine capsule.[100] Endochondral bone is dense and almost avascular, so that penetration of the tissue by antibiotics is difficult.

Treponema pallidum organisms apparently lie dormant or relatively inactive in the host for many years and then abruptly become reactivated. The process may be asymptomatic until it erodes the labyrinthine capsule with multiple

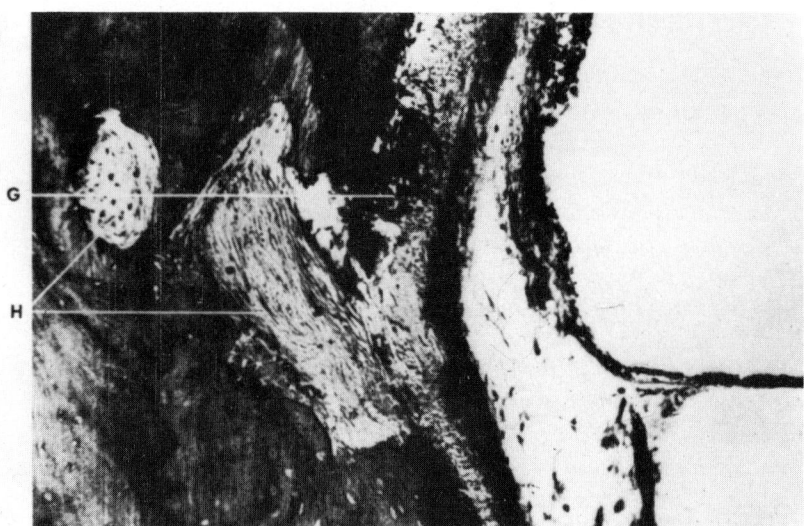

FIGURE 11–30 Osteomyelitis in the basal turn of the cochlear capsule, including an active syphilitic gumma (G) displacing the endosteum and healed, inactive osteolytic areas filled with connective tissue (H). (*From* Nager, F.: Pract. Otolaryngol., *17*:1, 1955.)

miliary gummata associated with arteritis. The spirochetes then invade the inner ear and slowly produce bouts of labyrinthitis, leading to the degeneration of cochlear and vestibular receptors. Different stages of activity in the gummatous lesions adjacent to the inner ear account for periods of quiescence and exacerbation of symptoms.

The labyrinthine capsule bone may be riddled with miliary gummata even in the region of the annular ligament. Invasion of the ossicles with secondary ankylosis of the incudomalleal joint may add an element of conduction to the deafness, but bony ankylosis of the stapes footplate apparently is not seen.

The inflammatory changes extend to the labyrinth to produce varying degrees of chronic labyrinthitis which account for the severe auditory and vestibular symptoms. When the gummatous process reaches the labyrinthine spaces, a rapid progression of symptoms may ensue, with profound loss of vestibular function together with total hearing loss in some cases, indicating an extensive, irreversible labyrinthine infection.[101, 102]

MANIFESTATIONS. There may be a rather abrupt onset of hearing loss in apparently healthy individuals between the ages of 8 and 20, with a predominance in females. However, onset may be delayed until the patient is 40 or even 50 years old. The involvement is bilateral, although initially it may be asymmetrical, producing confusion with Ménière's disease. Periods of exacerbation associated with pregnancy or intercurrent infection are frequently noted. Tinnitus may persist even after hearing is completely lost.[71, 103]

Rapid progression to complete bilateral cochlear and vestibular loss may occur despite antisyphilitic therapy. In many instances there is an association with a preceding interstitial keratitis, which had developed many years before. Various stages of activity in the gummatous lesions adjacent to the inner ear, with concurrent healing and growth of new active lesions, account for periods of quiescence and exacerbation of symptoms.[104-106]

A diagnostic test often considered pathognomonic of sensorineural hearing loss due to late congenital syphilis is the presence of Hennebert's sign. This is a positive fistula sign in the absence of a fistula, the tympanic membrane being intact. It indicates an erosion of the bony labyrinth with consequent transmission to the inner ear of middle ear pressure changes. In this test, the nystagmic response becomes more marked when negative pressure is applied.[107, 108]

Non-treponemal antigen blood serological tests for syphilis (i.e., VDRL, RPR, Kolmer-Wassermann) are frequently non-reactive in these cases, whereas the FTA–ABS test is positive. Spinal fluid serological findings are consistently negative.

TREATMENT. Assay of ampicillin concentration in perilymph has been carried out in both cats and humans. Concentrations of 0.032 mcg (or more) per ml,[91] believed to be required for immobilization of *Treponema pallidum*, have been found.[109] After treatment of late congenital syphilis with penicillin G is concluded, a four-week trial administration of 2 to 4 gm oral ampicillin daily in combination with prednisone has proved to be of benefit in some cases.[109] While the optimum dosage of steroid has not been determined, treatment commencing with 30 mg of prednisone daily for one week and continued at 25 mg daily for three more weeks is being used at present.[110-112] Morrison states that hearing improvement should occur within four weeks if it occurs at all.[112] In the absence of response, prednisone should be withdrawn as rapidly as possible. However, if the treatment brings improvement, it should be continued over the next five months, with prednisone prescribed in gradually diminishing doses and ampicillin maintained at its original dosage.

The pure tone audiogram is of little value in measuring response to therapy. In these cases, improvement in speech discrimination tends to accord with the patient's subjective sense of improvement in hearing and is associated with decreased tinnitus and vertigo.

REFERENCES

1. Blount, J. H., Darrow, W. W., and Johnson, R. E.: Venereal disease in adolescents. Pediatr. Clin. North Am., 20(4):1021, 1973.
2. V.D. Statistical Letter. Issue 125. Washington, D.C., U.S. Dept. of Health, Education and Welfare, 1976.
3. Schaudinn, F. R., and Hoffmann, E.: Preliminary report on the presence of spirochetes in syphilitic lesions and in papillomas. Arb. K. Gesundheitsamtes, 22:527, 1905.
4. Schaudinn, F. R., and Hoffmann, E.: Finding of spirochetes in the lymph node juice of persons with syphilis. Dtsch. Med. Wochenschr., 31:711, 1905.
5. Cumberland, M. C., and Turner, T. B.: The rate of multiplication of *Treponema pallidum* in normal and immune rabbits. Am. J. Syph., 33:201, 1949.
6. Ovcinnikov, N. M., and Delektorskij, V. V.: Morphology of *Treponema pallidum*. Bull. WHO, 35:223, 1966.
7. Davies, T. A.: Primary Syphilis in the Female. Oxford, Oxford University Press, 1931.
8. Wilkinson, A. E., and Cowell, L. P.: Immunofluorescent staining for the detection of *Treponema pallidum* in early syphilitic lesions. Br. J. Vener. Dis., 47:252, 1971.
9. Chandler, F. W., and Cannefax, G. R.: Evaluation of darkfield and immunofluorescent techniques for demonstrating *Treponema pallidum* in fluids with small numbers of organisms. Br. J. Vener. Dis., 45:1, 1969.
10. Edwards, E. A.: Detecting *Treponema pallidum* in primary lesions by the fluorescent antibody technique. Public Health Rep., 77:427, 1962.
11. Elsas, F. J.: Comparison of direct and indirect fluorescent antibody methods for staining *Treponema pallidum*. Br. J. Vener. Dis., 47:255, 1971.

12. Sachar, D. B., Klein, R. S., Swerdlow, F., et al.: Erosive syphilitic gastritis: Darkfield and immunofluorescent diagnosis from biopsy specimen. Ann. Intern. Med., 80:512, 1974.
13. Schwartz, I. R.: Gastroscopic observations in secondary syphilis. Gastroenterology, 10:227, 1948.
14. Calkins, E., Loudon, F., Mellinkoff, S. M., et al.: Isolation of *Treponema pallidum* from three patients with visceral syphilis by means of animal inoculation. Johns Hopkins Med. J., 87:61, 1950.
15. Vryonis, G., and Morgan, H.: Spirochete counts on fluid from the surface lesions in early human syphilis. Ven. Dis. Inform., 20:343, 1939.
16. Magnuson, H. J., Thomas, E. W., Olansky, S., et al.: Inoculation syphilis in human volunteers. Medicine, 35:133, 1956.
17. Stokes, J. H., Beerman, H., and Ingraham, N. R.: Modern Clinical Syphilology. 3rd ed. Philadelphia, W. B. Saunders, 1944.
18. Dismukes, W. E., Dalgado, D. G., Mallernee, S. V., and Myers, T. C.: Destructive bone disease in early syphilis. JAMA, 236:2646, 1976.
19. Bauer, M.F., and Caravati, C. M.: Osteolytic lesions in early syphilis. Br. J. Vener. Dis., 43:175, 1967.
20. Wile, U. J., and Senear, F. E.: A study of the involvement of the bones and joints in early syphilis. Am. J. Med. Sci., 152:689, 1916.
21. Reynolds, F., and Wassermann, H.: Destructive osseous lesions in early syphilis. Arch. Intern. Med., 69:263, 1942.
22. Baker, A. L., Kaplan, M. M., Wolfe, H. J., and McGowan, J. A.: Liver disease associated with early syphilis. N. Engl. J. Med., 284:1422, 1971.
23. Lee, R. V., Thornton, G. F., and Conn, H. O.: Liver disease associated with secondary syphilis. N. Engl. J. Med., 284:1423, 1971.
24. Turner, T. B., Hardy, P. H., and Newman, B.: Infectivity tests in syphilis. Br. J. Vener. Dis., 45:183, 1969.
25. Falls, W. F., Ford, K. L., Ashworth, C. T., and Carter, N. W.: The nephrotic syndrome in secondary syphilis. Ann. Intern. Med., 63:1047, 1965.
26. Bhorade, M. S., Carag, H. B., Lee, H. J., et al.: Nephropathy of secondary syphilis. JAMA, 216:1159, 1971.
27. Braunstein, G. D., Lewis, E. J., Galvanek, E. G., et al.: The nephrotic syndrome associated with secondary syphilis, an immune deposit disease. Am. J. Med., 48:643, 1970.
28. Frazier, C. N., and Pian, H. C.: Relative infectivity of blood and cerebrospinal fluid in secondary syphilis. Am. J. Med., 6:443, 1949.
29. Chesney, A. M., and Kemp, J. E.: Incidence of *Spirochaeta pallida* in cerebrospinal fluid during early stage of syphilis. JAMA, 83:1725, 1924.
30. Nadol, J. B.: Hearing loss of acquired syphilis: Diagnosis confirmed by incudectomy. Laryngoscope, 85:1888, 1975.
31. Willcox, R. R., and Goodwin, P. G.: Nerve deafness in early syphilis. Br. J. Vener. Dis., 47:401, 1971.
32. Feng, Y.: Acute syphilitic meningitis with multiple and unilateral involvement of cranial nerves. Chin. Med. J., 59:101, 1941.
33. Gamble, C. N., and Reardan, J. B.: Immunopathogenesis of syphilitic glomerulonephritis. N. Engl. J. Med., 292:449, 1975.
34. Bruetsch, W. L.: Neurosyphilis. *In*: Baker, A. B. (ed.): Clinical Neurology. New York, Harper & Row, 1955, pp. 799–845.
35. Duncan, W. P., Jenkins, T. W., and Parham, C. E.: Fluorescent treponemal antibody cerebrospinal fluid (FTA–CSF) test. Br. J. Vener. Dis., 48:97, 1972.
36. Garner, M. F., and Backhouse, J. L.: Fluorescent treponemal antibody tests on cerebrospinal fluid. Br. J. Vener. Dis., 47:356, 1971.
37. Duncan, W. P., and Kuhn, U. S.: Further studies of the FTA–CSF test with a monospecific anti-IgM conjugate. Br. J. Vener. Dis., 49:487, 1973.
38. Pangborn, M. C.: A new serologically active phospholipid from beef heart. Proc. Soc. Exp. Biol. Med., 48:484, 1941.
39. Wassermann, A.: Uber die Entwicklung und den gegenwartigen Stand der Serodiagnostik gegenuber Syphilis. Berl. klin. Wochenschr., 44:1599, 1634, 1907.
40. Kahn, R. L.: Micro-Kahn reactions. JAMA, 87:2092, 1926.
41. Harris, A., Rosenberg, A. A., and Riedel, L. M.: A microflocculation test for syphilis using cardiolipin antigen. J. Ven. Dis. Inform., 27:169, 1946.
42. Kolmer, J. A., and Lynch, E. R.: Cardiolipin antigens in the Kolmer complement fixation test for syphilis. Am. J. Clin. Pathol., 18:731, 1948.
43. Portnoy, J., Garson, W., and Smith, C. A.: A rapid plasma reagin test for syphilis. Public Health Rep., 72:761, 1957.
44. Portnoy, J., Brewer, J. H., and Harris, A.: Rapid plasma reagin card test for syphilis and other treponematoses. Public Health Rep., 77:645, 1962.

45. Cannefax, G. R., and Garson, W.: Reiter protein complement fixation test for syphilis. Public Health Rep., 72(14):335, 1957.
46. D'Alessandro, G., and Dardanoni, L.: Isolation and purification of the protein antigen of the Reiter treponeme. Am. J. Syph., 37:137, 1953.
47. Nelson, R. A., and Mayer, M. M.: Immobilization of *Treponema pallidum* in vitro by antibody produced in syphilitic infection. J. Exp. Med., 89:369, 1949.
48. Deacon, W. E., Falcone, V. H., and Harris, A.: A fluorescent test for treponemal antibodies. Proc. Soc. Exp. Biol. Med., 96:477, 1957.
49. Hunter, E. F., Deacon, W. E., and Meyer, P. E.: An improved FTA test for syphilis, the absorption procedure (FTA–ABS). Public Health Rep., 79:410, 1964.
50. Rathlev, T.: Haemagglutination test utilizing pathogenic *Treponema pallidum* for the serodiagnosis of syphilis: A preliminary report. Br. J. Vener. Dis., 43:181, 1967.
51. Tomizawa, T., and Kasamatsu, S.: Haemagglutination tests for the diagnosis of syphilis: A preliminary report. Jpn. J. Med. Sci. Biol., 19:305, 1966.
52. Scotti, A. T., and Logan, L. C.: A specific IgM antibody test in neonatal congenital syphilis. J. Pediatr., 73:242, 1968.
53. Logan, L. C., and Cox, P. M.: Evaluation of a quantitative automated micro-haemagglutination assay for antibodies to *Treponema pallidum*. Am. J. Clin. Pathol., 53:163, 1970.
54. Beelar, V. P., Zimmerman, H. J., and Manchester, B.: Prozone phenomenon in the serodiagnosis of syphilis. Am. J. Med. Sci., 217:658, 1949.
55. Nicholas, L., and Beerman, H.: Present day serodiagnosis of syphilis. Am. J. Med. Sci., 249:466, 1965.
56. Haserick, J. R., and Long, R.: Systemic lupus erythematosus preceded by false positive serologic tests for syphilis. Ann. Intern. Med., 37:559, 1952.
57. Catterall, R. D.: Systemic disease and the biological false positive reaction for syphilis. Br. J. Vener. Dis., 48:1, 1972.
58. Harvey, A. M., and Schulman, L. E.: Connective tissue disease and the chronic biologic false positive test for syphilis. Med. Clin. North Am., 50(5):1271, 1966.
59. Tuffanelli, D. L.: False positive reactions for syphilis. Arch. Dermatol., 98:606, 1968.
60. Doniach, D., and Walker, J. G.: A unified concept of autoimmune hepatitis. Lancet, 1:813, 1969.
61. Catterall, R. D.: The chronic biological false positive reaction. *In*: Morton, R. S., and Harris, J. R. (eds.): Recent Advances in Sexually Transmitted Diseases. New York, Longman, 1975.
62. Kraus, S. J.: Non-syphilitic FTA–ABS reactions in lupus erythematosus. *In*: Nicholas, L. (ed.): Sexually Transmitted Diseases. Springfield, Ill., Charles C Thomas, 1973.
63. Kraus, S. J., Haserick, J. R., and Logan, L. C.: Atypical fluorescence in the FTA–ABS test related to DNA antibodies. J. Immunol., 106:1665, 1971.
64. Garner, M. F., Backhouse, J. L., Daskalopoulos, G., and Walsh, J. L.: The *Treponema pallidum* haemagglutination test in biological false-positive and leprosy sera. J. Clin. Pathol., 26:258, 1973.
65. Johnston, N. A.: *Treponema pallidum* haemagglutination test for syphilis: Evaluation of a modified micro-method. Br. J. Vener. Dis., 48:474, 1972.
66. Blum, G., Ellner, P. D., McCarthy, L. R., and Papachristos, T.: Reliability of the treponemal haemagglutination test for the serodiagnosis of syphilis. J. Infect. Dis., 127:321, 1973.
67. Dorne, M., and Zakon, S.: Enlargement of one sternoclavicular articulation as a valuable clinical sign of late congenital syphilis. Arch. Dermatol., 32:602, 1935.
68. Higoumenakis, G. C.: Le signe de la clavicule et sa valeur diagnostique dans la syphilis hereditaire. Ann. Dermatol. Syphiligr., 8:939, 1937.
69. Dax, E. C., and Stewart, R. M.: The sign of the clavicle. Br. Med. J., 1:771, 1939.
70. Clutton, H. H.: Symmetrical synovitis of knee in hereditary syphilis. Lancet, 1:391, 1886.
71. Fiumara, N. J., and Lessell, S.: Manifestations of late congenital syphilis. Arch. Dermatol., 102:78, 1970.
72. Borella, L., Goobar, J., and Clark, G.: Synovitis of the knee joints in late congenital syphilis. JAMA, 180:190, 1962.
73. Karnosh, L. J.: Histopathology of syphilitic hypoplasia of teeth. Arch. Dermatol., 13:25, 1926.
74. Sarnat, B. J., and Shaw, N. G.: Dental development in congenital syphilis. Am. J. Dis. Child., 64:771, 1942.
75. Bernfield, W. K.: Hutchinson's teeth and early treatment of congenital syphilis. Br. J. Vener. Dis., 47:54, 1971.
76. Sicher, H., and Bhaskar, S. N. (eds.): OrBan's Oral Histology and Embryology. St. Louis, C. V. Mosby, 1972.
77. Bauer, W. H.: Tooth buds and jaws in patients with congenital syphilis: Correlation between distribution of *Treponema pallidum* and tissue reaction. Am. J. Pathol., 20:297, 1944.
78. Putkonen, T.: Does early treatment prevent dental changes in congenital syphilis? Acta Derm. Venereol., 43:240, 1963.

79. Hutchinson, J.: On the influence of hereditary syphilis on the teeth. Trans. Pathol. Soc., 10:287, 1858.
80. Friedenwald, J. S.: Ocular lesions in fetal syphilis. Johns Hopkins Med. J., 46:185, 1930.
81. Lennarson, V. E., and Jeans, P. C.: Congenital syphilis of the eye. Am. J. Syph., 21:90, 1937.
82. Klauder, J. V., and Meyer, G. P.: Chorioretinitis in congenital syphilis. Arch. Ophthalmol., 49:139, 1953.
83. Duke-Elder, S. (ed.): System of Ophthalmology. Vol. 8. St. Louis, C. V. Mosby, 1965, pp. 815–830.
84. Montenegro, E., Israel, C. W., Nicol, W. G., and Smith, J. L.: Histopathologic demonstration of spirochetes in the human eye. Am. J. Ophthalmol., 67:335, 1969.
85. Goldman, J. N., and Girard, K. F.: Intraocular treponemes in treated congenital syphilis. Arch. Ophthalmol., 78:47, 1967.
86. Klauder, J. V., and Cowan, A.: Corneal examination and slit lamp microscopy in diagnosis of late congenital syphilis, especially in adults. JAMA, 113:1624, 1939.
87. Klauder, J. V., and Vandoren, E.: Analysis of 532 cases of interstitial keratitis. Arch. Ophthalmol., 26:408, 1941.
88. Willcox, R. R.: A survey of problems in the antibiotic treatment of gonorrhea. Br. J. Vener. Dis., 46:217, 1970.
89. Langham, M.: Factors affecting the penetration of antibiotics into the aqueous humor. Br. J. Ophthalmol., 35:614, 1951.
90. Goldman, J. N.: Clinical experience with ampicillin and probenecid in the management of treponeme-associated uveitis. Trans. Am. Acad. Ophthalmol. Otolaryngol., 74:509, 1970.
91. Cottini, G. B., and Lazzaro, C.: L'ampicillina in dermovenerologica. Minerva Derm., 39:196, 1964.
92. Woods, A. C.: Cortisone in interstitial keratitis. Am. J. Syph., 35:517, 1951.
93. Hardy, P. H., Perine, P. L., Marino, J. T., et al.: Inapparent central nervous system infection in early congenital syphilis. Proceedings of the First Symposium on the Biology of Spirochetes. Minneapolis, June 1975.
94. Curtis, A. C., and Philpott, O. S.: Prenatal syphilis. Med. Clin. North Am., 48(3):707, 1964.
95. Peterson, J. C.: Congenital syphilis: A review of its present status and significance in pediatrics. South. Med. J., 66:257, 1973.
96. Paparella, M. M., and Shumrick, D. A. (eds.): Otolaryngology. Vol. 2. Philadelphia, W. B. Saunders, 1973, pp. 318 and 349.
97. Kerr, A. G., Smyth, G. D., and Cinnamond, M.: Congenital syphilitic deafness. J. Laryngol. Otol., 87:1, 1973.
98. Ballantyne, J., and Groves, J. (eds.): Scott-Brown's Diseases of the Ear, Nose and Throat. 3rd ed. Philadelphia, J. B. Lippincott, 1971, p. 443.
99. Wiet, R. J., and Milko, D. A.: Isolation of spirochetes in the perilymph despite prior antisyphilitic therapy. Arch. Otolaryngol., 101:104, 1975.
100. Mack, L. W., Smith, J. L., Walter, E. K., et al.: Temporal bone treponemes. Arch. Otolaryngol., 90:37, 1969.
101. Mayer, O., and Fraser, J. S.: Pathological changes in the ear in late congenital syphilis. J. Laryngol. Otol., 51:683, 755, 1936.
102. Nager, F. R.: Die Lues Hereditaria tarda des Innerohres—eine Folge chronischer Osteomyelitis des Felsenbeins. Pract. oto-rhino-laryng., 17:1, 1955.
103. Rodger, T. R.: Syphilis as seen by the aural surgeon. J. Laryngol. Otol., 55:168, 1940.
104. Karmody, C., and Schuknecht, H.: Deafness in congenital syphilis. Arch. Otolaryngol., 83:44, 1966.
105. Perlman, H. B., and Leek, J.: Late congenital syphilis of ear. Laryngoscope, 62:1175, 1952.
106. Perlman, H. B.: Late congenital syphilis. Proceedings of the Symposium on Sensorineural Hearing Processes and Disorders. Detroit, Henry Ford Hospital, 1967.
107. Keidel, A., and Kemp, J.: Deafness in late congenital syphilis. South. Med. J., 16:647, 1923.
108. Kerr, A. G.: The pathology, the audiogram, and the prognosis in perceptive deafness. J. Laryngol. Otol., 83:435, 1969.
109. Kerr, A. G., Smyth, G., and Landau, H.: Congenital syphilitic labyrinthitis. Arch. Otolaryngol., 91:474, 1970.
110. Patterson, M. E.: Congenital luetic hearing impairment: Treatment with prednisone. Arch. Otolaryngol., 87:378, 1968.
111. Hahn, R. D., Rodin, P., and Haskins, H. L.: Treatment of neural deafness with prednisone. J. Chronic Dis., 15:395, 1962.
112. Morrison, A. W.: Management of severe deafness in adults. Proc. R. Soc. Med., 62:959, 1969.

OTHER VENEREAL DISEASES

LOUISE E. TAVS, M.D.

CHANCROID

Chancroid is an autoinoculable disease, caused by *Hemophilus ducreyi* and characterized by one or more painful ulcerations of the genital region, with or without inguinal adenitis.

For more than 300 years there had been much confusion between syphilitic chancre and chancroid, until Bassereau delineated the two entities in 1852. Ducrey identified the bacterial agent of chancroid in 1889,[1] and Tomasczewski succeeded in reproducing chancroidal lesions in human subjects in 1903, using cultures of *H. ducreyi*.[2]

Chancroid is encountered worldwide, flourishing in the presence of sexual promiscuity and poor hygiene and occurring most commonly in uncircumcised males.[3] The disease is transmitted almost invariably by sexual contact, with the female often being an asymptomatic carrier.

ETIOLOGY

Hemophilus ducreyi bacilli are gram-negative, non-motile, plump, short rods (1 to 1.5 μ long and 0.6 μ wide), with rounded ends. They are usually arranged in couplets end to end and are often classified as streptobacilli because they tend to form chains. Their growth requirements in culture have been studied[4] and include preformed iron protoporphyrin (X factor) which is supplied by adding substantial amounts of freshly clotted blood to the usual laboratory media.

MANIFESTATIONS (Figs. 12–1 to 12–7)

The incubation period for chancroid is usually two to seven days but may be as long as two weeks. A minute abrasion appears to be necessary for *H.*

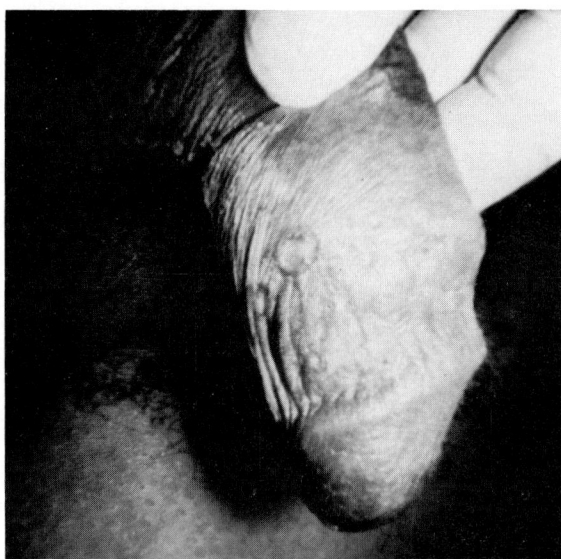

FIGURE 12-1 Early chancroid lesions. Note the scalloped edges, necrotic base, and narrow erythematous halo.

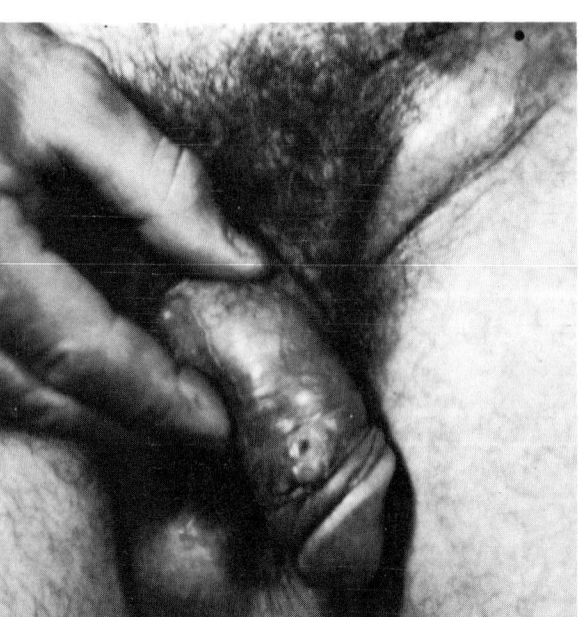

FIGURE 12-2 Chancroid ulceration and inflammatory regional bubo, producing a unilocular abscess.

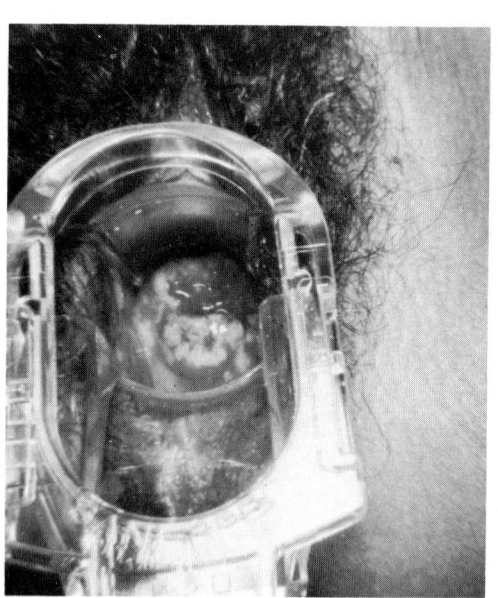

FIGURE 12-3 Chancroid ulcerations of cervix.

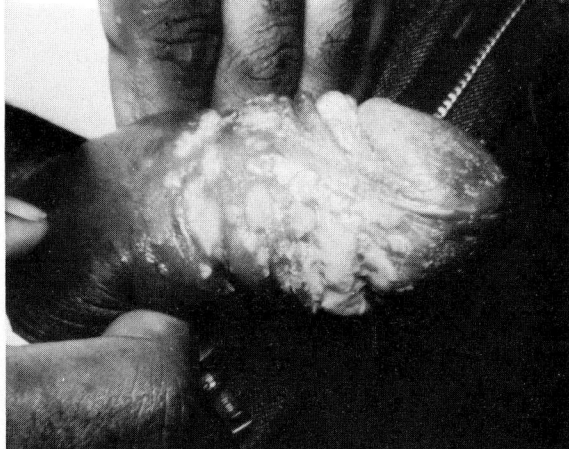

FIGURE 12-4 Multiple chancroid ulcers with secondary infection caused by fusospirochetosis.

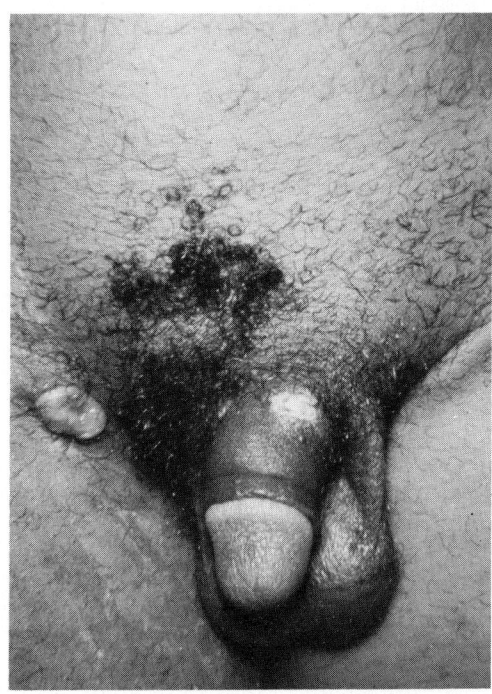

FIGURE 12-5 Penile chancroid ulcer with secondary ulceration at the site of spontaneous rupture of a unilateral bubo.

FIGURE 12-6 Syphilitic chancre that developed at the site of an untreated chancroid.

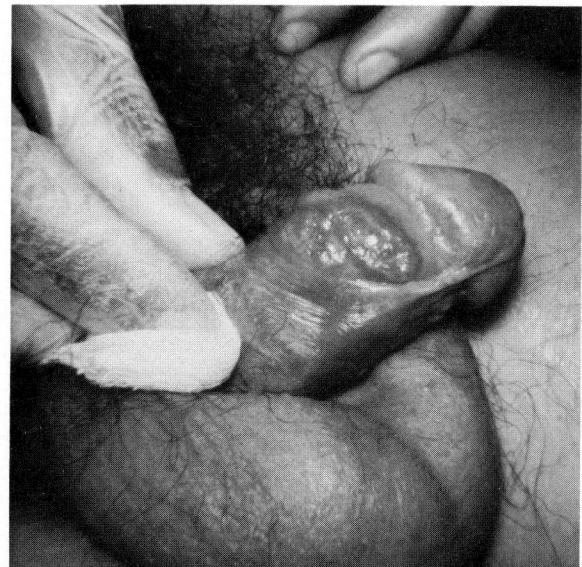

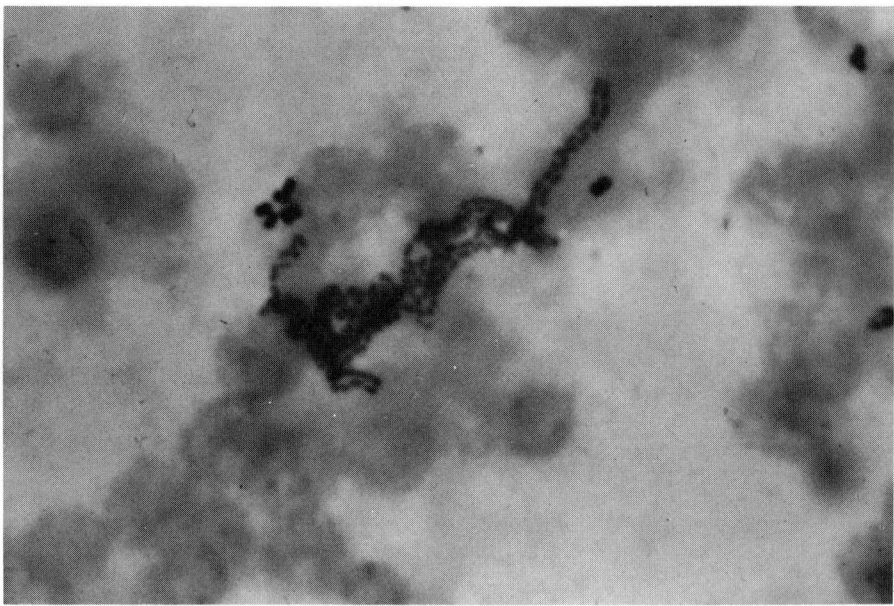

FIGURE 12–7 Gram-stained preparation of *Hemophilus ducreyi,* cultured on freshly clotted human blood. Two characteristics are shown: (a) long, tangled chain formation with the gram-negative rods end-to-end, and (b) tendency to parallelism.

ducreyi to enter the skin. The initial lesion is a vesicopustule, which ruptures to form a shallow ulcer. Unlike the chancre of syphilis, the chancroidal ulcer is painful, non-indurated, and bleeds easily on manipulation. The margins are scalloped, undermined, and outlined by a narrow erythematous halo.

When the small pustules are ruptured, the base becomes irregular, pebbled, and covered with a purulent, yellowish-gray exudate. Numerous hemorrhagic points in the base of the ulceration represent underlying dilated capillaries. The ulcer enlarges by contiguous spread, and additional multiple lesions may develop rapidly by autoinoculation.

H. ducreyi has a predilection for cutaneous surfaces; mucous membranes are seldom affected. Lesions in the male are frequently found on the prepuce, especially on the internal surface, coronal sulcus, frenulum, and shaft of the penis. The glans itself is rarely involved. Lesions in the balanopreputial groove usually occur on the cutaneous side, with no extension to the region covered by the mucous membrane.[5] The borders of the ulcerations tend to follow anatomical barriers, such as the frenulum.

In the female, the initial lesion of chancroid is most commonly seen at the fourchette.[6] Subsequent ulcers may be scattered over the labia majora, perineum, and perianal skin. Occasionally, lesions may develop on the labia minora or vestibule, but they rarely form on the introitus or cervix. The fact that the mucosa is less vulnerable to *H. ducreyi* infection than the skin may permit an asymptomatic carrier state to exist in the female.

Five to 14 days after the appearance of the lesion, an inguinal lymphadenitis is evident in approximately 50 per cent of male patients with chancroid, particularly if phimosis has occurred. The involvement of lymph nodes is unilateral in two thirds of these patients. Lymphadenitis is much less common in the female. The chancroidal bubo forms when one or two nodes enlarge, becoming fluctuant and markedly tender as an acute unilocular abscess develops. A periadenitis is also produced, with the overlying skin becoming red, thinned, and tender. The mass may rupture spontaneously through one ostium, with resulting inoculation of the skin around the drainage site. This may produce extensive and painful satellite chancroidal ulcerations, occasionally complicated by fusospirochetal infection. The ensuing constitutional manifestations are mild, except for occasional fever associated with the adenitis.

The adenitis may involute after two or three weeks, or the drainage may persist for months. In some cases, the lymphadenitis may subside spontaneously without external drainage. The ulcerations may last from a week to several months, depending on their size, location, and the treatment given. Phimosis, secondary infection with fusospirochetes, and coexistence with a syphilitic chancre prolong the duration.

Extragenital chancroidal lesions of the finger, tongue, lips, and breast have been reported but are rare.[7] The "mixed chancre," a chancroidal ulcer that evolves into a typical syphilitic chancre, was described by Rollet in 1859. Initially, this lesion has the clinical appearance of chancroid, and *H. ducreyi* can be recovered from it. However, as the syphilitic chancre develops, the characteristic induration, sharp margination, and clean base of the erosion become apparent. *Treponema pallidum* then can be identified in the ulcer, but usually *H. ducreyi* no longer can be found. Giant syphilitic chancres are often the result of "mixed chancres."

DIAGNOSIS

Smears for Hemophilus ducreyi. The chancroidal lesion should first be gently cleansed with saline-soaked gauze to reduce surface contaminants. After the edges of the ulcer have been compressed to release exudate from the undermined borders, the exudate is collected with a platinum loop or sterile cotton-tipped applicator. It is carefully transferred to a glass slide to preserve the morphological integrity of the chained organisms. After fixation with heat, the exudate is Gram-stained and examined for gram-negative rods. These are arranged in pairs end to end, in short chains, and frequently in a flotilla or "school of fish" formation. Smears can be made from pus aspirated from a bubo, but these are less likely to demonstrate the organism than the exudate from ulcerations.

Culture for Hemophilus ducreyi. Exudate from an ulcer is inoculated into 3 to 4 ml of freshly clotted human blood. (If the patient's own blood is used, it is advisable to inactivate the serum at 56° C for 30 minutes.) The sterile cotton-tipped applicator used to collect the exudate is left in the serum, which is promptly placed in an incubator at 37° C. Cultures must be examined after 24 hours and if negative should be reexamined 24 hours later. The colonies of *H. ducreyi*, viewed in oblique light, are barely perceptible as suspended, translucent, gray-white dots adhering to the sides of the tube. After the serum is gently stirred with a second sterile cotton-tipped applicator and the material obtained gently rolled on a slide, the specimen is air-dried, fixed with heat, and Gram-stained. This method of culture demonstrates two characteristics of *H. ducreyi*: (a) a tendency to form short or long, often tangled, chains, and (b) a marked propensity for parallelism. After 48 hours, however, contaminants in the culture proliferate to such an extent that *H. ducreyi* cannot compete.

Simple culture methods utilizing human or rabbit blood have proved to be valuable diagnostic tools.[8-10]

Autoinoculation. A small area of skin is scarified, and exudate from a chancroidal lesion rubbed into the abraded area. Tiny vesicopustules develop within 48 hours, in which *H. ducreyi* can be demonstrated more readily than by smear or culture methods. This procedure is rarely performed today.

Biopsy. Biopsy is indicated primarily in ulcers of long duration in order to rule out malignancy. Even if chancroid is diagnosed, it is essential to conduct darkfield examination and serological tests for syphilis. Other diseases, including lymphogranuloma venereum, granuloma inguinale, and fusospirochetosis, may also complicate chancroid. When superimposed on a chancroidal lesion, fusospirochetosis may produce a rapidly spreading, destructive, phagedenic ulceration that may cause mutilation.

THERAPY

The possibility of coexistent syphilis masked by chancroid must be of major concern in the treatment. In the presence of a chancroidal bubo for which tetracycline is particularly effective, the total dose administered should be sufficient to abort a possible incubating syphilitic infection.

Treatment Schedules

Sulfisoxazole: 4.0 gm daily for 12 to 15 days.
Tetracycline: 500 mg at 6-hour intervals (2 gm daily) for 15 to 20 days.
Streptomycin: 1 gm IM daily for 7 to 10 days.
Kanamycin: 500 mg IM twice daily for 7 to 10 days (if resistance to treatment is encountered).

Fluctuant buboes should be aspirated (not incised) with a large bore needle. If lesions are extensive or complicated by fusospirochetosis, a warm potassium permanganate compress (1:8000 dilution) may be helpful.

GRANULOMA INGUINALE

Granuloma inguinale is a chronic, mildly contagious, autoinoculable venereal disease that involves the genitalia and surrounding skin. It is characterized by red, velvety granulations and is caused by *Calymmatobacterium (Donovania) granulomatis*.

The disease was first described by McLeod in 1882,[11] and the etiological agent discovered by Donovan in 1905.[12] First identified in the United States by Grindon in 1913,[13] it was experimentally produced in humans by subcutaneous transplantation of infected tissue by McIntosh in 1926.[14] The organism was cultivated in the chick embryo yolk sac by Anderson in 1943.[15] Attempts to produce the disease in the usual laboratory animals have failed.

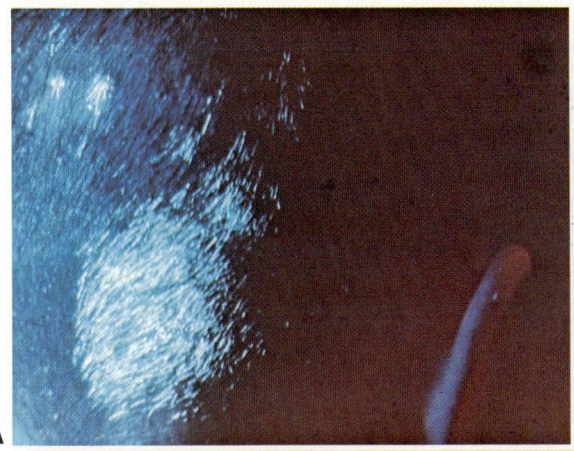
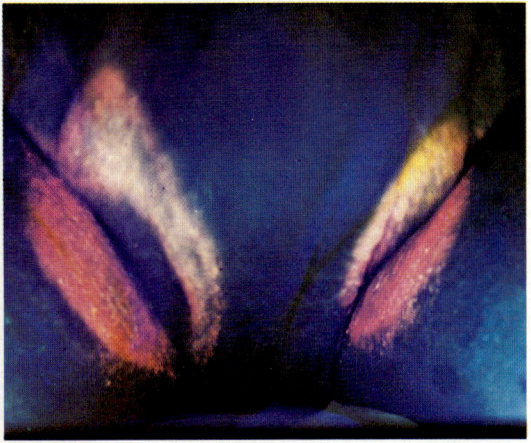
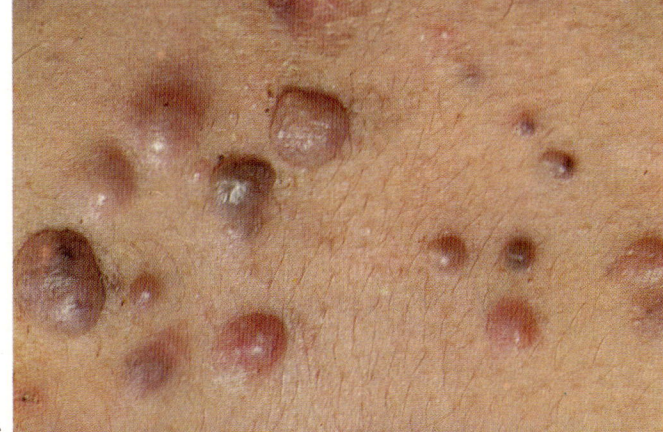
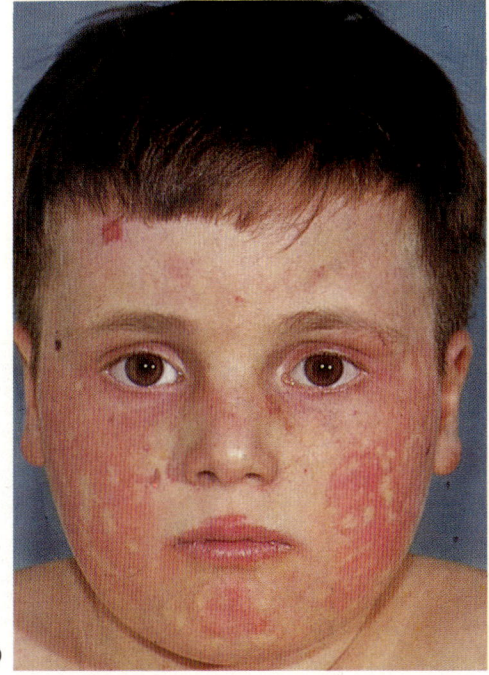
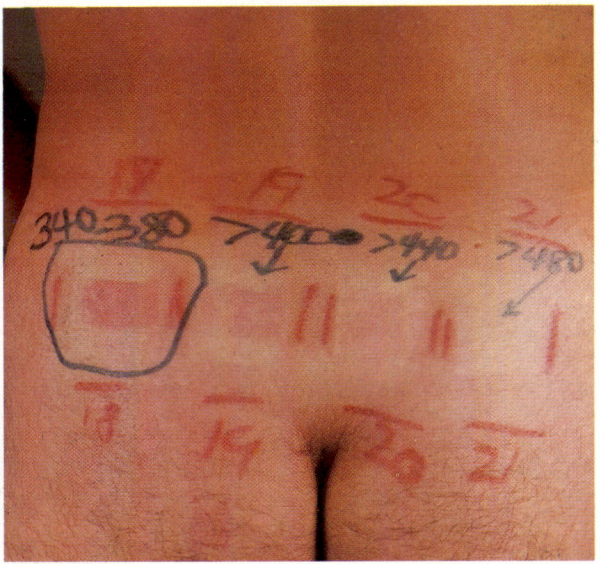

I–A Blue-green fluorescence of scalp tinea under the Wood's light.

I–B Coral-red fluorescence of erythrasma under Wood's light examination.

I–C Basal cell carcinomata manifest on the unexposed skin of a patient with basal cell nevus syndrome.

I–D Rothmund-Thomson syndrome.

I–E Demarcated redness and edema minutes after exposing low back of a patient with solar urticaria to indicated wavelengths of light.

PLATE I

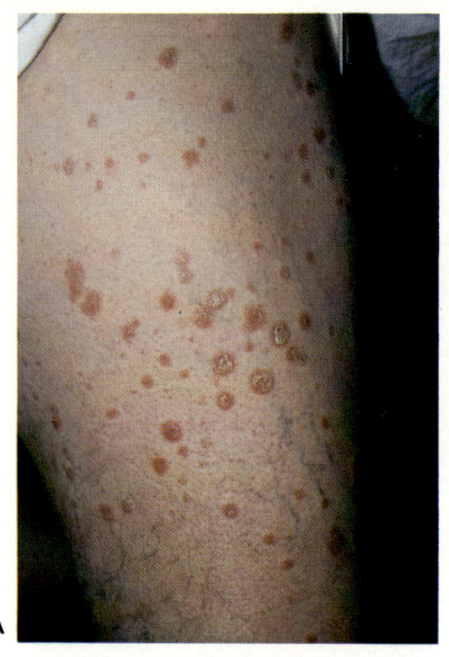
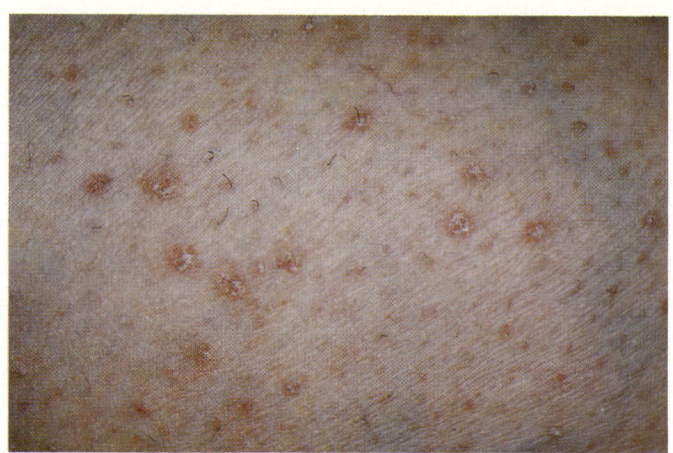
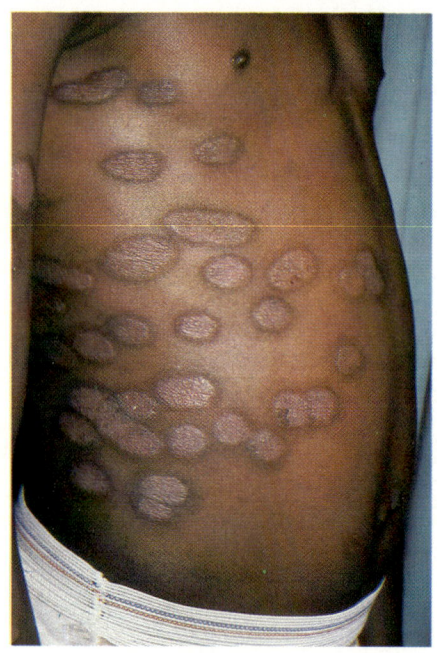
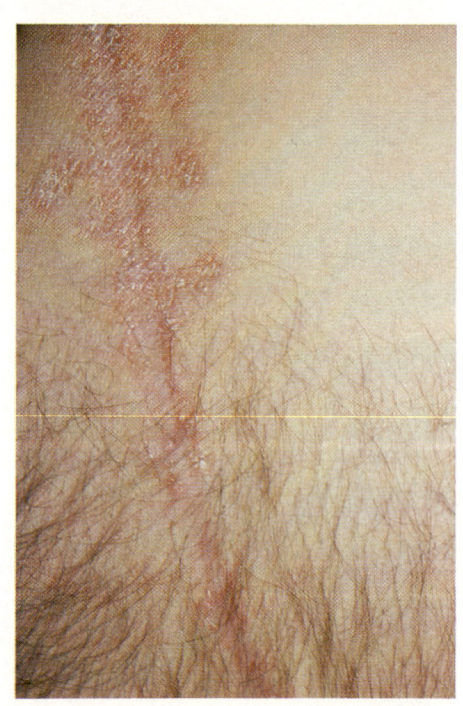
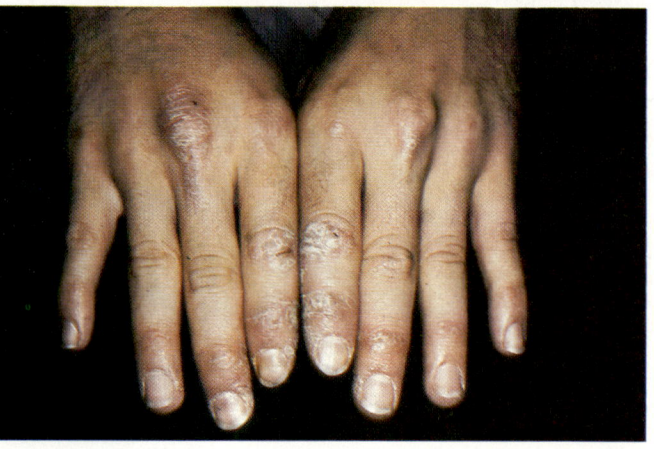

II–A Guttate psoriasis following streptococcal pharyngitis.

II–B Psoriasis occurring at site of injury caused by razor shaving (Koebner phenomenon).

II–C Psoriasis occurring in healing lesions of varicella (Koebner phenomenon).

II–D Psoriasis occurring in a scar (Koebner phenomenon).

II–E Psoriasis. Koebner phenomenon secondary to trauma caused by guitar strings and karate practice.

PLATE II

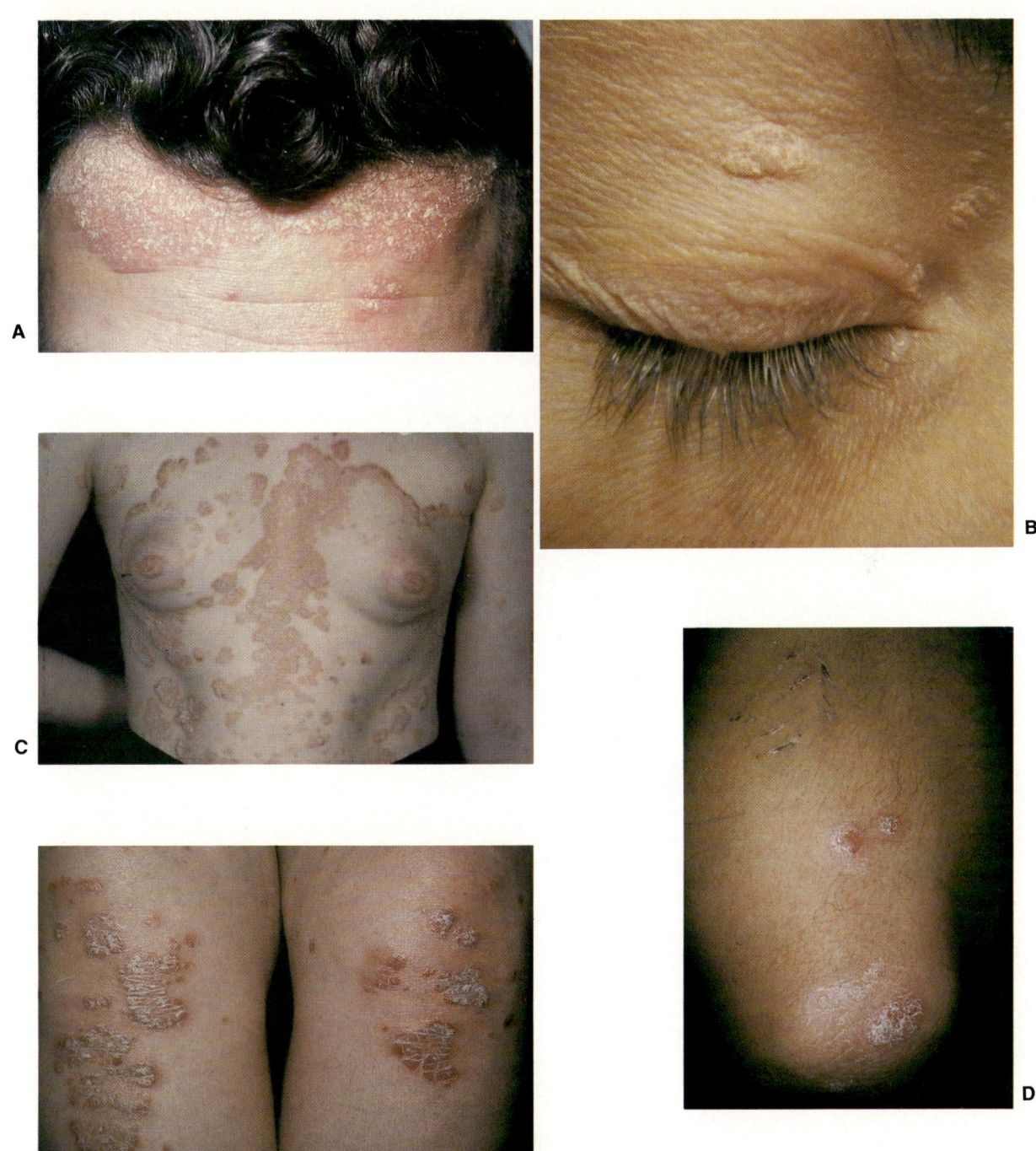

PLATE III

III–A Psoriasis of the scalp.

III–B Psoriasis of the eyelid and brow.

III–C Psoriasis may take many forms. Here it has a polycyclic form, which may resemble fungus infection of the skin.

III–D Psoriasis. Early lesion of the elbow.

III–E Psoriasis typically located on the knees.

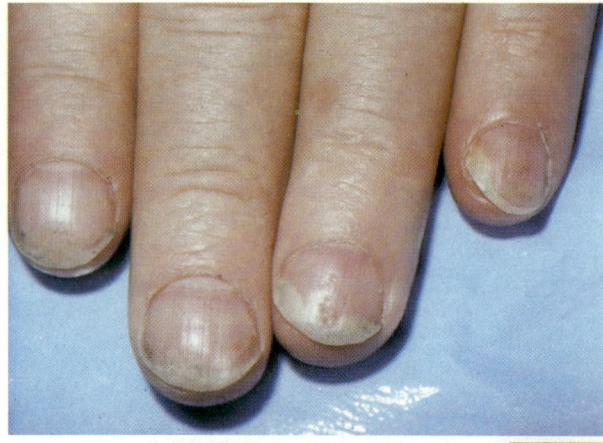

IV-A Psoriatic changes in the nails. There are little pits in the nail plate, which is detatching itself distally from an abnormal underlying bed.

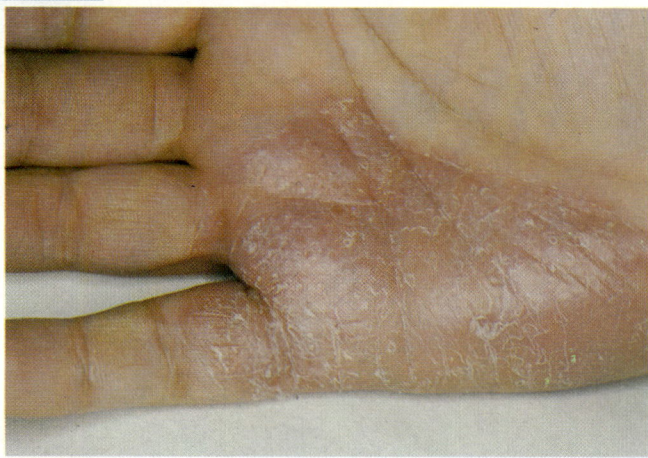

IV-B Psoriasis of the palm. Note the sharp margin.

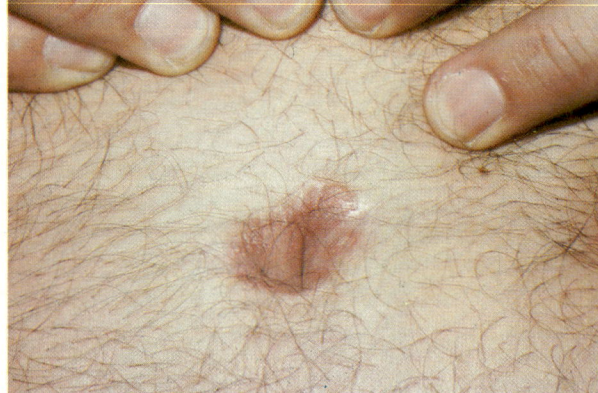

IV-C Psoriasis of the umbilicus—an example of "inverse" psoriasis.

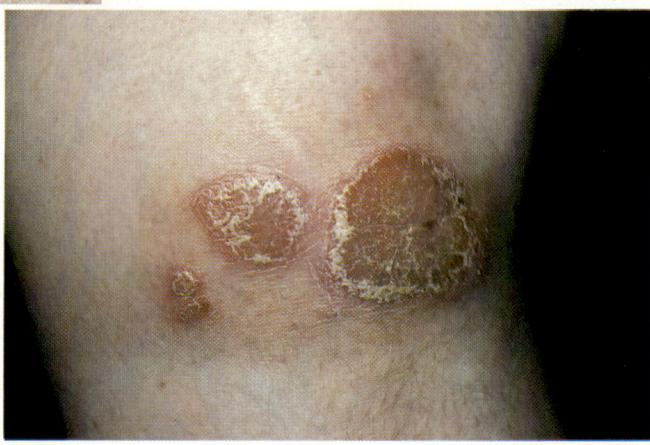

IV-D Secondarily infected (impetiginized) psoriasis.

PLATE IV

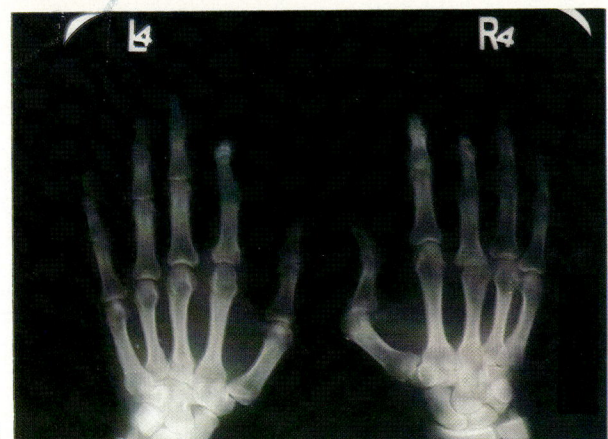

V–A Psoriatic arthropathy.

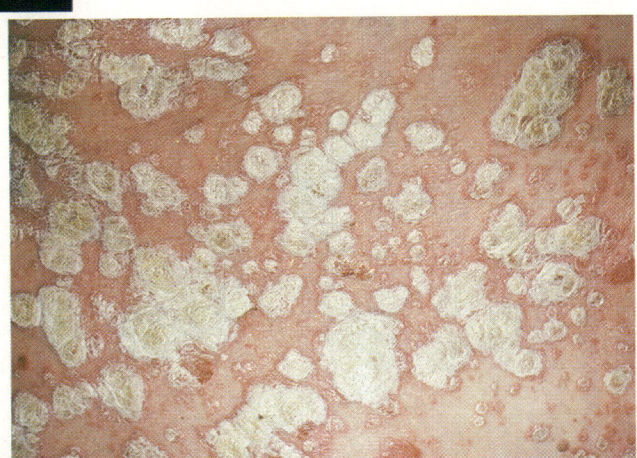

V–B-i and ii Psoriasis. Silvery plaques on an erythematous base.

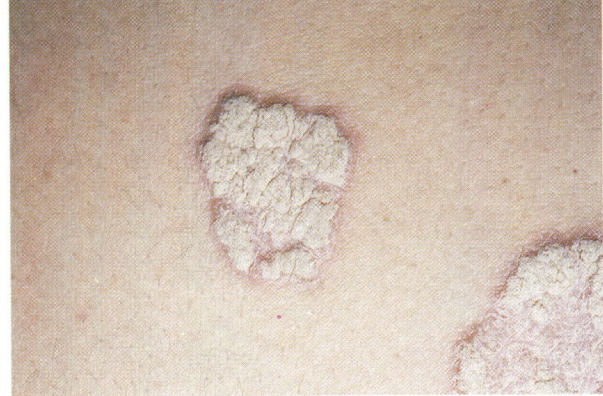

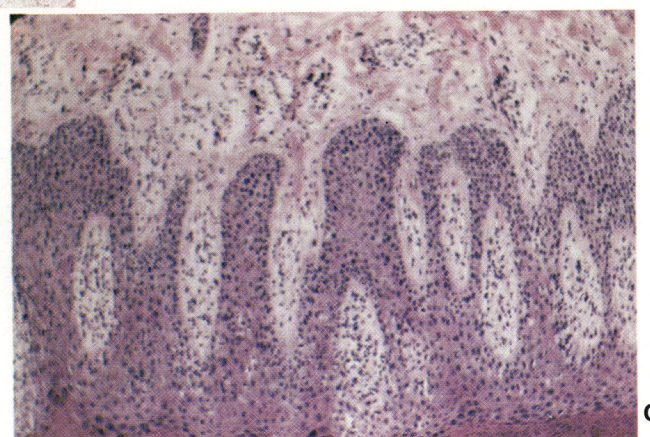

V–C Psoriasis. Histological section demonstrates elongation and clubbing of the rete pegs as well as inflammatory infiltrate.

PLATE V

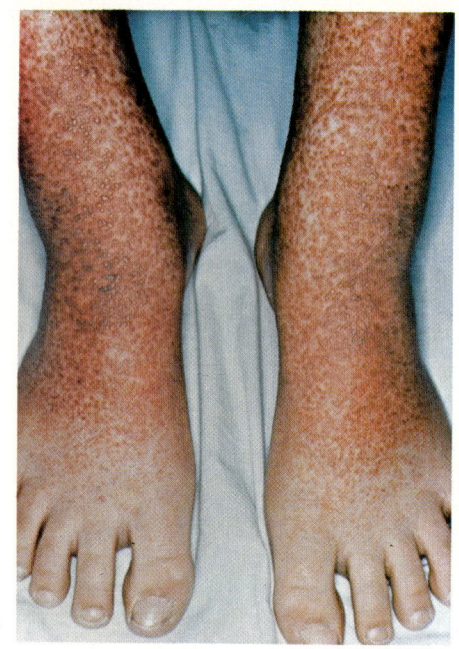

VI–A Atypical measles. (Courtesy of Dr. Adnan S. Dajani.)

VI–B Mucous patches of the tongue. The essential lesion is a flat papule whose surface has been eroded by moisture and friction, producing an erosion 5 to 10 mm in diameter, round or oval, painless, and slightly raised above the surrounding surfaces. On the dorsum of the tongue, the tough-surfaced structure permits no erosion, and the lesion remains a flat, smooth, reddish-pink papule denuded of lingual papillae.

VI–C Balanitis circinata of the Reiter syndrome. This geographical balanitis appears as scalloped, shallow, red erosions with slightly raised edges that assume an arciform outline by coalescence of adjacent superficial erosions within a circumscribed area of erythema. This 29-year-old male had a temperature of 101°F (38.64°C), weight loss of 15 pounds, and severe arthritic involvement of both knees and ankles, which were hot, tender, and swollen with effusion.

VI–D Benign juvenile melanoma.

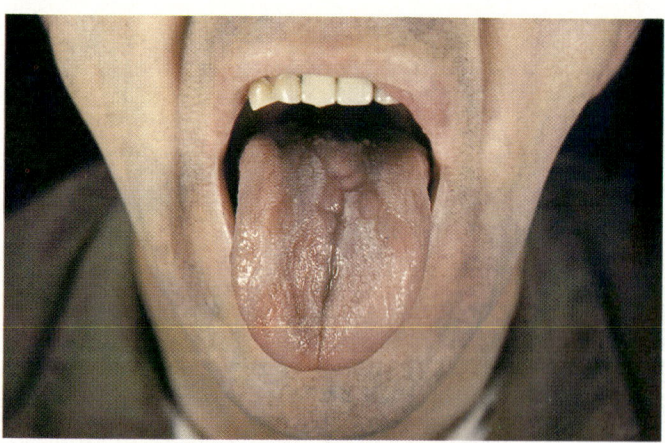

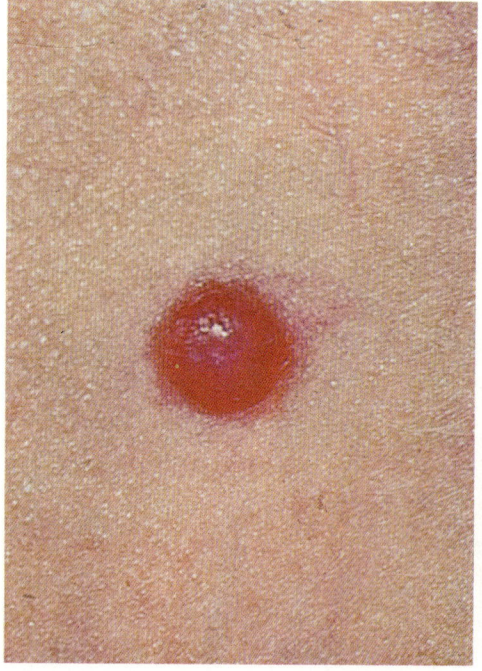

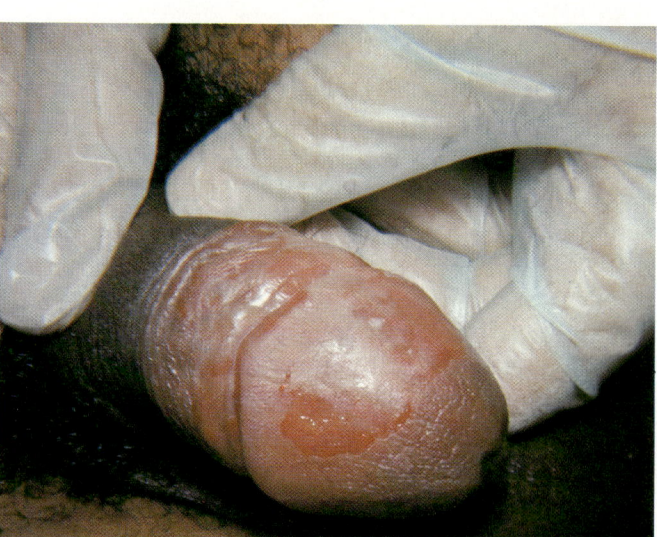

PLATE VI

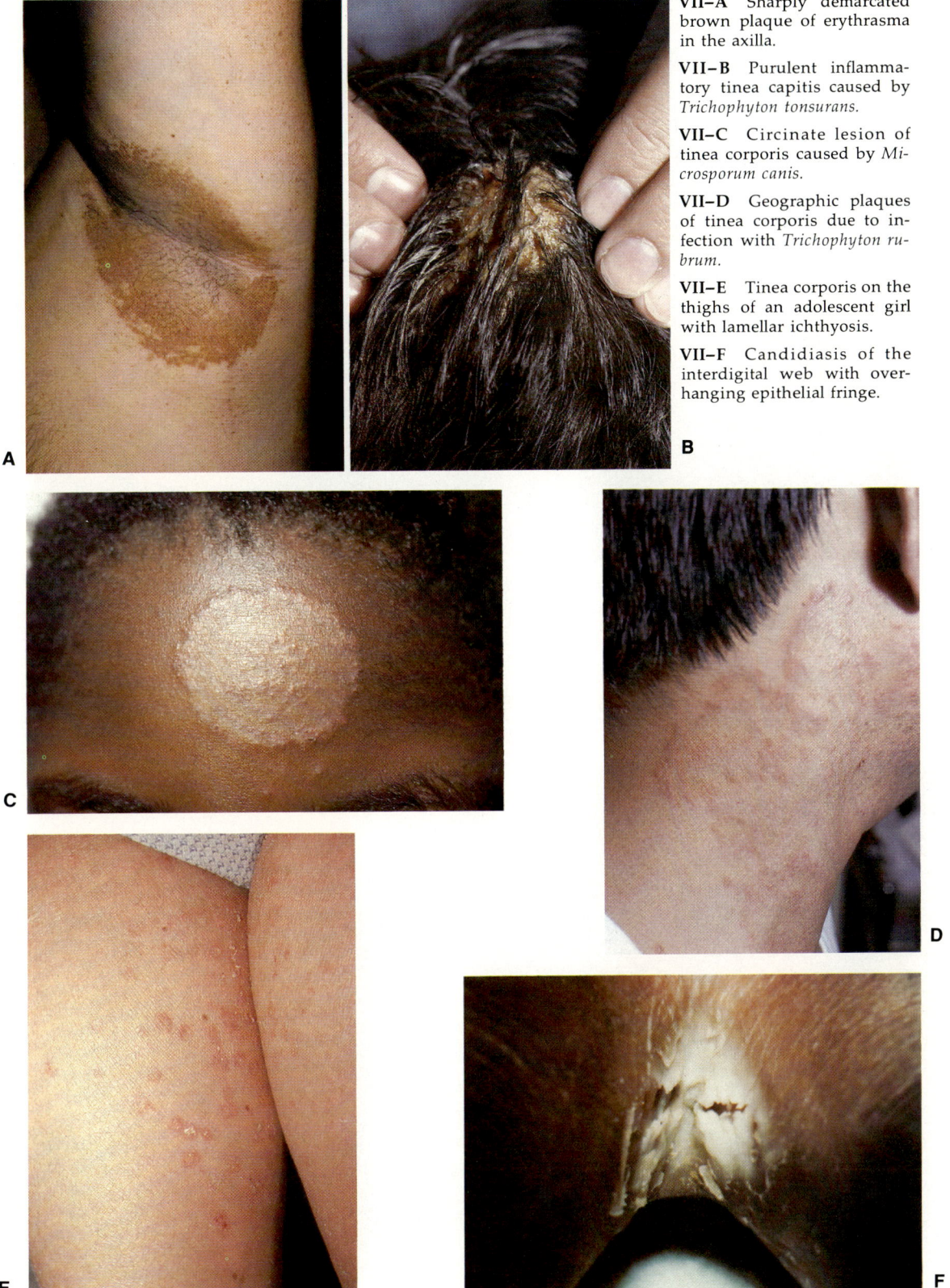

VII–A Sharply demarcated brown plaque of erythrasma in the axilla.

VII–B Purulent inflammatory tinea capitis caused by *Trichophyton tonsurans*.

VII–C Circinate lesion of tinea corporis caused by *Microsporum canis*.

VII–D Geographic plaques of tinea corporis due to infection with *Trichophyton rubrum*.

VII–E Tinea corporis on the thighs of an adolescent girl with lamellar ichthyosis.

VII–F Candidiasis of the interdigital web with overhanging epithelial fringe.

PLATE VII

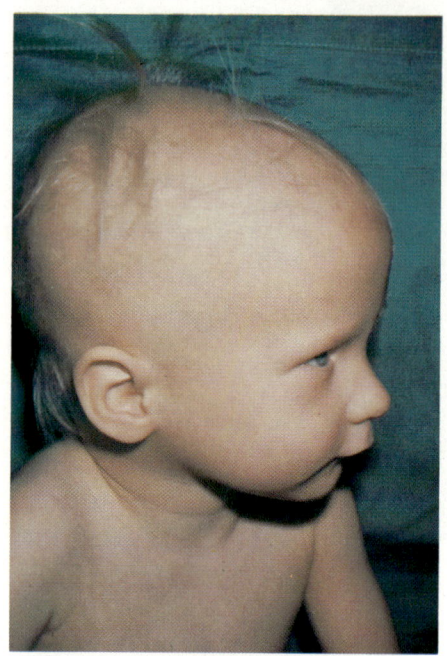

VIII–A Ectodermal defect. Scant, lusterless hair with lesions of trichorrhexis nodosa.

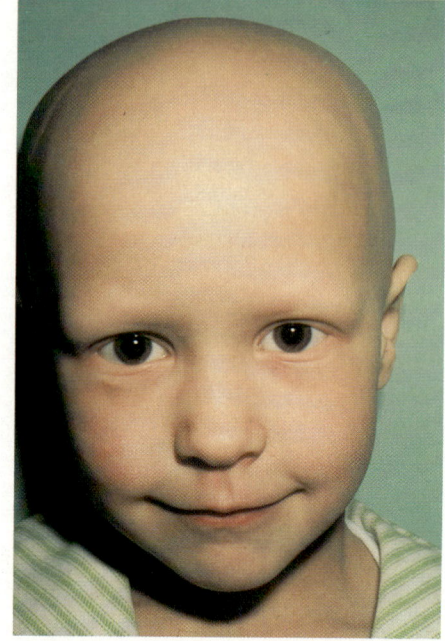

VIII–B Alopecia universalis. Anagen and telogen effluvium in a three-year-old child.

VIII–C Trichotillomania. Well-delineated patterned hair loss with fractured hair of normal density.

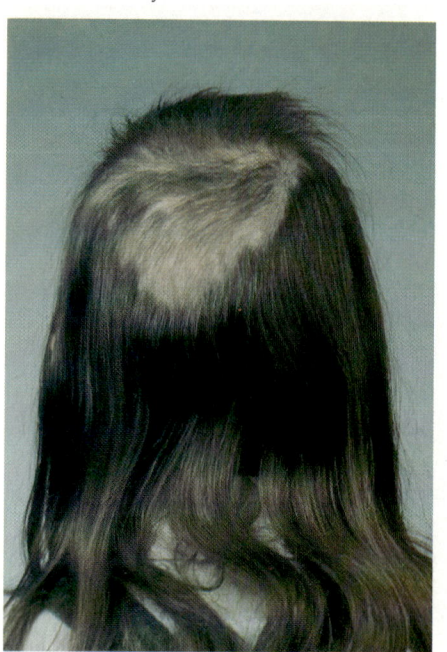

VIII–D Tinea capitis. Inflammatory kerion in a prepubertal male.

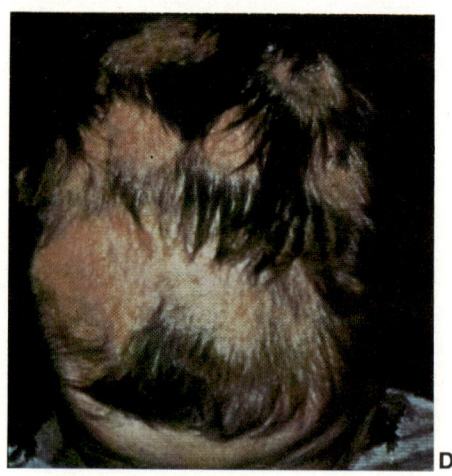

PLATE VIII

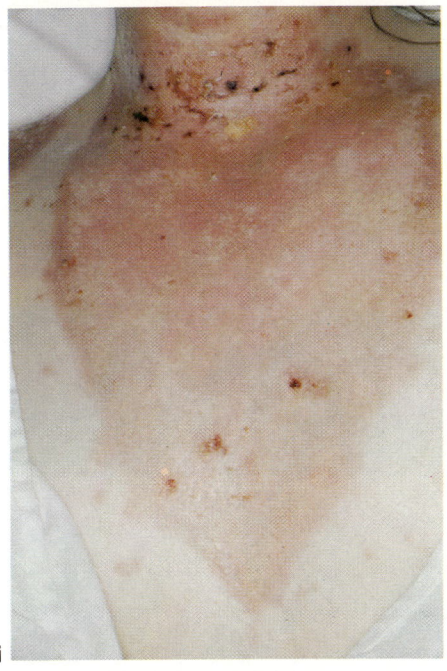
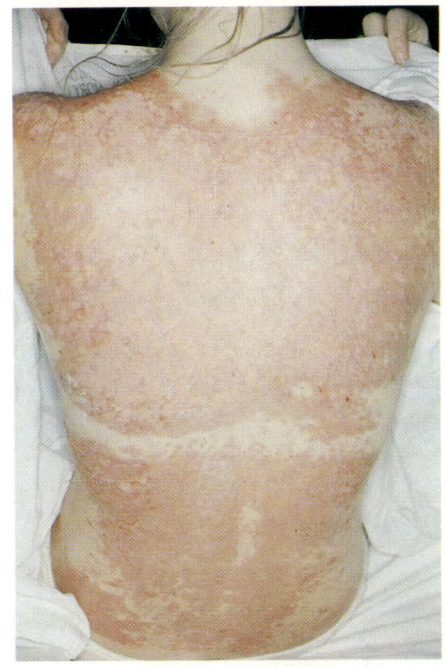

IX–A-i and ii Lupus erythematosus. Lesions limited to the light-exposed areas of the skin.

IX–B Systemic lupus erythematosus. Lesions on the dorsa of the hands and around the nails.

IX–C Photosensitive facial eruption in a patient with congenital absence of the second component of complement.

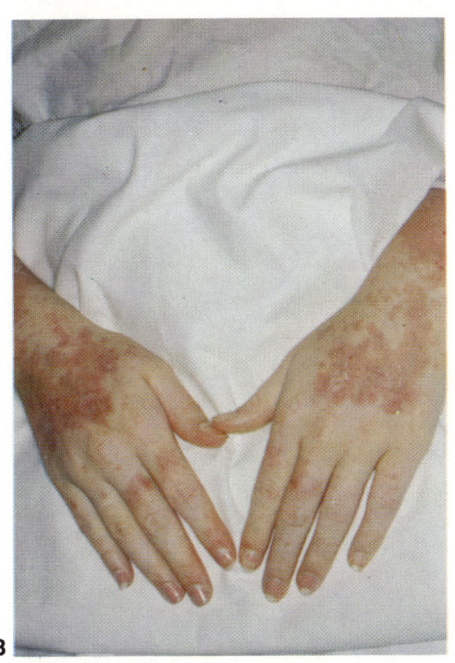
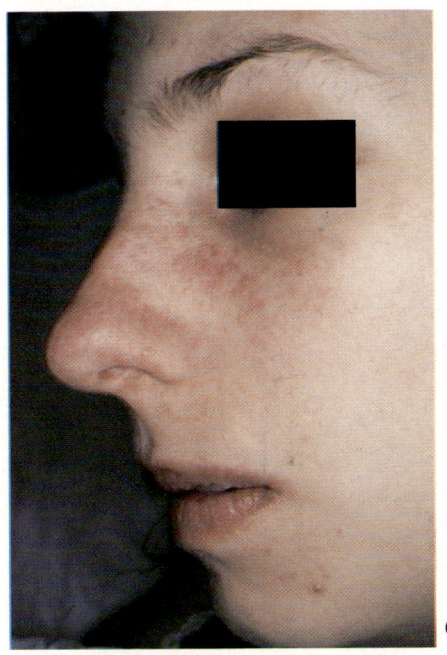

PLATE IX

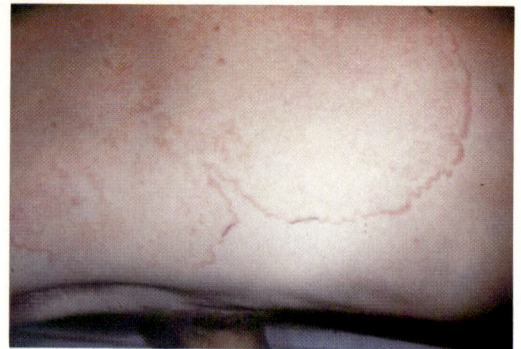

X–A Erythema marginatum.

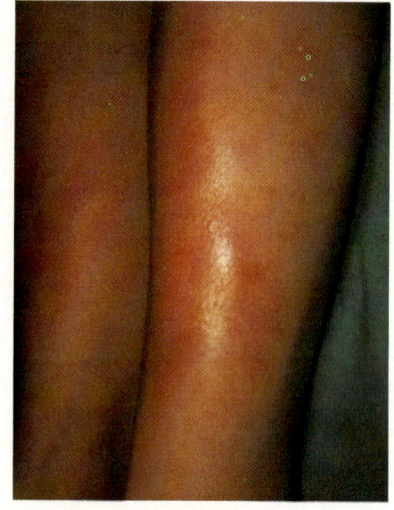

X–B Erythema nodosum.

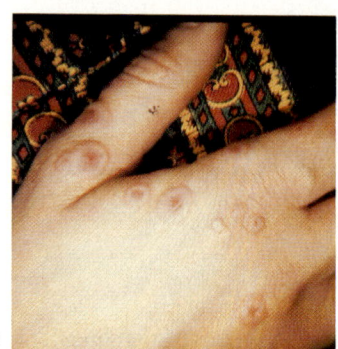

X–C Erythema multiforme. Papular, urticarial, and target lesions.

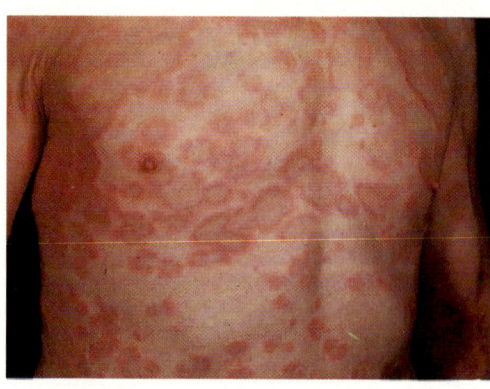

X–D-i and ii Erythema multiforme. Widespread lesions on the trunk.

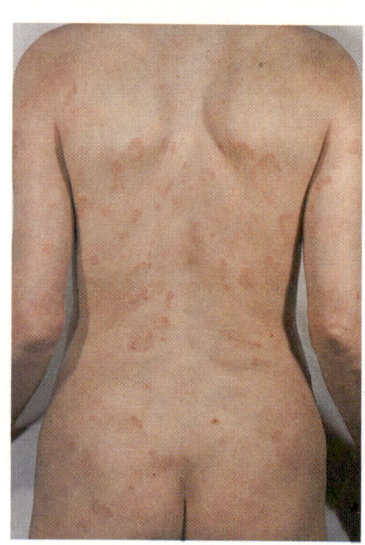

X–E Erythema multiforme. Target or iris lesions with central hemorrhage.

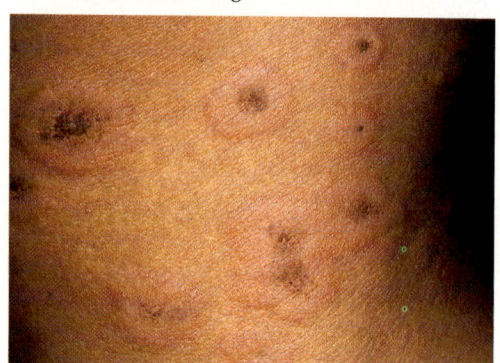

PLATE X

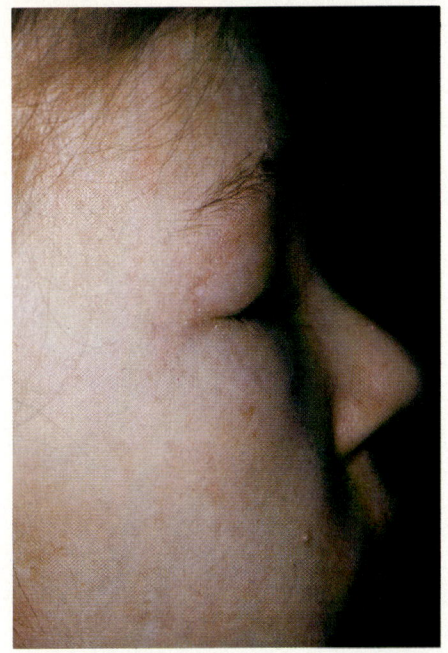

XI-A Dermatomyositis. Periorbital swelling and pinkish erythema.

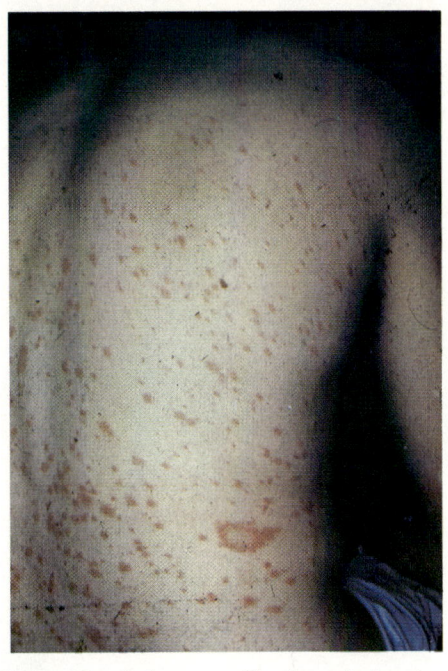

XI-B Pityriasis rosea. The large lesion is the "herald patch."

XI-D Lichen planus.

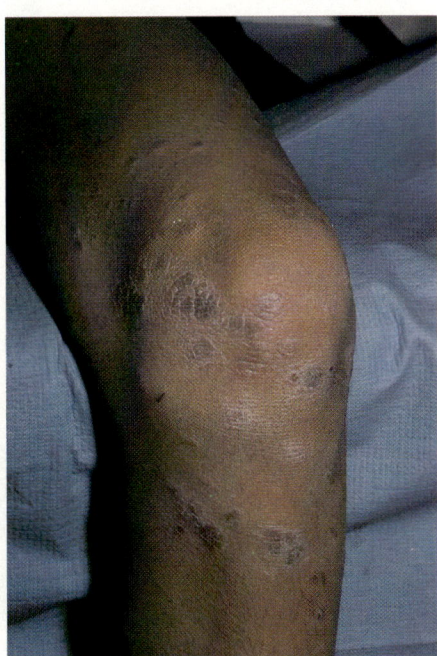

XI-C Pyoderma gangrenosum in a patient with granulomatous bowel disease.

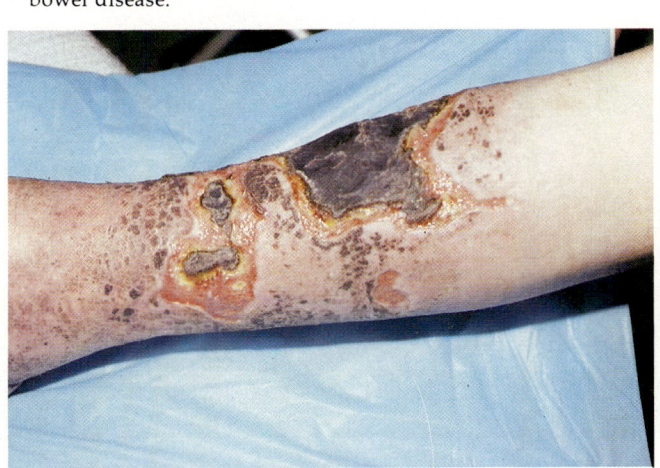

PLATE XI

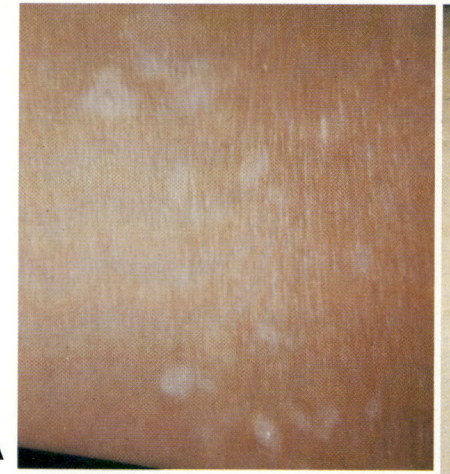

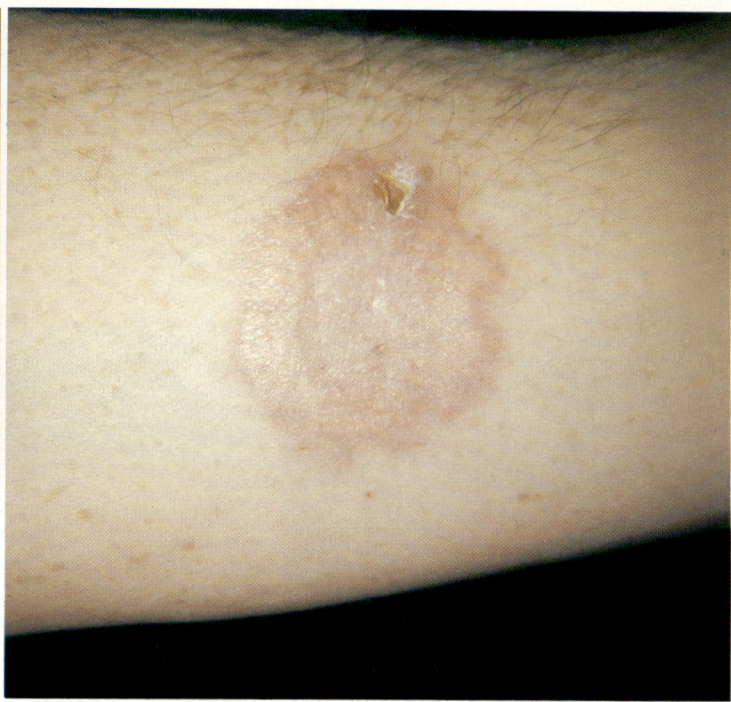

XII–A Lichen sclerosus et atrophicus.

XII–B Necrobiosis lipoidica diabeticorum.

XII–C Granuloma annulare.

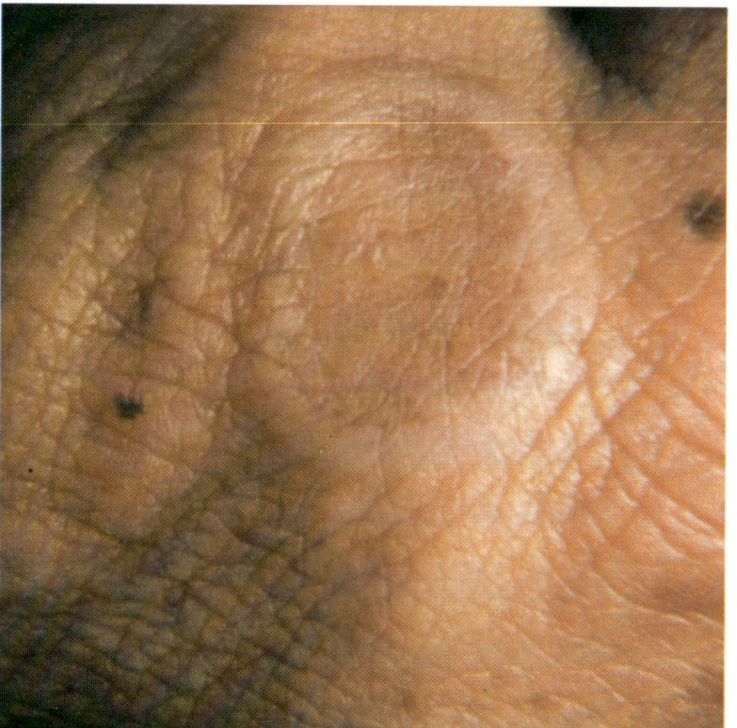

PLATE XII

ETIOLOGY

Donovania granulomatis is a gram-negative, non-motile, non-spore-forming, ovoid or lima bean-shaped bacillus that varies in size from 1 to 1.5 μ in length and 0.6 to 0.8 μ in width. It is encapsulated when mature. With Wright-Giemsa or silver preparations, the intense polar staining of chromatin granules may give the organism the appearance of a closed safety pin. The ultrastructure of *D. granulomatis* is typical of gram-negative bacteria.[16]

In the tissues of the host, *D. granulomatis* reproduces by a simple process. After the encapsulated mature bacillus is engulfed by a mononuclear cell, intracytoplasmic replication by binary fission yields many non-encapsulated, immature bacilli, often occupying vacuoles in the cytoplasm of the host cell. As the bacilli mature, they become encapsulated, and are released into the tissue when the mononuclear cell ruptures, at which point the cycle repeats itself. The organism can be cultured only with difficulty, using artificial media containing beef heart infusion agar with fresh yolk, which provides a peptide (such as vitellin) that is evidently essential for growth. *Donovania granulomatis* may be an intestinal inhabitant in some individuals,[17] which may account for the high proportion of recorded cases of granuloma inguinale in sodomists.[18,19]

MANIFESTATIONS

Granuloma inguinale is primarily a disease of moist, stratified squamous epithelium. The incubation period varies from 14 to 50 days, but may range from eight days to four months. The initial lesion is a soft, painless, flat-topped papule that enlarges into a beefy-red, dome-shaped nodule. It usually occurs on the external genitalia or in the perianal region. Within days, the nodule breaks down to form a painless ulcer with sharply defined border, vivid red and velvety base, and serosanguineous exudate. If the vaginal mucosa or cervix is involved, exuberant granulation tissue may be prominent.

The disease spreads along the folds of the groin, either directly through the dermis, producing coalescing satellite lesions, or by autoinoculation of adjacent or opposing surfaces. In about 90 per cent of reported cases, the inguinal manifestations are associated with or are secondary to genital or anal lesions.[20] Inguinal involvement also may result from subcutaneous granulomatous extension of the infection, producing localized soft and fluctuant masses or "pseudobuboes," which rupture subsequently to form the typical ulcerations. Involvement of the underlying lymph nodes is minimal.

The initial sites of infection are the prepuce, coronal sulcus, glans, penile shaft, and perianal region in the male, and the labia majora, labia minora, fourchette, cervix, and perineum in the female.[21-23] Extragenital lesions occur occasionally, particularly in the oral cavity, lips, or cheek, and almost invariably are associated with granuloma inguinale involving the groin.[20,24-28]

As classified by Halty,[29] granuloma inguinale can be divided into four clinical types (Figs. 12-8 to 12-12):

1. *Nodular:* A sharply defined, painless, soft, pink to beefy-red, dome-shaped granuloma that bleeds readily on manipulation.

2. *Ulcerovegetative:* The type of ulceration most frequently encountered. Satellite nodules develop, which ulcerate and coalesce with the original lesion,

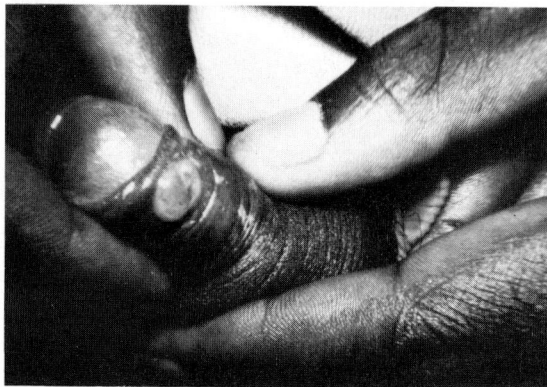

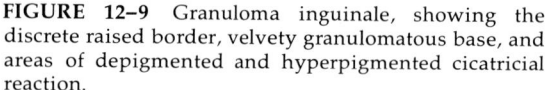

FIGURE 12–8 Dome-shaped nodular lesion of early granuloma inguinale.

FIGURE 12–9 Granuloma inguinale, showing the discrete raised border, velvety granulomatous base, and areas of depigmented and hyperpigmented cicatricial reaction.

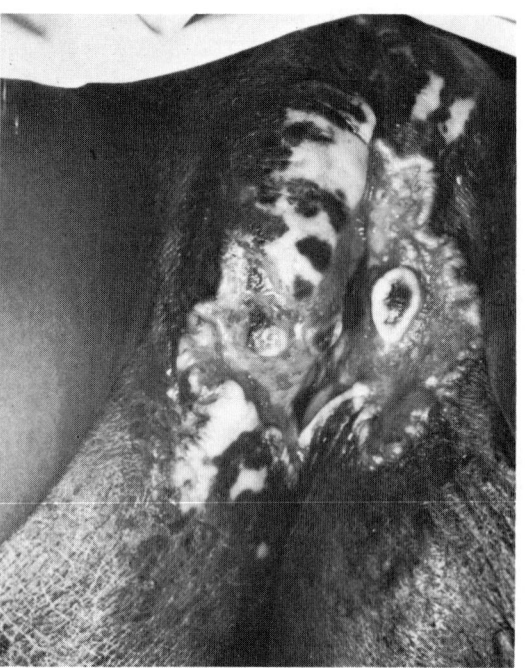

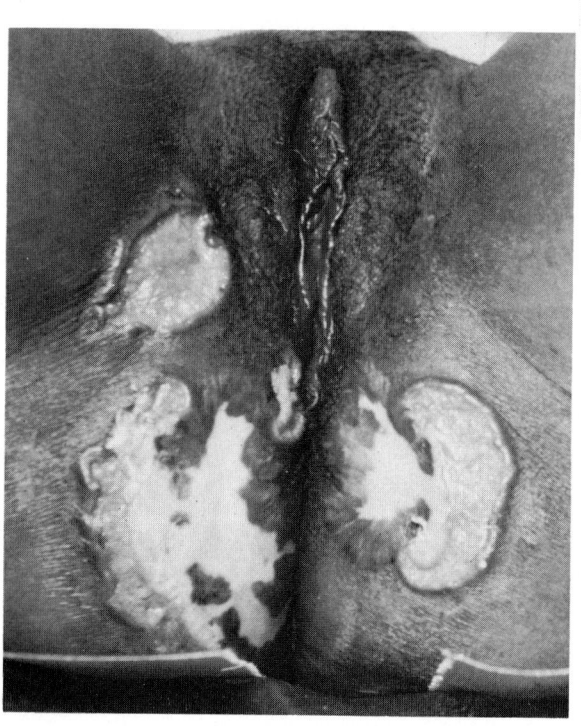

FIGURE 12–10 Granuloma inguinale, demonstrating the typical raised sharp margin, granulomatous, velvety base of the ulceration, and areas of depigmented scar.

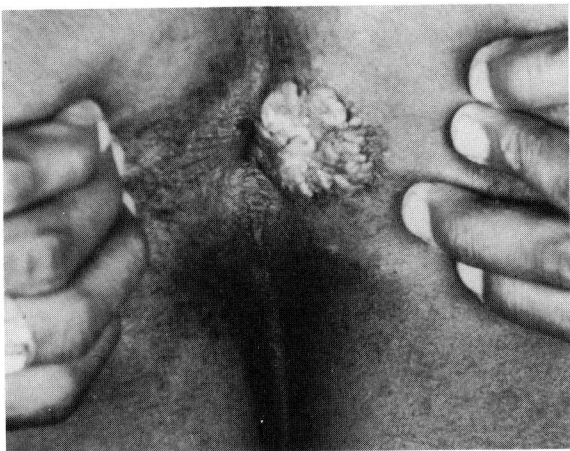

FIGURE 12-11 Hypertrophic granuloma inguinale. This patient also had extragenital granuloma inguinale of the gingiva.

producing serpiginous extension over the genitalia, inguinal folds, perineal, perianal, and intergluteal areas. In the male, the extension tends to be upward toward the inguinal groove. In the female it is downward toward the perineal and perianal areas.

3. *Hypertrophic:* Piled-up, vegetative, granulomatous masses, which may become several centimeters high.

4. *Cicatricial:* Caused by a peculiar host reaction that produces bands of rapidly-forming fibrosis that sequester islands of active infection. The resulting areas of scar tissue contain nests of inflammatory cells and *D. granulomatis* embedded in the dense collagenous fibrous tissue.

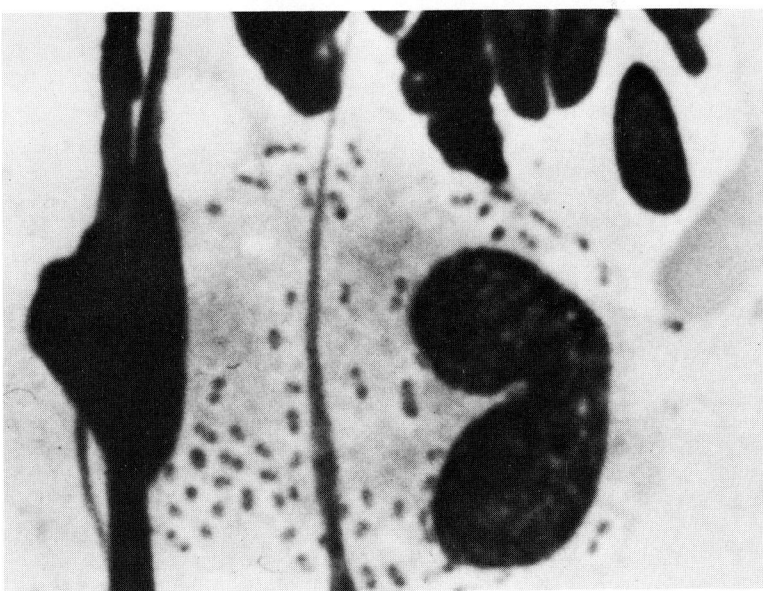

FIGURE 12-12 *Calymmatobacterium (Donovania) granulomatis* within cytoplasm of mononuclear cell. Giemsa stain of tissue teased from ulcer margin.

COMPLICATIONS

Fusospirochetosis is the most common complication of granuloma inguinale. A painful, rapidly spreading, necrotic ulceration results, which may progress to mutilating destruction of tissue. Rarely, granuloma inguinale may extend to the uterus, fallopian tubes, ovaries, bladder, and pelvic tissue; metastatic spread may extend to bone, liver, or lung. Pregnancy appears to facilitate dissemination.[20, 30-33] Partial stenosis of the urethral, vaginal, and anal orifices have been reported.[20, 34] Pseudoelephantiasis, caused by mechanical pressure on the lymphatics by fibrosis and by the dense cellular infiltrate, may develop. Evidence suggests that chronic granuloma inguinale may be a premalignant condition.[22, 35, 36]

DIAGNOSIS

As in all diseases associated with genital lesions, syphilis must first be excluded by darkfield examination and serological tests. The clinical diagnosis of granuloma inguinale, based on the history and morphology of the lesion, must be confirmed by demonstration of Donovan bodies (*Donovania granulomatis*) in tissue specimens. A fragment of friable granulation tissue may be removed from the margin of the lesion with an iris scissors, curet, or scalpel. Or it may be teased out between the edges of two microscopic slides.

After anesthetizing with lidocaine (Xylocaine), a larger specimen may be obtained by making a wedge-shaped excision or by using a biopsy punch. The clean undersurface of part of the tissue should be smeared along several glass slides or crushed between two glass slides. The remainder of the biopsy specimen should be sent for histopathological study. Material aspirated from fluctuant pseudobuboes is also suitable for the preparation of smears.

After staining, the smears are searched for the pathognomonic agent, which is a large mononuclear cell with a foamy, vacuolated cytoplasm (25 to 90 μ in diameter), containing Donovan organisms.

After drying in air, the smears are first flooded with 1 per cent pinacyanole dye in methyl alcohol for two minutes. The stain is then diluted with an equal amount of neutral distilled water for two minutes, and then washed with distilled water. Under the oil immersion lens, the Donovan bodies stain dark blue with a purplish-pink capsule.

Following fixation with methyl alcohol, a Giemsa or Wright stain may be used to equal advantage. The mature *Donovania granulomatis* stains purplish-rose with Giemsa and blue to deep purple with Wright, the latter also producing more intense staining of the polar bodies. The pale purplish-pink of the capsule can be decolorized by overwashing the slide with distilled water.

Paraffin tissue sections stained with hematoxylin and eosin demonstrate histological features compatible with the diagnosis of granuloma inguinale. A Giemsa or silver stain technique is essential to demonstrate the pathognomonic cell with its bacterial inclusions.

TREATMENT

Tetracycline administered in a dosage of 2 gm daily (500 mg orally at 6-hour intervals) for 20 to 25 days, with a total dose of 40 to 50 gm, is usually adequate to treat granuloma inguinale. Erythromycin in the same dosage may be used as an alternative. In the past, streptomycin (1 gm intramuscularly at 12-hour intervals for 10 to 15 days) has been employed but resistance to streptomycin may develop. Treatment should be continued for at least one week after the lesions appear to be healed. Since relapse may occur many months after apparently successful treatment, an examination periodically for 12 months after therapy is recommended.

Neither the sulfonamides nor penicillin is effective against *D. granulomatis,* but both may be helpful in the treatment of secondary infection. Local therapy with wet dressings of hydrogen peroxide or sodium perborate, or warm compresses of potassium permanganate in 1:8000 dilution, may be beneficial.

LYMPHOGRANULOMA VENEREUM
(Durand-Nicolas-Favre disease, Lymphopathia venereum, Lymphogranuloma inguinale)

Lymphogranuloma venereum is an infectious venereal disease caused by an agent of the genus *Chlamydia*. An inconspicuous initial genital lesion is followed by suppurative regional lymphadenitis, which is frequently associated with constitutional symptoms.

Although Wallace[37] is credited with the original description of the disease in 1833, the first definitive report was made by Durand, Nicolas, and Favre in 1913.[38] Frei introduced an intradermal skin test in 1925, using pus from a bubo as antigen.[39] Chlamydial inclusions were first observed in smears from the eye by Halberstaedter and Prowazek in 1907.[40] The culture of the organism in the chick embryo yolk sac by Rake, McKee, and Shaffer[41] led to the development of an antigen used in diagnostic tests. In 1957, Tang and his associates used the same method to culture the trachoma inclusion conjunctivitis (TRIC) agent.[42] In 1936, Bedson pioneered in the isolation and characterization of the chlamydial agent causing psittacosis.[43-45]

ETIOLOGY

Members of the genus *Chlamydia* are responsible for a wide range of infections in birds and mammals. In human beings, these include lymphogranuloma venereum, psittacosis, trachoma, inclusion conjunctivitis, cervicitis, proctitis, and a large proportion of non-gonococcal urethritis and ophthalmia neonatorum infections.

Chlamydia are obligate intracellular parasites. Lacking energy-generating mechanisms, they are dependent on the host cell for metabolic energy.[46] They have a characteristic developmental cycle and reproduce by binary fission. Chlamydia cells range in size from 0.2 μ to 1 μ in diameter, contain both RNA and DNA, have cell walls similar to those of bacteria, and possess group and specific complement-fixing antigens.

The inclusions of *Chlamydia* subgroup A contain glycogen and therefore stain with iodine, while those of *Chlamydia* subgroup B do not (Table 12–1). Chlamydial strains that are capable of synthesizing folic acid are inhibited by sulfonamides.

TABLE 12–1 DIVISION OF *CHLAMYDIA* INTO SUBGROUPS A AND B

Property	*Chlamydia* Subgroup A	*Chlamydia* Subgroup B
Presence of glycogen in the inclusion	Present	Absent
Susceptibility to sulfonamides	Sensitive	Resistant
Susceptibility to tetracycline	Sensitive	Sensitive
Susceptibility to streptomycin	Resistant	Resistant
Species	*C. trachomatis*	*C. psittaci*
Diseases produced	Trachoma Inclusion conjunctivitis TRIC ophthalmia neonatorum Lymphogranuloma venereum (most cases) Non-specific urethritis (many cases) The Reiter syndrome(?) Mouse pneumonitis	Ornithosis (psittacosis) Meningopneumonitis Lymphogranuloma venereum (occasional case) Numerous diseases in birds and mammals

MANIFESTATIONS (Figs. 12–13 to 12–15)

The primary lesion of lymphogranuloma venereum is painless, inconspicuous, and evanescent. It develops after an incubation period, usually of five to 21 days but occasionally as long as two months. Usually located on the genitalia, the initial, tiny, herpetiform vesicle or vesicopapule soon evolves into a shallow, non-indurated erosion, 2 to 3 mm in diameter, with sharp margination and a narrow, erythematous halo. Often going unnoticed, the lesion heals spontaneously without scar formation.

INGUINAL SYNDROME

The regional lymph nodes enlarge a week to several months after the healing of the initial lesion. The inguinal, femoral, and iliac chains are involved, since the primary lesion in the male is usually on the penis, coronal sulcus, prepuce, glans, or urethra. In approximately one third of patients, lymphadenopathy is bilateral.

The nodes are firm and rubbery, moderately tender, and adherent to the underlying and overlying tissues. They become matted together by periadenitis to form elongated, sausage-like inflammatory masses above and below the taut Poupart's ligament, producing the "pathognomonic" groove of Greenblatt.

Although in some patients the inflammatory process in the bubo may subside, alternating areas of fluctuation and induration usually develop as a

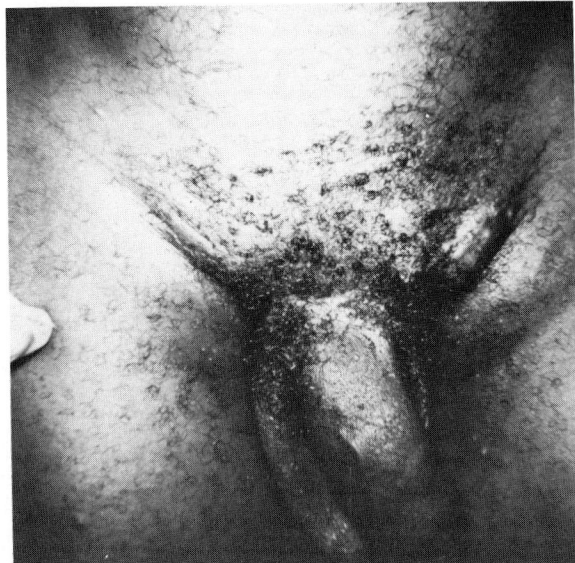

FIGURE 12-13 Lymphogranuloma venereum. Bilateral buboes above and below the inguinal ligament, producing the pathognomonic groove of Greenblatt. The chlamydial complement fixation test in this case was reactive to a titer of 1:240 dilutions.

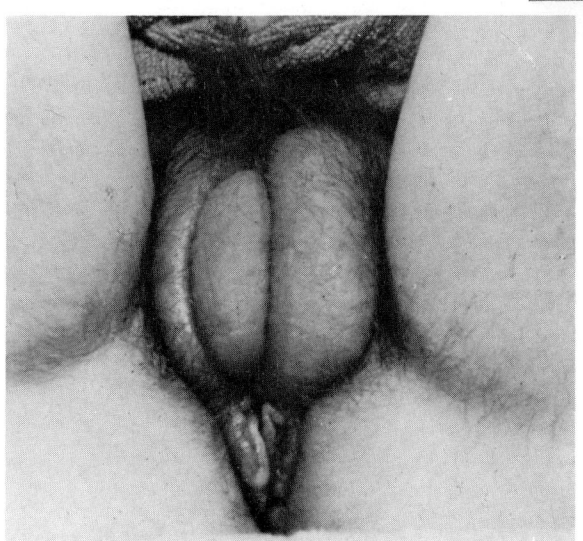

FIGURE 12-14 A late manifestation of lymphogranuloma venereum: esthiomene or vulvar elephantiasis.

FIGURE 12-15 Elephantiasis of the vulva in a patient with mixed infection: lymphogranuloma venereum and granuloma inguinale.

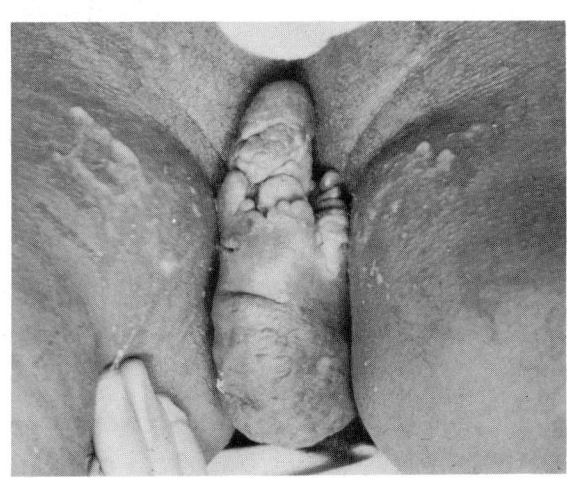

multilocular abscess forms. The overlying skin becomes dusky red, and soft areas soon rupture, discharging first a thick pus and later a milky fluid through multiple fistulous tracts. Chronic sinuses may persist.

RECTAL SYNDROME

Homosexual males may develop rectal lymphogranuloma, and females may be infected as a consequence of anal coitus.[35] However, in females the primary lesion often occurs near the fourchette or in the lower half of the vagina. The precise route by which the rectum becomes infected in these cases is not known. The lymphatics from the cervix and the major portion of the vagina drain into the external iliac, hypogastric, and common iliac lymphatic chains, while those in the portion of the vagina that is continuous with the vulva drain into the inguinal nodes. An additional lymphatic plexus exists, which drains the posterolateral vaginal walls, following the middle hemorrhoidal (rectal) artery through the tissue planes of the perineal body, where the vagina and rectum are in closest proximity. These terminate in the lacework of lymphatic anastomoses that surround the terminal rectum and anal canal,[47-49] in the area where proctitis usually begins and strictures eventually form.

As lymphadenitis develops in the anorectal, pararectal, rectosigmoidal, and hypogastric lymph node chains, a matted inflammatory mass forms. The resulting multilocular abscesses rupture into the bowel, with drainage of infectious pus, blood, and mucus. This purulent proctocolitis may persist for weeks or for many months. As healing proceeds, an encircling, tubular, fibrous stricture may form, with its lowest edge situated 4 to 5 cm from the anal margin. About one third of women with rectal strictures also have rectovaginal fistulae originating distal to the stricture, fistulae-in-ano, or fistulae opening into the perineum, rectum, or gluteal area.

Infiltrative, ulcerative, and subsequently fibrotic lesions of the vulva and vagina may produce a fenestrated or "buttonhole" labia or cicatricial stenosis of the vagina or urethra. A soft, puffy swelling of the labia and clitoris, with normal overlying skin, may occur as well as polypoid, lobulated anal growths resembling hemorrhoids.[27, 50]

Constitutional symptoms may include headache, meningismus, chills, fever, night sweats, malaise, weight loss, migratory joint pains, polyarthritis, hyperglobulinemia, and splenomegaly. The most common skin manifestation is erythema nodosum, but erythema multiforme, scarlatiniform eruption, or papulopustular lesions may also be encountered.

Urethritis, cystitis, pneumonitis, meningitis, and meningoencephalitis also can be caused by the lymphogranuloma venereum agent. Eye manifestations may include conjunctivitis uveitis, sclerokeratitis, iridocyclitis and keratoconjunctivitis associated with preauricular adenopathy, simulating Parinaud's oculoglandular syndrome.[51, 52, 53]

DIAGNOSIS

Several tests and procedures are of value in confirming a diagnosis of lymphogranuloma venereum (Table 12–2).

TABLE 12–2 DIFFERENTIAL DIAGNOSIS OF LYMPHOGRANULOMA VENEREUM

Findings	Lymphogranuloma Venereum	Chancroid	Granuloma Inguinale	Herpes Genitalis
Etiological agent	*Chlamydia*, subgroup A	*Hemophilus ducreyi*	*Donovania (Calymmatobacterium) granulomatis*	Herpes simplex virus, usually type II
Incubation period	5 to 21 days; up to 2 months	2 to 7 days	14 to 50 days; up to 4 months	2 to 6 days, up to 2 weeks
Tissue primarily involved	Lymphatic tissue of inguinal, genital, and rectal regions.	Skin of genitalia, regional lymph nodes.	Moist, stratified squamous epithelium of genital and oral regions.	Cutaneous and mucosal surfaces.
Initial lesion	Evanescent single herpetiform erosion.	Vesicopustule; thereafter, a painful ulcer.	Flat-topped or dome-shaped papule or nodule.	Grouped vesicles; later, minute painful erosions.
Sex predilection	More common in males	More common in males	More common in males	Equal sex distribution
Adenopathy	*Male*: Enlargement of multiple nodes in inguinal and femoral areas, moderately tender and matted together. Separated by taut Poupart's ligament producing groove of Greenblatt. Minimal inflammation of overlying tissues. *Female*: Involvement of anorectal, sacral, and hypogastric nodes with rupture into rectum.	After 5 to 14 days one or two regional nodes enlarge. Often unilateral, acutely inflammatory and tender. Develops in 50% of males with chancroidal ulcers.	Subcutaneous extension of granulomatous process may produce a pseudo bubo. Minimal involvement of the underlying lymph-nodes.	1 to 2 enlarged, tender regional nodes, usually unilateral.
Suppuration	Slow development into a *multilocular* abscess.	Rapid development into a *unilocular* abscess.	None	None

Table continued on following page

TABLE 12-2 DIFFERENTIAL DIAGNOSIS OF LYMPHOGRANULOMA VENEREUM—*Continued*

Findings	Lymphogranuloma Venereum	Chancroid	Granuloma Inguinale	Herpes Genitalis
Course of adenopathy	Periadenitis develops. Matted nodes become adherent to overlying tissue; bubo retains shape after rupture, since suppuration does not involve entire gland. Ruptures occur at intervals through multiple ostia, followed by slow involution.	Uniform enlargement of 1 or 2 nodes; suppuration involves entire gland; acute inflammation of the overlying skin. May involute after 2 to 3 weeks or months or spontaneously rupture through one ostium, after which abscess collapses. Rapid healing follows.	Pseudobuboes erupt to surface, producing typical ulceration. Gradual extension of ulceration over months or years; occasional areas of cicatricial reaction.	Spontaneous involution as eruption subsides.
Discharge	Initially, thick, purulent and usually free of blood. Later, thin, milky fluid.	Purulent discharge mixed with blood.	Serosanguineous exudate	Serous exudate
Presence of pain	Initial lesion is painless; buboes are moderately tender.	Painful ulcers; buboes are painful and tender.	Painless unless secondarily infected.	Painful erosions; bubo moderately tender.
Sinus and fistula formation	Ruptured buboes produce multiple sinuses and fistulae.	Ulcerative lesion may develop at site of rupture and drainage.	None	None
Elephantiasis	Esthiomene produced by lymphangitis, fibrosis, and lymphostasis.	None	Pseudoelephantiasis secondary to cellular infiltrate and fibrosis.	None
Stricture formation and other late manifestations	Inflammatory rectal stricture, followed by tubular stricture due to scar; labial fenestration.	Scars at sites of ulcerations or bubo breakdown.	Partial stenosis of urethral, vaginal, or anal orifices (rare).	None
Toxic skin manifestations	Erythema nodosum; erythema multiforme; scarlatiniform eruption; papulopustular lesions.	None	None	None

Extragenital lesions	Primary inoculation of eye may produce keratoconjunctivitis and Parinaud's oculoglandular syndrome.	Extragenital lesions are seldom primary and rarely found on finger, tongue or lips because of autoinoculation.	May occur on gingiva or cheek as a result of autoinoculation; rarely primary.	May occur on finger, eye, or oral mucosa. Usually primary infection.
Changes in blood chemistry	Hyperglobulinemia; hyperproteinemia; reversed albumin-globulin ratio.	None	None	None
Constitutional symptoms	Headache, meningismus, fever, malaise, weight loss, arthralgia, polyarthritis, uveitis, iridocyclitis, proctocolitis.	Low-grade fever may accompany bubo formation.	Absent	Low-grade fever, headache, malaise, dysuria. Occasional twinges of pain in groin may be noted.
Dissemination	Meningitis and meningoencephalitis (rare).	None	Metastatic lesions on bone, liver, lung, ovary, lymph nodes, usually associated with pregnancy.	HSV may exist in sensory spinal ganglia during remissions. Meningitis due to HSV type II; meningoencephalitis due to type I.
Complications	Ulcerations secondary to elephantiasis; labial fenestration; urethral or rectal strictures; perirectal abscess and fistulae.	Fusospirochetosis, mixed infection with syphilis or herpes genitalis, phimosis, paraphimosis.	Fusospirochetosis, partial stenosis of urethra, vagina, or anus, pseudoelephantiasis.	Kaposi's varicelliform eruption in presence of atopic eczema or thermal burns. Pneumonia in immunologically compromised patient.
Complement fixation tests	Serum fixes complement in presence of chlamydial antigen demonstrating *group* antibody. Micro-immunofluorescence test under study. Low incidence of false positive reactions to non-treponemal antigen tests for syphilis.	None	Serum fixes complement in the presence of antigen prepared from *Donovania granulomatis*. Poor specificity.	Complement-fixing antibodies present; neutralizing antibody assays; micro-immunofluorescent test.
Propensity to congenital infection	None recorded. However, chlamydial antibodies are passively transferred in utero.	None	None	Exposure to HSV in birth canal may produce localized or disseminated infection.

Table continued on following page

TABLE 12-2 DIFFERENTIAL DIAGNOSIS OF LYMPHOGRANULOMA VENEREUM—Continued

Findings	Lymphogranuloma Venereum	Chancroid	Granuloma Inguinale	Herpes Genitalis
Modes of cultivation	Isolation in irradiated McCoy or HeLa tissue cells; lethal to mice on intracerebral inoculation. Can be isolated on embryonic chick yolk sac.	Exudate cultured on freshly clotted human or rabbit blood.	Yolk sac of chick embryo. Special artificial media containing fresh yolk.	Tissue culture on diploid human fibroblast cells, primary rabbit kidney cells.
Oncogenic status	Controversial. Premalignant role for vulvar, cervical, and anorectal lesions claimed.	None	Chronic lesions believed potentially oncogenic.	Association with risk of cervical or nasopharyngeal neoplasia under evaluation.
Diagnosis	Chlamydial complement fixation test. Culture on tissue cells or yolk sac of chick embryo. Lethal effect on intracerebral inoculation of mice.	Demonstration of organism on Gram stained smear of exudate. Culture on fresh clotted human or rabbit blood. Syphilis ruled out by darkfield examination and serological tests.	Demonstration of *Donovania granulomatis* in cytoplasm of mononuclear cells in tissue smears or biopsy sections. Compatible histopathology.	Tzanck test: demonstration of multinucleated epithelial cells and intranuclear inclusions from vesicle fluid or cells from base of erosion. Culture of virus.
Treatment	Sulfonamides, tetracycline, erythromycin. Aspiration of fluctuant buboes. Dilation or resection of stricture.	Sulfonamides, tetracycline, erythromycin, streptomycin. Aspiration of fluctuant bubo. Cleansing of ulcerations with pHisoHex.	Tetracycline, erythromycin; streptomycin, occasionally ampicillin. Hydrogen peroxide local compresses.	Unsatisfactory at present: astringents, drying lotions; antibiotic creams; idoxuridine ointment; autovaccine; gamma globulin; heterocyclic dye and photoinactivation; interferon inducers; oral antimetabolites; use of liquid nitrogen during first 48 hours of the eruption.

Complement fixation test. The lymphogranuloma complement fixation (LGV–CF) test is a chlamydial group-specific test. It uses antigen obtained from the agents causing either enzootic abortion in ewes (EAE) or lymphogranuloma venereum. These are grown in the yolk sacs of embryonated chicken eggs. Titers of 1:32 or greater are regarded as significant, particularly if an increased titer occurs after two weeks. The complement fixation test attains its maximum positivity three to six weeks after the appearance of the bubo. However, many patients with lymphogranuloma venereum do not show titer change. In early infections, positivity falls off rapidly after effective treatment,[54] but in chronic cases titers may remain high.[50]

The radioisotope precipitation (RIP) test. The RIP test is more sensitive than the complement fixation tests and also detects chlamydial *group* antibody.[55]

Isolation of Chlamydia in cell culture. The most conclusive proof of the diagnosis is isolation of the agent from aspirates of lymph nodes, pus, or rectal discharge. A sensitive, simplified one-passage chlamydial cultural technique in irradiated McCoy tissue cells[56] can be used for diagnosis, epidemiological studies, and assessment of the results of treatment.[57,58] HeLa 229 tissue cells are also used successfully for chlamydial isolation,[59] the cultures being examined microscopically for glycogen-containing inclusions.

Isolation of Chlamydia in yolk sac. Isolation of the agent by inoculation of material into yolk sacs of embryonated chicken eggs has been used for the past three decades, but superior recovery is obtained by tissue cell culture procedures.

Micro-immunofluorescence (micro-IF) test. The micro-immunofluorescence test, pioneered by Wang,[60] is a sensitive test that can distinguish the TRIC agent from the lymphogranuloma venereum agent and can detect antibodies to individual chlamydial serotypes.[61,62] The micro-IF test has facilitated serotyping of chlamydial agents from ocular, genital, and rectal infections and has separated the lymphogranuloma venereum agent into three distinctive serotypes.

Biopsy. Biopsy of involved lymph nodes may be useful in doubtful cases,[22] but the histopathological findings are not diagnostic of the disease.

TREATMENT

Sulfisoxazole: 1 gm four times daily for 10 days may give satisfactory results in the early stages of bubo formation, although repeated courses may be required.

Tetracycline: 500 mg administered orally every six hours (2 gm daily) for 21 to 30 days is usually effective.

Erythromycin: In the same dosage as that of tetracycline, erythromycin is usually an effective alternative.

Fluctuant buboes should be aspirated, using a large bore needle. Rectal strictures, which are about 10 times more frequent in the female than in the male, may be relieved by repeated dilatations, although surgical resection may be required.

THE REITER SYNDROME (Oculo-genital-synovial syndrome)

The syndrome of polyarthritis, non-gonococcal urethritis, conjunctivitis, and less commonly, keratosis and dysentery, was originally described by Brodie in 1818[63] and a century later by Reiter in 1916.[64]

ETIOLOGY

The search for the etiological agent of the Reiter syndrome has been pursued by many investigators. Significant evidence has been compiled relating *Chlamydia* to the Reiter syndrome, including isolation of *Chlamydia* from the synovial fluid, synovial membrane, conjunctiva, and urethra of patients with this disease.[65-68] Intradermal tests with chlamydia antigens also produce positive findings,[69] and the chlamydial complement fixation[70] and micro-immunofluorescence tests[71] are reactive in many patients with the disorder. Experimentally, rabbits have been shown to develop chlamydia-positive arthritis after inoculation of the eye with *Chlamydia*.[72]

Isolation of *Chlamydia* from the lesions of the Reiter syndrome does not necessarily establish a causal relationship between the agent and the disease. Therefore, further attempts to isolate the agent are essential to detect members of *Chlamydia* subgroup B as well as subgroup A in patients and control groups.

The roles of other organisms in initiating the disease or in producing relapses of the Reiter syndrome also have been considered. These include *Mycoplasma,* pleuropneumonia-like organisms, adenoviruses, and enterococci. Autoimmune phenomena have also been postulated, and genetic susceptibility to develop the Reiter syndrome may be a contributing factor. A circulating antibody to prostatic antigen can be detected in a majority of patients by a hemagglutination test.[73]

In a study of 110 relatives and 20 spouses of 35 patients, Lawrence[74] found that while rheumatoid arthritis and rheumatoid factor were no more frequent in the families of affected patients, psoriasis was 14 times more common in male relatives than in the general population. Ankylosing spondylitis occurred eight times more often, and bilateral sacroiliitis (discovered radiographically) was nearly three times as frequent, suggesting that heredity plays a part in the predisposition.

HL-A, the major human histocompatibility system, is a complex blood group system, inherited as a simple autosomal dominant characteristic, with antigens that can be detected in peripheral blood lymphocytes. A susceptibility to reactive arthritis after certain infections may be linked closely with possession of HL-antigen 27. Approximately 60 per cent of patients with the Reiter syndrome who have been tissue-typed have demonstrated HL-A27,[75-79] with a high proportion containing the HL-A27/W10 combination. HL-antigen 27 is also associated with ankylosing spondylitis and sacroiliitis occurring with iritis.[80]

MANIFESTATIONS (Fig. 12–16)

The Reiter syndrome is chiefly a disease of young male adults, although it may occur in women and children.[81] Sexual exposure or an episode of diarrhea may precede the symptoms by several days to three or four weeks. The syndrome usually begins as a non-gonococcal urethritis, often associated with prostatitis. The urethritis may be mild and detectable only in smears obtained in the early morning, or acute, with prostatitis and occasionally hemorrhagic cystitis.[82] The condition may also follow a gonococcal urethritis if a "double infection" was acquired. The urethral discharge varies from scant and serous to profuse, purulent, and blood-tinged.

Soon after the appearance of the urethritis, bilateral conjunctivitis develops in about half of the patients. The severity varies from a mild, fleeting inflammation to marked conjunctival injection with purulent exudate. Anterior uveitis may also appear during the initial attack of conjunctivitis, but more frequently develops during relapses occurring weeks or months later.

One or more joints become involved within days or weeks or sometimes several months after onset of the syndrome, and thereafter arthritis dominates the clinical findings in both severity and duration. The knees, ankles, metatarsophalangeal joints, and wrists are most commonly affected, becoming swollen, painful, tender, and warm to palpation. The synovial fluid appears yellowish and turbid and contains polymorphonuclear leukocytes and a few lymphocytes. It may be sterile or may yield *Chlamydia* or *Mycoplasma* on selective culture. A high hemolytic complement activity in the synovial fluid has been described.[83]

A calcaneal spur associated with plantar fasciitis, demonstrable in most

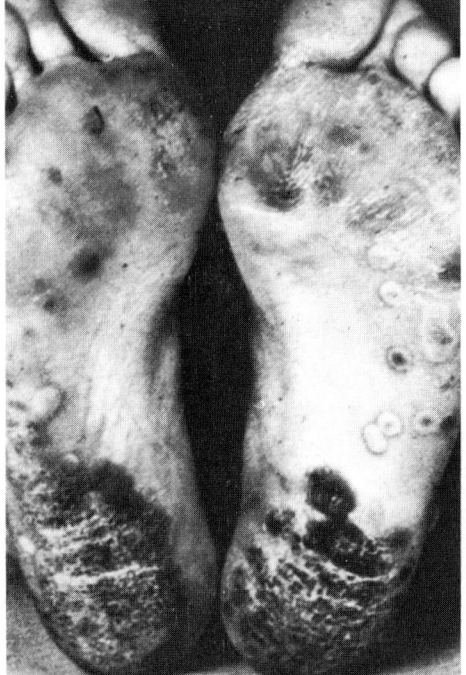

FIGURE 12–16 The Reiter syndrome with typical keratoderma blennorhagicum of soles. (An example of balanitis circinata is shown in Plate VI–C.)

cases by radiographic studies, may produce a painful heel and difficulty in walking. Bilateral sacroiliac arthritis with low back pain occurs with particular frequency in patients with anterior uveitis and recurrent attacks of Reiter's disease.[84]

The arthritis may last for two or more months, occasionally persisting for more than a year, with characteristic periods of spontaneous remissions and recurrences. Various joints may become involved in succession, or relapses in previously affected joints may occur. Most patients apparently recover after one or more episodes, but residual joint damage may occur, including ankylosing spondylitis.

Mucocutaneous lesions may precede or follow the arthritis or exist alone. They develop most commonly on the glans penis, oral mucosa, soles, and palms, but may have a disseminated distribution. The circinate or gyrate pattern seen on the palate or penis is produced by the coalescence of small, superficial erosions with slightly raised edges that occur at the periphery of a circumscribed area of erythema. Occasionally, the circinate lesions are confined to the perimeatal mucosa. Several types of lesions may be found on the oral mucosa: transient small vesicles with surrounding erythema, shallow, painless erosions with whitish borders, or patches of bright erythema (Plate VI–B).

Skin lesions are found in about 10 per cent of patients with Reiter's disease.[82] These develop primarily on the soles but may occur on the palms, extremities, torso, and scalp. The lesions start as red macules, develop into vesicopustules, then become markedly hyperkeratotic. Rupioid (heaped-up) lesions may coalesce to form psoriasiform plaques with gyrate or more complex "geographic" configurations characteristic of keratosis blennorrhagica. The nails become thick and brittle with subungual accumulations of keratotic material. Ultimately, the crusts and horny masses of the various lesions become detached, leaving a pigmentary residue.

Severe cases of the Reiter syndrome may be manifested by fever, malaise, secondary anemia, weight loss, and raised erythrocyte sedimentation rate. Parotitis has been observed,[85] and the chronic, relapsing form of the disease may lead to pericarditis, conduction defects, aortic valve incompetence,[86] and localized neuropathy.[87]

When the primary triad of polyarthritis, non-gonococcal urethritis, and conjunctivitis is present, the Reiter syndrome is easily identified. However, less clear-cut cases require a careful history and further observation before an accurate diagnosis is possible. Serological tests for syphilis should be made at intervals for three months to rule out syphilis.

TREATMENT

Treatment of the disease should be individualized, depending upon the signs and symptoms. Because of the possible etiological role of *Chlamydia*, oral tetracycline should be administered in doses of 500 mg at six-hour intervals (2 gm daily) for 15 to 20 days.

Complete bed rest and immobilization of acutely affected joints is recommended. Gentle passive movement twice daily is essential to prevent stiffness. For an acute arthritic episode, hospitalization with orthopedic consultation is advisable. Aspiration of large joint effusions may appreciably relieve pain;

aspirin, phenylbutazone (Butazolidin), or indomethacin may be used with caution, depending on age of the patient.

Conjunctivitis usually resolves spontaneously, but the application of 4 per cent sulfisoxazole eyedrops, or 0.5 per cent prednisolone eyedrops may be helpful. Anterior uveitis is best treated in collaboration with an ophthalmologist.

The skin lesions of Reiter's disease may be treated with tar and salicylic acid ointment or topical steroids. In recalcitrant, disabling cases, both skin and arthritic manifestations have responded favorably to methotrexate.

GONORRHEA

Gonorrhea is an acute infectious disease caused by *Neisseria gonorrhoeae* and transmitted almost exclusively by sexual contact. It is localized primarily in the genitourinary tract. It is not only the most common venereal disease but also the most prevalent bacterial infection of adults in the United States. *The highest incidence of gonorrhea occurs in the age group between 15 and 29.*

ETIOLOGY

The gonococcus, observed by Neisser in 1879 in urethral exudate,[88] was the first member of the genus *Neisseria* to be described. The genus includes two pathogenic gram-negative species: the gonococcus (*Neisseria gonorrhoeae*) and the meningococcus (*N. meningitidis*). Several other species that are occasionally pathogenic may inhabit the upper respiratory tract or the female genital tract and are differentiated by colony morphology, antigenic structure, chromogenesis, and characteristic fermentation pattern (Table 12–3).

N. gonorrhoeae are round or coffee-bean shaped, gram-negative cocci, 0.8 by 0.6 μ in size. They are usually paired, non-encapsulated and non-motile, and are usually found within the cytoplasm of polymorphonuclear leukocytes.

In common with other species of *Neisseria,* gonococci elaborate indophenol oxidase, which can rapidly oxidize the dye tetramethyl-*p*-phenylenediamine. This capacity is the basis for the useful oxidase test. In fermentation tests, the gonococcus catabolizes glucose to produce acid (acetic acid and possibly a small amount of lactic acid) but not gas.[89]

The traditional medium used to culture gonococci is chocolate agar, which

TABLE 12–3 FERMENTATION PATTERNS OF *NEISSERIA* SPECIES

Organism	Growth in Agar Devoid of Blood	Fermentation			
		GLUCOSE	MALTOSE	SUCROSE	LACTOSE
N. gonorrhoeae	−	+	−	−	−
N. meningitidis	−	+	+	−	−
N. lactamicus	+	+	+	−	+
N. catarrhalis	+	−	−	−	
N. sicca	+	+	+	+	
N. flavescens	+	−	−	−	

is blood agar heated to 80° to 90° C. In 1964[90] Thayer and Martin introduced selective media that incorporated vancomycin, sodium colistimethate, and nystatin into the basic chocolate agar medium to inhibit gram-positive, gram-negative, and yeast-like organisms, while permitting growth of gonococci and meningococci in the primary culture. Most species of *Proteus,* which is an important contaminant in specimens obtained from the rectum, can be suppressed by the addition of trimethroprim to the medium.

When it is grown on agar media, *N. gonorrhoeae* forms four distinct types of colonies.[91] On primary isolation, only colony types 1 and 2 are found after 18 to 24 hours of incubation. Mutation occurs after prolonged incubation or following repeated, non-selective subcultures, giving rise to the relatively non-virulent colony types 3 and 4. Laboratory-adapted strains of gonococci are usually clones of types 3 and 4.

Colony types 1 and 2 are small, dark brown-to-deep gold in color, and have a glistening convexity; clonal types 3 and 4 are large, with a granular surface, and are beige to cream in color. Types 1 and 2 have been shown to be more virulent in experimental intraurethral inoculation in humans,[91] more virulent for chick embryo,[92] and more resistant to phagocytosis by polymorphonuclear leukocytes.[93,94] Clonal types 1 and 2 also differ in their filamentous, hair-like pili, composed of single protein subunits having a molecular weight of about 23,000. These are antigenically identical among various strains of gonococci. Experimental evidence suggests that pili may be important in the attachment of gonococci to mucosal surfaces. An antigen prepared from purified gonococcal pili quantitatively to measure anti-pilar antibody, using radioimmunoassay technique, is under study.[95]

Antigenic heterogeneity and distinctive nutritional profiles among various strains of gonococci have been demonstrated.[96] Gonococcal isolates from patients with disseminated gonococcal infection often show greater clinical virulence, increased antibiotic susceptibility, and a characteristic nutritional profile.[97] A gonococcal lipopolysaccharide endotoxin has also been isolated,[98] which may be responsible for the erosive balanitis and cervicitis associated with acute gonococcal infection.

GONORRHEA IN THE MALE (Figs. 12–17 to 12–20)

The gonococcus has a distinct predilection for surfaces lined with columnar, and to a lesser extent, transitional, epithelium. The incubation period for gonococcal urethritis averages from two to five days but is occasionally as long as two weeks. Electron microscopic studies have shown that gonococci attached closely to the surface of urethral epithelial cells, producing a zone of adhesion.[99] Eventually, gonococci and neutrophils accumulate in the subepithelial connective tissue, and epithelial cells are desquamated. A purulent urethral discharge develops, composed of desquamated epithelial cells, polymorphonuclear leukocytes, and serum. The urethral orifice may appear red and puffy, and there may be superficial balanitis or sufficient edema of the foreskin to produce phimosis.

The mucus-producing glands of Littre, which open into the anterior urethra, become infected in almost every case of gonococcal urethritis. The threads found in the first glass of urine in the traditional two-glass test are casts

GONORRHEA 281

FIGURE 12–17 Condyloma acuminatum (associated with an acute gonococcal urethritis).

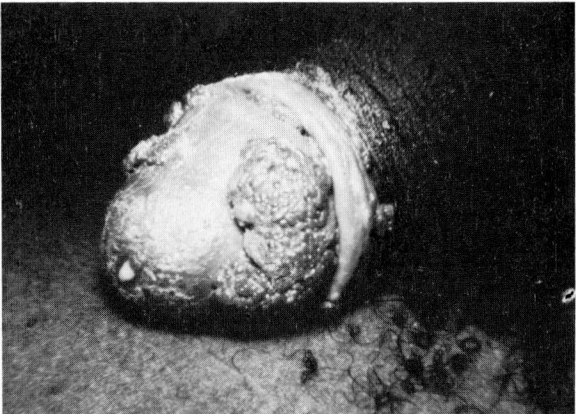

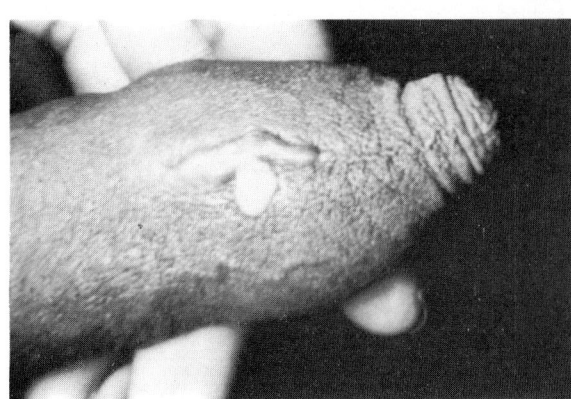

FIGURE 12–18 This patient had a periurethral abscess and cellulitis, with rupture through the penile skin and drainage of gonococcal purulent discharge.

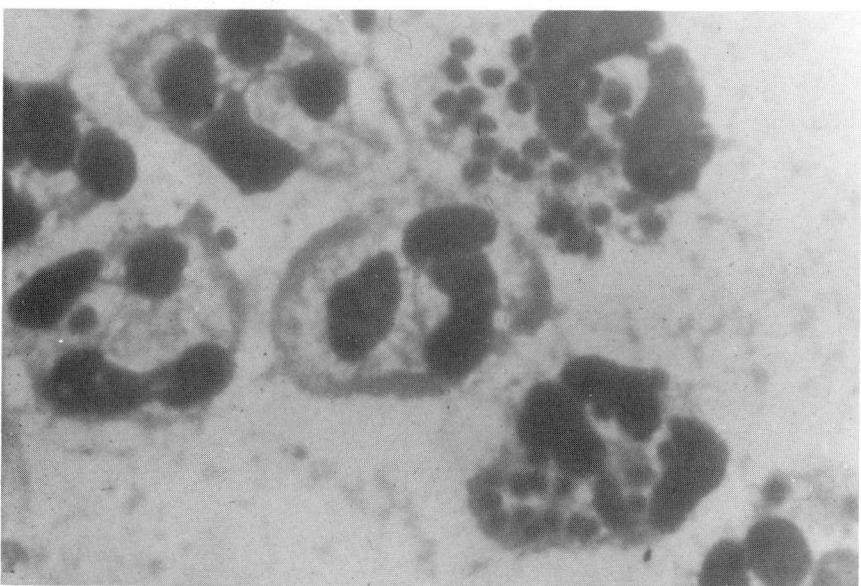

FIGURE 12–19 *Neisseria gonorrhoeae*. Gram-negative diplococci within cytoplasm of polymorphonuclear leukocytes.

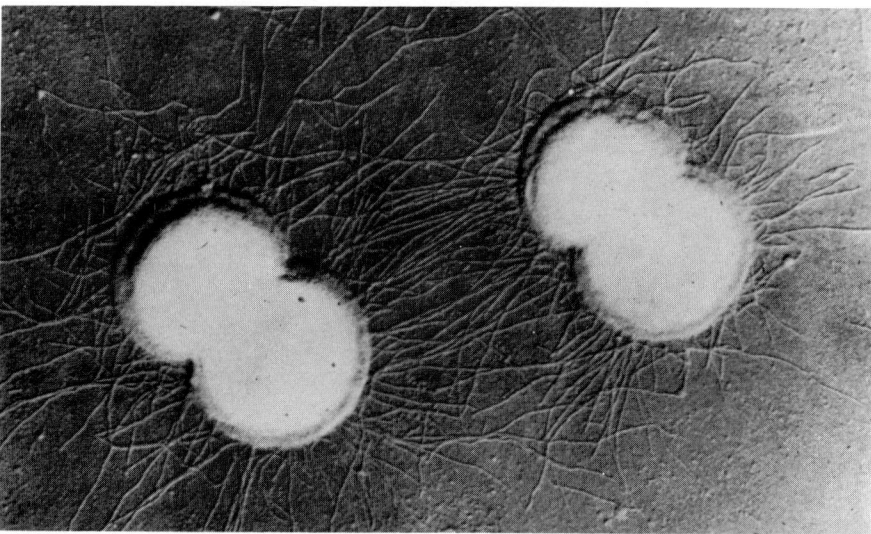

FIGURE 12–20 Filamentous pili present on *Neisseria gonorrhoeae*, Types 1 and 2. (Courtesy of Drs. Sam To and Charles C. Brinton, University of Pittsburgh.)

of the Littre ducts, composed of epithelial and pus cells. Occasionally, the infection extends beyond littritis to produce a hot, tender periurethral abscess with swelling and cellulitis. Thrombosis and phlebitis of the dorsal vein may ensue. The periurethral abscess later may rupture to form a sinus draining purulent, gonococcal discharge into the urethra or through the skin of the penis. When the posterior urethra is involved, urinary frequency and dysuria become more marked, and a few drops of blood may be seen at the end of urination. Untreated gonorrhea may extend to Cowper's glands, prostate, trigone of the bladder, seminal vesicles, and epididymis (Fig. 12–21). The asymptomatic carrier infections that may occur in males, together with minimally symptomatic infections, constitute a reservoir of potential gonococcal infection in the community.[100, 101]

GONORRHEA IN THE FEMALE

In the female, the endocervical glands are lined with columnar epithelium and are the primary site of gonococcal infection. About half of the female patients who have gonorrhea seek medical attention not because of symptoms but because a male sexual partner contracted the disease from them. Other women complain of increased vaginal discharge or urinary frequency and mild dysuria. Clinically, the cervix may appear normal except for slight redness and puffiness about the cervical os. There also may be varying degrees of erosive cervicitis with mucopurulent discharge flowing from the os. In some cases, purulent material can be expressed from the orifices of Skene's ducts and the urethra by gentle, manual, outward pressure along the urethra. Sometimes an acute bartholinitis may develop.

An estimated 10 to 15 per cent of women with gonorrhea develop some degree of acute pelvic inflammatory disease. Transient endometritis may occur,

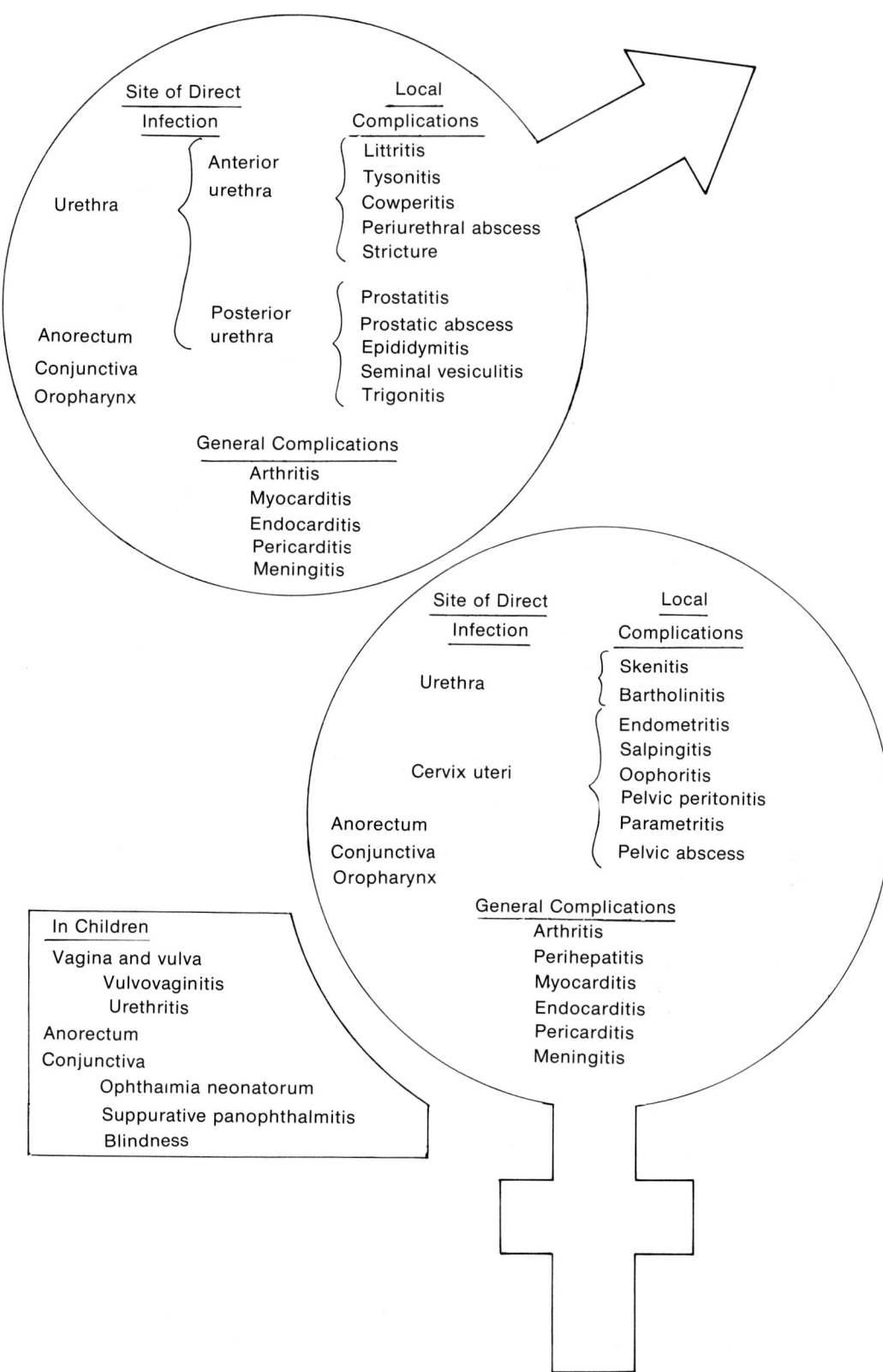

FIGURE 12–21 Complications of gonococcal infection in the male and female.

with contiguous spread of gonococci from the cervix to the endometrial cavity and thereafter to the columnar epithelium of the fallopian tubes. The endometritis may resolve spontaneously during monthly shedding of endometrial cells. Intermenstrual bleeding or increased or prolonged menstrual flow are common occurrences in patients with acute infection. Lymphatic or hematogenous spread of gonorrhea from the uterus to the parametrial area is uncommon except in pregnant patients.[120]

Approximately 65 per cent of females with gonococcal salpingitis develop symptoms within seven days after onset of menstruation. Salpingitis probably results from the reflux of menstrual blood into the fallopian tubes. During menses, there is endocervical shedding of gonococci; pH changes in the cervical mucus favor gonococcal growth. The use of an intrauterine device increases the probability of developing salpingitis.[103] Studies have indicated that gonococci tend to attach themselves to spermatozoa and so could ride "piggyback" into the fallopian tubes.[104, 105]

The gonococci adhere to the mucosal cells of the endosalpinx, penetrate the epithelial cells, and produce primary destruction of the mucosa, with resulting partial or complete occlusion. Purulent exudate may escape from the patent fimbriated ends of the tubes, and pelvic peritonitis usually follows, with subsequent formation of "violin string" adhesions. Complications also include pyosalpinx, hydrosalpinx, and pelvic or tubo-ovarian abscess.

One of the most reliable symptoms of acute pelvic infection is bilateral lower abdominal pain, which may be constant or cramping, give a "bearing down" feeling, and increase with movement. Adnexal tenderness and pain elicited by gentle movement of the cervix result from stretching the broad ligament. Fever, nausea and vomiting, elevated erythrocyte sedimentation rate, and leukocytosis may also occur, depending on the severity of the infection. The pain probably is caused by distention of the fallopian tubes. Since the pain impulse is carried by autonomic nerves it may feel diffuse and deep and be difficult for the patient to localize.[106]

Gonococcal perihepatitis of Fitz-Hugh and Curtis results from the spread of gonococcal peritonitis into the upper abdominal cavity. The acute onset of severe right upper quadrant pleuritic pain and tenderness is accompanied by some degree of abdominal wall rigidity and fever. In some cases the gallbladder may initially not be seen on radiographic examination owing to the presence of dense pericholecystitis.[107, 108]

Gonococcal Proctitis

In homosexual males, gonococcal infection may involve the urethra, anorectal canal, or pharynx. In both males and females, rectal gonorrhea is usually the result of direct implantation. Over 90 per cent of males with this infection have had homosexual contact. In the female, direct spread to the anal area from infected vaginal discharge may also occur. The incidence of anal gonorrhea in infected females varies from 22 to 40 per cent, with the anorectum as the only site of involvement in 5 to 6 per cent.[109, 110]

At the time of diagnosis, about 65 per cent of males and 85 per cent of females with anorectal infection are asymptomatic. Others may experience anal itching or burning, sticky crusting, rectal fullness and painful defecation, tenesmus, low back pain, and mucopurulent or blood-tinged anal discharge.

The diagnosis is made by culturing N. gonorrhoeae in specimens taken from anorectal crypts on Thayer-Martin selective media, identifying those colonies of gram-negative diplococci as oxidase-positive.

Pharyngeal Gonorrhea

Prior to 1967,[111] only one case of proved oral gonococcal infection had been reported.[112] Oropharyngeal gonococcal infection occurs in approximately 20 per cent of homosexual men and 10 per cent of women who have practiced fellatio on a male with gonococcal urethral infection.[113] Correlation between symptoms and the presence of pharyngeal gonococci is inconsistent, since patients practicing fellatio complain of sore throat more often than those who do not, whether or not gonococci are present.

Most of the oral cavity is lined with stratified squamous epithelium. Columnar epithelium lines the secretory and excretory ducts of mucous, serous, and salivary glands and occurs in the nasopharynx and adjacent to the ostia of the eustachian tubes. Primary infection with gonococci probably occurs in these areas and then spreads to the rest of the oropharynx.[114]

The majority of gonococcal pharyngeal infections are asymptomatic and show no clinical signs of pharyngitis. However, some may have diffuse pharyngeal edema and redness, punctate pustules in the tonsillar area, or patchy erythema of the tonsillar area, palate, and uvula.

The diagnosis of gonococcal pharyngitis is made by culturing cells of the pharynx on Thayer-Martin medium. Unlike specimens obtained from anogenital sites, growth of gram-negative diplococci with oxidase-positive colonies is not adequate confirmation of gonococcal pharyngeal infection, since N. meningitis and N. lactamicus, relatively common inhabitants of the pharynx, also fulfill these criteria. Fermentation tests that produce acid in glucose but not in maltose, lactose, or sucrose are required to identify the gonococcus.

DISSEMINATED GONOCOCCAL INFECTION (Figs. 12–22 and 12–23)

Disseminated gonococcal infection results from hematogenous spread of gonococci from the site of primary infection. Morbidity ranges from a self-limited bacteremia to destructive arthritis, endocarditis, or meningitis.

Prolonged infectivity, associated with gonococcal pharyngitis,[113] anorectal gonorrhea,[115] or an asymptomatic genital tract source, increases the risk of dissemination. Pregnancy, particularly the second and third trimesters, may be a precipitating factor in 25 to 40 per cent of females with gonococcemia.[116] Menstruation is associated with both blood-borne dissemination and localized spread from a primary site.

The most common manifestation of gonococcemia is the gonococcal arthritis-dermatitis syndrome, which has become the leading cause of acute polyarthritis in young adults. Typically, it develops in two stages. In the first stage, positive blood cultures can be obtained in about 50 per cent of patients.[116] The patient is usually febrile, and skin lesions, or occasionally mucosal lesions[117] characteristic of septic vasculitis, appear. The skin lesions are

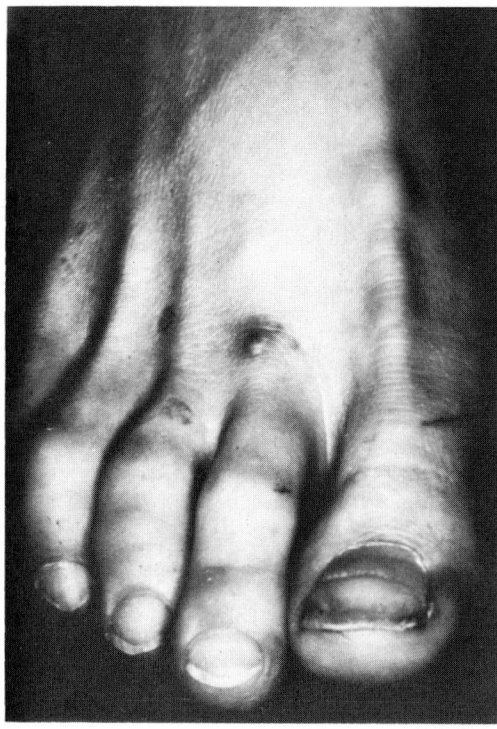

FIGURE 12–22 Hemorrhagic papule of disseminated gonococcal arthritis-dermatitis syndrome.

located principally over joints on the distal portions of the extremities, number from three to 20, and heal spontaneously in four to six days. They are usually small erythematous or hemorrhagic papules, petechiae, or vesicopustules on a hemorrhagic base, which may become necrotic. During the first two to three days, gonococci may be demonstrated by specific immunofluorescent staining

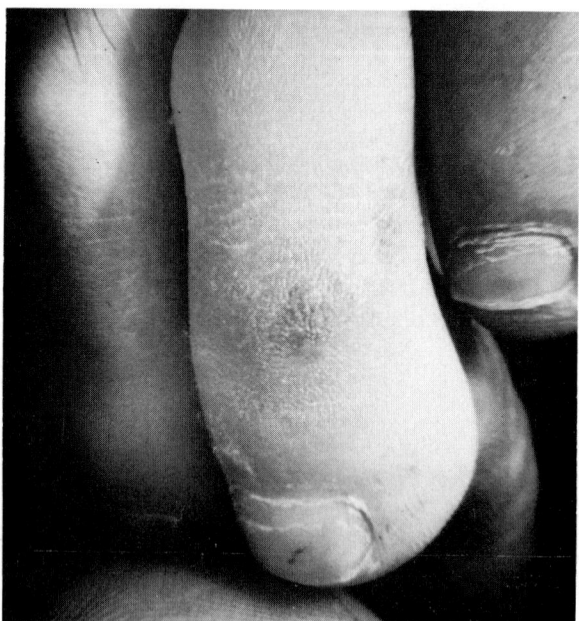

FIGURE 12–23 Maculopapule with necrotic center in patient with disseminated gonococcal arthritis-dermatitis syndrome. An erythematous macular lesion is nearby.

of material obtained from vesicopustular lesions.[116, 118, 119] Much less frequently, gonococci may be found with Gram-stained smear technique.[118]

A characteristic polyarticular arthritis and tenosynovitis may involve knees, ankles, wrists, elbows, and small joints of the hands and feet. Low back pain also may be present. The pain of migratory joint symptoms is often disproportionate to the objective findings, and the greatest tenderness may be related to a localized area of the joint that shows no evidence of effusion.[120] In this stage, minimal effusion occurs, and a positive culture is obtained from affected joints in less than 10 per cent of patients.

The second stage of disseminated infection evolves about one week later if treatment is delayed. Blood cultures by now usually become negative, and no new skin lesions appear. The polyarthritis and periarticular inflammation disappear, but a purulent synovial effusion with septic arthritis develops in one or two joints. *N. gonorrhoeae* can be recovered in about half of these patients, but a negative culture of synovial fluid does not exclude the diagnosis of gonococcal arthritis. In some cases, gonococci in synovial fluid may be demonstrated by Gram or immunofluorescent stain.

Sometimes, a patient may present features of both stages, such as active skin lesions associated with a purulent synovitis that is positive on culture. From a pragmatic viewpoint, a diagnosis of gonococcal arthritis is justified if three criteria are met: (a) acute arthritis in one or more joints, (b) positive culture for *N. gonorrhoeae* from the endocervix, urethra, pharynx, rectum, joint, or blood, and (c) prompt therapeutic response to penicillin.

Although Thayer-Martin and Transgrow selective media are appropriate for culture of material from sites that are heavily colonized by mixed flora, strains of *N. gonorrhoeae* may be inhibited by the concentration of vancomycin or trimethoprim used in these media. Therefore, plain chocolate agar should be used to culture synovial fluid or exudate of skin lesions of disseminated gonococcal infection. Clinical virulence, manifested by the capacity to cause disseminated gonococcal infection, may be linked to low antibiotic resistance in a specific strain or strains of *N. gonorrhoea*.

TREATMENT OF DISSEMINATED GONOCOCCAL INFECTION

The recommended treatment is 6 to 10 million units of aqueous crystalline penicillin G, given intravenously daily for two to three days (or until acute symptoms subside), followed by oral ampicillin in doses of 2 gm daily for 10 to 14 days. A rapid therapeutic response to conventional high-dose penicillin therapy is useful in confirming the diagnosis of gonococcal arthritis and dermatitis. The occasional occurrence of endocarditis or meningitis associated with gonococcemia argues against the use of lower penicillin dosages.[121] Overt endocarditis or meningitis requires much longer courses of high-dose intravenous therapy.

It has been suggested that the administration of intravenous penicillin in high doses may not be necessary for effective treatment.[122] An alternative treatment program consists of 4.8 million units of aqueous procaine penicillin G given intramuscularly with 1 gm probenecid orally, followed by 2.4 million units of aqueous procaine penicillin G IM daily for 10 to 14 days (Table 12–4).

In the presence of penicillin allergy, an initial oral dose of 1.5 gm

TABLE 12-4 TREATMENT OF UNCOMPLICATED GONORRHEA

Medication	Schedule
Aqueous procaine penicillin G (APPG)	4,800,000 APPG IM (one-half dose in each buttock), plus 1 gm probenecid orally one-half hour before or at the time of the injection.
Tetracycline	1.5 gm (6 capsules of 250 mg each) tetracycline orally stat. Thereafter, 500 mg tetracycline every 6 hours for a total of 9.5 gm.
Spectinomycin*	2 gm IM
Ampicillin	1 gm probenecid orally, followed in one-half hour by 3.5 gm ampicillin. Thereafter, 500 mg probenecid after 6, 12, and 18 hours.
Doxycycline	200 mg doxycycline orally stat. Thereafter, 100 mg doxycycline every 12 hours for a total of 900 mg.
Erythromycin	1.5 gm erythromycin orally stat. Thereafter, 500 mg erythromycin orally every 6 hours for a total of 9.5 gm.
Trimethoprim plus sulfamethoxazole (Bactrim, Septra)	4 tablets every 12 hours for 2 days. Total: 16 tablets

*Note: If penicillinase-producing strain of gonococci is encountered, use spectinomycin as first alternative.

tetracycline, followed by 2 gm tetracycline daily for 10 to 12 days, can be used to treat disseminated gonococcal infection. With these regimens, most patients become afebrile within 24 hours and within three days show significant reduction in joint inflammation. Following treatment, "test of cure" cultures are required to determine whether the initial focus of infection in the pharynx, urogenital tract, or rectum has been eradicated.

PREPUBESCENT GONOCOCCAL INFECTION

This disorder is manifest in girls as a diffuse vaginitis with secondary vulvitis (often associated with dysuria) labial redness and swelling, and purulent discharge. Infrequently, it may be complicated by endocervicitis, salpingitis, and peritonitis. A Gram stain of the discharge demonstrating gram-negative intracytoplasmic diplococci may be helpful, but a positive culture on Thayer-Martin selective medium is necessary for diagnosis. Urogenital gonococcal infection in boys follows the pattern of gonorrhea in the adult male. Cultures from the pharynx and anorectum also may be indicated in many of these cases.

GONOCOCCAL OCULAR INFECTION

Along with the rising incidence of gonorrhea, there has been an increase in reported instances of primary gonococcal ocular infection in neonates, teenagers, and young adults.

Gonococcal conjunctivitis results from the direct inoculation of the gonococcus onto the conjunctiva either by the fingers, or by contact of the infant's conjunctiva with the infected cervix at birth. Unlike the bulbar conjunctiva, which contains stratified squamous epithelium, the tarsal conjunctiva is composed of columnar epithelium and is therefore vulnerable to primary gonococcal infection.

After an incubation period of two to four days, a purulent conjunctival discharge develops, initially in one eye, with associated edema and hyperemia of the bulbar and tarsal conjunctiva. Without treatment, the disease may become bilateral and may progress rapidly to corneal ulceration, iridocyclitis, and blindness. Other types of ophthalmia can also occur, such as inclusion conjunctivitis caused by *Chlamydia*. Gonococcal conjunctivitis in the neonate or in older individuals can usually be diagnosed by Gram stain of the purulent exudate. However, cultures are essential for confirmation.

The incidence of gonococcal ophthalmia neonatorum can be reduced by at least 90 per cent with the prophylactic Credé technique of instilling 1 per cent solution of silver nitrate eyedrops into the conjunctival sac. Treatment of gonococcal ophthalmia in the infant or older patient requires hospitalization and consultation with an ophthalmologist.

REFERENCES

1. Ducrey, A.: Experimentelle Untersuchungen über den Ansteckungsstoff des weichen Schankers und über die Bubonen. Monatschr. Prakt. Derm., *9*:387, 1889.
2. Tomasczewski, E.: Bakteriologische Untersuchungen über den Erreger des Ulcus Molle. Z. Hyg. Infektions KR, *42*:327, 1903.
3. Asin, J.: Chancroid: Report of 1402 cases. Am. J. Syph., *36*:483, 1952.
4. Ajello, G., Deacon, W. E., Paul, L., and Walls, K. W.: Nutritional studies of virulent strain of *Hemophilus ducreyi*. J. Bacteriol., *72*:802, 1956.
5. Sullivan, M.: Chancroid. Am. J. Syph., *24*:482, 1940.
6. Strakosch, E. A., Kendell, H. W., Craig, R., and Schwemlein, G.: Clinical and laboratory investigation of 370 cases of chancroid. J. Invest. Dermatol., *6*:95, 1945.
7. Hart, G.: Chancroid, Donovanosis, and Lymphogranuloma Venereum. CDC 75–8302. Washington, D.C., U.S. Dept. of Health, Education and Welfare, 1964.
8. Beeson, P. B., and Heyman, A.: Studies on chancroid: Efficiency of the cultural method of diagnosis. Am. J. Syph., *29*:633, 1945.
9. Deacon, W. E., Albritton, C. C., Olansky, S., and Kaplan, W.: A simple procedure for the isolation and identification of *Hemophilus ducreyi*. J. Invest. Dermatol., *26*:399, 1956.
10. Borchardt, K. A., and Hoke, A. W.: Simplified laboratory technique for the diagnosis of chancroid. Arch. Dermatol., *102*:188, 1970.
11. McLeod, K.: Serpiginous ulceration of the genitals. Indian Med. Gaz., *17*:121, 1882.
12. Donovan, C.: Ulcerating granuloma of the pudenda. Indian Med. Gaz., *40*:411, 1905.
13. Grindon, J.: Granuloma inguinale tropicum: A report of three cases. J. Cutan. Dis., *31*:236, 1913.
14. McIntosh, J. A.: A study of the etiology of granuloma inguinale. J. Tenn. Med. Assoc., *19*:190, 1926.
15. Anderson, K.: The cultivation from granuloma inguinale of a microorganism having the characteristics of Donovan bodies in the yolk-sac of chick embryos. Science, *97*:560, 1943.
16. Davis, C. M., and Collins, C.: Granuloma inguinale: An ultrastructural study of *Calymmatobacterium granulomatis*. J. Invest. Dermatol., *53*:315, 1969.
17. Goldberg, J., and Bernstein, R.: Two cases of perianal granuloma inguinale in male homosexuals. Br. J. Vener. Dis., *40*:137, 1964.
18. Marmell, M.: Donovanosis of the anus in the male. Br. J. Vener. Dis., *34*:213, 1958.
19. Davis, C. M.: Granuloma inguinale. JAMA, *211*:632, 1970.
20. Rajam, R., and Rangiah, P.: Donovanosis. WHO Monograph Series #24, 1954.
21. Arnell, R. E., and Potekin, J.: Granuloma inguinale of the cervix. Am. J. Obstet. Gynecol., *39*:626, 1940.
22. Greenblatt, R. B., Pund, E., Sanderson, E., et al.: Management of Chancroid, Granuloma

Inguinale and Lymphogranuloma Venereum in General Practice. USPHS publication #255. Washington, D.C., U.S. Dept. of Health, Education and Welfare, 1958.
23. Lal, S., and Nicholas, C.: Epidemiological and clinical features in 165 cases of granuloma inguinale. Br. J. Vener. Dis., 46:461, 1970.
24. Pariser, H., and Beerman, H.: Granuloma inguinale. Am. J. Med. Sci., 208:547, 1944.
25. Greenblatt, R. B., Torpin, R., and Pund, E.: Extragenital granuloma inguinale. Arch. Dermatol., 38:358, 1938.
26. Garg, B. R., Lal, S., Bedi, B., et al.: Donovanosis (granuloma inguinale) of the oral cavity. Br. J. Vener. Dis., 51:136, 1975.
27. Greenblatt, R. B., Dienst, R., and Baldwin, K.: Lymphogranuloma venereum and granuloma inguinale. Med. Clin. North Am., 43:1493, 1959.
28. Weiner, A., Gaynon, I., and Osherwitz, M.: Granuloma inguinale of the eyelid. Am. J. Ophthalmol., 26:13, 1943.
29. Halty, M.: Les formes cliniques du granuloma venerien. Ann. Dermatol. Syphiligr., 4:1101, 1933.
30. Cherny, W., Jones, C., and Peete, C.: Disseminated granuloma inguinale and its relationship to granuloma of the cervix and pregnancy. Am. J. Obstet. Gynecol., 74:597, 1957.
31. Sieber, P. E.: Granuloma inguinale with bone involvement. Am. J. Roentgenol. Radium Ther. Nucl. Med., 95:515, 1965.
32. Palik, E., and Schenken, J.: Disseminated granuloma venereum. Am. J. Clin. Pathol., 15:419, 1945.
33. Packer, H., Turner, H., and Dulaney, A.: Granuloma inguinale of the vagina and cervix uteri with bone metastases. JAMA, 136:327, 1948.
34. Gould, W. M., and Clark, E.: Granuloma inguinale. Calif. Med., 104:392, 1966.
35. Stewart, D. B.: The gynecological lesions of lymphogranuloma venereum and granuloma inguinale. Med. Clin. North Am., 48:773, 1964.
36. Alexander, L. J., and Shields, T.: Squamous cell carcinoma of the vulva secondary to granuloma inguinale. Arch. Dermatol., 67:395, 1953.
37. Wallace, W.: A Treatise on Venereal Disease and its Varieties. London, Burgess and Hill, 1833, p. 371.
38. Durand, M., Nicolas, J., and Favre, M.: Lymphogranulomatose inguinale: Subaiguë d'origine génitale probable, peut-être vénérienne. Bull. Mem. Soc. Med. Hosp. Paris, 35:274, 1913.
39. Frei, W.: Eine Neue Hautreaktion bei Lymphogranuloma Inguinale. Wochenschr. Klin., 4:2148, 1925.
40. Halberstaedter, L., and von Prowazek, S.: Über Zelleinschlüsse Parasitärer Natur beim Trachom. Arb. K. Gesundheitsamtes, 26:44, 1907.
41. Rake, G. W., McKee, C. M., and Shaffer, M. F.: Agent of lymphogranuloma venereum in the yolk-sac of the developing chick embryo. Proc. Soc. Exp. Biol. Med., 43:332, 1940.
42. Tang, F., Chang, H., Huang, Y., and Wang, K.: Isolation of trachoma virus in chick embryo. J. Hyg. Epidemiol. Microbiol. Immunol., 1:109, 1957.
43. Bedson, S. P.: Observations bearing on the antigenic composition of psittacosis virus. Br. J. Exp. Pathol., 17:109, 1936.
44. Bedson, S. P.: The nature of the elementary bodies in psittacosis. Br. J. Exp. Pathol., 13:65, 1932.
45. Bedson, S. P.: Immunological studies with the virus of psittacosis. Br. J. Exp. Pathol., 14:162, 1933.
46. Chang, R. S.: Attributes of microorganisms. In: Hoeprich, P. D. (ed.): Infectious Diseases. New York, Harper & Row, 1972.
47. Martin, C., and Bacon, H. E.: Lymphogranuloma venereum. Int. Clin., 4:250, 1935.
48. Lee, H., and Staley, R.: Inflammatory strictures of the rectum and their relation to lymphogranuloma inguinale. Ann. Surg., 100:486, 1934.
49. Gray, H., and Goss, C. M.: Anatomy of the Human Body. 29th ed. Philadelphia, Lea & Febiger, 1973.
50. Sigel, M. M. (ed.): Lymphogranuloma Venereum: Epidemiological, Clinical, Surgical, and Therapeutic Aspects. Miami, University of Miami Press, 1962.
51. Coutts, W.: Lymphogranuloma venereum lesions of the eye. Am. J. Ophthalmol., 25:916, 1942.
52. Curth, W., and Curth, H.: Chronic conjunctivitis due to the virus of venereal lymphogranuloma. JAMA, 115:445, 1940.
53. Thygeson, P.: Observations on uveitis associated with viral disease. Trans. Am. Ophthalmol. Soc., 55:333, 1957.
54. Becker, L. E.: Lymphogranuloma venereum. Int. J. Dermatol., 15(1):26, 1976.
55. Gerloff, R. K., and Watson, R.: The radioisotope precipitation test for psittacosis group antibody. Am. J. Ophthalmol., 63:1492, 1967.
56. Magruder, G. B., Gordon, F., Quan, A., and Dressler, H.: Accidental human trachoma with rapid diagnosis by a cell-culture technique. Arch. Ophthalmol., 69:300, 1963.

57. Darougar, S., Kinnison, J., and Jones, B.: Simplified irradiated McCoy cell culture for isolation of *Chlamydia*. *In:* Nichols, R. L. (ed.): Trachoma and Related Disorders. Excerpta Medica, 1971, p. 63.
58. Darougar, S., Jones, B., Kinnison, J., and Vaughan-Jackson, J.: Chlamydia infection: Advances in the diagnostic isolation of *Chlamydia*, including TRIC agent, from the eye, genital tract, and rectum. Br. J. Vener. Dis., *48*:416, 1972.
59. Smith, T. F., Weed, L. A., Segura, J., et al.: Isolation of *Chlamydia* from patients with urethritis. Mayo Clin. Proc., *50*:105, 1975.
60. Wang, S. P., and Grayston, J. T.: Classification of TRIC and related strains with micro-immunofluorescence. *In*: Nichols, R. L. (ed.): Trachoma and Related Disorders. Excerpta Medica, 1971, p. 305.
61. Dwyer, R., Treharne, J., Jones, B., and Herring, J.: Results of micro-immunofluorescence tests for the detection of type-specific antibody in certain chlamydial infections. Br. J. Vener. Dis., *48*:452, 1972.
62. Treharne, J., Davey, S., Gray, S., and Jones, B.: Immunological classification of TRIC agents and of some recently isolated lymphogranuloma venereum agents by the micro-immunofluorescence test. Br. J. Vener. Dis., *48*:18, 1972.
63. Brodie, B. C.: Pathological and Surgical Observations on Diseases of the Joints. London, Longman, 1818.
64. Reiter, H.: Über Eine Bisher Unerkannte Spirochaeten Infektion. Deutsch Med. Wochenschr., *42*:1535, 1916.
65. Vaughan-Jackson, J. D., Dunlop, E., Darougar, S., et al.: Chlamydial infection: Results of tests for *Chlamydia* in patients suffering from acute Reiter's disease compared with results of tests of the genital tract and rectum in patients with ocular infection due to TRIC agent. Br. J. Vener. Dis., *48*:445, 1972.
66. Schachter, J.: Isolation of *Bedsonia* from human arthritis and abortion tissues. Am. J. Ophthalmol., *63*:1082, 1967.
67. Schachter, J., Barnes, M., Jones, J., et al.: Isolation of *Bedsonia* from the joints of patients with Reiter's syndrome. Proc. Soc. Exp. Biol. Med., *122*:283, 1966.
68. Dunlop, E., Freedman, A., Garland, J., et al.: Infection by *Bedsonia* and the possibility of spurious isolation: Genital infection, disease of the eye, Reiter's disease. Am. J. Ophthalmol., *63*:1073, 1967.
69. Barwell, C., Dunlop, E., and Race, J.: Results of complement-fixation and intradermal tests for *Bedsonia* in genital infection, disease of the eye, Reiter's disease. Am. J. Ophthalmol., *63*: 1527, 1967.
70. Ostler, H., Dawson, C., Schachter, J., and Engleman, E.: Reiter's syndrome. Am. J. Ophthalmol., *71*:986, 1971.
71. Dwyer, R., Treharne, J., Jones, B., and Herring, J.: Chlamydial infection: Results of micro-immunofluorescence tests for the detection of type-specific antibody in certain chlamydial infections. Br. J. Vener. Dis., *48*:452, 1972.
72. Ostler, H., Schachter, J., and Dawson, C.: Ocular infection of rabbits with a *Bedsonia* isolated from a patient with Reiter's syndrome. Invest. Ophthalmol., *9*:256, 1970.
73. Grimble, A.: Auto-immunity in Reiter's syndrome. Br. J. Vener. Dis., *39*:246, 1963.
74. Lawrence, J. S.: Family survey of Reiter's disease. Br. J. Vener. Dis., *50*:140, 1974.
75. Brewerton, D., Caffrey, M., Nicholls, A., et al.: Reiter's disease and HL–A27. Lancet, *2*:996, 1973.
76. Aho, K., Ahvonen, P., Lassus, A., et al.: HL-antigen 27 and reactive arthritis. Lancet, *2*:157, 1973.
77. Arnett, F., McClusky, O., and Schacter, B.: Incomplete Reiter's syndrome: Discriminating features and HL–A–W27 in diagnosis. Ann. Intern. Med., *84*:8, 1976.
78. Morris, R., Metzger, A., Bluestone, R., and Terasaki, P.: HL–A–W27—A clue to the diagnosis and pathogenesis of Reiter's syndrome. N. Engl. J. Med., *290*:554, 1974.
79. McClusky, O., Lordon, R., and Arnett, F.: HL–A27 in Reiter's syndrome and psoriatic arthritis: A genetic factor in disease susceptibility and expression. J. Rheumatol., *1*:263, 1974.
80. Brewerton, D., Hart, F., and Nicholls, A.: Ankylosing spondylitis and HL–A27. Lancet, *1*:904, 1973.
81. Moss, I. S.: Reiter's disease in childhood. Br. J. Vener. Dis., *40*:166, 1964.
82. Schofield, C. B. S.: Sexually Transmitted Diseases. 2nd ed. New York, Longman, 1975.
83. Pekin, T. J., Malinin, T., and Zvaifler, N.: Unusual synovial fluid findings in Reiter's syndrome. Ann. Intern. Med., *66*:677, 1967.
84. Grainger, R. G., and Nicol, C. S.: Pelvic infection as a cause of bilateral sacro-iliac arthritis and ankylosing spondylitis. Br. J. Vener. Dis., *35*:92, 1959.
85. Reckless, J. P.: Reiter's syndrome with parotitis in the female. Br. J. Vener. Dis., *48*:207, 1972.
86. Collins, P.: Aortic incompetence and active myocarditis in Reiter's disease. Br. J. Vener. Dis., *48*:300, 1972.
87. Catterall, R. D., Rooney, K. J., and Kirby, B.: Neuralgic amyotrophy in Reiter's disease. Br. J. Vener. Dis., *41*:62, 1965.

88. Neisser, A.: Die Mikrokokken der Gonorrhoe; referirende Mittheilung. Dtsh. Med. Wochenschr., 8:279, 1882.
89. Morse, S. A., Stein, S., and Hines, J.: Glucose metabolism in *Neisseria gonorrhoeae*. J. Bacteriol., 120:702, 1974.
90. Thayer, J. D., and Martin, J. E.: A selective medium for the cultivation of *N. gonorrhoeae* and *N. meningitidis*. Public Health Rep., 79:49, 1964.
91. Kellogg, D. S., Peacock, W. L., Deacon, W. E., et al.: *Neisseria gonorrhoeae:* Virulence genetically linked to clonal variation. J. Bacteriol., 85:1274, 1963.
92. Buchanan, T. M., and Gotschlich, E. C.: Correlation between gonococcal colony morphology and infectivity for the chick embryo. J. Exp. Med., 137:196, 1973.
93. Thongthai, C., and Sawyer, W.: Resistance to phagocytosis and colonial morphology of *N. gonorrhoeae*. Bacteriol. Proc., 71:110, 1971.
94. Holmes, K.: Gonococcal infection: Clinical, epidemiologic, and laboratory perspectives. Adv. Intern. Med., 19:259, 1974.
95. Buchanan, T. M., Swanson, J., Holmes, K., et al.: Quantitative determination of antibody to gonococcal pili. J. Clin. Invest., 52(11):2896, 1973.
96. Catlin, B. W.: Nutritional profiles of *N. gonorrhoeae, N. meningitidis* and *N. lactamica* in chemically defined media and the use of growth requirements for gonococcal typing. J. Infect. Dis., 128:178, 1973.
97. Morello, J., Lerner, S., and Bohnhoff, M.: Characteristics of atypical *N. gonorrhoeae* from disseminated and localized infections. Infect. Immun., 13:1510, 1976.
98. Tauber, H., and Garson, W.: Isolation of lipopolysaccharide endotoxin. J. Biol. Chem., 234:1391, 1959.
99. Ward, M., and Watt, P.: Adherence of *N. gonorrhoeae* to urethral mucosal cells: An electron-microscopic study of human gonorrhea. J. Infect. Dis., 126:601, 1972.
100. Pariser, H., Farmer, A., and Marino, A.: Asymptomatic gonorrhea in the male. South. Med. J., 57:688, 1964.
101. Handsfield, H., Lipman, T., Harnisch, J., et al.: Asymptomatic gonorrhea in men. N. Engl. J. Med., 290:117, 1974.
102. Eschenbach, D. A., and Holmes, K.: Acute pelvic inflammatory disease: Current concepts of pathogenesis, etiology, and management. Clin. Obstet. Gynecol., 18(1):35, 1975.
103. Noonan, A., and Adams, J.: Gonorrhea screening in an urban hospital family planning program. Am. J. Public Health, 64:701, 1974.
104. James, A., Knox, J., and Williams, R.: Attachment of gonococci to sperm. Br. J. Vener. Dis., 52:128, 1976.
105. James-Holmquest, A., Swanson, J., Buchanan, T., et al.: Differential attachment by piliated and nonpiliated *N. gonorrhoeae* to human sperm. Infect. Immun., 9:897, 1974.
106. Rees, E., and Annela, E.: Gonococcal salpingitis. Br. J. Vener. Dis., 45:205, 1969.
107. Reichert, J., and Valle, R.: Fitz-Hugh-Curtis syndrome. JAMA, 236:266, 1976.
108. Vickers, F., and Maloney, P.: Gonococcal perihepatitis. Arch. Intern. Med., 114:120, 1964.
109. Pariser, H.: Asymptomatic gonorrhea. Med. Clin. North Am., 56(5):1127, 1972.
110. Dans, P. E.: Gonococcal anogenital infection. Clin. Obstet. Gynecol., 18(1):103, 1975.
111. Fiumara, N. J., Wise, H., and Many, M.: Gonorrheal pharyngitis. N. Engl. J. Med., 276:1248, 1967.
112. Frazer, A., and Menton, J.: Gonococcal stomatitis. Br. Med. J., 1:1020, 1931.
113. Wiesner, P., Tronca, E., Bonin, P., et al.: Clinical spectrum of pharyngeal gonococcal infection. N. Engl. J. Med., 288:181, 1973.
114. Ratnatunga, C.: Gonococcal pharyngitis. Br. J. Vener. Dis., 48:184, 1972.
115. Handsfield, H. H.: Disseminated gonococcal infection. Clin. Obstet. Gynecol., 18(1):131, 1975.
116. Holmes, K. K., Counts, G., and Beaty, H.: Disseminated gonococcal infection. Ann. Intern. Med., 74:979, 1971.
117. Cowan, L.: Gonococcal ulceration of the tongue in the gonococcal dermatitis syndrome. Br. J. Vener. Dis., 45:228, 1969.
118. Tronca, E., Handsfield, H., Wiesner, P., and Holmes, K.: Demonstration of *N. gonorrhoeae* with fluorescent antibody in patients with disseminated gonococcal infection. J. Infect. Dis., 129:583, 1974.
119. Barr, J., and Danielsson, D.: Septic gonococcal dermatitis. Br. Med. J., 1:482, 1971.
120. Bennett, R. M.: Disseminated gonococcal infection: The problems of diagnosis and management. J. Reprod. Med., 11:99, 1973.
121. Wiesner, P., Handsfield, H., and Holmes, K.: Low antibiotic resistance of gonococci causing disseminated infection. N. Engl. J. Med., 288:1221, 1973.
122. Trentham, D., McCravey, J., and Masi, A.: Low-dose penicillin for gonococcal arthritis. JAMA, 236:2410, 1976.

13

FUNGAL INFECTIONS

PRUDENCE B. STEWARDSON-KRIEGER, M.D.
and NANCY B. ESTERLY, M.D.

INTRODUCTION

Some bacterial infections cause a reaction in the skin similar to that seen in many fungal infections. The fungal-like bacterial skin infections include diseases caused by the *Corynebacterium* species termed "diphtheroids," and infections caused by certain members of the bacterial order Actinomycetales. Most of these conditions occur with greater frequency in adolescence and adulthood than in infancy and childhood.

Mycotic diseases of the skin and subcutaneous tissue are often classified according to the depth at which they involve the integument and the type of response that they elicit in the host. The first group of such diseases is caused by a number of heterogeneous species of fungi and consists of mild superficial infections of the stratum corneum that do not provoke an inflammatory response in the host. These include tinea nigra, the black and white piedras, and tinea versicolor.

The second and more commonly encountered group of fungal skin infections is caused by the dermatophytes. These organisms also remain localized to the stratum corneum but usually elicit an inflammatory response in the infected host. The names of the individual dermatophytoses contain the word tinea (Latin for moth) followed by the Latin term for the anatomical region infected (e.g., tinea pedis).

The third group of mycotic soft tissue infections includes diseases caused by agents that primarily invade the subcutaneous tissue by inoculation through a damaged epidermis. Of these rarely encountered infections, only sporotrichosis and chromoblastomycosis will be discussed.

The last group of mycotic diseases included in this chapter will be classified under the heading "opportunistic infections" and will include candidal disease (although superficial candidiasis may also occur in persons who are not debilitated). The number of normally non-pathogenic mycotic species that can be opportunistic invaders of immunodeficient patients is large, but this chapter will be limited to candidiasis, aspergillosis, and phycomycosis. Some systemic mycotic conditions, such as North American blastomycosis, will not be discussed because they rarely affect the adolescent. A more complete discussion of mycological characteristics of these diseases may be found in a textbook of medical mycology.[1]

DIPHTHEROID SKIN INFECTIONS

The genus of gram-positive bacilli called *Corynebacterium* includes the species *Corynebacterium diphtheriae* and a large number of ordinarily nonpathogenic species called diphtheroids, which are the predominant constituents of the normal skin flora. The cutaneous diphtheroids are a very heterogeneous group of organisms with widely varying nutritional and biochemical characteristics, which makes their precise classification both difficult and controversial.[2] The specific skin infections caused by these agents are usually minor and harmless and are more often seen in adolescence and adulthood than in childhood.

ERYTHRASMA

Erythrasma is a benign, chronic, superficial infection of the stratum corneum caused by the fluorescent filamentous diphtheroid *Corynebacterium minutissimum*.[3] It is characterized by the presence of brownish-red, dry, well-defined, scaly-to-shiny macular patches that vary widely in size and cause only minimal pruritus (Plate VII–A). These patches occur most frequently in moist intertriginous areas, such as the groin, axillae, and toe webs, but they can become more generalized, particularly in obese individuals living in tropical climates. The commonest sites of involvement are the genitocrural region and the toe web spaces of adult males, where erythrasma may coexist with tinea cruris and tinea pedis.[4,5]

The incidence of erythrasma increases with age, being unusual in childhood and relatively common in adolescence.[6,7] Erythrasma is transmissible and can become endemic in confined populations.[8,9] However, the causative agent is part of the normal cutaneous flora in a substantial portion of the general population who show no evidence of the disease.[3,4]

Laboratory Findings. The etiological organisms and the lesions of erythrasma fluoresce a bright coral-red color when examined under a Wood's light. The organisms appear as gram-positive, pleomorphic coccobacilli with numerous filamentous forms in a Gram-stained smear. Although the causative agent can be grown on routine laboratory media, cultures are not helpful or necessary for the diagnosis of the disease.

Differential Diagnosis. Erythrasma may be confused with the dermatophyte infections with which it may coexist. Erythrasma, however, does not elicit an inflammatory response in the host and does not progress to vesiculation. It must also be differentiated from tinea versicolor, which is not erythematous and generally occurs on the upper trunk rather than in the intertriginous areas. The moist, macerated lesions of intertrigo, which become secondarily infected with common skin bacteria or fungi, occur in the same sites as erythrasma but are different in appearance. Erythrasma is easily distinguished from other entities by its characteristic fluorescence under a Wood's light.

Treatment. The lesions of erythrasma may respond to local therapy with a number of topical agents, including tolnaftate and Whitfield's ointment.[10, 11] Severe or chronic erythrasma usually requires the use of oral systemic antibiotic therapy. Erythromycin is the drug of choice,[3] although tetracycline is also effective. The incidence of the disease is reduced by frequent thorough cleansing of affected areas with an antibacterial soap.[12]

TRICHOMYCOSIS AXILLARIS

Trichomycosis axillaris is a relatively innocuous infection of the hair shaft, caused by keratinophilic diphtheroids, most commonly *Corynebacterium tenuis*.[13] The infection, which is usually in the axillae and occasionally in the pubic area, is characterized by the presence of tiny nodules distributed along the hair shaft. These nodules are most often yellow but may be red or black.[13] The disease is most prevalent in patients with hyperhidrosis, particularly in warm, humid weather. Patients feel no discomfort but frequently complain of offensive axillary odor and staining of light-colored clothing. The hair becomes brittle and dull, and actual damage to the hair shaft can be seen under the electron microscope.[14]

This infection occurs only following puberty, with the advent of axillary and pubic hair, but thereafter is found with equal frequency in all age groups.[15] The disease is apparently quite common, and in one study of various populations, it occurred in 27 to 42 per cent of adult males.[15] It is considerably less common in adult females, probably owing to the practice of shaving axillary hair. The use of a deodorant may deter its development.[15]

Laboratory Findings. The disease can often be diagnosed clinically, but a microscopic examination of a potassium hydroxide (KOH) preparation of an infected hair shaft will reveal the causative organisms, which appear as fine, short coccobacilli. These bacteria may be cultured on special laboratory media, but cultures are not necessary for diagnosis of the infection.

Differential Diagnosis. Trichomycosis axillaris may be distinguished from white and black piedra by microscopic examination of a KOH preparation of the hair shaft. The yellow variety of the infection also often gives a golden fluorescence under Wood's light, while piedra does not. Infection of the hair shaft with a dermatophyte fungus and infestation with lice may both be confused initially with trichomycosis axillaris but should be easy to differentiate.

Treatment. The infection may be treated by shaving the axillary hair, improving hygienic measures, and using a deodorant. The disease tends to recur repeatedly in some individuals.

PITTED KERATOLYSIS

Pitted keratolysis is a common infection of the stratum corneum of the plantar surface of the foot. It is thought to be caused most often by a species of

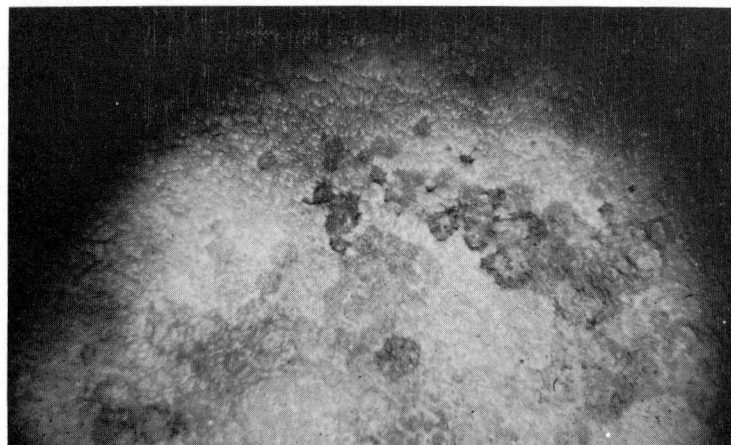

FIGURE 13-1 Pitted keratolysis on the sole.

keratinophilic diphtheroid,[16] but the identity of the etiological agent remains controversial. The infection is characterized by the presence of irregularly shaped superficial erosions of various sizes, which are usually mild and asymptomatic but may become quite severe and debilitating (Fig. 13-1). Secondary infection with other bacteria may complicate the clinical picture. In mild cases, hyperhidrosis occurs, but in more severe disease the lesions become anhidrotic. When the disease becomes extensive, patients complain of exquisitely tender feet and the inability to bear weight. As with most diphtheroid infections, it is more common in warm, moist weather and in tropical climates, especially in persons who wear occlusive footgear.[17] The disease can occur at any age but has been described primarily in adults.

Laboratory Findings. A KOH preparation of scrapings from the lesions will frequently reveal filamentous coccobacilli. However, the diagnosis may be made clinically.

Treatment. The infection may occasionally be severe enough to require hospitalization.[17] Topical therapy with 20 to 40 per cent formalin in Aquaphor has been shown to be effective.[5] In mild or asymptomatic disease, discontinuing the use of occlusive footgear may lead to resolution of the lesions without medical therapy.

ACTINOMYCETES INFECTIONS

The bacteria that belong to the order Actinomycetales include both the mycobacteria and the agents commonly referred to as the actinomycetes. The two most frequent agents of human actinomycetes infection, the anaerobic *Actinomyces* and the aerobic *Nocardia,* were once thought to be closely related to the fungi because of their tendency to grow in branches, or mycelia, in culture and in infected tissue. However, both their structural composition and their susceptibility to commonly used antibacterial agents have established them as true bacteria. They are gram-positive, filamentous organisms that tend to grow slowly and to break into segments that resemble pleomorphic coccobacilli.

Neither actinomycosis nor nocardiosis is particularly common, and both are found more frequently in debilitated or immunodeficient persons. Although these diseases can occur at any age, most of the reported cases are in adults. Primary cutaneous infection is rare,[18, 19] and involvement of the skin and subcutaneous tissues is generally a result of contiguous spread from other sites or of secondary infection of injured skin and subcutaneous tissue.

ACTINOMYCOSIS

Actinomycosis is a chronic infection occurring most often in the cervicofacial, thoracic, and abdominal regions. It is caused commonly by the anaerobe *Actinomyces israelii* (a frequent resident of the dental and tonsillar crypts of the mouth) and rarely by other species of *Actinomyces*. It is characterized by suppuration, painful induration, and the formation of multiple draining sinuses.

Cervicofacial actinomycosis begins when the infecting organism invades a traumatized mucous membrane in the oral cavity, often in persons with poor oral hygiene and carious teeth. Hard, slowly enlarging, mildly tender, erythematous nodules appear on the jaw, then suppurate centrally, and subsequently discharge their purulent contents onto the skin surface through sinus tracts. Patients often exhibit trismus but experience only mild pain and rarely develop signs of systemic illness. The infection may remain localized but if left untreated shows a propensity for invading bone and may spread contiguously to involve other tissues, such as the tongue, the middle ear, the eye, and the meninges.

Actinomyces infection of the thoracic region begins as a pulmonary infection, most often secondary to aspiration of the organism from the oropharynx. Initially, the patient is mildly to moderately ill. The disease progresses slowly, with the eventual formation of multiple small pulmonary abscesses and the contiguous spread of infection through the pleura and the tissues of the thorax. Subsequently, multiple draining sinus tracts appear on the chest wall. By this time, the patient is chronically ill.

In abdominal actinomycosis, the initial infection usually develops in the ileum, the colon, or the appendix. The disease can spread contiguously to involve a number of organs, including the kidney and the liver, and often secondarily involves the abdominal wall, causing multiple draining sinuses to appear on the surface as in the cervicofacial and thoracic forms of the disease.

Primary *Actinomyces* infection of other body sites, including the urinary tract, the central nervous system, and the bones and joints, occurs infrequently. Anorectal infection, giving rise to recurrent draining fistulas in ano, may be more common than is generally recognized.[20]

Localized *Actinomyces* infection of the skin can occur and causes a clinical syndrome known as mycetoma. However, mycetoma is more often caused by one of many other actinomycetes and fungal agents.[21] This condition is rare in the United States but prevalent in many tropical regions. It occurs most often on the feet or ankles of persons who work barefoot. It is characterized by the appearance of chronic, slowly enlarging, painless subcutaneous nodules that develop central suppuration and form multiple draining sinuses. The infection usually remains localized to the extremity, often involving connective tissue and bone as well as the skin and subcutaneous tissues in the infected area.

Laboratory Findings. The purulent exudate of *Actinomyces* infections often contains tiny yellowish-white particles called "sulfur granules," which are composed of small tangles of actinomyces filaments with club-shaped ends. On Gram stain, this material is found to contain both gram-positive filamentous structures and pleomorphic coccobacilli. The organism can be cultured on special media under strict anaerobic conditions, but isolation of the *Actinomyces* is usually difficult.

Differential Diagnosis. The presence of typical sulfur granules in the purulent exudate obtained from draining sinuses greatly aids in the diagnosis of *Actinomyces* infections that involve the skin and subcutaneous tissues. Other bacterial species may rarely produce similar-appearing granules in exudate, but these organisms can be differentiated on Gram stain. Pulmonary nocardiosis may give rise to draining sinuses of the chest wall and cause a clinical disease very much like thoracic actinomycosis. Cervicofacial actinomycosis must be differentiated from mycobacterial disease. When *Actinomyces* gives rise to mycetoma, numerous other actinomycotic and fungal pathogens must be considered in the differential diagnosis.

Treatment. Penicillin is the drug of choice for the treatment of actinomycosis. Therapy is initiated with aqueous penicillin G given intravenously at a dosage of 1 to 10 million units per day until the patient's condition is improved. It is recommended that therapy be continued for one year with oral phenoxymethyl penicillin. Surgical debridement or resection may be indicated for extensive disease but should only be performed after antibiotic therapy has been administered for a period of four to six weeks.[22] Alternate antibiotic choices for use in the penicillin-allergic patient include tetracycline and clindamycin.

NOCARDIOSIS

Human infection with *Nocardia* most frequently results in a primary pulmonary infection that may give rise to draining sinuses of the chest wall and may metastasize to distant body sites, especially the brain. Approximately 15 per cent of cases in a recent survey were localized skin and subcutaneous infections.[23] The most common cause of both pulmonary and extrapulmonary nocardiosis is *Nocardia asteroides,* although approximately one third of skin and subcutaneous infections are caused by *Nocardia brasiliensis*.[23] Soft tissue disease may be limited to suppurative wound infections or may result in the chronic painless nodules and draining sinuses of mycetoma. Lymphocutaneous infection indistinguishable from that caused by *Sporothrix schenckii* has also been described.[24, 25]

Over one half of the cases of nocardiosis occur in patients with a significant, underlying, debilitating condition.[23] Most patients are adult males, with a ratio of three males to every female patient.[23] *Nocardia* as a cause of extrapulmonary skin and subcutaneous infection in the normal child and adolescent is rare.

Laboratory Findings. A Gram stain of purulent exudate from a *Nocardia* infection reveals the presence of gram-positive, long, branching filaments and bacillary forms. An acid-fast stain is helpful, since *Nocardia* is the only actinomycetes that is acid-fast. The organism grows easily on common laboratory media under aerobic conditions, but it grows slowly, and culture results may not be available for up to two weeks.

Differential Diagnosis. Pulmonary nocardiosis resulting in draining sinuses of the chest wall must be differentiated from pulmonary actinomycosis. Skin and subcutaneous infection must be differentiated from disease caused by *Sporothrix schenckii,* as well as the numerous actinomycotic and fungal causes of the clinical syndrome known as mycetoma.

Treatment. The preferred treatment for nocardiosis is the administration of trisulfapyrimidines orally for at least six weeks and usually six months or longer. Surgical debridement or excision of infected tissue may also be indicated.

SUPERFICIAL FUNGAL INFECTIONS

The superficial fungal infections are caused by organisms that infect the stratum corneum or hair shaft without eliciting an inflammatory response, so that the only symptoms are cosmetic. The only widely encountered superficial fungal infection in the United States is tinea versicolor, a disease that is even more prevalent in tropical countries. Tinea versicolor is unusual in young children and the elderly and is most often seen in adolescents and young adults.[26] The other superficial fungal diseases, tinea nigra and piedra, occur predominantly in tropical countries and only occasionally in the United States. Tinea nigra is a chronic infection, with onset most often during childhood or adolescence. Black piedra is not confined to a particular age group, while white piedra usually occurs in post-pubescent persons.

TINEA VERSICOLOR

Tinea versicolor is an innocuous, chronic infection of the stratum corneum of glabrous skin caused by the dimorphic fungus *Pityrosporum orbiculare.* This organism is an extremely common resident of normal human skin and has been found on one or more surface sites in over 90 per cent of persons studied.[27] Although the microbe is a common skin inhabitant of all age groups after infancy, the number of organisms is relatively small until puberty, when it increases substantially, perhaps because of heightened sebaceous gland activity.[28] The disease is characterized by the presence of slightly scaly, discolored, macules of irregular size that tend to coalesce into large patches (Fig. 13-2). The upper trunk, neck, and proximal arm are the most frequently affected sites although other areas may become involved (Fig. 13-3). Facial involvement is not unusual, particularly during adolescence. The lesions vary in color according to the natural pigmentation of the patient, and both hypopigmented and hyperpigmented macules can occur.[29] Hypopigmented lesions fail to darken or tan after exposure to sunlight. The mechanism for this phenomenon is not known, but recent evidence suggests that the organism may suppress the formation of melanin.[30] Lesions may cause mild pruritus or may be asymptomatic.

Pityrosporum orbiculare exists predominantly in the yeast phase on normal skin and causes the clinical lesions of tinea versicolor only when substantial numbers of filamentous forms develop.[31] The increased susceptibility of some persons to this disease may be related to decreased epithelial cell turnover

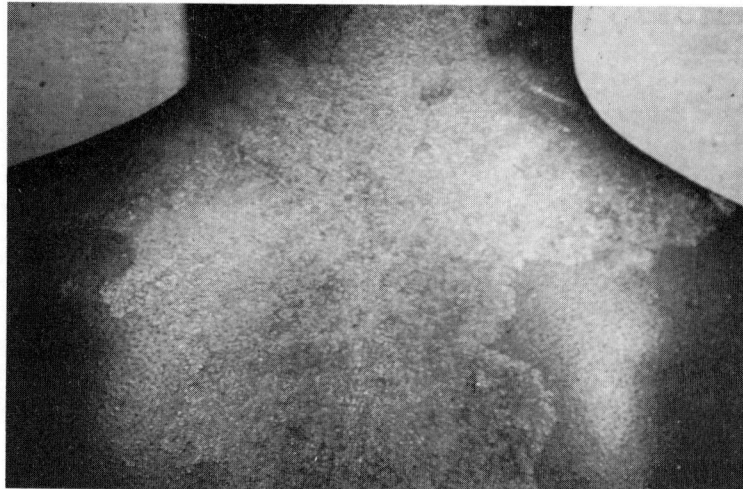

FIGURE 13-2 Coalescent plaque of tinea versicolor on the back of an adolescent male.

induced by such factors as excessive sweating and warm, moist weather.[26] Other possible predisposing factors include poor general health, treatment with corticosteroid medications, and genetically determined susceptibility.[32]

The disease is seen rarely in childhood or late adulthood but is frequently seen in persons between the ages of 15 and 30.[26] The average age of onset is in the early twenties, and males and females are affected equally.[26] Tinea versicolor is common worldwide but is especially prevalent in warm or tropical climates.

Laboratory Findings. Microscopic examination of a KOH preparation of skin scrapings from a tinea versicolor lesion will reveal small groups of budding thick-walled yeast cells intermingled with short, thick, occasionally branched hyphae. Examination of the patient's lesions with a Wood's lamp will show a characteristic bronze or yellow fluorescence. Culture of the causative agent is not helpful, since the organism is present as normal flora on the skin of most persons. Furthermore, special culture techniques not routinely available are required to grow the organism.

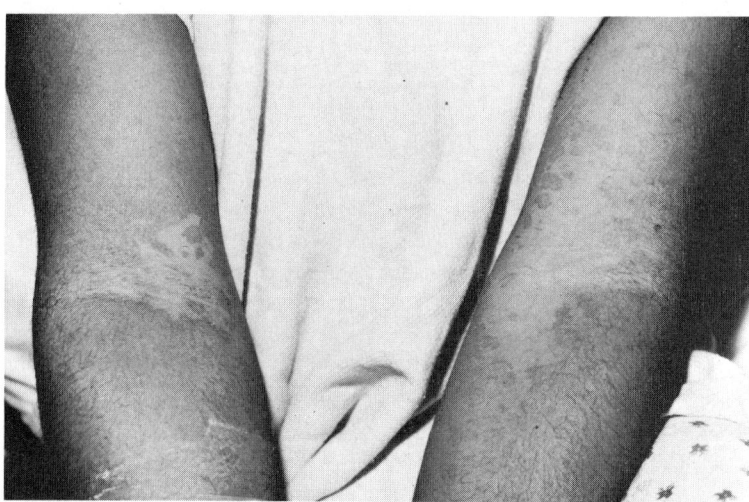

FIGURE 13-3 Tinea versicolor involving the antecubital fossae and lower arms.

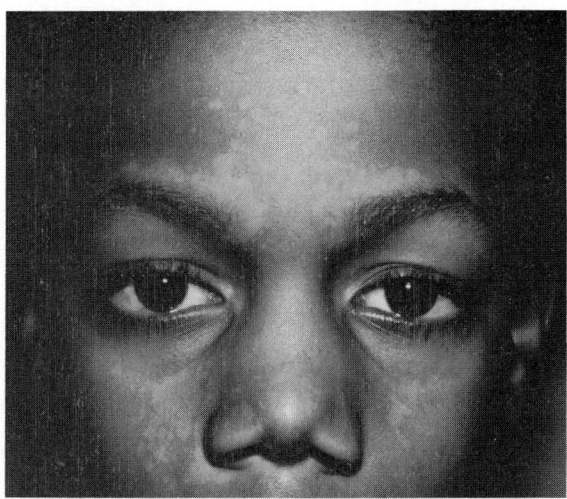

FIGURE 13-4 Tinea versicolor on the face of a 13-year-old boy, mimicking seborrheic dermatitis.

Differential Diagnosis. Tinea versicolor must be differentiated from non-scaling disorders of pigmentation, such as vitiligo and post-inflammatory change and from dermatophyte infections of glabrous skin. Tinea versicolor may mimic non-infectious scaling disorders, such as seborrheic dermatitis and pityriasis alba, especially when it affects the face (Fig. 13-4). Erythrasma may also resemble tinea versicolor but is usually restricted to the intertriginous areas. The typical findings on microscopic KOH examination and the bronze fluorescence of lesions under a Wood's lamp serve to identify the disease.

Treatment. Tinea versicolor may be treated relatively easily by a number of therapeutic agents. Many mild antifungal preparations and keratolytic agents, if applied regularly, will cause the lesions to regress within three to four weeks. A common procedure is the application of a 2 1/2 per cent selenium sulfide suspension shampoo to affected areas for 10 minutes during a shower or as a lotion overnight for four days. This procedure may be repeated one week later. Time of application can be adjusted if the skin becomes irritated. A 25 per cent solution of sodium hyposulfite or thiosulfate applied twice daily for two to four weeks is also an effective treatment. Antifungal agents, such as haloprogin, miconazole nitrate, and clotrimazole, are acceptable means of therapy but are more expensive than the other preparations. Pruritus and scaling will clear promptly, but pigmentary changes may persist for longer periods. Response to therapy can be assessed by a repeated KOH preparation or examination under a Wood's lamp. The patient should be advised that recurrences are frequent. However, rapid resolution should follow with reinstitution of an appropriate therapeutic regimen.

TINEA NIGRA

Tinea nigra is a mild infection of the stratum corneum of the palms and less often of the soles or other skin surfaces; it is caused by the dimorphic fungus *Cladosporium wernecki* in the Western hemisphere and by *Cladosporium mansoni* in Africa and Asia. The disease is characterized by grayish-brown-to-black macular patches with distinct borders and without erythema or scales. The infection is harmless, painless, and non-pruritic.

Unlike tinea versicolor, the etiological agent is not part of the normal skin flora but is probably a common inhabitant of the soil in tropical or subtropical climates. The infection occurs in the southeastern part of the United States[33] and may occur in persons who have vacationed in regions of the world where *Cladosporium* is common.[34] In contrast to the equal sex distribution of tinea versicolor, the lesions of tinea nigra are diagnosed more frequently in females.[34] No inherited predisposition or factors increasing susceptibility to the disease have been identified. In most reported patients, the onset of infection was during childhood or adolescence.[34]

Laboratory Findings. Skin scrapings from the lesions should be prepared with KOH and examined by low power microscopy. The examiner should look for the presence of dark brown, septate, branching hyphae mixed with occasional budding yeast cells. The *Cladosporium* may be cultured from epidermal scrapings on routine fungal media.

Differential Diagnosis. Tinea nigra has been confused with junctional nevus of the palm[35] and with malignant melanoma.[36] The lesions must also be differentiated from disorders associated with increased pigmentation, such as Addison's disease.[35]

Treatment. The lesions of tinea nigra are easily treated with fungistatic keratolytic agents, such as Whitfield's ointment or undecylenic acid ointment. The topical medication should be applied daily until the lesions resolve.

PIEDRA

Black and white piedra are mycotic infections of the superfollicular portion of the hair shaft. Black piedra is caused by the ascomycete mold *Piedraia hortae* and white piedra by the yeast *Trichosporon beigelii*. Black piedra usually infects the hair of the scalp and rarely the pubic and axillary hair. It is characterized by the presence of hard, firmly adherent, dark brown, variously sized nodules growing along the superfollicular portions of the hair shafts. The infection causes localized damage to the hair shaft, which may exhibit breakage. White piedra infects the hair of any body region, but the scalp is less commonly affected than the axillae, beard, and pubic areas. It is characterized by the appearance of soft, beige-to-yellow, loosely adherent accretions distributed along the hair shaft, which often breaks at these points of infection.

Black piedra and to a lesser extent white piedra are common in tropical South America and the Far East.[34] Both infections may occur in animals as well as in human beings. Neither disease is native to the United States. In some primitive societies, black piedra may be a desired condition for cosmetic or cultural reasons.[37] All age groups are equally affected by black piedra, whereas white piedra, because of its predilection for pubic, axillary, and facial hair, is more common in post-adolescence.

Laboratory Findings. On microscopic examination of KOH preparations, the hair shaft nodule of black piedra is seen to consist of a mass of tightly arranged, pigmented, branched, and septate mycelia. The center of the nodule contains oval cells or asci that have eight spindle-shaped ascospores at maturity. The soft nodules of white piedra tend to grow in a sheath-like fashion along the hair shaft and consist of translucent, irregularly arranged mycelia mixed with occasional arthrospores. Both *Piedraia hortae* and *Trichosporon beigelii* can be cultured on ordinary fungal media in the laboratory, but microscopic examination of wet mount preparations is sufficient for specific diagnosis of these two diseases.

Differential Diagnosis. Piedra must be differentiated from pediculosis, trichomycosis axillaris, and occasionally from dermatophytosis. Wet mount microscopic preparations of these organisms have very different appearances from the piedras. In addition, the nodules of piedra do not demonstrate fluorescence under a Wood's light.

Treatment. The piedras are easily treated by cutting or shaving the infected hair.

THE DERMATOPHYTOSES (Ringworm)

The mycotic species known as dermatophytes consists of a unique group of closely related filamentous fungi with a propensity for invading the keratinized surfaces of humans and other mammals. Most of these organisms are worldwide in distribution and sometimes inhabit healthy skin without causing disease.[38] The three principal genera responsible for human dermatophytoses are *Trichophyton, Microsporum,* and *Epidermophyton,* but each of the species has its own epidemiological characteristics. The *Trichophyton* species cause lesions of all keratinized surfaces, including skin, nails, and hair, while *Microsporum* species primarily invade the hair, and *Epidermophyton* species the intertriginous skin surfaces. However, the clinical syndromes and histopathology of human dermatophyte infections are related more closely to the anatomical site involved than to the causative agent. The clinical dermatophytic diseases are designated as "tinea," followed by the Latin word for the anatomical site of infection. Seven dermatophytoses of humans will be discussed in this chapter: tinea capitis, tinea barbae, tinea corporis, tinea manus, tinea unguium, tinea cruris, and tinea pedis.

The environmental origin of a dermatophyte infection varies with the infecting species. Dermatophytes acquired from the soil are termed geophilic, those acquired from animals, zoophilic, and those acquired from humans, anthropophilic. *Epidermophyton* species infections are acquired from human sources, but various species of both *Trichophyton* and *Microsporum* can be transmitted by both human and non-human sources.

Anthropophilic dermatophytes apparently elicit a delayed-type hypersensitivity response in the infected host, although some dermatophytes, most notably the zoophilic species, tend to elicit a more severe suppurative inflammation when they infect humans.[39] Increased susceptibility to chronic or recurrent *Trichophyton* infection has been demonstrated in some persons and may be related to a specific deficit of cell-mediated immunity.[40, 41] A family history of atopy is found in a large proportion of these chronically infected patients.[40] Some degree of resistance to reinfection seems to be acquired by most infected persons and may be associated with a positive delayed hypersensitivity response.[42, 43] Clinical observations suggest that resistance develops in early life. For example, only American soldiers and Vietnamese children acquired *Trichophyton mentagrophytes* infections during the Vietnamese war, whereas adult Vietnamese were apparently resistant to this fungus, which is indigenous to rats in Vietnam.[44] Although humoral immunity to dermatophytes can be detected by serological techniques, no relationship between circulating antibody and resistance to dermatophyte disease has been demonstrated.[45]

A unique, immunologically based, secondary skin eruption termed the dermatophytid or "id" reaction occasionally appears in hypersensitized persons, presumably due to circulating antigens originating from the primary infection site.[39] The eruption occurs most frequently on the fingers of persons with tinea pedis and in this circumstance is characterized by the appearance of grouped papules, vesicles, and occasionally sterile pustules. Symmetrical urticarial lesions and a more generalized maculopapular eruption may occur as well. Dermatophytid reactions also are seen in children with tinea capitis, usually manifested as symmetrically distributed, scattered follicular lesions of the trunk.

The important diagnostic procedures for the various dermatophyte diseases include Wood's lamp examination of infected hairs, microscopic examination of KOH wet mount preparations of infected material, and cultural identification of the etiological agent on special laboratory media. Under Wood's lamp examination, hairs infected by the most common *Microsporum* species fluoresce a bright green color; most *Trichophyton*-infected hairs do not fluoresce. The Wood's lamp is also useful for the diagnosis of the non-dermatophyte infections such as tinea versicolor, erythrasma, and trichomycosis axillaris.

Material for KOH preparation is best obtained from skin lesions by first cleansing the site with alcohol and then scraping adherent scales from the actively spreading border of the infection. Infected hairs should be selected from the margin of a lesion, epilated with a forceps, and examined under the microscope with particular attention to the follicular portion of the shaft. Specimens also should be sent to the microbiology laboratory in a dry, sterile envelope or Petri dish for implantation on special culture media. For a more detailed discussion of the diagnosis of dermatophyte infections, the reader should consult a textbook of medical mycology.[1]

The most frequent dermatophyte infections in adolescents are tinea cruris and tinea pedis, both of which affect males more often than females.[38, 39] Tinea unguium usually is seen in association with tinea pedis. Tinea capitis is prevalent largely in prepubescent children, while tinea corporis is not limited to a particular age group. Tinea barbae is a relatively rare disease seen only in adult males.

TINEA CAPITIS

Tinea capitis is a dermatophyte infection of the scalp and scalp hair follicles, most often produced by the species *Microsporum audouini, Microsporum canis,* and *Trichophyton tonsurans* and much less often by other *Microsporum* and *Trichophyton* species.[39] In *Microsporum* and some *Trichophyton* infections, the organisms form spores in a sheathlike fashion around the hair shaft, referred to as an ectothrix infection. *Trichophyton tonsurans* produces an infection within the hair shaft, referred to as an endothrix infection.

Several clinical presentations of tinea capitis may occur. The most common or "gray patch" syndrome, produced by *Microsporum* species, is characterized initially by the appearance of a small papule at the base of a hair follicle. Subsequently, a widening annular area of the scalp surface becomes erythematous and scaly, and the hairs of the involved skin lose their pigmentation and become brittle and broken. Multiple confluent areas of alopecia develop. Patients may complain of severe pruritus of the involved scalp. Endothrix infections, such as those caused by *Trichophyton tonsurans,* produce a syndrome referred to as "black dot ringworm." This is characterized initially by multiple, much smaller, circular patches with only a few involved hairs, which are broken off very close to the hair follicle, giving a polka dot appearance (Fig. 13–5). Subsequently, this type of involvement tends to produce a chronic, more diffuse alopecia.

When a significant inflammatory response to an infecting organism occurs, raised, boggy, granulomatous masses, often studded with sterile pustules, appear at sites of infection; these lesions are called kerions (Plate VII–B). Permanent scarring and alopecia may follow such a host response, which is elicited most often by *Microsporum canis* and *Trichophyton tonsurans.* Favus, a form of tinea capitis rare in the United States, is caused by the fungus *Trichophyton schoenleini* and characterized by the development of scaly erythematous patches with honeycomb yellow crusts and a dull-green fluorescence under a Wood's lamp.

In the United States and Puerto Rico, the most frequent etiological agents of tinea capitis are *Microsporum audouini* and *Microsporum canis*.[46] In Mexico and some South American countries (hence among persons emigrating from these countries), infections with *Trichophyton tonsurans* are common.[46] *Microsporum audouini* and *Trichophyton tonsurans* are anthropophilic species acquired most often by contact with infected hairs and epithelial cells shed on environmental surfaces such as theater seats and on hats and combs. It has been shown that infected children disperse dermatophyte spores into their immediate environment and that their non-infected classmates demonstrate significantly higher carriage rates than age-matched controls.[47] *Microsporum canis* is a zoophilic species whose preferred hosts are cats and dogs; it is transmitted by direct contact with domestic pets.[48]

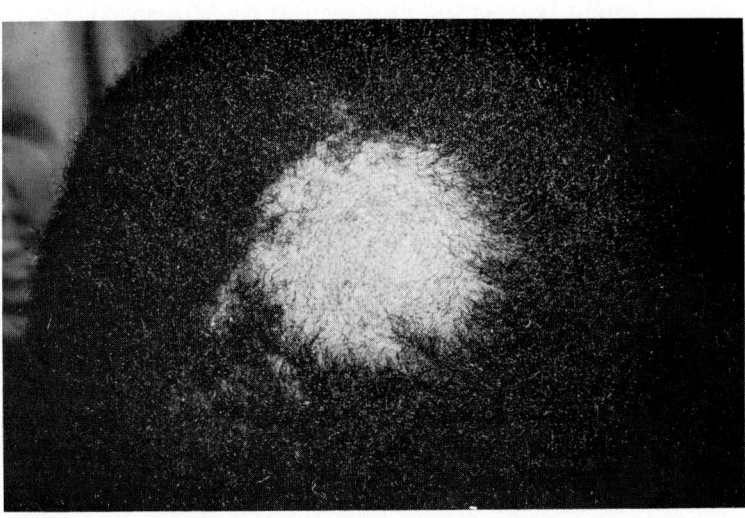

FIGURE 13–5 Tinea capitis due to *T. tonsurans*. Note the "black dots" (broken-off hairs) in the area of alopecia.

Tinea capitis caused by the *Microsporum* species is restricted to the preadolescent population, and, in fact, chronic tinea capitis has been shown to spontaneously regress with the onset of puberty.[49] It has been suggested that this phenomenon may be the result of an increased fungistatic capacity of sebum.[49] The affliction also is diagnosed much more often in boys. Infection with *Trichophyton tonsurans* is not confined to a particular age group and does not show a tendency to resolve spontaneously at puberty.

Laboratory Findings. Wood's lamp examination of *Microsporum*-infected lesions gives a characteristic bright green fluorescence, whereas lesions caused by *Trichophyton tonsurans* fail to fluoresce. Microscopic examination of a KOH preparation of an infected hair will reveal tiny arthrospores surrounding the hair shaft in *Microsporum* disease and chains of arthrospores within the hair shaft in *Trichophyton tonsurans* infections. A specific etiological diagnosis of tinea capitis may be obtained by planting infected hairs or epidermal scales on specially prepared laboratory media containing antibacterial antibiotics. Although identification of the culture may require several weeks, this adjunctive diagnostic procedure may be useful in some cases of tinea capitis.

Differential Diagnosis. Tinea capitis initially may be confused with seborrheic dermatitis, psoriasis, alopecia areata, trichotillomania, folliculitis decalvans, or certain dystrophic hair disorders. When the inflammation is pronounced, as in kerion, primary or secondary bacterial infection of the scalp must also be considered. In adolescents and adults, the patchy, moth-eaten type of alopecia associated with secondary syphilis (alopecia syphilitica) may resemble tinea capitis. Wood's lamp examination or microscopic examination of a KOH preparation of infected hair should differentiate these diseases from dermatophytosis. A serological test for syphilis should be performed if the diagnosis is in doubt.

Treatment. Oral systemic antibiotic therapy with griseofulvin microcrystalline is currently recommended for all forms of tinea capitis. Treatment may be necessary for several weeks and should be continued for two weeks after Wood's lamp examination or KOH preparations have become negative. Adverse reactions to griseofulvin include gastrointestinal disturbances and headache, in addition to hepatotoxicity and rare cases of blood dyscrasia. Unconfirmed reports about the possible carcinogenicity of this antibiotic require that the drug be reserved for strictly indicated diseases.[50]

Topical therapy alone is ineffective, since the medication cannot penetrate to the depths of the hair follicle where the fungus is situated. Nevertheless, it may be important as an adjunctive measure to reduce the shedding of spores. For this purpose, vigorous shampooing with antiseborrheic preparations and application of mild keratolytic agents may be recommended. It is not necessary to shave the scalp.

TINEA BARBAE (Barber's itch)

Tinea barbae is an uncommon dermatophyte infection of the bearded region of men. The most frequent etiological agents are the zoophilic species *Trichophyton mentagrophytes* and *Trichophyton verrucosum,* which tend to produce a severe, suppurative, deep folliculitis. The lesion is generally singular or confluent and confined to one side of the face. Patients may manifest mild systemic symptoms.[39] Occasionally they may develop a less inflammatory type of tinea barbae and, in these instances, the anthropophilic species *Trichophyton rubrum* may be the causative agent.[39] This form of the disease is characterized by localized erythematous patches with central scaling and a raised vesiculopustular margin resembling the lesions of tinea corporis. Both forms of tinea barbae are accompanied by localized alopecia, and the severe form results in permanent scarring. Other species of dermatophytes, including *Microsporum canis*, may rarely cause tinea barbae, the severity of involvement depending on both the specific fungal agent and the response of the individual host.[39]

Tinea barbae is more common in men from rural areas who work with farm animals that transmit the disease. Rarely, *Trichophyton rubrum* infection is transmitted by contaminated equipment in barber shops.[39]

Laboratory Findings. Microscopic examination of a KOH preparation of either infected epidermal scales scraped from the margin of the lesion or of the base of an infected hair epilated from the border of the lesion will often reveal the fungal nature of the infection. Infected material should be transported to the laboratory for implantation on specific fungal media.

Differential Diagnosis. Tinea barbae must be differentiated from sycosis vulgaris, a bacterial folliculitis of the beard, which usually involves both sides of the face and the upper lip, as opposed to the unilateral distribution of tinea barbae. Tinea barbae also may be confused with pseudofolliculitis of the beard and occasionally with cystic acne. Microscopic demonstration of the etiological fungus should establish the diagnosis.

Treatment. Oral griseofulvin microcrystalline is recommended for the treatment of tinea barbae, although the more inflammatory lesions resolve spontaneously after a period of weeks without specific systemic antifungal therapy. Griseofulvin is especially useful in the therapy of the more chronic, less inflammatory, superficial form of the disease. Local measures, such as daily application of warm saline compresses, epilation of infected hairs, and shaving of the uninvolved beard, are also recommended.

TINEA CORPORIS

Tinea corporis refers to dermatophytic infection of glabrous skin, most often of the face, trunk, and proximal extremities. It can be caused by almost any of the dermatophyte species, although *Trichophyton rubrum* and *Trichophyton mentagrophytes* are the usual agents in adults. In children, *Microsporum canis* infections are seen frequently. The most typical clinical lesion of tinea corporis begins as a dry, mildly erythematous, elevated, scaling patch that spreads centrifugally as it clears centrally, so that it forms the characteristic annular lesions that have given the dermatophyte infections the name "ringworm" (Plate VII–C). At times, gyrate or figurate plaques with advancing borders may spread over large areas (Plate VII–D). Most lesions clear spontaneously within several months, but the infection may become chronic. In some instances, the tissue reaction to the invading fungus is more pronounced, the advancing border of the lesion is vesiculated, and the central portion of the lesion becomes hyperpigmented and crusted. Such lesions are somewhat more common in infection with zoophilic species such as *Microsporum canis* and tend to resolve spontaneously. Lesions do not always demonstrate central clearing (Plate VII–E), and variations in host response may produce a variety of clinical appearances of tinea corporis, including granulomatous lesions and the kerion-like lesions referred to as tinea profunda. Invasion of lanugo hair follicles by the fungus contributes to the increased inflammatory response in some infections.[39]

Tinea corporis can be acquired through direct contact with infected persons or through indirect contact with infected scales or hairs deposited on environmental surfaces. *Microsporum canis* infections are usually seen in children who have had close contact with infected pets, and other mammals also have been shown to provide a reservoir of infection for humans.[44] Not infrequently, dermatophyte infection of another anatomical site, such as the scalp, leads to secondary infection of the glabrous skin. Tinea corporis occurs throughout the world but is more widespread in tropical countries. The role of a warm, wet climate in the production of epidemic tinea corporis in susceptible hosts has been demonstrated in the markedly increased prevalence of *Trichophyton mentagrophytes* disease contracted by servicemen in Vietnam.[44] All age groups are affected by tinea corporis.

Laboratory Findings. Since the lesions of tinea corporis have a variable appearance and may resemble a number of other cutaneous diseases, microscopic examination of KOH wet mount preparations and diagnostic fungal cultures should always be obtained when fungal skin infection is a possibility.

Differential Diagnosis. Many non-dermatophytic skin lesions, both infectious and non-infectious, must be differentiated from the lesions of tinea corporis. The most frequently confused entities are nummular eczema, pityriasis rosea, psoriasis, seborrheic dermatitis, tinea versicolor, erythrasma, and secondary syphilis. The lesions of these diseases tend to be more symmetrically and widely distributed than in the usual case of tinea corporis. A positive KOH preparation or fungal culture of skin scrapings will confirm the diagnosis.

Treatment. Most patients with tinea corporis will respond to treatment with one of the topical antifungal agents (haloprogin, tolnaftate, miconazole nitrate, or clotrimazole) twice daily for two to four weeks. In unusually severe or extensive disease, a course of therapy with oral griseofulvin microcrystalline for over several weeks may be required.[39]

TINEA CRURIS

Tinea cruris ("jock itch") is a very common dermatophyte infection of the groin, almost always of adolescent and adult males[51]; it is caused most often by the anthropophilic species *Epidermophyton floccosum* and *Trichophyton rubrum* and occasionally by the zoophilic species *Trichophyton mentagrophytes*. The usual initial lesion is a small, raised, scaly, erythematous patch on the inner aspect of the thigh, which spreads peripherally, often developing multiple tiny vesicles at the advancing margin. Irregular, sharply bordered patches with hyperpigmented scaly centers evolve (Fig. 13–6). Lesions are usually bilateral and initiated at the point of contact between the scrotum and the thigh. In some instances, particularly in infections due to *Trichophyton mentagrophytes,* the inflammatory reaction is more severe, and the infection may spread to skin beyond the crural region.[44] Such infections generally show a greater involvement of the hair follicles. Subcutaneous abscesses have been reported to

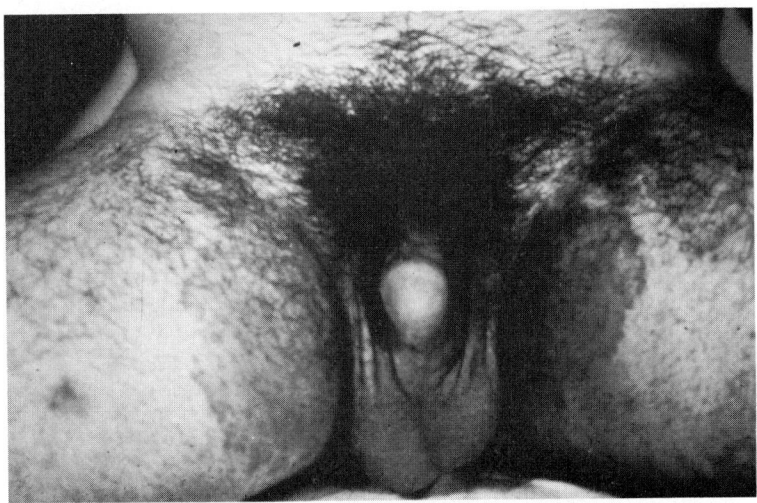

FIGURE 13–6 Tinea cruris in a teenage male. Note the sharply demarcated borders of the lesion.

occur.[52] Pruritus may be severe initially but abates as the inflammatory reaction subsides. Bacterial superinfection may alter the clinical appearance of the lesions,[44] and erythrasma or candidiasis may coexist with the dermatophytosis.[4]

Tinea cruris is seen worldwide, but like many mycotic skin diseases, it occurs with greater frequency in wet, hot climates. It is more prevalent in obese persons and in those who perspire excessively and wear tight-fitting clothing. The disease occurs with great frequency in adolescent and young adult males and is very uncommon in children and females.[39, 51] It may occur in epidemic proportions in crowded, relatively enclosed populations, such as military personnel or athletic teams,[39, 44] especially where bath and bed linens may be shared.

Laboratory Findings. An examination of a KOH preparation of epidermal scrapings will usually reveal the septate hyphae and arthrospores characteristic of a fungal skin infection. Confirmation by culture of the organism should also be sought. Coral-red fluorescence on Wood's lamp examination is indicative of the diphtheroid skin infection, erythrasma.

Differential Diagnosis. Tinea cruris must be differentiated from erythrasma, intertrigo, and superficial candidiasis. Bacterial superinfection of primary dermatophytosis must be excluded in patients with severe inflammatory reactions. Irritant and allergic contact dermatitis may also mimic tinea cruris.

Treatment. Since tinea cruris is exacerbated by increased perspiration and the friction produced by tight-fitting underclothing, the patient should be advised to use a bland absorbent powder and to wear loose cotton underwear.

Topical therapy with either clotrimazole or miconazole nitrate is recommended for severe infection, especially since these agents are effective in mixed candidal-dermatophyte infections.[53] Superinfection with bacteria, especially with Group A streptococci, requires appropriate oral antibiotic therapy. Pure dermatophyte infections also may be treated with haloprogin or tolnaftate; the latter is available without a prescription.[53]

TINEA PEDIS (Athlete's foot)

Tinea pedis refers to dermatophyte infection of the toe webs and soles of the feet and is the most common dermatophyte infection. The etiological agents usually implicated are *Trichophyton rubrum*, *Trichophyton mentagrophytes*, and *Epidermophyton floccosum*. Fungal foot infection affects between one fourth to three fourths of the adult population,[38, 39] although dermatophyte species are often isolated from the feet of persons with no apparent infection.

The most common expression of disease is the appearance of moist intertriginous fissures accompanied by maceration and peeling of the surrounding skin. This type of infection has a predilection for the third and fourth interdigital spaces and the subdigital spaces (Fig. 13-7). Patients frequently complain of severe tenderness and itching and a persistent foul foot odor. Such lesions tend to become chronic but can usually be treated effectively. Somewhat less commonly, patients develop a chronic, patchy, diffuse hyperkeratosis on the sole, characterized by very thickened skin covered by fine white scales (Fig. 13-8). This type of chronic infection is more resistant to treatment.

An inflammatory vesicular type of reaction may be seen in response to infection with *Trichophyton mentagrophytes* (Fig. 13-9). Lesions may involve all areas of the foot, including the dorsal surface, but are usually patchy in distribution. They begin as papules and progress to vesicles and bullae that may become pustular. Despite the severity of the inflammation, this type of infection tends to resolve spontaneously. Occasionally, a very severe from of athlete's foot occurs as a result of secondary bacterial infection, which may be exacerbated by topical antifungal therapy. This infection is characterized by a severe vesicopustular reaction and ulceration with underlying cellulitis and frequently lymphangitis. Pronounced exfoliatation may ensue, and patients may manifest systemic symptoms and become quite disabled.

All forms of tinea pedis are uncommon in childhood. However, when the infection occurs, the lesions are more often of the inflammatory type. In one study, the mean age at onset of dermatophytosis was 15 years, with over two

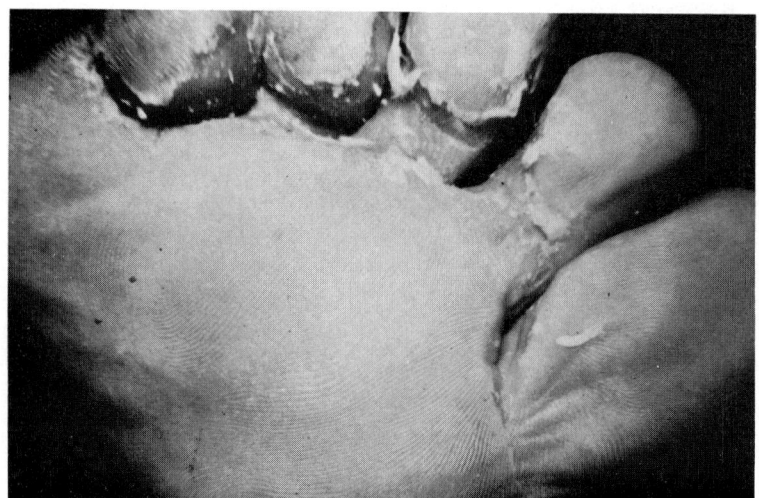

FIGURE 13-7 Chronic tinea pedis with marked scaling of the interdigital and subdigital spaces.

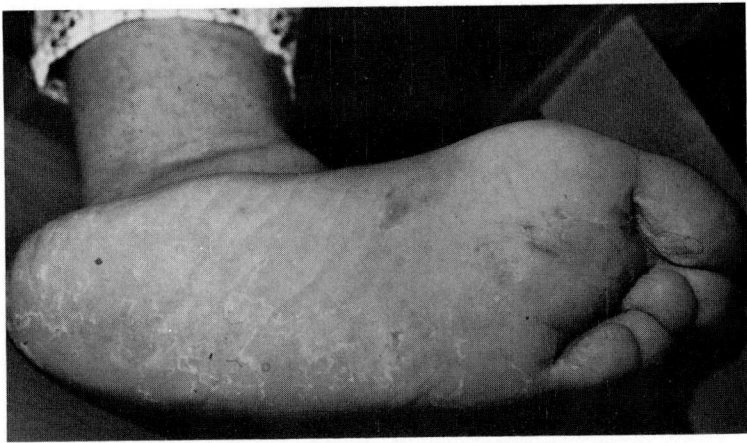

FIGURE 13–8 Diffuse hyperkeratotic tinea pedis of the sole in an adolescent male.

thirds of the patients studied manifesting tinea pedis.[42] The disease is seen in both men and women, but the incidence of infection is much higher among males. In one survey of adolescent boys, one third were shown to have the disease, with the incidence increasing so sharply with age that more than half of the young men over 17 were affected.[54]

A number of factors predispose to infection, most prominently tight-fitting, occlusive footwear and warm, humid weather. The disease may be transmitted through shared bath and shower facilities and swimming pool areas[55] and hence is very prevalent among members of athletic teams and military personnel.

Laboratory Findings. In the vast majority of cases, the fungal etiology may be demonstrated by microscopic examination of a KOH preparation of infected material. The fourth toe web provides a high yield of infected scales. In instances of vesicobullous eruption, the blister top should be removed and examined with KOH. Identification of the causative agent should be established by culture. Wood's light examination will differentiate tinea pedis from erythrasma of the toe webs.

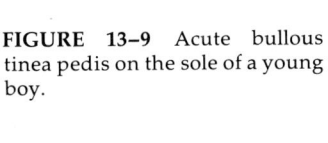

FIGURE 13–9 Acute bullous tinea pedis on the sole of a young boy.

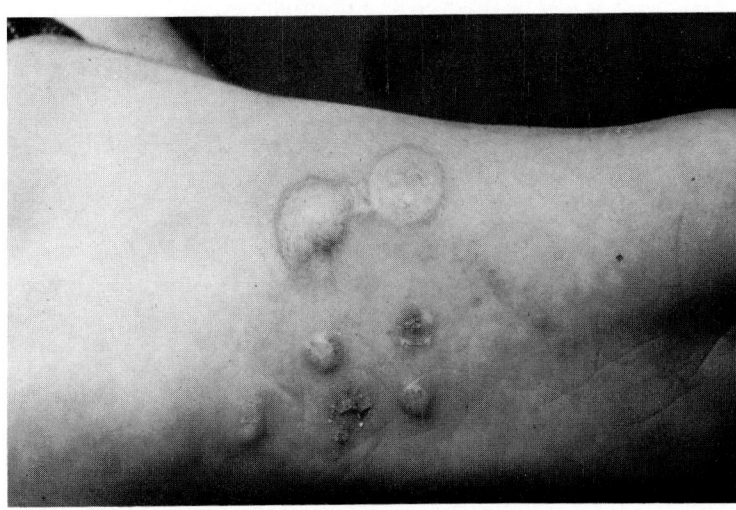

Differential Diagnosis. Tinea pedis must be differentiated from simple maceration of the interdigital spaces and from erythrasma, which may be clinically indistinguishable from dermatophyte toe web infection. Foot infections with *Candida albicans* and with a variety of bacterial organisms may cause confusion or may coexist with primary tinea pedis, especially the inflammatory type. Contact dermatitis, dyshidrotic eczema, and atopic dermatitis may simulate tinea pedis or tinea manuum but are distinguished by the absence of fungal elements on KOH examination.

Treatment. Simple measures may suffice for milder infections, such as avoidance of occlusive footwear, use of an absorbent antifungal powder such as zinc undecylenate, and careful drying between the toe webs after bathing. Topical therapy with clotrimazole or miconazole nitrate is effective in most cases, and both of these agents are also effective against candidal infection or superinfection.[53, 56, 57] Haloprogin and tolnaftate can be used in uncomplicated dermatophyte infections. Several weeks of therapy may be necessary, and some low-grade chronic infections, especially those caused by *Trichophyton rubrum*, fail to respond even then. In such cases, systemic therapy with griseofulvin may effect a cure. However, reservations about this drug, due to its potential carcinogenicity, warrant its use only in severe cases that have not responded to topical therapy. Response to treatment may be temporary in any case, since recurrent infections are common in a certain percentage of the population.

TINEA MANUUM

Tinea manuum is a dermatophyte infection of the hand, most often unilateral, involving the interdigital spaces and the palmar surfaces. It is most commonly caused by the same agents involved in dermatophyte foot infections, including *Trichophyton rubrum, Trichophyton mentagrophytes,* and *Epidermophyton floccosum,* and it is usually secondary to tinea pedis. Clinical expressions of this infection range from a diffuse hyperkeratosis involving both fingers and palm to a less common patchy, inflammatory, vesicular type of reaction. Intermediate forms with discrete erythematous papules or with severe scaling and exfoliation are also seen.[39] As is true for tinea pedis infections, the more chronic, less inflammatory lesions are likely to be caused by *Trichophyton rubrum,* whereas the more acute inflammatory reactions are most often secondary to *Trichophyton mentagrophytes*. Tinea manuum is seen in adolescents or young adults with primary dermatophyte infection of the feet and is diagnosed and treated in the same manner as tinea pedis.

TINEA UNGUIUM

Tinea unguium (onychomycosis) is a dermatophyte infection of the nail plate that is seen most often in patients with tinea pedis but may occur in association with other dermatophytoses or as a primary infection. It can be caused by a number of dermatophyte agents, of which *Trichophyton rubrum* is the most common and *Trichophyton mentagrophytes* the next most common. Since *Trichophyton mentagrophytes* seldom involves the hands, *Trichophyton rubrum* is the most frequent cause of tinea unguium of the fingernails.[58] The most superficial form of tinea unguium is often caused by *Trichophyton mentagrophytes* and is manifested by irregular, single or multiple white patches on the surface of the nail, unassociated with paronychial inflammation or deep infection. *Trichophyton rubrum* generally causes a more invasive, subungual infection, initiated at the sides of the distal tip of the nail and often preceded by mild paronychia. The middle and ventral layers of the nail plate and perhaps the nail bed are the sites of infection.[58] The nail first develops a yellowish discoloration and slowly becomes thickened, brittle, and loosened from the nail bed because of the accumulation of subungual keratin. In advanced infection, the nail may turn dark brown to black in color and may crack or break off (Fig. 13-10). Often several nails are involved, but single nail involvement is not unusual. The affliction is usually painless and is more a cosmetic problem than a truly debilitating disorder.

Laboratory Findings. Thin shavings taken from the infected nail, preferably from the deeper areas in cases of severe involvement, should be examined microscopically with KOH and submitted to the laboratory for culture. Fungus may not be easy to demonstrate, and repeated attempts may be required. It is essential to sample the more ventral nail layers near the nail bed, except in very superficial disease, since the fungus is not viable on the distal dead portion of the nail.[58] The diagnosis of tinea unguium is less difficult when the disease occurs in conjunction with chronic tinea pedis.

Differential Diagnosis. Tinea unguium must be differentiated from a variety of dystrophic nail disorders.[39] Both psoriatic nails and the nail lesions of lichen planus can be confused with tinea unguium, but the identification of typical lesions elsewhere on the body provides invaluable information for diagnosis. Nails infected with *Candida albicans* have several distinguishing features, most notably, pronounced paronychial swelling.

Treatment. The therapy of tinea unguium is very difficult and frequently disappointing. Avulsion or nearly complete removal of the nail combined with prolonged griseofulvin therapy and the application of topical fungistatic agents to the nail bed may be effective in a fair percentage of cases.[59, 60] The topical

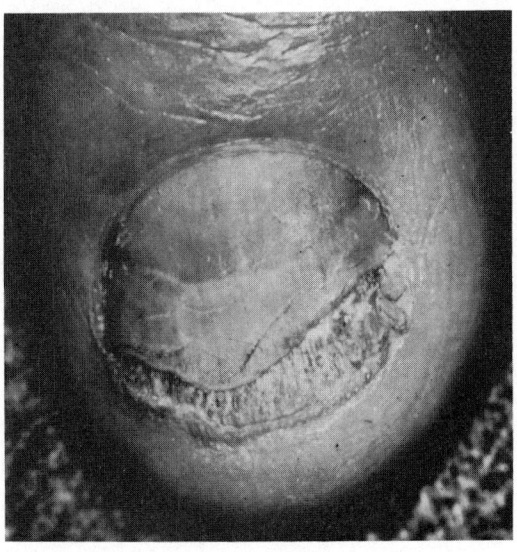

FIGURE 13-10 *Tinea unguium.* Dermatophyte infection of the nails, demonstrating partial loss of the nail plate.

application of 10 per cent aqueous glutaraldehyde has been useful in some toe infections, which may not respond to griseofulvin therapy.[61] When it is employed, griseofulvin therapy may be required for more than a year and should be reserved for especially severe disease for which the patient is motivated to obtain a cure.

SUBCUTANEOUS MYCOSES

Subcutaneous mycotic infections are caused by a number of fungi that are normally soil saprophytes of low virulence. They give rise to relatively localized infections in humans when they are implanted in subcutaneous tissues through damaged epidermis. These infections are more prevalent in underdeveloped regions of the world, especially in the rural areas of subtropical and tropical countries. Subcutaneous mycoses are infrequent in the United States, especially in urban populations. Only two entities will be discussed in this chapter: sporotrichosis and chromoblastomycosis, both of which occur in the United States.[62, 63] These infections are found most often in adults with occupational exposure to soil and plant saphrophytes, but all age groups are potentially susceptible.

Primary cutaneous and subcutaneous infections with the "deep" mycoses, i.e., histoblastosis, coccidioidomycosis, blastomycosis, and cryptococcosis, are rare and will not be discussed in this chapter. The reader is referred to a textbook of medical mycology[1] or to one of many reviews that have been written about the deep mycoses.[39, 64]

SPOROTRICHOSIS

Sporotrichosis is an uncommon, chronic, subcutaneous infection caused by the dimorphic fungus *Sporothrix schenckii,* which exists in the soil and on both living and decaying vegetation. In its most common form, the disease is acquired by contact of injured skin with the organism in its natural habitat. The ensuing infection is characterized by the appearance of a small, painless, subcutaneous nodule or ulcer some weeks after exposure. Subsequently, the nodule ulcerates through the overlying skin and then heals very slowly and with scarring. The infection spreads along lymphatic channels in an indolent fashion, and multiple nodules and ulcers develop as the disease progresses. This form of the infection is termed lymphocutaneous sporotrichosis and accounts for approximately three fourths of reported cases.[65]

The second most common form of the disease is fixed cutaneous sporotrichosis, which occurs mainly in endemic areas where individuals demonstrate a high frequency of positive delayed-type hypersensitivity reactions to the organism. Infection in a previously sensitized person usually remains localized to the site of entrance of the organism and does not spread along lymphatic channels. The localized lesions can demonstrate variable morphology, ranging from scaly maculopapular lesions to verrucous and weeping ulcers. Small satellite lesions are common. This type of sporotrichosis often becomes chronic and is resistant to local treatment.[66]

A third rare form of cutaneous sporotrichosis occurs when the infection is restricted to mucocutaneous surfaces, giving rise to suppurative, ulcerating lesions that evolve to form painful vegetative or granulomatous lesions, often with significant involvement of the regional lymphatics.[66]

Sporotrichosis occurs as an occupational disease in gardeners and florists.[67] It is more common in warm, humid climates. The greatest number of infections occur in Central and South America and Mexico,[66] although the disease has been noted in various regions of the United States.[62, 68] A number of reports of childhood sporotrichosis have appeared in the American literature,[68, 69, 70] and 50 per cent of these infections have occurred in children aged 10 years or older. Over two thirds of the patients were male, and the most common sites of infection were the upper and lower extremities, although lesions of the face and trunk were relatively frequent.[68, 69, 70] As in adults, the lymphocutaneous type of disease is the most common, and many patients come from rural environments.

Laboratory Findings. The disease must be diagnosed definitively by cultural isolation of the causative agent. *Sporothrix schenckii* grows well on commonly used fungal media and can be isolated from aspirates of nodules or swabs from ulcerative lesions. Although the organism will usually grow in less than a week, several weeks may occasionally be required. Direct examination of the clinical material is usually unrewarding, but a fluorescent antibody staining technique may be an aid to rapid diagnosis.[71]

Cultured extracts of the fungus may be used to detect delayed-type hypersensitivity reactions to the organism, and this skin test may be useful for diagnosing the disease in non-endemic areas. However, in endemic areas, a high percentage of individuals without infection show positive reactions.[66] Serological procedures have yielded inconsistent results in persons with cutaneous and subcutaneous sporotrichosis, and although these procedures may be useful in some instances, they are not widely available.[72]

Differential Diagnosis. The lymphocutaneous form of sporotrichosis is sufficiently unique to allow a clinical diagnosis to be made. Occasionally, this type of infection may be confused with cutaneous tuberculosis, primary cutaneous coccidioidomycosis, or blastomycosis. Leishmaniasis, syphilis, furunculosis, and tularemia should also be considered in the differential diagnosis.[73] A clinically indistinguishable disease has been reported as a manifestation of infection with *Nocardia brasiliensis*.[24, 25] The differential diagnosis of fixed cutaneous sporotrichosis, which is rare in the United States, is more difficult. The lesions in this form of the infection may resemble cutaneous tuberculosis, chromoblastomycosis, some candidal lesions, and some cutaneous syphilitic lesions, among others. Anthrax, impetigo, furunculosis, cutaneous cancer, and cat-scratch disease also may be considered.[74] Sporotrichoid infections confined to mucous membrane surfaces may initially resemble aphthous ulcers or oral lichen planus.[66]

Treatment. The treatment of choice for cutaneous sporotrichosis is orally administered potassium iodide, given in an initial dosage of 5 drops three times a day, to be gradually increased to 30 to 40 drops three times a day over the first four days of therapy in an adolescent or adult patient. Treatment is continued for four to six weeks after resolution of the lesions. Some localized forms of disease may respond to topical application of 2 per cent potassium iodide solution in 0.2 per cent iodine.[66] A number of distressing side reactions may follow orally administered potassium iodide. These include gastrointestinal discomfort, soreness of the mouth, increased salivation and lacrimation, swelling of the salivary glands, and a variety of drug rashes.[75] Gradual increase in the dosage, as well as tapering when side effects are intolerable, is therefore recommended, as is close patient supervision. Most adverse reactions will abate within a few days of discontinuing the drug. Some patients may exhibit allergic reactions, including both serum sickness and anaphylaxis.[75] In some patients with severe or relapsing cutaneous sporotrichosis, amphotericin B therapy may prove effective.[66]

CHROMOBLASTOMYCOSIS

Chromoblastomycosis is an uncommon, localized infection of the cutaneous and subcutaneous tissue caused by one of a group of fungi belonging to the family Dematiaceae, which are soil saprophytes. The most frequently isolated agents from this type of infection are *Cladosporium carrioni, Fonsecaea pedrosi, Phialophora verrucosa,* and *Fonsecaea compactum,* all of which are common inhabitants of soil and decaying vegetation. The disease occurs most frequently among barefoot laborers in rural subtropical or tropical countries but has been reported in the United States.[63] It is characterized by small papular or verrucous lesions, usually on the foot or ankle. The infection spreads to the adjacent skin and subcutaneous tissue by satellite lesions that appear to form along the lymphatic channels. The lesions are slightly scaly and have a dull red-gray color. Occasionally, lesions show peripheral spread with central healing, resulting in a scar or keloid. Trauma and secondary bacterial infection may alter the clinical appearance of lesions. Usually, uncomplicated lesions are relatively asymptomatic, but superinfection may lead to blockage of local lymph channels and swelling of the affected limb.

Differential Diagnosis. The disease must be differentiated from a number of other mycotic infections characterized by localized cutaneous and subcutaneous lesions, including primary cutaneous blastomycosis, eumycotic mycetoma, superficial candidiasis, and sporotrichosis. Several bacterial agents may cause similar lesions, such as the spirochetes of syphilis and yaws, the mycobacteria, and the actinomycotic agents of mycetoma. The parasitic disease cutaneous leishmaniasis must also be distinguished but does not usually affect the lower extremities.

Laboratory Findings. Chromoblastomycosis can be diagnosed by microscopic examination of a potassium hydroxide preparation of material obtained from a clinical lesion, which reveals the presence of pigmented, segmented hyphae and thick-walled, round, granular fungal cells. Confirmation by culture should be obtained but may take some weeks.[76]

Although both serological and delayed-type hypersensitivity tests have been described, they have not been shown to be helpful diagnostically and are not generally available.[76]

Treatment. The treatment of choice in early cases is surgical removal of infected tissue, either by excision, electrodesiccation, or cryosurgery.[76] In advanced cases, the use of amphotericin B injections locally rather than systemically may effect a cure,[77] as systemic amphotericin B therapy does not result in sufficient local concentrations to kill the causative fungus reliably. Both thiabendazole and 5-fluorocytosine have been used in extensive cases, and initial trials indicate that these agents may be of benefit.[76]

OPPORTUNISTIC MYCOTIC INFECTIONS

The term "opportunistic" used in association with infections is somewhat misleading, as any agent that produces human infection may correctly be called an opportunist. A number of the entities discussed earlier, such as tinea versicolor and some dermatophytoses might also be considered opportunistic mycotic infections. However, the designation is ordinarily reserved for infections caused by microbial agents that are ubiquitous in distribution and very low in pathogenic potential. These agents cause infection only when substantial alteration or breakdown of host defenses permits them to become invasive. Although this situation is most typical of immunodeficient or debilitated patients, breakdown of local or "barrier" defenses occurs in healthy persons with relative frequency, giving rise to localized cutaneous infection with agents such as *Candida albicans*. In addition to superficial candidiasis, this section will also discuss cutaneous aspergillosis and phycomycosis.

CANDIDIASIS

The yeast-like fungi of the genus *Candida* are ubiquitous in the environment and may be isolated from intertriginous areas of healthy human skin. Although other candidal species can be responsible for human infections, *Candida albicans* is the most frequent etiological agent of candidiasis. Experiments have shown that *Candida albicans* is more virulent than all other candidal species.[78] This organism is not a member of the normal skin flora but is a frequent skin transient and a member of the microflora of the alimentary tract and vagina.[79] Certain environmental conditions, notably increased temperature and humidity, are associated with an increased frequency of isolation of *Candida albicans* from cutaneous sites.[78] Many bacterial species are known to inhibit the growth of *Candida albicans*, and alteration of normal flora by the use of antibiotics has been shown to lead to an overgrowth of the yeast.[80, 81] Candidal infections usually occur when a significant alteration of the host defenses, either local or generalized, allows the organism to become invasive.[81] Studies have indicated that susceptibility to candidal infection may be related in some instances to a specific or generalized deficit of cellular immunity.[82]

Candidal infection may be acute or chronic, superficial or systemic. Systemic and disseminated candidiasis almost always occur in persons debilitated by underlying disease, but localized forms of mucocutaneous candidiasis are seen with relative frequency in otherwise normal individuals.

ORAL CANDIDIASIS (Thrush)

Oral candidiasis is commonly seen in newborn infants who acquire the organism from the maternal vagina during birth. Thrush is uncommon in older children, adolescents, and adults, in whom its presence indicates either an underlying predisposing condition, such as chronic corticosteroid therapy or diabetes, or a prolonged usage of antibiotics.[78, 83, 84] The lesions of chronic oral candidiasis in older children and adolescents are usually deeper and more adherent than the lesions in infants.[84] Thrush is characterized by dirty-white, plaque-like lesions of the tongue, buccal mucosa, and soft palate. When the friable surface material is removed, the inflamed underlying mucosa often bleeds easily in the eroded sites.

Vaginal Candidiasis

Candida albicans inhabits the vagina in at least 5 per cent of adult females,[79] and vaginal candidiasis is a relatively common disease. A number of factors predispose to this infection, including antibiotic therapy, corticosteroid therapy, diabetes mellitus, pregnancy, and the use of oral contraceptives.[78, 83, 84, 85] The infection is manifested by cheesy white plaques on an erythematous mucosa and a thick, white-yellow discharge. The disease may be relatively mild or it may be accompanied by pronounced inflammation and scaling of the entire external genitalia and surrounding skin, with progression to vesiculation and ulceration in some cases. Patients often complain of severe itching and burning.

Intertriginous and Interdigital Candidiasis

Intertriginous candidiasis is seen most often in the axillae, in the groin, under the breasts, under overhanging abdominal fat folds, in the umbilicus, and between the buttocks. The lesions are characterized by large confluent areas of moist, denuded, erythematous skin with an irregular, macerated, scaly border. Satellite lesions consist of small vesicles or pustules (Fig. 13–11). In time, intertriginous candidal lesions may become lichenified, resulting in a dry, scaly appearance. The lesions develop on skin subjected to irritation and maceration from friction caused by constant apposition. Candidal superinfection is more likely to occur in moist, warm weather under conditions that lead to excessive perspiration. Candidal intertrigo occurs more frequently in obese persons and in those with underlying disorders (such as diabetes mellitus) that predispose to candidal infection.[83]

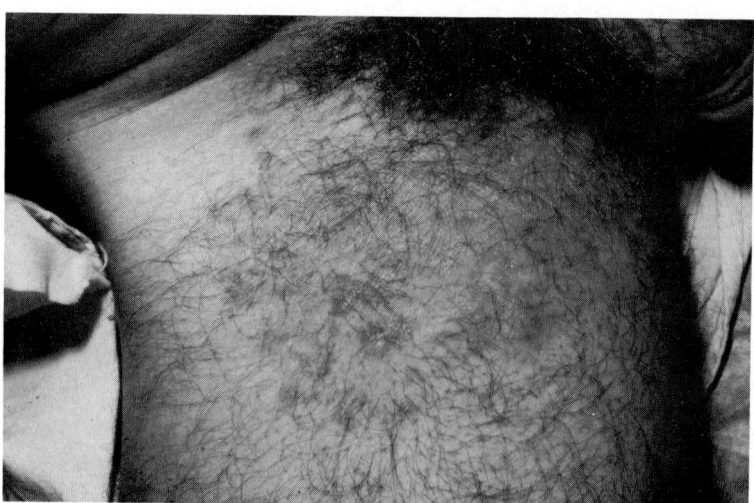

FIGURE 13–11 Candidiasis. Candidal infection of the groin, showing erythema, scaling, and satellite pustules.

A similar condition, interdigital candidiasis, commonly occurs when hands are constantly immersed in water. It is characterized by fissures between the fingers with red, denuded centers and an overhanging white epithelial fringe (Plate VII–F). Similar lesions can occur between the toes in persons who wear occlusive footgear.

PERIANAL CANDIDIASIS

Pruritus ani is an irritative dermatitis of the perianal skin, characterized by erythematous, excoriated skin and symptoms of severe pruritus. It is aggravated by occlusive, moist underclothing, poor hygiene, anal fissures, and pinworms. Occasionally, this dermatitis may become superinfected with *Candida albicans*, especially in persons receiving oral antibiotic therapy or corticosteroid medication who carry large numbers of the organism in their alimentary tract. The involved skin becomes denuded and macerated, and the lesions are identical to the lesions of candidal intertrigo or candidal diaper rash. However, colonization of the perianal skin with *Candida albicans* is frequent, and isolation of the organism from this area is not proof of superinfection.

CANDIDAL PARONYCHIA AND ONYCHIA

Candidal nail infection is characterized by a tender, erythematous swelling at the base of the nail (posterior nail fold) that occasionally discharges purulent material. If the lesion becomes chronic, the nail is secondarily invaded and becomes brittle and thickened, initially in the proximal portion and subsequently over the entire nail plate. The nail develops a brownish discoloration and prominent transverse ridges or grooves and may be completely destroyed (Fig. 13–12). Associated infection with *Pseudomonas* may impart a green color to the nail plate, particularly at the lateral margins.

This type of onychia is much more common on the fingers than on the toes,

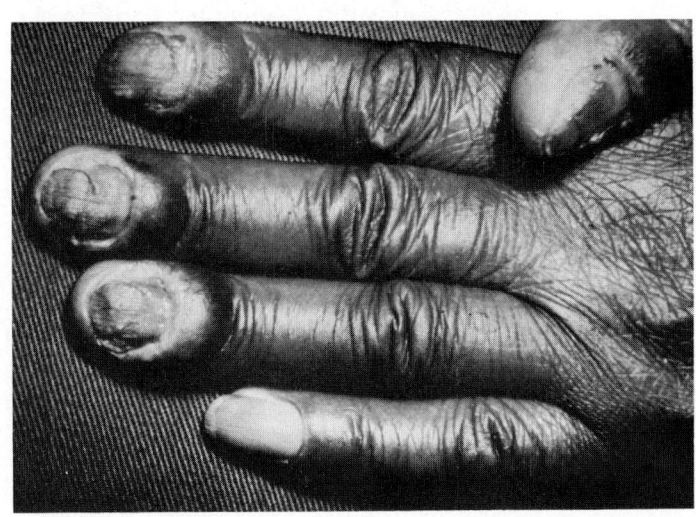

FIGURE 13–12 Candidiasis. Multiple nail involvement in candidal onychia.

although *Candida paropsilosis* of the toenails has been reported.[58] Fingernail onychia occurs in persons whose hands are frequently immersed in water. Like other mucocutaneous candidal diseases, this affliction is seen more often in persons with underlying debilitating conditions such as diabetes mellitus.

Laboratory Findings. Material such as mucosa, skin, or nail scrapings should be examined under the microscope. Either a potassium hydroxide wet mount preparation or a Gram-stained preparation may be used. An infected specimen will contain mycelia and yeast forms, both of which are strongly gram-positive. If mycelial forms are absent, only candidal colonization can be presumed.

The organism is easily grown on laboratory media, but the interpretation of cultures obtained from cutaneous sites must be tempered by the knowledge that the organism can be found as a transient on healthy skin and mucous membranes. *Candida albicans* may be easily identified in that it is the only yeast to develop pseudomycelia (germ tubes) after two hours of incubation in serum.[86]

Candidal delayed-type hypersensitivity tests are positive in most persons,[83] and although negative skin tests are found in persons with disseminated candidiasis, a negative skin test does not necessarily indicate increased susceptibility to candidal disease.[83] A number of serological techniques will demonstrate the presence of humoral immunity to *Candida,* but serodiagnosis is not useful in assessment of superficial candidiasis.[83]

Differential Diagnosis. Oral and vaginal mucosal lesions secondary to *Candida albicans* in adolescents and adults must be differentiated from similar lesions representing leukoplakia, lichen planus, and syphilis. Trichomonas vaginitis may be difficult to distinguish from candidiasis clinically.

Intertriginous and interdigital candidiasis must be differentiated from uncomplicated, uninfected intertrigo and simple interdigital maceration, as well as from intertrigo superinfected with other microorganisms, particularly *Staphylococcus*. The lesions of interdigital candidiasis may be clinically indistinguishable from tinea pedis and occasionally from erythrasma of the toe webs. Tinea cruris and erythrasma of the groin area may also resemble candidiasis of this region, especially when the candidal infection is chronic and lichenified, or when the tinea cruris is of the more acute, inflammatory type.

Candidal paronychia must be differentiated from pyogenic paronychia, which is usually of staphylococcal origin. Occasionally, *Candida* and staphylococci are responsible for a mixed infection. Candidal onychia can be differentiated from tinea unguium by the presence of soft tissue swelling or paronychia at the base of the nail and by its progression from the nail base rather than from the distal free edge of the nail plate. In addition, candidal onychia is not accompanied by significant subungual accumulation of keratinous debris.[87]

Treatment. Oral candidiasis may be effectively treated with nystatin oral suspension. A dose of 400,000 units (equivalent to 4 cc) should be rinsed in the mouth for one minute four to six times a day for a period of one to two weeks.[88] The application of 1 per cent gentian violet to the lesions is effective but cosmetically unattractive and may be a cause of mucosal necrosis if overused.

Vaginal candidiasis is best treated by the insertion of nystatin vaginal tablets twice a day for approximately two weeks.[88] If this therapy is ineffective, oral nystatin tablets, which reduce the number of *Candida* in the alimentary tract, may be helpful. When there is substantial involvement of the vulva and perineal skin, the topical application of nystatin ointment two or three times a day is recommended.[88] Although nystatin cream is also effective, its use may result in significant burning discomfort.

The treatment of intertriginous and interdigital candidiasis is best accomplished by modifying aggravating conditions, such as excessive moisture and tight-fitting clothing. Patients should be urged to wear loose-fitting, absorbent clothing and to bathe frequently. The application of nystatin powder to the affected areas several times a day is helpful.[88] When significant inflammation is present, a combination corticosteroid-nystatin ointment may be applied several times daily for at least a week.[88] Topical application of clotrimazole, miconazole nitrate and amphotericin B is also effective in the treatment of superficial candidiasis.[53] In the treatment of candidal infection of the perineal area, the reduction of alimentary candidal carriage by the use of oral nystatin tablets or nystatin oral suspension may be a necessary adjunct to the topical medication.

Patients with chronic candidal paronychia should be advised to avoid continual immersion of their hands in water. The topical application of nystatin ointment or cream is recommended. If the infection is a mixed candidal-bacterial one, oral antibiotic therapy should also be employed, and incision and drainage may occasionally be necessary. Candidal onychia should be treated by trimming the nail back to the point of infection two or three times a month, in combination with the application of topical medication. Therapy may be required for several months.[88]

ASPERGILLOSIS

Primary cutaneous aspergillosis is a rarely reported infection and is usually associated with significant underlying chronic disease.[89] The most frequent *Aspergillus* species is *Aspergillus fumigatus,* although *Aspergillus niger* has been implicated in cases of primary cutaneous aspergillosis.[90] The various *Aspergillus* species are ubiquitous in the environment and are normally non-pathogenic. Primary cutaneous aspergillosis is characterized by the appearance of multiple, discolored, cutaneous nodules and may resemble such diseases as actinomycosis or lepromatous leprosy.[89, 90] Hyphae may be demonstrated in the cutaneous granuloma, and positive cultures from carefully obtained specimens confirm the diagnosis. This condition has been reported to be responsive to topically applied nystatin.[90]

The role of *Aspergillus* in the causation of infectious or inflammatory conditions of the external ear canal is controversial.[91, 92] The species *Aspergillus niger* has been grown in almost pure culture from specimens obtained from the ear canal, although its role in provoking an inflammatory response is uncertain.[91] An underlying disorder such as seborrheic dermatitis or psoriasis may be responsible for the inflammation and the fungal organism may be only an opportunistic colonizer.[91] If "otomycosis" does not respond to topical antifungal therapy,[93] another cause for the lesions should be sought.

PHYCOMYCOSIS (Mucormycosis)

Infections caused by the fungal organisms of the genera *Rhizopus, Absidia,* and *Mucor* occur with some frequency in patients in all age groups with a variety of underlying debilitating conditions. The classification and taxonomy of the causative agents are disputed. Some mycologists prefer the designation "mucormycosis," after the order Mucorales, but the terms "phycomycosis" and "mucormycosis" are generally synonymous in the clinical literature.[94] The agents are ubiquitous in the environment and normally non-pathogenic.

Cutaneous or subcutaneous infection with one of these agents may be characterized by the appearance of a slowly enlarging, painless subcutaneous nodule.[95] Other reported clinical manifestations include chronic indolent ulcers and papular lesions.[94] Mucocutaneous infection of the nasal and paranasal area is one of the most frequently encountered signs of this disease. Most infections probably are preceded by some form of trauma that allows inoculation of the fungus into the tissues. Infection is established by these normally non-pathogenic species only when the patient's host defenses are severely disturbed.[96]

The specific fungal etiology of the lesions is established by laboratory culture, but the ubiquitous distribution of the organisms should be kept in mind. Direct examination of tissue may or may not be helpful, but the presence of typical fungal elements in biopsy specimens is strong evidence of infection.

Amphotericin B is the drug of choice in most forms of mucormycosis; however, primary cutaneous disease is rare, and not much therapeutic experience has been accumulated. Surgical debridement or excision may be useful adjuncts to specific antifungal drugs.

REFERENCES

1. Rippon, J. W.: Medical Mycology: The Pathogenic Fungi and the Pathogenic Actinomycetes. Philadelphia, W. B. Saunders, 1974.
2. Somerville, D. A.: The microbiology of the cutaneous diphtheroids. Br. J. Dermatol., 86(8):16, 1972.
3. Sarkany, I., Taplin, D., and Blank, H.: The etiology and treatment of erythrasma. J. Invest. Dermatol., 37:283, 1961.
4. Temple, D. E., and Boardman, C. R.: The incidence of erythrasma of the toe webs. Arch. Dermatol., 86:518, 1962.
5. Rippon, J. W.: Other actinomycetous infections. In; Medical Mycology: The Pathogenic Fungi and the Pathogenic Actinomycetes. Philadelphia, W. B. Saunders, 1974, pp. 40–47.
6. Somerville, D. A., Seville, R. H., Cunningham, R. C., et al.: Erythrasma in a hospital for the mentally subnormal. Br. J. Dermatol., 82:355, 1970.
7. Munro-Ashman, D., Wells, R. S., and Clayton, Y. M.: Erythrasma in adolescence. Br. J. Dermatol., 75:401, 1963.
8. Kooistra, S. A.: Prophylaxis and control of erythrasma of the toe webs. J. Invest. Dermatol., 45:399, 1965.
9. Somerville, D. A.: Erythrasma in normal young adults. J. Med. Microbiol., 3:57, 1970.
10. Ayres, S., and Mihan, R.: Erythrasma. Response to tolnaftate, an antifungal medication. Arch. Dermatol., 97:173, 1968.
11. Seville, R. H., and Somerville, D. A.: The treatment of erythrasma in a hospital for the mentally subnormal. Br. J. Dermatol., 82:502, 1970.
12. Somerville, D. A., Seville, R. H., and Noble, W. C.: A 'soap-trial' for the treatment of erythrasma. Trans. St. Johns Hosp. Dermatol. Soc., 56:172, 1970.
13. Crissey, J. T., Rebell, G. C., and Laskas, J. J.: Studies of the causative organism of trichomycosis axillaris. J. Invest. Dermatol., 19:187, 1952.
14. Orfanos, C. E., Schloesser, E., and Mahrle, G.: Hair-destroying growth of *Corynebacterium tenuis* in the so-called trichomycosis axillaris. Arch. Dermatol., 103:632, 1971.
15. Savin, J. A., Somerville, D. A., and Noble, W. C.: The bacterial flora of trichomycosis axillaris. J. Med. Microbiol., 3:352, 1970.
16. Taplin, D., and Zaias, N.: The etiology of pitted keratolysis. Proceedings of the XIIIth International Congress Dermatology, 1:593, 1968.
17. Lamberg, S.: Symptomatic pitted keratolysis. Arch. Dermatol., 100:10, 1969.

18. Long, P. I., and Campana, H. A.: An unusual mycetoma. Arch. Dermatol., 93:341, 1966.
19. Vasarinish, P.: Primary cutaneous nocardiosis. Arch. Dermatol., 98:489, 1968.
20. Brewer, N. S., Spencer, R. J., and Nichols, D. R.: Primary anorectal actinomycosis. JAMA, 228:1397, 1974.
21. Rippon, J. W.: Mycetoma. In: Medical Mycology: The Pathogenic Fungi and the Pathogenic Actinomycetes. Philadelphia, W. B. Saunders, 1974, pp. 48-69.
22. Rippon, J. W.: The pathogenic actinomycetes. In: Medical Mycology: The Pathogenic Fungi and the Pathogenic Actinomycetes. Philadelphia, W. B. Saunders, 1974, pp. 13-30.
23. Beaman, B. L., Burnside, J., Edwards, B., and Causey, W.: Nocardial infections in the United States, 1972-1974. J. Infect. Dis., 134:286, 1976.
24. Bates, R. R., and Rifkind, D.: *Nocardia brasiliensis* lymphocutaneous syndrome. Am. J. Dis. Child., 121:246, 1971.
25. Mitchell, G., Wells, G. M., and Goodman, J. S.: Sporotrichoid *Nocardia brasiliensis* infection: Response to potassium iodine. Am. Rev. Respir. Dis., 112:721, 1975.
26. Roberts, S. O. B.: Pityriasis versicolor: A clinical and mycological investigation. Br. J. Dermatol., 81:315, 1969.
27. Roberts, S. O. B.: Pityrosporum orbiculare: Incidence and distribution on clinically normal skin. Br. J. Dermatol., 81:264, 1969.
28. Roberts, S. O. B.: The mycology of the clinically normal scalp. Br. J. Dermatol., 81:626, 1969.
29. Allen, H. B., Charles, C. R., and Johnson, B. L.: Hyperpigmented tinea versicolor. Arch. Dermatol., 112:1110, 1976.
30. Jung, E. G., and Bohnert, E.: Mechanism of depigmentation in pityriasis versicolor alba (PVA). Arch. Dermatol., 256:333, 1976.
31. McGinley, K. J., Lantis, L. R., and Marples, R. R.: Microbiology of tinea versicolor. Arch. Dermatol., 102:168, 1970.
32. Burke, R. C.: Tinea versicolor: Susceptibility factors and experimental infection in human beings. J. Invest. Dermatol., 36:389, 1961.
33. Van Velsor, H., and Singletary, H.: Tinea nigra palmaris. A report of 15 cases from coastal North Carolina. Arch. Dermatol., 90:59, 1964.
34. Rippon, J. W.: Superficial infections. In: Medical Mycology: The Pathogenic Fungi and the Pathogenic Actinomycetes. Philadelphia, W. B. Saunders, 1974, pp. 84-95.
35. Smith, J. G., Sams, W. M., and Roth, F. J.: Tinea nigra palmaris: A disorder easily confused with junctional nevus of the palm. JAMA, 167:312, 1958.
36. Vaffee, A. S.: Tinea nigra palmaris resembling malignant melanoma. N. Engl. J. Med., 283:1112, 1970.
37. Moyer, D. G., and Keeler, C.: Note on culture of black piedra for cosmetic reasons. Arch. Dermatol., 89:436, 1964.
38. Noble, W. C., and Somerville, D. A.: Microbiology of Human Skin. Philadelphia, W. B. Saunders, 1974, pp. 206-224.
39. Rippon, J. W.: Dermatophytosis and dermatomycosis. In: Medical Mycology: The Pathogenic Fungi and the Pathogenic Actinomycetes. Philadelphia, W. B. Saunders, 1974, pp. 96-174.
40. Jones, H. E., Reinhardt, J. H., and Rinaldi, M. G.: Immunologic suceptibility to chronic dermatophytosis. Arch. Dermatol., 110:213, 1974.
41. Sorenson, G. W., and Jones, H. E.: Immediate and delayed hypersensitivity in chronic dermatophytosis. Arch. Dermatol., 112:40, 1976.
42. Jones, H. E., Reinhardt, J. H., and Rinaldi, M. G.: A clinical, mycological, and immunological survey for dermatophytosis. Arch. Dermatol., 108:61, 1973.
43. Jones, H. E., Reinhardt, J. H., and Rinaldi, M. G.: Model dermatophytosis in naturally infected subjects. Arch. Dermatol., 110:369, 1974.
44. Allen, A. M., and Taplin, D.: Epidemic *Trichophyton mentagrophytes* infections in servicemen: Source of infection, role of environment, host factors and susceptibility. JAMA, 226:864, 1974.
45. Reyes, A. C., and Friedman, L.: Concerning the specificity of dermatophyte-reacting antibody in human and experimental animal sera. J. Invest. Dermatol., 47:27, 1966.
46. Ajello, L.: Geographic distribution and prevalence of the dermatophytes. Ann. N. Y. Acad. Sci., 89:30, 1960.
47. Midgley, G., and Clayton, Y. M.: Distribution of dermatophytes and *Candida* spores in the environment. Br. J. Dermatol., 86(8):69, 1972.
48. English, M. P.: The epidemiology of animal ringworm in man. Br. J. Dermatol., 86(8):78, 1972.
49. Rothman, S., Smiljanic, A. M., and Whitkamp, A. W.: Mechanism of spontaneous cure in puberty of ringworm of the scalp. Science, 104:201, 1946.
50. *The Medical Letter on Drugs and Therapeutics.* 18:17, 1976.
51. Blank, F., and Mann, S. J.: *Trichophyton rubrum* infections according to age, anatomical distribution and sex. Br. J. Dermatol., 92:171, 1975.
52. Convit, J., de Albornoz, M. B., and Viso, R. F.: Subcutaneous abscesses produced by *Trichophyton rubrum*. Med. Cutan., 4:501, 1970.

53. *The Medical Letter on Drugs and Therapeutics, 18*:101, 1976.
54. Munro-Ashman, D.: Tinea pedis in adolescence. Proc. R. Soc. Med., *55*:551, 1962.
55. Gentles, J. C., Evans, E. G. V., and Jones, G. R.: Control of tinea pedis in a swimming bath. Br. Med. J., *2*:577, 1974.
56. Fulton, J. E.: Miconazole therapy for endemic fungal disease. Arch. Dermatol., *111*:596, 1975.
57. Gentles, J. C., Jones, G. R., and Roberts, D. T.: Efficacy of miconazole in the topical treatment of tinea pedis in sportsmen. Br. J. Dermatol., *93*:79, 1975.
58. English, M. P.: Nails and fungi. Br. J. Dermatol., *94*:697, 1976.
59. Russell, B., Frain-Bell, W., Stevenson, C. J., et al.: Chronic ringworm infection of the skin and nails treated with griseofulvin: Report of a therapeutic trial. Lancet, *1*:1141, 1960.
60. Davies, R. R., Ewerall, J. D., and Hamilton, E.: Mycologic and clinical evaluation of griseofulvin for chronic onychomycosis. Br. J. Med., *3*:464, 1967.
61. Suringa, D. W.: Treatment of superficial onychomycosis with topically applied glutaraldehyde. Arch. Dermatol., *102*:163, 1970.
62. Park, C. H., Greer, C. L., and Cook, C. B.: Cutaneous sporotrichosis: Recent appearance in northern Virginia. Am. J. Clin. Pathol., *57*:23, 1971.
63. Howles, J. K., Kennedy, C. B., Garvin, W. H., et al.: Chromoblastomycosis: Report of nine cases from a single area in Louisiana. Arch. Dermatol., *69*:83, 1954.
64. Riley, H. D.: Systemic mycoses in children. Parts I and II. Curr. Probl. Pediatr., *2*:12, 13, 1972.
65. Wilson, D. E., Mann, J. J., Bennett, J. E., and Utz, J. P.: Clinical features of extracutaneous sporotrichosis. Medicine, *46*:265, 1967.
66. Rippon, J. W.: Sporotrichosis. *In:* Medical Mycology: The Pathogenic Fungi and the Pathogenic Actinomycetes. Philadelphia, W. B. Saunders, 1874, pp. 248–267.
67. Foerster, H. R.: Sporotrichosis: Occupational dermatosis. JAMA, *87*:1605, 1926.
68. Dahl, B. A., Silberfarb, P. M., Sarosi, G. A., et al.: Sporotrichosis in children. Report of an epidemic. JAMA, *215*:1980, 1971.
69. Orr, E. R., and Riley, H. D.: Sporotrichosis in childhood: Report of ten cases. J. Pediatr., *78*:951, 1971.
70. Linch, P. J., and Botero, F.: Sporotrichosis in children. Am. J. Dis. Child., *122*:325, 1971.
71. Kaplan, W., and Ivens, M. S.: Fluorescent antibody staining of *S. schenckii* in cultures and clinical materials. J. Invest. Dermatol., *35*:151, 1960.
72. Blumer, S. D., Kaufman, L., Kaplan, W., et al.: Comparative evaluation of five serologic methods for the diagnosis of sporotrichosis. Appl. Microbiol., *26*:4, 1973.
73. Chandler, J. W., Kriel, R. L., and Tosh, F. E.: Childhood sporotrichosis. Am. J. Dis. Child., *115*:368, 1968.
74. Conkwright, D. D.: Case of sporotrichosis confused as cat-scratch fever. Amer. Practit., *10*:1751, 1959.
75. Peach, M. J.: Anions: Phosphate, iodine, fluoride, and other anions. *In:* Goodman, L. S., and Gilman, A. (eds.): The Pharmacological Basis of Therapeutics. New York, Macmillan, 1975, pp. 798–808.
76. Rippon, J. W.: Chromomycosis. *In:* Medical Mycology: The Pathogenic Fungi and the Pathogenic Actinomycetes. Philadelphia, W. B. Saunders, 1974, pp. 229–247.
77. Hughes, W. T.: Chromoblastomycosis: Successful treatment with topical amphotericin B. J. Pediatr., *71*:351, 1967.
78. Maibach, H. I., and Kligman, A. M.: The biology of experimental human cutaneous moniliasis. (*Candida albicans*). Arch. Dermatol., *85*:233, 1962.
79. Noble, W. C., and Somerville, D. A.: The fungal flora. *In:* Microbiology of Human Skin. Philadelphia, W. B. Saunders, 1974, pp. 206–224.
80. Paine, T. F.: The inhibitory actions of bacteria on *Candida* growth. Antibiot. Chemother., *8*:273, 1958.
81. Seelig, M. S.: Mechanisms by which antibiotics increase the incidence and severity of candidiasis and alter the immunological defenses. Bacteriol. Rev., *30*:442, 1966.
82. Kirkpatrick, C. H., and Smith, T. K.: Chronic mucocutaneous candidiasis: Immunologic and antibiotic therapy. Ann. Intern. Med., *80*:310, 1974.
83. Rippon, J. W.: Candidosis. *In:* Medical Mycology: The Pathogenic Fungi and the Pathogenic Actinomycetes. Philadelphia, W. B. Saunders, 1974, pp. 175–204.
84. Dobias, B.: Moniliasis in pediatrics. Am. J. Dis. Child., *94*:234, 1957.
85. Porter, P. S., and Lyle, J. S.: Yeast vulvovaginitis due to oral contraceptives. Arch. Dermatol., *93*:402, 1966.
86. Taschdijan, C. L., Burchall, J. J., and Kozinn, P. J.: Rapid identification of *Candida albicans* by filamentation on serum and serum substitutes. Am. J. Dis. Child., *99*:212, 1960.
87. Zaias, N.: Onychomycosis. Arch. Dermatol., *105*:263, 1972.
88. Witten, V. H., and Katz, S. I.: Nystatin. Med. Clin. North Am., *54*:1329, 1970.
89. Caro, I., and Dogliotti, M.: Aspergillosis of the skin: Report of a case. Dermatologica, *146*:244, 1973.

90. Cahill, K. M., El Mofty, A. M., and Kawaguchi, T. P.: Primary cutaneous aspergillosis. Arch. Dermatol., *96*:545, 1967.
91. Kingery, F. A. J.: The myth of otomycosis. JAMA, *191*:141, 1965.
92. McGonigle, J., Jr., and Jilson, O.: Otomycosis, an entity. Arch. Dermatol., *95*:45, 1967.
93. Rippon, J. W.: Mycotic infections of the eye and ear. *In:* Medical Mycology: The Pathogenic Fungi and the Pathogenic Actinomycetes. Philadelphia, W. B. Saunders, 1974, pp. 475–490.
94. Rippon, J. W.: Mucormycosis. *In:* Medical Mycology: The Pathogenic Fungi and the Pathogenic Actinomycetes. Philadelphia, W. B. Saunders, 1974, pp. 430–447.
95. Harris, J. S.: Mucormycosis. Report of a case. Pediatrics, *16*:857, 1955.
96. Straatsma, B. R., Zimmerman, L. F., and Gass, J. P. M.: Phycomycosis, a clinical-pathological study of 51 cases. Lab. Invest., *11*:963, 1962.

14
CUTANEOUS NEVI

ALEXANDER A. FONDAK, M.D.
DAVID L. RAMSAY, M.D., M.Ed.

Several types of nevi commonly encountered in the practice of adolescent dermatology are described in this chapter. The discussion will focus primarily on epidermal and nevocytic nevi. The inclusion of certain dermatological entities in the category of nevus and the exclusion of others is a matter of opinion, because the term nevus may be defined in a variety of ways. A broad definition of nevus is "anything, especially anything odd, abnormal, or faulty, that is related to gestation, conception, and postnatal development and stems from hereditable or embryogenic fault, abnormality, or oddity."[1] More commonly, however, the term is used to refer to a localized benign growth that is present at birth or appears during development and is composed either of nevus cells or of an excess of one or more of the normal components of the skin.

THE ORIGIN OF NEVI

Until recent times, birthmarks were thought to be the result of psychological or physical trauma to the fetus. A birthmark, therefore, was a reflection in the child of a traumatic event that occurred before birth. This "maternal impression" theory is no longer considered valid; however, a pathophysiological mechanism for nevus formation has yet to be established. One hypothesis concerning the origin of nevi suggests a relationship to genetic mutation.[2] Another involves an interrelationship between nerves and nerve growth and the production of nevi. A possible influence of the nervous system on the origin of nevi is occasionally suggested by the dermatomal distribution of certain nevi, which may be associated with underlying somatic abnormalities.

TABLE 14-1 TYPES OF CUTANEOUS NEVI

KERATINOCYTIC EPIDERMAL NEVI	NEVOCYTIC NEVI	MELANOCYTIC NEVI

Differentiation toward epidermis:
1. Verrucous epidermal nevi
   A. Localized and linear verrucous epidermal nevi
   B. Inflammatory linear verrucous epidermal nevi
2. Ichthyosis hystrix (localized epidermolytic hyperkeratosis)
3. Becker's giant pigmented hairy nevus (not a true nevus)
 	
Differentiation toward hair follicle:
  Nevus comedonicus
 	
Differentiation toward sebaceous glands:
  Nevus sebaceus
	Junctional
	Intradermal
	Compound
	Benign juvenile melanoma (spindle and epithelioid cell nevus)
	Halo nevus
	Congenital giant nevocytic nevus (garment nevus, bathing trunk nevus)
		Mongolian spot
		Nevus of Ota and Ito
		Blue nevus

CLASSIFICATION OF CUTANEOUS NEVI

No universally accepted classification of cutaneous nevi is available. Nevi are most frequently classified by cell type. A secondary classification may be devised according to the degree of cellular maturation and apparent tissue differentiation.[3] The classification of cutaneous nevi presented in Table 14–1 is based primarily upon cell type. The epidermal nevi are further subdivided according to degree of cellular differentiation. Melanocytic and nevocytic nevi are grouped separately for the purposes of this discussion.

KERATINOCYTIC EPIDERMAL NEVI

The nomenclature used to refer to keratinocytic epidermal nevi may be confusing, since it often reflects an admixture of clinical and histopathological opinion. In the literature, at least 50 terms have been used to describe these nevi.[4] In the following discussion we will try to clarify this situation by defining the terms chosen.

VERRUCOUS EPIDERMAL NEVI

Verrucous epidermal nevi may be subdivided into two distinct entities: localized and linear verrucous epidermal nevi (non-inflammatory) and inflammatory linear verrucous epidermal nevus (*Ilven*).

LOCALIZED AND LINEAR VERRUCOUS EPIDERMAL NEVI (Non-Inflammatory)

These conditions may be present at birth or may develop during childhood or adolescence. The localized form is a fairly well demarcated lesion with

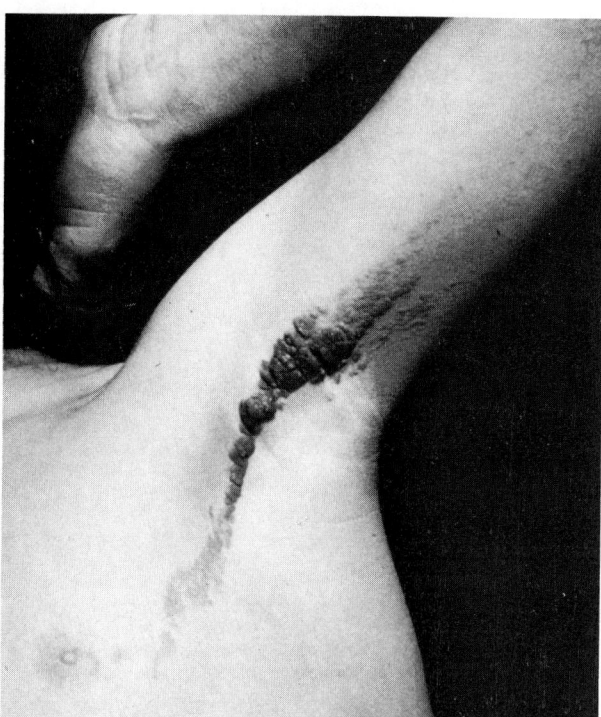

FIGURE 14–1 Linear epidermal nevus.

discrete or confluent skin-colored or light brown hyperkeratotic papules. The surface of the lesion varies from nodular to verrucoid. Multiple lesions arranged in a linear fashion are called linear verrucous epidermal nevi (non-inflammatory) (Fig. 14–1).[5] Both types of nevus may be found almost anywhere on the body. When one extremity or one side of the body is involved, the clinical term *nevus unius lateris* is used.

Histopathological Findings. Both types of non-inflammatory verrucous epidermal nevi contain varying degrees of hyperkeratosis, acanthosis, papillomatosis, and elongation of the rete ridges.

INFLAMMATORY LINEAR VERRUCOUS EPIDERMAL NEVUS
(Ilven, Liven, or Nevil)

This entity was first described by Unna in 1896.[6] He noted that on histological examination, certain linear nevi resembled chronic lichenified dermatitis or psoriasis (Fig. 14–2). In 1971, Kaidbey and Kurban described five patients with this condition, which they called "dermatitic epidermal nevus."[7] A study of 15 patients with *Ilven* was reported by Altman and Mehregan in 1971.[8] In patients from both studies, the onset of lesions had usually occurred in childhood. All of the patients of Kaidbey and Kurban were male; in Altman and Mehregan's series, there was a 4:1 female to male ratio.

The patchy or linear lesions are composed of grouped, erythematous, slightly verrucous, scaly papules. Areas of lichenification and excoriation may be superimposed. Lesions are usually unilateral and are most commonly found in the buttock area, although the legs are also frequently involved. Most

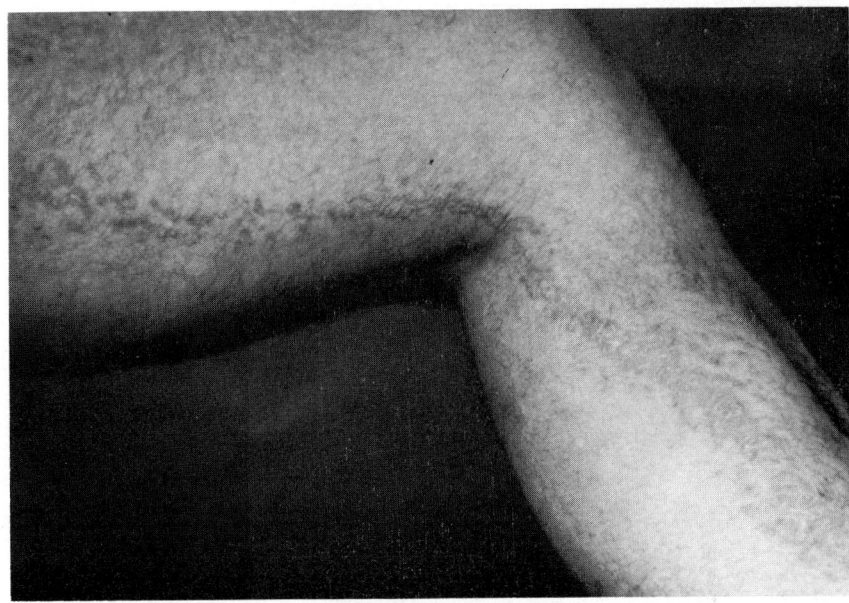

FIGURE 14-2 Inflammatory linear verrucous epidermal nevus.

patients experience mild to moderate pruritus. The lesions tend to be persistent, regardless of therapy.

Histopathological Findings. These lesions are characterized by hyperkeratosis, with moderate acanthosis, papillomatosis, and elongation of the rete ridges. The dermis contains a lymphohistiocytic infiltrate.

ICHTHYOSIS HYSTRIX

Until recently, the term ichthyosis hystrix frequently was used interchangeably with *nevus unius lateris*. As we have indicated, the latter term is generally reserved to describe a distinct clinical lesion, linear verrucous epidermal nevus (non-inflammatory). So too, the term ichthyosis hystrix currently is used to describe a distinct morphological form of epidermal nevus (Fig. 14–3). Ichythyosis hystrix refers to localized lesions of congenital epidermolytic hyperkeratosis (intraepidermal microvesiculation), which are also found in congenital ichthyosiform erythroderma.[9] Clinically, the lesions may resemble other forms of non-inflammatory linear verrucous epidermal nevi, with linear bands of brownish, verrucous, hyperkeratotic papules. The bands usually are arranged in a parallel configuration, often having a whorl-like pattern.

Ichythyosis hystrix may be dominantly inherited. In its most severe form, it results in a condition known to the layman as "porcupine man."

Histopathological Findings. The diagnosis of ichthyosis hystrix depends on the histopathological findings in the affected skin.[10] The epidermis shows marked hyperkeratosis, papillomatosis, and acanthosis. In addition and most important, there is epidermolytic hyperkeratosis, which is characterized by hypergranulosis and vacuolization of the cells of the granular layer.[11]

330 CHAPTER 14—CUTANEOUS NEVI

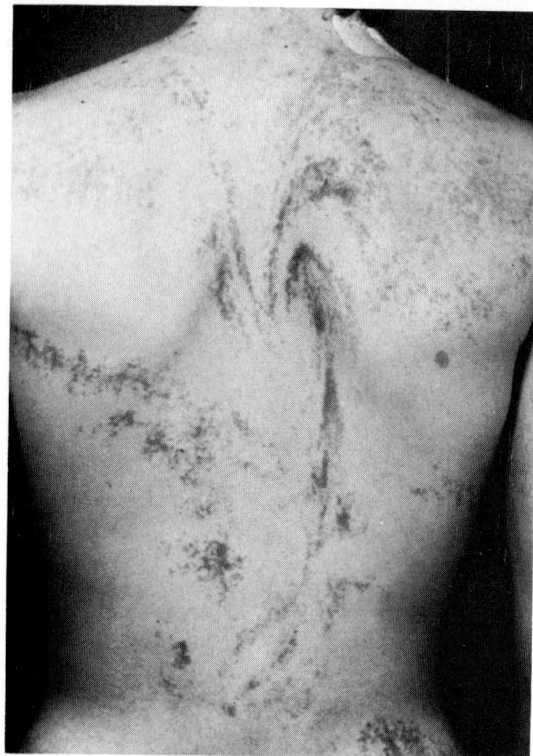

FIGURE 14–3 Ichthyosis hystrix.

TREATMENT OF KERATINOCYTIC EPIDERMAL NEVI

For the most part, treatment of these lesions is unsatisfactory. Superficial removal of the warty lesions usually is followed by recurrence.[12] The only definitive treatment* is complete excision, which may be postponed until adolescence to allow for the full development of the lesion. If the lesion is extensive, grafting may be necessary.

Solomon and Esterly[13] recommend topical application of salicylic acid (3 per cent in cold cream) or lactic acid (3 to 6 per cent in cold cream) for the treatment of hyperkeratotic lesions in older children. Tretinoin cream, in 0.05 per cent concentration, applied topically three times a day, also has been shown to be effective in reducing hyperkeratosis in patients with epidermolytic hyperkeratosis.[14] Since ichthyosis hystrix is a localized form of epidermolytic hyperkeratosis, tretinoin cream might prove helpful in this disease also.

Whenever an extensive epidermal or organoid nevus is found in a child, a thorough history should be obtained and a physical examination performed periodically. The procedures are necessary to ascertain the presence of any associated abnormalities, especially of the skeletal, nervous, and vascular systems.

---

*"Definitive" here does not imply cosmetic success.—Ed.

BECKER'S NEVUS

The pigmented, hairy, epidermal nevus of Becker (Becker's melanosis) is a poorly circumscribed area of hyperpigmentation with hypertrichosis.[15] This lesion is not really a nevus, since there is no apparent overgrowth of either keratinocytes or melanocytes, as the clinical appearance would suggest. However, both its clinical presentation and its occurrence in adolescence lead most dermatologists to think of it as a nevus.

The lesion usually appears in pubescent males, although it is occasionally found in women.[16] It is often first noted after exposure to strong sunlight. In fact, the two cases reported by Becker were preceded by severe sunburn. The nevus is usually located unilaterally on the upper half of the trunk, especially around the shoulder.

The areas of hyperpigmentation and hypertrichosis tend to persist for life. However, the intensity of pigmentation may decrease as the patient ages. This lesion, unlike a congenital giant nevocytic nevus, has no increased potential for malignant degeneration.

Histopathological Findings. Mild to moderate acanthosis is usually found in histological sections of Becker's nevus. The basal cell layer in the affected areas may be diffusely hyperpigmented, as compared with unaffected areas, and melanophages are often present in the papillary dermis. The number of epidermal melanocytes is either normal or slightly increased and the number of pilosebaceous structures may be increased.

NEVUS COMEDONICUS

Nevus comedonicus is a rare condition manifested as a linear array of comedone-like papules. The central crater of the papule is usually almost black and is surrounded by a slight scale (Fig. 14–4). Two forms of nevus comedonicus may be seen: lesions containing predominantly comedone-like structures, and lesions containing pustules and cysts. The linear lesions are usually unilateral, but bilateral involvement has been reported to occur.[17] Males and females are equally affected. The usual sites are the face, neck, arm, and chest. There is apparently no association with acne vulgaris. Treatment for nevus comedonicus, as for other epidermal nevi, is unsatisfactory. Excision of the lesion, including the underlying dermis, is definitive but leaves a scar.

Histopathological Findings. Many keratinous plugs are seen within immature pilosebaceous follicles. Occasionally, rudimentary hair shafts and sebaceous gland lobules are contained in the sections.

NEVUS SEBACEUS (of Jadassohn)

Nevus sebaceus (of Jadassohn) usually appears on the scalp or face as a yellowish, well-circumscribed, slightly raised, oval plaque. Its color varies from reddish-yellow to yellowish-brown, and its surface tends to be hairless and either verrucoid or slightly nodular (Fig. 14–5). Occasionally, it is present in a linear form, especially behind the ear. In a series of 140 patients, the incidence in males and females was found to be approximately equal.[18] In this series, 82

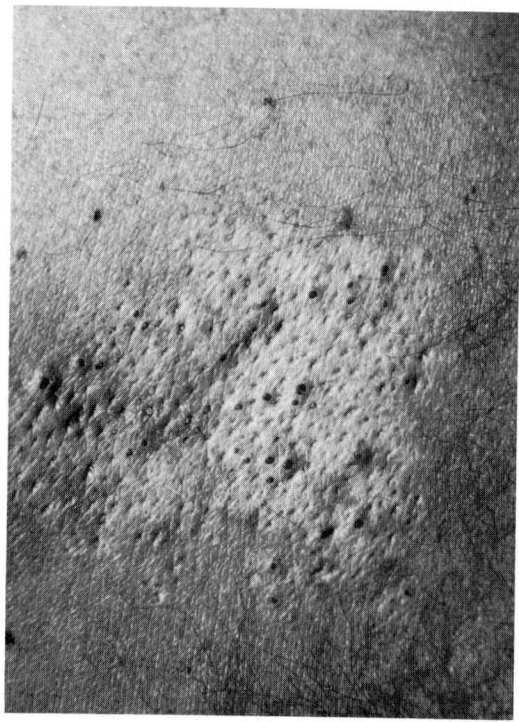

FIGURE 14–4 Nevus comedonicus.

patients had had lesions since birth. In 37 cases, the nevi had developed later, usually during early childhood or rarely during adolescence. The lesion grows relatively slowly during childhood, but progresses more rapidly during puberty, reflecting the response of the glandular structures to hormonal stimuli.[19]

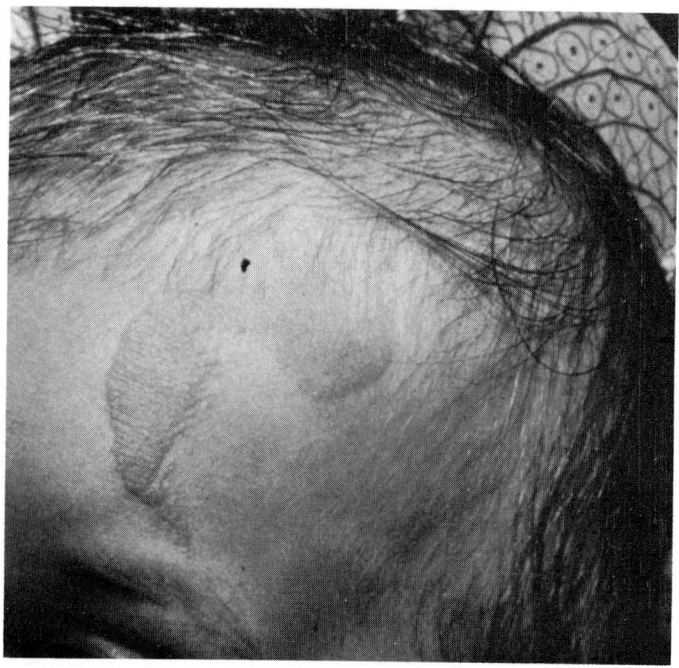

FIGURE 14–5 Nevus sebaceus.

Although an increase in both the number and size of sebaceous glands is evident in most lesions during adolescent years and later, these glands may be diminished or even absent. Therefore, some investigators[19] believe that this lesion may not be totally of sebaceous gland origin. Ectopic apocrine glands are frequently present[18] as well as an admixture of various cystic glandular structures. The term "organoid nevus" describes more accurately the multifaceted malformation represented by this lesion.

The various malformations within a nevus sebaceus (organoid nevus) are far from stable. Mehregan and Pinkus[19] divide the life cycle of the nevus sebaceus into three phases. In early childhood, the lesion is relatively quiescent, and the sebaceous glands are underdeveloped. During adolescence, the nevus grows rapidly, sebaceous glands enlarge, and ectopic apocrine glands appear, enlarge, and become cystic. During the third and least predictable phase, which occurs in adulthood, secondary neoplasia may develop. In a series of 150 cases,[19] 33 patients developed 52 tumors. Twenty-one were basal cell epitheliomas, and eight were benign sweat gland adenomas (syringocystadenoma papilliferum).

The development of basal cell carcinoma in nevus sebaceus is difficult to assess because of the incongruent reports in the literature. Estimates range from between 5 and 14 per cent[20] to 22 per cent.[21] Wilson Jones and Heyl[18] believe that basal cell carcinomas occur in approximately 6.5 per cent of cases of nevus sebaceus. They point out the relative frequency of basaloid proliferation present in these lesions, which may be mistaken for malignant change.

Histopathological Findings. The histological findings in nevus sebaceus depend on the age of the lesion.[19] In early lesions, there is mild papillomatous hyperplasia of the epidermis, which becomes more prominent as the patient ages. During childhood, sebaceous glands are relatively underdeveloped and are smaller and fewer in number than those found in adolescents or in adults. Hair follicles in early lesions also are underdeveloped. Normal hair follicles and hair shafts can be seen in older lesions. Ectopic apocrine glands are also found in adult cases.

During adult life, the lesions of nevus sebaceus begin to undergo pseudo-epitheliomatous hyperplasia and secondary neoplasia. Syringocystadenoma papilliferum is a sweat gland adenoma most frequently contained in an area of nevus sebaceus, but other types of benign tumors as well as basal cell carcinomas may develop.

TREATMENT

Excision is the treatment of choice for nevus sebaceus. A surgical solution to the problem should be sought even if the lesion is quiescent in order to prevent the occurrence of malignancy. Even in the adult with pseudo-epitheliomatous hyperplasia, complete conservative surgical excision usually prevents further difficulties.

EPIDERMAL NEVUS SYNDROME

In 1962, Feuerstein and Mims[22] reported two patients who had linear nevus sebaceus lesions on the face associated with convulsions and mental retardation. Since that time, many other patients with various linear epidermal or organoid (nevus sebaceus) nevi associated with seizures, mental retardation, and multiple developmental abnormalities have been reported.[23, 24]

In 1975, Solomon and Esterly[25] described their findings in 60 patients with this neurocutaneous syndrome. Thirty-six (60 per cent) had lesions of *nevus unius lateris,* frequently involving the limbs. Another 20 per cent had lesions of ichythyosis hystrix, generally on the trunk. Linear nevus sebaceus, usually of the scalp and face, was present in 10 per cent of patients. Approximately 33 per cent had an admixture of lesions.

Associated with the skin lesion was a variety of skeletal abnormalities, including incomplete formation of bony structures, hypoplasia and hypertrophy of bones, and bony cysts. Of the 60 patients described in this series, 50 per cent had severe to moderate neurological involvement and 40 per cent demonstrated mental retardation. A fourth group of developmental abnormalities was vascular in nature and included cerebral hemangiomas and cutaneous and renal vascular malformations.

In addition to the major developmental anomalies of skin, central nervous system, bone, and blood vessels, various ocular and renal abnormalities occur in the epidermal nevus syndrome.[26, 27]

As children with this syndrome reach maturity, they must be carefully followed medically to ascertain whether they have an increased susceptibility to develop internal malignancy. Several systemic malignancies have been reported in patients with this syndrome,[12, 28] although a causal relationship has not been proved.

If a patient is suspected of having the epidermal nevus syndrome, the guidelines of Solomon and Esterly[25] are helpful in delineating any abnormalities. A careful history, including the patient's developmental pattern, must be obtained. A complete physical examination also must be performed. The cutaneous, neurological, musculoskeletal, and cardiovascular systems should carefully be examined for the presence of abnormalities.

NEVOCYTIC NEVI

ORIGIN OF THE NEVUS CELL

An early theory concerning the development of the nevus cell was proposed by Unna in 1894. Called the "Abtropfung" theory, it held that dermal nevus cells were epidermal cells that had "dropped off" from the epidermis into the dermis. A later theory was formulated in 1951 by Masson,[29] who believed that junctional nevus cells (epidermal nevus cells) resulted from an "overproliferation of melanoblasts," leading to an increase in the number of melanocytes. The nevus cells in the dermis were thought to be derived from two origins: (1) epidermal melanocytes that had migrated downward, and (2) Schwannian cells of intradermal nerves that had migrated upward. The fact that both epidermal melanocytes and Schwann cells share a common ancestry in the neural crest lent credence to this theory.

Another investigator has postulated that nevus cells are not derived from normal epidermal melanocytes or Schwann cells but are misdirected embryonic cells arising from "nevoblasts."[30] Still other investigators consider nevus cells to be true melanocytes.[31]

Setting aside the debate concerning the origin of the nevus cell, some dermatopathologists believe nevus cells may be differentiated from melanocytes by light microscopy, since nevus cells are arranged in clusters and, more important, do not contain dendritic processes. We have accepted this histological differentiation for the purpose of classification, recognizing that the issue is still unresolved, and that there may indeed be no difference between the nevus cell and the melanocyte.

LIFE CYCLE OF COMMON NEVUS CELL NEVI

The percentage of infants born with nevus cell nevi has been estimated to be 2.7 per cent among Caucasians and 15.6 per cent among blacks. These data were based upon clinical diagnoses rather than biopsy findings and have since been challenged. Although 3.9 per cent of 1,058 Caucasian infants studied[33] were found to have had pigmented lesions at the time of birth, only 1 per cent had nevus cell nevi proved by histological examination of the lesions.

Nevus cell nevi increase during adolescence, remain quiescent during adulthood, and involute after the age of 60. Nevus cell nevi, therefore, are an infrequent finding in patients over the age of 80.

CLINICAL APPEARANCE OF THE COMMON NEVUS CELL NEVI

The three most common types of nevocytic nevi, classified according to their histopathological characteristics, are junctional, compound, and intradermal nevi.

A *junctional* nevus is a flat or slightly elevated, well-demarcated, brown to brownish-black round or ovoid lesion. Its surface is usually smooth with preserved skin markings. Junctional nevus cell nevi may appear anywhere on the skin or on mucous membranes. Most nevi found in infants and children are of this type (Fig. 14–6).

Compound nevi appear clinically as either moderately raised or papillomatous lesions. They are usually round or oval and are light brown in color, with the hyperpigmented area extending beyond the raised portion of the lesion and often forming a halo. They may have brown stippling and coarse hair on the surface. Compound nevi tend to enlarge and darken during puberty and pregnancy.

A third clinical variety is a firm, dome-shaped lesion, which is usually an *intradermal* nevus. Generally, it first appears on the face or neck during middle age as a light brown or flesh-colored lesion, possibly with coarse hair. A variant of the intradermal type is the pedunculated nevus. It is soft, usually flesh-colored, and may be found on the arms, legs, trunk, or in the skin folds.[35]

Histopathological Findings. The nevus cell nevus is distinguished by the histological presence of "nests" or collections of nevus cells in the lower epidermis, the dermis, or both. In the junctional nevus, nevus cells are present in discrete nests in the lower portion of the epidermis. Occasional nests also are present in the upper papillary dermis, but most maintain close contact with the

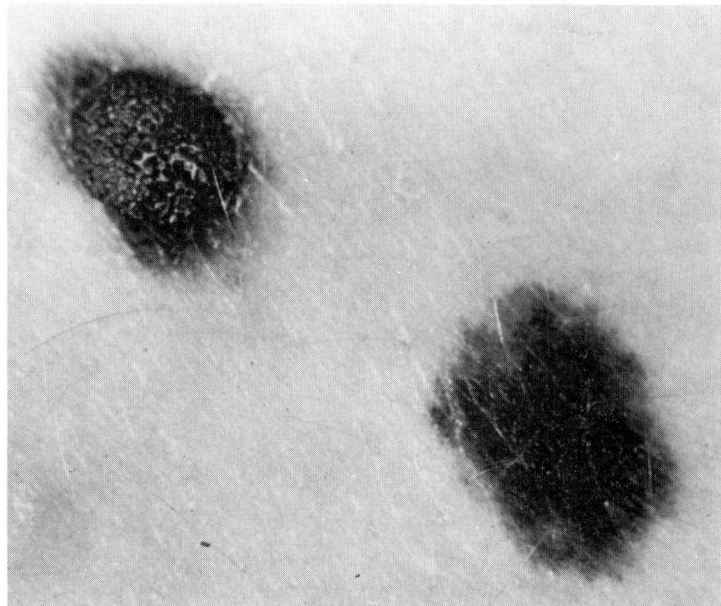

FIGURE 14–6 Lesion on left is a compound melanocytic nevus; lesion on right is a junctional lesion.

epidermis. Nevus cells are cuboidal or oval in appearance and contain varying amounts of melanin. Unless the nevus has been irritated, there are usually very few inflammatory cells in the dermis.

A compound nevus is intermediate between a junctional and an intradermal nevus and combines the histological features of both. Nests of nevus cells are present in the lower portion of the epidermis and in the upper portion of the dermis.

In the intradermal nevus cell nevus, the nevus cells are confined to the dermis where they are arranged in nests and cords. The nevus cells in the upper dermis are epithelioid in shape and have varying amounts of melanin. Those in the mid-dermis are smaller and have little or no melanin. The nevus cells present in the lowest portion of the dermis are often spindle-shaped and are frequently arranged in bundles, perhaps reflecting a neuroid origin. As in the junctional nevus, an inflammatory infiltrate is minimal unless the nevus has been irritated.

TREATMENT OF COMMON NEVUS CELL NEVI

Patients usually request treatment of a pigmented lesion for one of two reasons: cosmetic improvement or fear of malignancy. The method of removing the lesion depends upon both the indication for and the location of the lesion.

Most nevus cell nevi in which there is no clinical suspicion of malignancy, i.e., no surrounding erythema, tenderness, ulceration, or disorderly variation in shape or color (especially the simultaneous coloration of red, white, and blue), can be removed best by shave excision parallel to and just below the surface of the skin.[36] Bleeding can be stopped by light electrodesiccation. Nonetheless all nevi removed in this fashion should be submitted for histological examination in order to confirm the clinical diagnosis.

Even though occasional nevi are not completely removed by the scalpel shave excision method, studies have shown no increased incidence of malignancy in these lesions.[37, 38] In rare instances, however, recurrence of a pigmented lesion after partial removal can *simulate* the histological picture of malignant melanoma.[39, 40]

Although most nevus cell nevi can be removed by the scalpel shave excision method, certain types should be totally excised. In addition to those nevi suspected of malignancy, small hairy nevus cell nevi as well as congenital giant pigmented hairy nevi (garment or bathing trunk nevi) are best treated by total excision.[36] Macular nevi in children and adolescents tend to recur after scalpel shave excision and probably also should be totally excised.

Malignant Transformation Of The Common Nevus Cell Nevi

Pigmented nevi of the palms and soles were once thought to be potentially malignant and were often prophylactically removed. The malignant potential of these nevi is no longer believed to be any greater than that of nevi in other locations. However, 20 to 30 per cent of melanomas (approximately 25 per cent a year in the United States) are thought to arise from nevus cell nevi. The physician should be alert to changes in shape, size, or color of these lesions as well as to any recent episodes of itching or bleeding.

Balloon Cell Nevus

The balloon cell nevus is a rare variant of a compound or intradermal nevus. The first case was reported in 1935 by Miescher,[41] who thought the balloon cells were nevus cells that had become sebaceous gland cells. Recent electron microscopic studies have shown that balloon cells have the same origin as nevus cells.[42, 43]

Most patients who develop balloon cell nevi do so during the first three decades of life.[44] The lesions may be found on almost any part of the body but are usually located on the head, neck, or trunk. They are light brown or flesh-colored papules less than 5 mm in diameter and are usually indistinguishable from the common compound nevocellular nevus. They may be differentiated by using histological criteria. There does not appear to be any increased incidence of malignant change in this type of nevus, although a rare balloon cell type of malignant melanoma does exist.

Treatment of balloon cell nevi corresponds to treatment of other nevus cell nevi. Scalpel shave excision with light electrodesiccation of the base is usually adequate for removal.

Histopathological Findings. Balloon cell nevi are either compound or intradermal in type.[44] The balloon cells are large, polyhedral, and pale-staining. They can be found either in nests or arranged singly among the more common variety of nevus cells. Transitional cells between common nevus cells and balloon cells have been reported in cases of balloon cell nevi.[45]

BENIGN JUVENILE MELANOMA (Spindle Cell and Epithelioid Nevus, Spitz's Nevus)

The benign juvenile melanoma is a rare but very important histological variant of the compound nevus cell nevus. It was first described in 1948 by Spitz,[46] who noted that certain compound nevus cell lesions of children, which histologically resemble malignant melanoma, usually follow a benign clinical course and do not form metastases.

Benign juvenile melanomas generally occur in children between the ages of three and 13,[47] although they may also develop in adulthood.[48] The lesion is usually solitary, appearing in children as an oval, smooth, dome-shaped, reddish to reddish-purple papule or nodule (Plate VI–D). In adults, the lesions are usually more brown than red in color. They are located predominantly on the face, head, and neck of children and on the face, arms, and legs of adults.

The treatment of choice is conservative local excision, especially in children, in whom incomplete removal usually leads to recurrence.

Histopathological Findings. The overall histological pattern of a benign juvenile melanoma in most cases is similar to that of a compound nevus cell nevus, but the cellular atypia may cause confusion with malignant melanoma. The nevus cells are usually either epithelioid or spindle-shaped. Some lesions may contain both types of cells. Lesions composed predominantly of epithelioid cells are found more frequently in children, while the pure spindle-cell type is found most often in adults.

In benign juvenile melanoma, the nevus cells tend to form nests in both the epidermis and dermis. Multinucleated giant cells are frequently found in the epithelioid type and when present help to confirm the diagnosis. Mitotic figures may be numerous, especially in the spindle-cell type. Lesions in adults usually have more melanin in the dermis than lesions found in children. Both edema and dilated blood vessels are frequently found in the upper dermis.

HALO NEVUS (Sutton's Nevus, Leukoderma Acquisitum Centrifugum)

Halo nevus is a clinical term used to describe a zone of depigmentation (leukoderma) surrounding a pigmented lesion (Fig. 14–7). Most patients who develop halo nevi are either in late adolescence or early adulthood.

In most cases, a solitary lesion is present on the trunk, usually on the back. On clinical examination, one may find a centrally located reddish-brown papule surrounded by a whitish halo. The halo varies in width from 1 to 5 mm.[49] The center of the lesion is usually a nevus cell nevus of the intradermal or compound type, but halo formation has also been reported around blue nevi, malignant melanomas,[50] and giant congenital nevi.

From long-term observation of 14 patients with a total of 34 nevi, Frank and Cohen[51] concluded that most of these pigmented lesions would eventually involute and disappear. Electron microscopy studies have supported their postulation that the presence of a halo indicated destruction of the nevus cells in the lesion.[52]

Patients with resolving halo nevi have been found to possess circulating

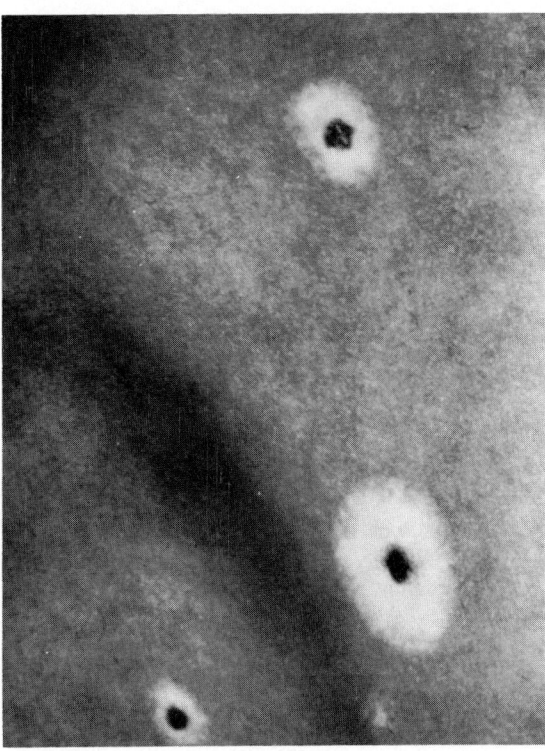

FIGURE 14–7 Halo nevi.

antibodies against the cytoplasm of melanoma cells, antibodies similar to those found in patients with malignant melanoma.[53] This finding has led to speculation that the halo nevus represents an attempt by the body to reject a pigmented lesion undergoing malignant change.

Since most halo nevi involute and disappear, usually no treatment is required. However, if there is any question about the exact diagnosis of the central pigmented lesion, complete conservative surgical excision is advised.

Histopathological Findings. In the early stage, the lesion is typical of a compound or intradermal nevus, with nevus cells in nests present at the epidermal junction. In the dermis, nevus cells are present either singly or in nests. The most striking feature of the halo nevus is the dense inflammatory infiltrate in the dermis, often in a band-like pattern. This infiltrate is composed mostly of lymphocytes, with occasional histiocytes and plasma cells. These inflammatory cells are present throughout the dermis, intermingled with the nevus cells and, sometimes even obscuring them. In the later stage, few nevus cells can be detected.

CONGENITAL GIANT PIGMENTED HAIRY NEVUS
(Garment Nevus, Bathing Trunk Nevus)

The congenital giant pigmented hairy nevus is a rare malformation of nevus cells and pilar complexes. Because of the cosmetic disfigurement it produces and because of its tendency toward malignant degeneration (approximately 10 per cent[54]) it is of great clinical significance.

The lesion, usually referred to as a congenital giant pigmented hairy nevus, is a large one, measuring many centimeters in diameter (Fig. 14–8). Because it may be so extensive that it covers the entire back, chest, bathing trunk area, or extremity, it is called "garment nevus." Recently, congenital nevi much smaller than the typical garment nevus have been found to have a similar histological pattern. These too may have a significant incidence of malignant degeneration, but the exact percentage is not known.[55]

The congenital giant pigmented hairy nevus is usually brown, with coarse, dark hairs on the surface. The surface is papillated or nodular, and the border is usually well defined. However, smaller satellite nevi may be present both at the periphery of the main lesion and distant from it. The lesion becomes darker, thicker, and more hairy as the patient matures. Giant pigmented hairy nevi may occur in a neurocutaneous syndrome known as neurocutaneous melanosis.[56, 57]

Affected infants have giant pigmented nevi (Fig. 14–9), often in the occipital or posterior nuchal areas or back, and melanotic tumors of the central nervous system (leptomeningeal melanosis). The presence of pigmented tumors in the central nervous system can lead to hydrocephalus, seizures, and mental retardation. Like skin lesions, these central nervous system tumors may undergo malignant change.

Changes resembling those of neurofibromatosis are seen occasionally in patients with congenital giant pigmented hairy nevi. Usually, these patients do not have a family history of neurofibromatosis;[56] nor do they have café au lait spots or axillary freckling.

The treatment of choice for congenital giant pigmented hairy nevi is

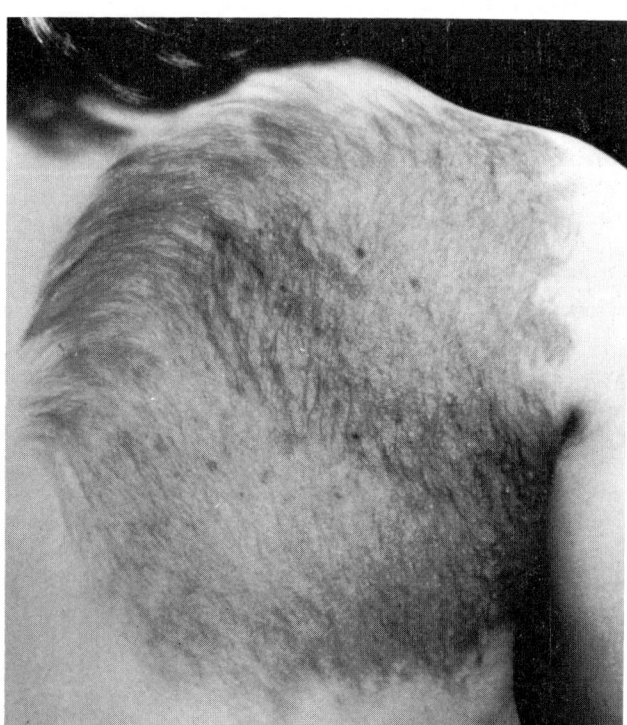

FIGURE 14–8 Giant congenital melanocytic nevus.

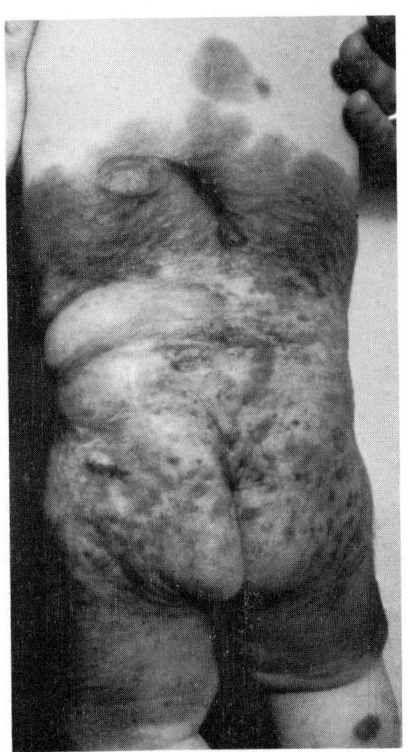

FIGURE 14-9 Bathing trunk nevus. Note that the lesion may be pendulous.

surgical excision.[54] This task is sometimes difficult because of the size of the lesion. When a large area of the body must be treated, surgical excision can be performed in stages at intervals of several months. A split thickness skin graft may be needed for large lesions.

Histopathological Findings. Hyperkeratosis and epidermal hyperplasia may be present. Nevus cells are found in nests in the lower epidermis and in the papillary dermis. In the papillary and reticular dermis, the nests of nevus cells of congenital nevi are often arranged in a band-like pattern or in single file between collagen bundles. They are also present around skin appendages and around nerves and blood vessels in the dermis. Extension of nevus cells into the reticular dermis and subcutaneous fat helps to differentiate congenital pigmented nevi from acquired nevus cell nevi.[34, 55]

MELANOCYTIC NEVI

Three nevoid conditions involve dermal melanocytes. These are the Mongolian spot, the nevus of Ota, and the common blue nevus. All three represent accumulations of melanocytes in the dermis.

Melanocytes originate in the neural crest of the embryo. It is presumed that the melanocytes present in the epidermis at birth arrived there by migration through the dermis during embryonic life. Melanocytes "held up" in the dermis on their way to the epidermis may remain in the dermis and appear at birth or afterward as either Mongolian spot, nevus of Ota, or blue nevus. These three conditions represent true nevi[3] because they are stable malformations composed of cells normally found in the skin (although their presence in the dermis is normal only during fetal development).

MONGOLIAN SPOT

The Mongolian spot is a poorly circumscribed, bluish-gray, macular area of hyperpigmentation found on the lower aspect of the back and over the buttocks. It usually is present at birth or becomes visible soon after. Mongolian spots fade as the child grows and tend to disappear by adolescence.

In a 1976 study, Jacobs and Walton[23] found Mongolian spots in 9.6 per cent of Caucasian, 70 per cent of Latin, 81 per cent of Asiatic, and 95 per cent of black infants. These data suggest that the incidence of Mongolian spots varies directly with the degree of natural pigmentation.

Since most Mongolian spots eventually fade, and since the lesions usually are not associated with an underlying abnormality, no therapeutic measures are required beyond reassurance to the patient.

Histopathological Findings. In a Mongolian spot, the only pathological change is in the dermis. Here, elongated, spindle-shaped melanocytes are scattered between the collagen bundles. Melanin granules are usually present within these cells. Because of the relatively small number of melanocytes present, the disorder may escape notice without specific clinical diagnosis.

NEVUS OF OTA

The nevus of Ota was first described in 1939.[58] The patient with this condition usually has a unilateral area of bluish-gray discoloration of the skin around an eye as well as hyperpigmentation of the sclera of the eye on the same side. In approximately 60 per cent of cases, the lesions are present at birth.[59] The remainder usually become visible during the first decade of life. There may be a higher predilection for this condition among females. Orientals appear to have the highest incidence of nevus of Ota, but the condition may also be seen in black patients and to a lesser degree in Caucasians.

The nevus of Ota is a unilateral, macular, hairless, blue-gray, poorly demarcated area (or areas) of discoloration involving the periorbital skin (Fig. 14–10). The skin of the temple, forehead, or malar area may also be involved. In approximately 5 per cent of cases, the discoloration is bilateral. In two thirds of cases, there is an associated bluish stain of the sclera of the eye around which the nevus is present.

The lesions of both the skin and eye persist for life. They may even have a tendency to enlarge as the patient ages. Malignant degeneration of these lesions is very rare but has occurred.[60]

The nevus of Ito is a similar discoloration of the skin of the supraclavicular, deltoid, or suprascapular areas. Treatment of both types of nevus is relatively unsuccessful. The discoloration of the skin can usually be masked by cosmetics.

Histopathological Findings. The discolored area of skin contains elongated melanocytes scattered among collagen bundles in the dermis in a pattern and concentration similar to those of the Mongolian spot. However, a fairly

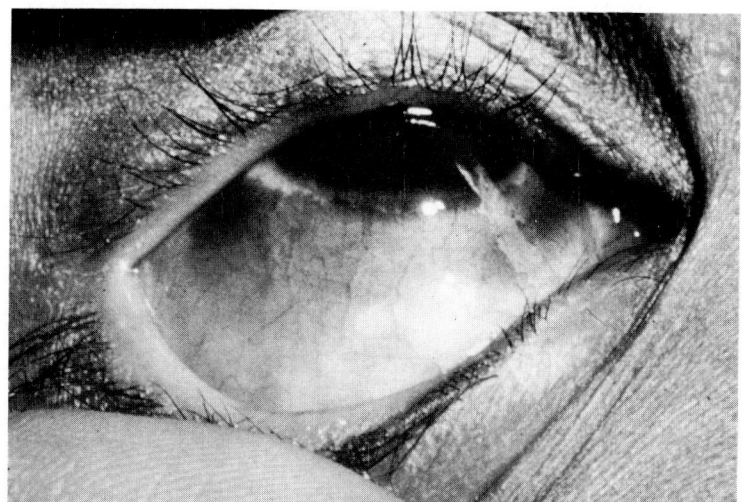

FIGURE 14–10 Nevus of Ota: Scleral melanosis.

dense group of melanocytes is occasionally seen, especially in biopsies obtained from those areas of discoloration that are somewhat indurated.

BLUE NEVUS

There are two types of blue nevus—the common type and the cellular type. The common blue nevus is usually a dark blue, smooth-surfaced, dome-shaped papule. Most common blue nevi measure less than 1 cm in diameter and are found on the face, buttocks, and dorsum of the hands and feet (Fig. 14–11). They

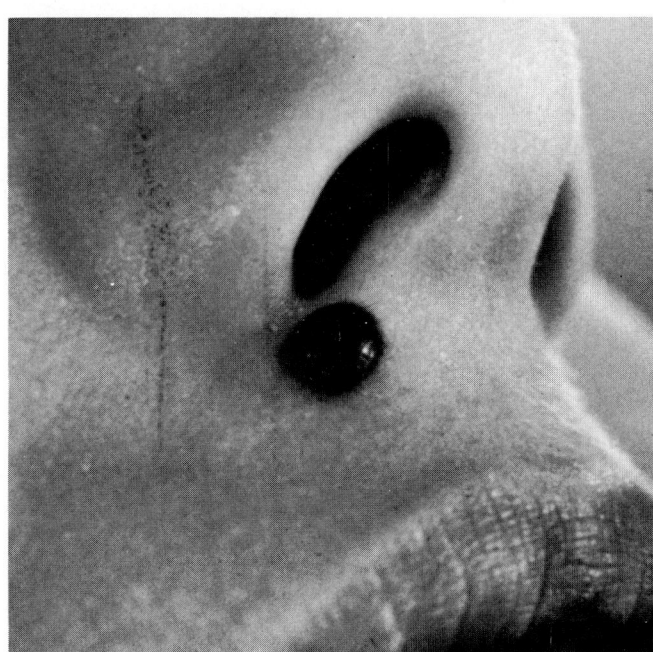

FIGURE 14–11 Blue nevus.

may be present at birth but are often first discovered in childhood. Unlike the cellular type, the common blue nevus rarely, if ever, undergoes malignant degeneration.

The cellular blue nevus is much less common. It is usually a blue-black nodule, larger than the common type, measuring more than 1 cm in diameter. More than half of cellular blue nevi are located on the buttocks and sacrococcygeal region,[61] and most are found in women. Malignant transformation of the cellular type of blue nevus may occur, but such a change is rare.

The treatment of choice for both types of blue nevus is conservative surgical excision. Patients who have a cellular blue nevus should be examined for the presence of regional lymphadenopathy and postoperatively should be studied regularly for a period of five years for signs of recurrence of the skin lesion.

Histopathological Findings. In the common blue nevus, many spindle-shaped, elongated melanocytes are present in the lower dermis and occasionally also in the subcutaneous fat. Fine granules of melanin usually are found within the melanocytes. Larger melanin granules are contained within dermal melanophages, which are frequently seen among the melanocytes. Compared with melanocytes, melanophages are shorter, thicker, and lack dendritic processes.

The cellular blue nevus contains not only isolated spindle-shaped melanocytes, which are also found in the common type, but also aggregations or islands of larger spindle-shaped cells with pale cytoplasm. The microscopic picture is frequently biphasic, with some areas typical of the common blue nevus and others composed totally of large, pale, spindle cells arranged in islands.[61]

REFERENCES

1. Leider, M., and Rosenblum, M.: A Dictionary of Dermatological Words, Terms and Phrases. New York, McGraw-Hill, 1968, p. 297.
2. Nicholls, E. M.: Genetic susceptibility and somatic mutation in the production of freckles, birthmarks, and moles. Lancet, 1:71, 1968.
3. Pinkus, H., and Mehregan, A. H.: Malformation and neoplasia. In: Guide to Dermatohistopathology. 2nd ed. New York, Appleton-Century-Crofts, 1976, pp. 435–440.
4. Adam, J. E., and Richards, R. N.: Ichthyosis hystrix versus linear verrucous epidermal nevus. Cutis., 5:1253, 1969.
5. Mehregan, A. H., and Rahbari, H.: Benign epithelioid tumors of the skin. I: Epidermal tumors. Cutis., 19:43, 1977.
6. Unna, P. G.: The Histopathology of the Diseases of the Skin. New York, Macmillan, 1896, p. 1148.
7. Kaidbey, K. H., and Kurban, A. K.: Dermatitic epidermal nevus. Arch. Dermatol., 104:166, 1971.
8. Altman, J., and Mehregan, A. H.: Inflammatory linear verrucous epidermal nevus. Arch. Dermatol., 104:385, 1971.
9. Zeligman, I., and Pomeranz, J.: Variations of congenital ichthyosiform erythroderma. Arch. Dermatol., 91:120, 1965.
10. Adams, J. E., and Richards, R. N.: Ichthyosis hystrix. Epidermolytic hyperkeratosis; discordant in monozygotic twins. Arch. Dermatol., 107:278, 1973.
11. Ackerman, A. B.: Histopathologic concept of epidermolytic hyperkeratosis. Arch. Dermatol., 102:253, 1970.
12. Pack, G. T., and Sunderland, D. A.: Naevus unius lateris. Arch. Surg., 43:341, 1941.
13. Solomon, L. M., and Esterly, N. B.: Neonatal Dermatology. Philadelphia, W. B. Saunders, 1973, pp. 60–64.
14. Schorr, W. F., and Pap, C. M.: Epidermolytic hyperkeratosis. Effect of tretinoin therapy on the clinical course and the basic defects in the stratum corneum. Arch. Dermatol., 107:556, 1973.

15. Becker, S. W.: Concurrent melanosis and hypertrichosis in distribution of nevus unius lateris. Arch. Dermatol., 60:155, 1949.
16. Copeman, P. W. M., and Wilson Jones, E.: Pigmented hairy epidermal nevus (Becker). Arch. Dermatol., 92:249, 1965.
17. Paige, T. N., and Mendelson, C. G.: Bilateral nevus comedonicus. Arch. Dermatol., 96:172, 1967.
18. Wilson Jones, E., and Heyl, T.: Naevus sebaceus. A report of 140 cases with special regard to the development of secondary malignant tumors. Br. J. Dermatol., 82:99, 1970.
19. Mehregan, A. H., and Pinkus, H.: Life history of organoid nevi. Arch. Dermatol., 91:574, 1965.
20. Rook, A.: Naevi and other developmental defects. In: Rook, A. J., Wilkinson, D. S., and Ebling, F. J. (eds.); Textbook of Dermatology. 2nd ed. Oxford, Blackwell, 1972, pp. 137–138, 152–153.
21. Michalowski, R.: Naevas sebace de Jadassohn—Un état precancereux. Dermatologica, 124:326, 1962.
22. Feuerstein, R. C., and Mims, L. C.: Linear nevus sebaceus with convulsions and mental retardation. Am. J. Dis. Child., 104:675, 1962.
23. Solomon, L. M., Fretzin, D. F., and Dewald, R. L.: The epidermal nevus syndrome. Arch. Dermatol., 97:273, 1968.
24. Lovejoy, F. H., Jr., and Boyle, W. E., Jr.: Linear nevus sebaceous syndrome: Report of two cases and a review of the literature. Pediatrics, 52:382, 1973.
25. Solomon, L. M., and Esterly, N. B.: Epidermal and other congenital organoid nevi. Curr. Probl. Pediatr., 6:3, 1975.
26. Lantis, S., Leyden, J., Thew, M., and Heaton, C.: Nevus sebaceus of Jadassohn—Part of a new neurocutaneous syndrome? Arch. Dermatol., 98:117, 1968.
27. Lansky, L. L., Funderbunk, S., Cuppage, F. E., et al.: Linear sebaceous nevus syndrome. Hamartoma variant. Am. J. Dis. Child., 123:587, 1972.
28. Dimond, R. L., and Amon, R. B.: Epidermal nevus and rhabdomyosarcoma. Arch. Dermatol., 112:1424, 1976.
29. Masson, P.: My conception of cellular nevi. Cancer, 4:9, 1951.
30. Mishima, Y.: Macromolecular changes in pigmentary disorders. III. Cellular nevi: Subcellular and cytochemical characteristics with reference to their origin. Arch. Dermatol., 91:536, 1965.
31. Clark, W. H., Jr., From, L., Bernadino, E. A., and Mihm, M. C.: The histogenesis and biologic behavior of primary human malignant melanomas of the skin. Cancer Res., 29:705, 1969.
32. Pratt, A. G.: Birthmarks in infants. Arch. Dermatol., 67:302, 1953.
33. Jacobs, A. H., and Walton, R. G.: The incidence of birthmarks in the neonate. Pediatrics, 58:218, 1976.
34. Sanderson, K. V.: Melanocytic naevi. In: Rook, A. J., Wilkinson, D. S., and Ebling, F. J. (eds.): Textbook of Dermatology. 2nd ed. Oxford, Blackwell, 1972, pp. 158–167.
35. Shaffer, B.: Pigmented nevi: Arch. Dermatol., 72:120, 1955.
36. Stegmaier, O. C.: Cosmetic management of nevi. JAMA, 199:167, 1967.
37. Walton, R. G., Sage, R. D., and Farber, E. M.: Electrodesiccation of pigmented nevi. Biopsy studies: Preliminary report. Arch. Dermatol., 76:193, 1957.
38. Cox, A. J., and Walton, R. G.: Introduction of junctional changes in pigmented nevi. Arch. Pathol., 79:428, 1965.
39. Kornberg, R., and Ackerman, A. B.: Pseudomelanoma. Arch. Dermatol., 111:1588, 1975.
40. Schoenfeld, R. J., and Pinkus, H.: The recurrence of nevi after incomplete removal. Arch. Dermatol., 78:30, 1958.
41. Miescher, G.: Umwandlung von Naevuszellen in Talgdruesenzellen? Arch. Dermat. Syph., 171:119, 1935.
42. Hashimoto, K., and Bale, G. F.: An electron microscopic study of balloon cell nevus. Cancer, 30:530, 1972.
43. Okun, M. R., Donnellan, B., and Edelstein, L.: An ultrastructural study of balloon cell nevus. Cancer, 34:615, 1974.
44. Schrader, W. A., and Helwig, E. B.: Balloon cell nevi. Cancer, 20:1502, 1967.
45. Wilson Jones, E., and Sanderson, K. V.: Cellular naevi with peculiar foam cells. Br. J. Dermatol., 74:47, 1963.
46. Spitz, S.: Melanomas of childhood. Am. J. Pathol., 24:591, 1948.
47. Kopf, A. W., and Andrade, R.: Benign juvenile melanoma. In: Year Book of Dermatology. Chicago, Year book Medical Publishers, 1965–1966, p. 7.
48. Echevarria, R., and Ackerman, L. V.: Spindle and epithelioid cell nevi in the adult. Cancer, 10:175, 1967.
49. Wayte, D. M., and Helwig, E. B.: Halo nevi. Cancer, 22:69, 1968.
50. Kopf, A. W., Morrill, S. D., and Silberling, I.: Broad spectrum of leukoderma acquisition centrifugum. Arch. Dermatol., 92:14, 1965.
51. Frank, S. B., and Cohen, H. J.: The halo nevus. Arch. Dermatol., 89:367, 1964.

52. Jacobs, J. B., Edelstein, L. M., Snyder, L. M., and Fortier, N.: Ultrastructural evidence for destruction in the halo nevus. Cancer Res., *35*:352, 1975.
53. Copeman, P. W. M., Lewis, M. G., Phillips, T. M., and Elliot, P. G.: Immunological associations of the halo nevus with cutaneous malignant melanoma. Br. J. Dermatol., *88*:127, 1973.
54. Greeley, P. W., Middleton, A. G., and Curtin, J. W.: Incidence of malignancy in giant pigmented nevi. Plast. Reconstr. Surg., *36*:26, 1965.
55. Mark, G. J., Mihm, M. C., Liteplo, M. G., et al.: Congenital melanocytic nevi of the small and garment type. Hum. Pathol., *4*:395, 1973.
56. Reed, W. B., Becker, S. W., Sr., Becker, S. W., Jr., et al.: Giant pigmented nevi, melanoma, and leptomeningeal melanocytosis. Arch. Dermatol., *91*:100, 1965.
57. Slaughter, J. C., Hardman, J. M., Kempe, L. G., et al.: Neurocutaneous melanosis and leptomeningeal melanomatosis in children. Arch. Pathol., *88*:298, 1969.
58. Ota, M.: Nevus fusco-caeruleus ophthalmo-maxillaris. Jpn. J. Dermatol., *46*:369, 1939.
59. Kopf, A. W., and Weidman, A. I.: Nevus of Ota. Arch. Dermatol., *85*:75, 1962.
60. Dorsey, C. S., and Montgomery, H.: Blue nevus and its distinction from Mongolian spot and the nevus of Ota. J. Invest. Dermatol., *22*:225, 1954.
61. Rodriguez, H. A., and Ackerman, L. V.: Cellular blue nevus. Cancer, *21*:393, 1968.

HAIR DISORDERS | 15

WILMA F. BERGFELD, M.D.

CLASSIFICATION AND PROPERTIES OF HAIR
(References 1–10)

Hair disorders in children are a visible marker of genetic, systemic, and cutaneous disease. Clinically, hair loss disorders can be divided into two major groups: non-scarring and scarring alopecia (Table 15–1). Causes of non-scarring alopecia include structural abnormalities of hair, alterations of hair growth cycle, and inflammatory cutaneous disease (Table 15–2). Causes of scarring alopecia include a variety of inflammatory diseases that displace and destroy the hair follicle and its appendages because of intense dermal inflammation. Diseases that cause scarring alopecia are lupus erythematosus, scleroderma, and localized infectious disorders, such as fungal kerions (Table 15–3). Physical or chemical trauma to the scalp usually injures the hair shaft but may also produce a severe inflammatory reaction within the skin, resulting in a scarring alopecia.

The evaluation of all hair disorders requires an extensive history with special reference to onset, duration, hair growth, and hair shedding counts. Hair pulls, clippings, and plucks are done to obtain specimens for examination of hair bulbs by light microscopy, to determine the hair growth cycle, and to delineate structural abnormalities. In children and prepubertal adolescents, the KOH preparation and Wood's light examination are essential for excluding tinea capitis. A skin biopsy specimen may be diagnostic in diseases that alter

TABLE 15–1 ALOPECIA

Non-scarring

Structural hair abnormalities
Alteration of hair growth cycles
Inflammatory scalp disorders

Scarring

Inflammatory scalp disorders
Physical and chemical scalp damage

TABLE 15-2   CAUSES OF NON-SCARRING ALOPECIA

Structural Abnormalities

Monilethrix
Trichorrhexis invaginata
Trichorrhexis nodosa
Pili torti
Pili annulati

Alteration of Growth Cycle

Anagen effluvium
Chemotherapeutic agents
Alopecia areata

Telogen Effluvium

Androgenic alopecia
Postpartum hair loss
Drugs
Malnutrition
Systemic disease
Neoplasia, local and systemic

TABLE 15-3   CAUSES OF SCARRING ALOPECIA

Inflammatory Scalp Disorder

Discoid lupus erythematosus
Lichen planopilaris
Pseudopelade
Localized scleroderma

Cutaneous Infections

Bacterial
Fungal

Cutaneous Injury due to Physical or Chemical Agents

Traction
Trichotillomania
Chemical burns
Radiation damage

the hair growth cycle, in inflammatory cutaneous disorders, and in neoplastic proliferative disease. Hair evaluation techniques, such as hair pulls, plucks, clippings, shedding counts, and scalp biopsy, may aid the physician in the diagnosis and the prediction of a prognosis. Special laboratory tests may also be indicated, depending on the patient's history and on the results of hair examination.

For a proper understanding of hair disorders, it is necessary for the clinician to be aware of the normal physiology of scalp hair growth. Scalp hair grows at an average rate of 0.35 mm per day; female hair grows faster than male hair, and hair grows faster in summer than in winter. In addition, there appears to be a diurnal variation in hair growth. The average number of scalp hairs is 100,000, and the average daily loss of scalp hair is from 25 to 100 hairs. Scalp hair grows in a dyssynchronous cycle, with 80 to 90 per cent of the hair in the anagen, or growing, phase, 10 to 15 per cent in the telogen, or resting, phase and 5 per cent in a transitional phase. Any alteration in this pattern will produce increased shedding of scalp hair. In children, 95 to 100 per cent of scalp hair is in the anagen phase during the first five years of life. After this period, hair growth assumes a dyssynchronous pattern.

CONGENITAL AND FAMILIAL ALOPECIA
(References 11–29)

ECTODERMAL DYSPLASIA

Ectodermal dysplasia is a term used to describe a variety of genodermatoses that present with abnormalities of the skin, appendages, hair, teeth, and neural tissue (Fig. 15–1, Table 15–4, Plate VIII–A).

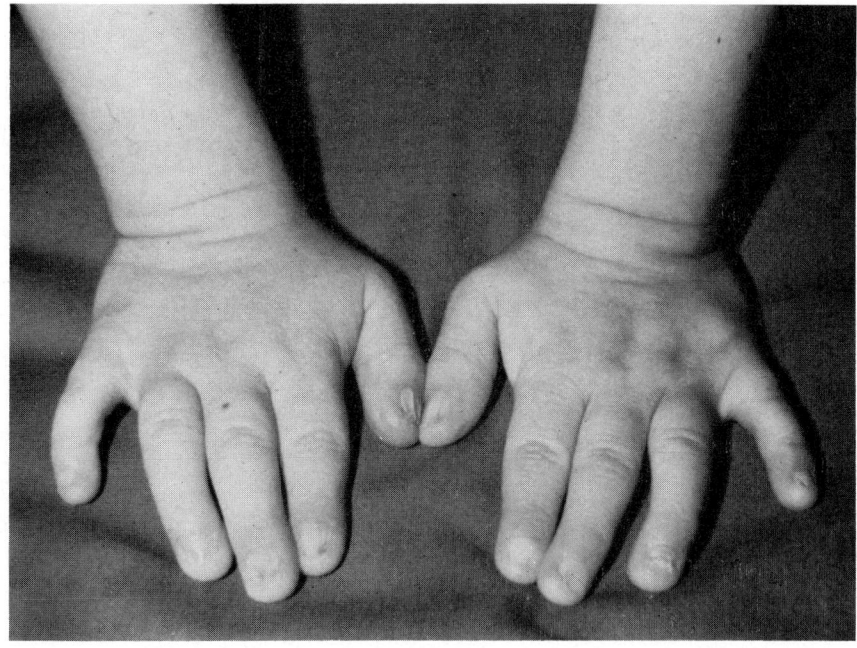

FIGURE 15–1 Ectodermal defect. Dystrophic nails.

TABLE 15-4 COMMON ECTODERMAL DYSPLASIAS

Type	Inheritance	Hair Abnormalities	Associated Abnormalities
Anhidrotic	X-linked	Hypotrichosis	Skin Teeth Breast
Hidrotic	Autosomal recessive	Hypotrichosis or atrichia	Skin Nails
Netherton's syndrome	Autosomal recessive	Trichorrhexis invaginata	Ichthyosis Atopy
Congenital trichorrhexis nodosa	Autosomal recessive	Trichorrhexis nodosa	Seizures Mental retardation Aminoaciduria
Familial pili torti	Autosomal recessive	Pili torti	Nails Teeth Deafness
Menkes' syndrome	X-linked	Pili torti Trichorrhexis nodosa	Mental retardation

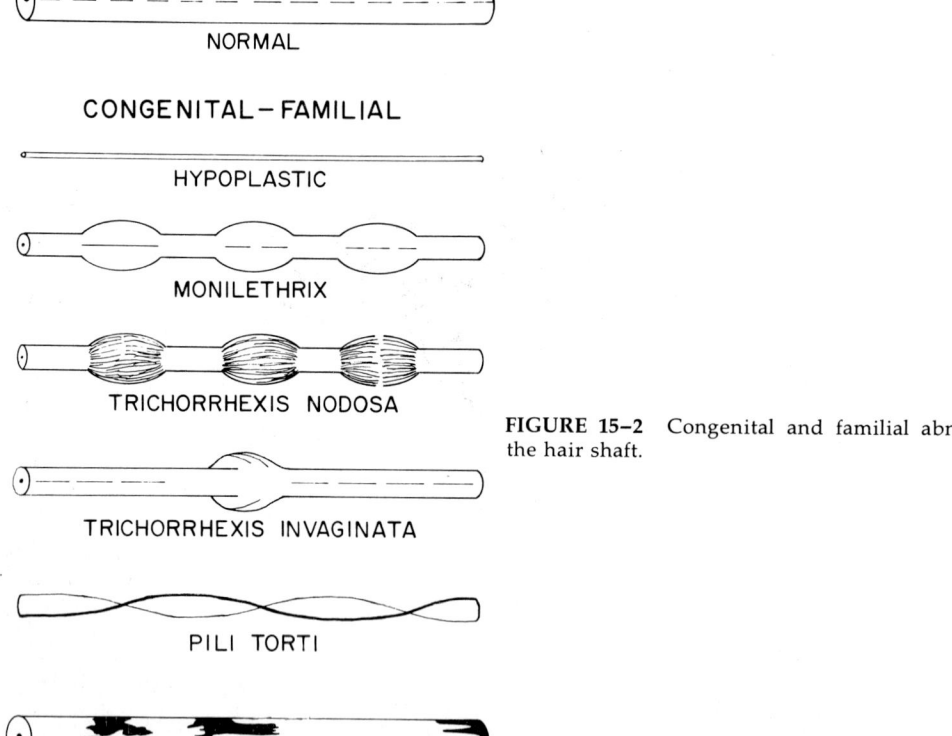

FIGURE 15-2 Congenital and familial abnormalities of the hair shaft.

Hair defects appear to be a primary genetic marker of congenital ectodermal dysplasia, indicated by decreased density of scalp hair, lightly pigmented hair, and abnormalities of the hair shaft. Other ectodermal defects include aplastic or dystrophic nails and diminished numbers of scalp appendages. Skeletal abnormalities, defects of carbohydrate, protein, and lipid metabolism, hormonal disturbances, and central nervous system disorders, such as mental retardation, allow the physician to classify the condition as well as to anticipate neurological dysfunction. Thus, the hair marker appears to open a Pandora's box for further medical and neurological investigation. Patients with ectodermal defects usually have either atrichia or hair that is described as sparse, poorly textured, and lusterless with a peculiar optical highlight. The density of scalp hair and its ability to reach appreciable length is often abnormal. In children with ectodermal dysplasia, the common structural abnormalities of hair shown on light microscopy are pili torti, pili annulati, trichorrhexis invaginata, trichorrhexis nodosa, and monilethrix (Fig. 15–2).

MONILETHRIX (Beaded Hair)

Monilethrix is a rare hair shaft abnormality that is inherited as a dominant trait with variable expression. The affected hair appears beaded, owing to the constriction of the hair matrix as a result of defective alpha-keratin formation. Examination of plucked or clipped hair by light microscope reveals beaded hair and other structural abnormalities, such as trichorrhexis nodosa. The beads, which appear singly or in groups, represent the normal hair shaft, while the shaft between the nodes is easily fractured. This condition may improve at puberty, during pregnancy, or with the use of oral contraceptives.

The hair appears normal at birth; however, early in infancy it becomes dry, lusterless, and brittle and fails to grow to any appreciable length. The condition is seen mainly in scalp hair but may also affect body hair. This disorder is not associated with any systemic disease or metabolic defect. It is, however, frequently associated with cutaneous disorders, such as keratosis pilaris (which may be noted prior to the scalp hair defect), cataracts, dental abnormalities, and brittle nails.

TRICHORRHEXIS INVAGINATA (Bamboo Hair)

Trichorrhexis invaginata is a rare autosomal recessive ectodermal disorder of hair with a bamboo-like abnormality of the hair shaft. It is more common in female than in male infants and may involve all the body hair. Clinically, the hair is dry, lusterless, easily fractured, sparse, and short. Improvement or disappearance of the condition may occur at puberty.

The disorder is caused by an abnormal invagination along the hair shaft, which resembles a ball-and-cup orthopedic prosthetic joint. Light microscopy of the affected hair demonstrates the cup at the proximal portion of the shaft. This defect is apparently caused by abnormal keratinization of the internal root sheath. The structural defect in trichorrhexis invaginata is a nodal lesion and should be differentiated from the defect in trichorrhexis nodosa, another nodal hair abnormality.

Trichorrhexis invaginata was first described by Netherton and was associated with a cutaneous disorder, ichthyosis linearis circumflexa or possibly lamellar ichthyosis. Since that time, other cutaneous disorders, including atopic diathesis, urticaria, angioneurotic edema, and anaphylactoid reactions, have been associated with the condition.

TRICHORRHEXIS NODOSA

Trichorrhexis nodosa is the most common abnormality of the hair shaft. It frequently results from a variety of physical and chemical processes that induce structural defects of the intercellular cement of the cuticle and defective keratinization of the external root sheath. Rarely, trichorrhexis nodosa may be associated with aminoaciduria, an inborn error of metabolism.

Trichorrhexis nodosa is characterized by dry, lusterless, short hair that is easily fractured. On examination of the hair by light microscope, single and multiple nodular swellings with the appearance of interlocking brushes can be demonstrated. These represent the site of fracture of the hair shaft.

Congenital Trichorrhexis Nodosa

Congenital trichorrhexis nodosa may be a familial disorder of hair and is occasionally associated with abnormalities of nails. This nodal defect may be the first genetic marker in patients with mental retardation due to a metabolic error, namely, argininosuccinicaciduria. The amino acid arginine can be easily identified in the urine, blood, and cerebral spinal fluid of the affected patient.

Acquired Trichorrhexis Nodosa

The most common cause of acquired hair loss secondary to structural hair abnormalities is acquired trichorrhexis nodosa. There are two clinical varieties: proximal shaft defects and distal nodal lesions. Proximal trichorrhexis nodosa is a distinctive disorder of blacks; distal nodal lesions are observed mainly in Caucasians. The scalp hair is usually of good density but fails to develop to any appreciable length. A past history of hair care reveals indulgence in a variety of techniques, such as hair straightening, hot combing, reverse permanent waving, and hair coloring procedures. Characteristically, the hair begins to break off suddenly and become strikingly short in either a patchy or diffuse pattern. If all thermal and chemical trauma to the hair is discontinued, the condition may reverse itself in approximately four years.

PILI TORTI (Twisted Hair)

Pili torti is a rare autosomal dominant disorder with variable expression. It affects females more often than males and is generally observed in infancy as a patchy or diffuse hair loss. It may also involve all the body hair, including eyebrows, eyelashes, beard, and axillary and pubic hair. The affected hair is brittle, dry, and lusterless and has a striking spangled appearance from reflected light.

Light microscopic examination of involved scalp hair demonstrates a flattened twisted hair shaft with a rotation of 180° to 360°. X-ray diffraction displays a normal alpha-keratin pattern within the affected hairs. These hairs fracture in the twisted section, producing short hair or diffuse alopecia. Occasionally, other ectodermal defects of hair and nails may be present, including monilethrix, keratosis pilaris, and ichthyosis. In a few instances, pili torti has been associated with mental retardation.

MENKES' KINKY HAIR SYNDROME (Pili Torti)

Menkes' kinky hair syndrome is a rare, sex-linked, recessive condition associated with neurodegeneration. The cause of this disorder is a defect in copper absorption and metabolism. Affected infants have kinky, light-colored hair, severe physical and mental retardation, failure to thrive, seizures, and hypothermia. The sparse, kinky hair usually has the structural defects of pili torti and less frequently those of trichorrhexis nodosa.

All major features of the disease appear to be a direct or indirect reflection of copper deficiency. Since hair is copper-dependent for its sulfhydryl and tyrosine activity, the lack of copper results in a defective and poorly pigmented hair shaft.

PILI ANNULATI (Ringed Hair)

Pili annulati is a rare familial defect of the hair shaft. When reviewed in reflected light the hair shaft demonstrates strikingly bright bands or rings along its entire length. Although the hair shaft has a uniform diameter, there is an irregular distribution of air-filled cavities interspersed in the keratin of the hair cortex. These air spaces or holes appear light by reflected light or dark by transmitted light. The hair shaft is structurally strong, and the bright rings tend to produce attractive highlights.

Pseudopili annulati is an unusual variant of normal hair in which bright rings appear to be secondary to periodic twisting or curling of the hair shaft.

ALTERATIONS OF HAIR GROWTH CYCLE
(References 30–54)

Scalp hair grows in a dyssynchronous pattern, normally demonstrating with 80 to 90 per cent of hair in the anagen (growing) stage and 10 to 15 per cent in the telogen (resting) phase. Any alteration of this growth pattern may produce an effluvium or increased shedding of scalp hair. The matrix of the anagen hair is metabolically very active and as a result is sensitive to many stimuli or insults. A minimal insult will initiate an early conversion to telogen hair; a more severe insult will completely interrupt functioning of the active anagen hair to produce anagen arrest, with subsequent abrupt shedding of

TABLE 15–5 CAUSES OF ANAGEN ARREST (EFFLUVIUM)

Thallium
Colchicine
Cyclophosphamide
6-Mercaptopurine
Methotrexate

Anticoagulants (heparin, heparinoids)

Dextran sulfate

Thiouracil
Carbimazole
Salicylate

Vitamin A

Triparanol

Corticosteroids (high-dose)

Alopecia areata

---

dystrophic hair (Table 15–5). Anagen effluvium may be reversible if the insulting factor(s) is removed.

ALOPECIA AREATA

Alopecia areata is a classic example of an anagen effluvium and is thought to be an autoimmune disease (Fig. 15–3). The acute onset of alopecia areata usually follows an abrupt anagen effluvium. As the disease becomes chronic, the hair loss gradually becomes a telogen effluvium. Clinically, patients with alopecia areata have a variety of patterned hair loss, which includes patchy discoid, marginal, totalis, universalis, and diffuse types. Most often the onset is abrupt, with initial patchy discoid loss of scalp hair, which may proceed to a totalis (total loss of scalp hair) or universalis (loss of scalp and body hair) condition. Pitting of the nail plate is observed in all forms of the disease; however, severely dystrophic nails are more commonly associated with alopecia universalis. The onset of alopecia areata may occur at any age and has a familial incidence of 20 per cent. The prognosis in children appears to be poorer than that in adults, especially in the case of alopecia universalis (Plate VIII–B). In contrast to alopecia universalis, the limited discoid form of alopecia areata has an excellent prognosis.

The diagnosis of alopecia areata is established by clinical presentation of patterned hair loss, hair plucks that demonstrate dystrophic hair, and an early anagen effluvium with a late telogen effluvium. A skin biopsy specimen of active alopecia areata displays a classic peribulbar inflammation with decreased numbers of anagen hairs.

Treatment modalities are many, but only limited success has been reported with the use of intralesional corticosteroids, systemic corticosteroids, zinc therapy, dinitrochlorobenzene (DNCB) sensitization, and topical use of phenolic irritants and ultraviolet light.

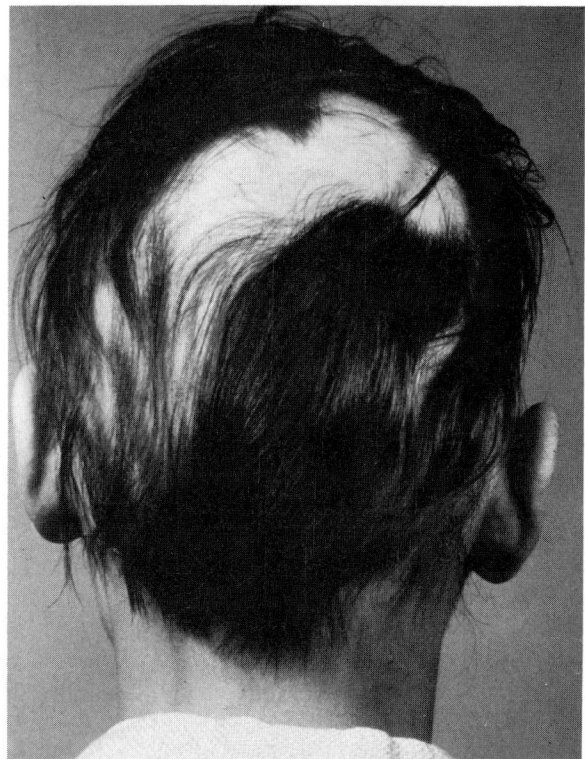

FIGURE 15–3 Alopecia areata. Diffuse patterned hair loss, anagen arrest, and telogen effluvium.

TELOGEN EFFLUVIUM

Telogen effluvium is the most common form of hair loss. The condition may be short-lived or long-lasting (Table 15–6). Telogen effluvium is the result of the premature conversion of anagen hair to telogen hair because of a stimulus or insult to the sensitive active matrix. The type of insult determines whether the

TABLE 15–6 CAUSES OF TELOGEN EFFLUVIUM

Acute or Early Onset (8 to 16 weeks)

Postpartum effluvium
Physiological effluvium of neonates
Androgenic alopecia
Postfebrile effluvium
Surgical shock
Drugs
Alopecia areata

Chronic (lasting longer than 16 weeks)

Nutritional and metabolic deficiency
Endocrinopathy
Collagen vascular disorders
Chronic infectious disorders
Psychological and neurological disorders
Androgenic alopecia

effluvium will be of early onset (two to four months) or of late onset (occurring more than four months following the stimulus). The prognosis of a telogen effluvium depends on its etiology. A telogen effluvium may either be self-limited, with total or partial reversibility, or irreversible, as seen in androgenic alopecia.

ANDROGENIC ALOPECIA

Androgenic alopecia occurs in both males and females and appears to be inherited as an autosomal dominant trait with variable expression. The onset of androgenic alopecia has been noted as early as 14 years of age. The earlier the onset, the more severe the alopecia. Characteristic of the condition is the sudden or insidious onset of telogen effluvium, with a patterned hair loss that differs in males and females. Females have diffuse hair loss over the central scalp as well as thinning of other body hair. Males develop a patterned hair loss, commonly with areas of frontal baldness, vertex baldness, total central baldness, or combinations of all three. Both males and females demonstrate a mild to marked receding frontal hairline. In the areas of hair loss, there is decreased density of hair, replacement of anagen terminal hair by short fine vellus hair, and a shortening of the anagen growth cycle. The short hair fails to grow to any appreciable length (Fig. 15-4).

The medical treatment of this condition has been unsatisfactory. However, cosmetic surgery, such as hair transplantation, has been successful in selected patients. The use of topical preparations containing testosterone, progesterone, and estrogens has been of little help. Psychological support with reassurance about the hereditary nature of the hair loss has been of some benefit in helping the patient accept the condition. Discontinuation of damaging cosmetic procedures and chemicals coupled with loose hair styling and the use of hair conditioners may reduce shedding or fracturing of scalp hair and improve the cosmetic appearance.

PHYSIOLOGICAL ALOPECIA

Neonatal infants may demonstrate an acute telogen effluvium that is abrupt or insidious. The onset occurs during the first few weeks of life, with gradual replacement of hair over the ensuing months. The new hair growth, however, may be of different color and texture. The cause of this effluvium is unknown but may be related to that of the postpartum effluvium seen in the mother.

PHYSICAL AND CHEMICAL DAMAGE
(References 55-66)

Repetitive chronic tension on the hair shaft produces hair shaft abnormalities, follicular damage, and subsequent hair loss. Common causes in children are braids, ponytails, elastic hair bands, and hair rollers. This type of alopecia is initially reversible, but continued tension on the hair and continued damage to the hair follicles may result in a scarring alopecia. Traction alopecia should be

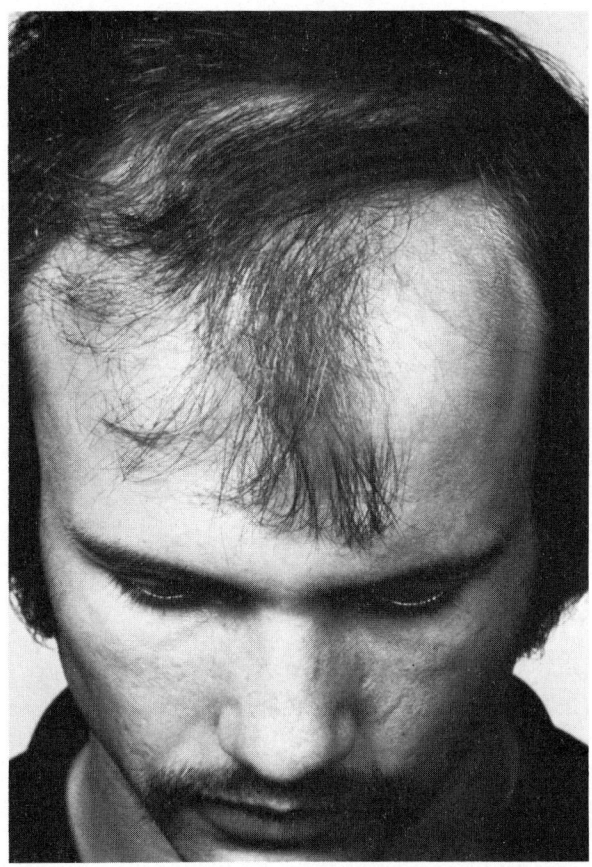

FIGURE 15–4 Androgenic alopecia. Male pattern alopecia with receding hairline in an 18-year-old.

suspected when there is peripheral alopecia and expanding or thinning of parted areas of hair.

Light microscopy of plucked or clipped hair demonstrates thinning of the hair cuticle, fractured hair, and lesions of trichorrhexis nodosa. When traction is discontinued, the scalp hair should be reversed in two to four years. However, once scarring has ensued, hair growth probably will permanently cease in the involved areas.

HOT COMB ALOPECIA

In black patients, cosmetic procedures to straighten the scalp hair are often initiated in adolescence and continued throughout adult life. These techniques employ hot combing, petrolatum, permanent waving, and reverse permanent waving. Hair loss is frequently first observed on the peripheral areas of scalp and on the vertex. In the chronic state, the entire scalp may be involved. Clinically, the presenting sign is traction alopecia or scarring alopecia, the latter being seen more commonly in older patients. The diagnosis is made by history, clinical presentation, light microscopy of clipped hair, and scalp biopsy. The scalp biopsy specimen demonstrates scarring alopecia with destruction of hair follicles.

As in traction alopecia, the prognosis is good if the condition is diagnosed early and straightening procedures are discontinued. If scarring has already occurred, the prognosis for hair regrowth is poor.

TRICHOTILLOMANIA

Trichotillomania is a self-induced traction alopecia produced by plucking, pulling, or cutting the hair in a bizarre pattern (Plate VIII-C). The condition is generally associated with psychological disorders and occurs more frequently in children than in adults. The patient is observed to have incomplete hair loss with a short stubble of scalp hair. If the eyelashes and eyebrows are involved, total loss of hair in these areas may occur. Diagnosis can be confirmed by light microscopic examination of clipped hair, which demonstrates fractured normal hair shafts. A scalp biopsy specimen is frequently helpful in identifying increased numbers of catagen hairs, follicular cysts, and perifollicular fibrosis. An occlusive bandage can be applied to the area of alopecia for four to six weeks to encourage regrowth of scalp hair. Because of the association with emotional disturbance, most patients with a diagnosis of trichotillomania should be evaluated by a psychologist or psychiatrist.

INFLAMMATORY SCALP DISORDERS

Some skin disorders that involve predominantly the epidermis and have only minimal dermal inflammation produce a reversible, temporary alopecia of scalp hair. This type of hair loss can be observed in patients with seborrheic dermatitis, psoriasis vulgaris, and pityriasis rubra pilaris. These papulosquamous disorders have a classic clinical appearance as well as characteristic skin biopsy findings. Increased shedding of scalp hair appears to be secondary to hyperkeratosis of the follicular orifices, with mild to moderate dermal inflammation that may focally involve the hair follicle. This form of alopecia is limited and reversible with treatment of the cutaneous disorder.

TINEA CAPITIS

Tinea capitis clinically may be observed as a scaly, non-inflammatory disorder or as an indurated suppurative plaque with folliculitis, known as a kerion. The more intense the dermal inflammation, the greater the incidence of dermal fibrosis and permanent alopecia (Plate VIII–D). The diagnosis is established by KOH examination of plucked hair for spores and hyphae, Wood's light examination, and fungal culture.

Papulosquamous tinea capitis is most frequently caused by *Microsporum canis* or *M. audouini*. The former demonstrates blue-green fluorescence on Wood's light examination. The suppurative form of tinea capitis (kerion) is frequently caused by *Trichophyton tonsurans* and less often by *T. mentagrophytes, Microsporum gypseum, M. ferrugineum,* and *Trichophyton schoenleini*. The treatment of choice for both disorders is local cleansing and debriding agents, topical antifungal agents, and oral griseofulvin.

SCARRING ALOPECIA (References 67–72)

Any cutaneous disorder that results in destruction of the hair follicles or replacement of normal dermis by neoplastic proliferation or fibrosis will produce irreversible alopecia.

LUPUS ERYTHEMATOSUS

The discoid type of lupus erythematosus, with or without systemic disease may be characterized by alopecic, indurated, papulosquamous plaques on the scalp and on sun-exposed areas of skin. A skin biopsy specimen of the active lesion demonstrates an intense inflammatory reaction around hair follicles, with ultimate destruction. Biopsy specimens of older lesions demonstrate dermal fibrosis and obliteration of dermal appendages, including hair follicles. The diagnosis of lupus erythematosus can be made by clinical presentation, skin biopsy, and direct immunofluorescence (see Chapter 16). Serological testing for collagen vascular disease may be negative.

LICHEN PLANOPILARIS

Lichen planopilaris is a rare, patchy, scarring alopecia of the scalp that is more common in adults than in children. Clinically and histologically, it is difficult to distinguish from discoid lupus erythematosus. However, direct immunofluorescence techniques can differentiate between the two disorders. Discoid lupus erythematosus demonstrates a band of fluorescence at the dermal-epidermal junction owing to deposition of IgG and C3, while lichen planopilaris demonstrates a globular deposition of IgG, IgA, and fibrinogen in the papillary dermis.

The treatment of discoid lupus erythematosus and lichen planopilaris of the scalp is similar. The use of antimalarial drugs and systemic and topical steroids is of some help in limiting the progression of the disease. The prognosis for regrowth of scalp hair in scarred alopecic areas is poor, and only cosmetic procedures, such as hair transplantation, will be helpful.

PSEUDOPELADE

This scarring alopecia is an uncommon disorder of the scalp characterized by asymptomatic, non-inflammatory patchy areas of scarring. It occurs more frequently in adults than in children, and its etiology is unknown. The diagnosis is made primarily by clinical presentation and a skin biopsy specimen showing a scarring alopecia with loss of scalp appendages. This disorder may be the end result of lichen planopilaris or other types of inflammatory scalp disease.

SCLERODERMA

Localized scleroderma (morphea) of the scalp or forehead is a rare cutaneous disorder characterized by scarred and atrophic skin (Fig. 15–5). The clinical and histological presentation is classic and demonstrates a scarring alopecia when hairy skin is involved. This condition is rarely associated with

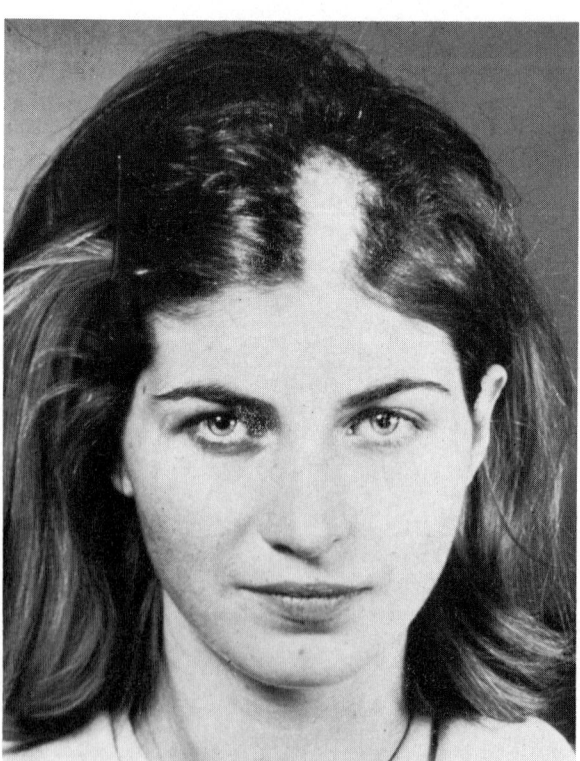

FIGURE 15–5 Coup de sabre. Localized scleroderma.

progressive systemic scleroderma. Active lesions have been treated with parenteral antimalarial drugs, with limited success. The disease is generally self-limiting, and the old quiescent lesions can be cosmetically treated by hair transplantation.

NEOPLASIA

Neoplastic proliferation, benign or malignant, that involves the scalp will interrupt the growth of scalp hair and possibly displace or destroy hair follicles. The patient will have an area of alopecia that may or may not contain a palpable tumor. Histopathological examination of a skin biopsy specimen obtained from the involved area is generally diagnostic. The most common benign neoplasms of the scalp are pilar cysts, nevocytic nevi, and nevus sebaceus of Jadassohn (Fig. 15–6). Malignant neoplastic lesions of the scalp are usually metastatic tumors of the breast, lung, or gastrointestinal tract, or the result of lymphoma cells, which are all rare in adolescence.

HIRSUTISM (References 73–85)

Hypertrichosis and hirsutism are both defined as an increase of body hair. Hirsutism, which includes hypertrichosis, is a disorder of women or children (mostly female) characterized by extensive body hair tending toward masculine distribution. Hypertrichosis refers mainly to localized excessive body hair.

HYPERTRICHOSIS

Localized hypertrichosis is secondary to trauma, chemical irritation, and hormonal or corticosteroid stimulation of the skin. Frequently, hamartomatous

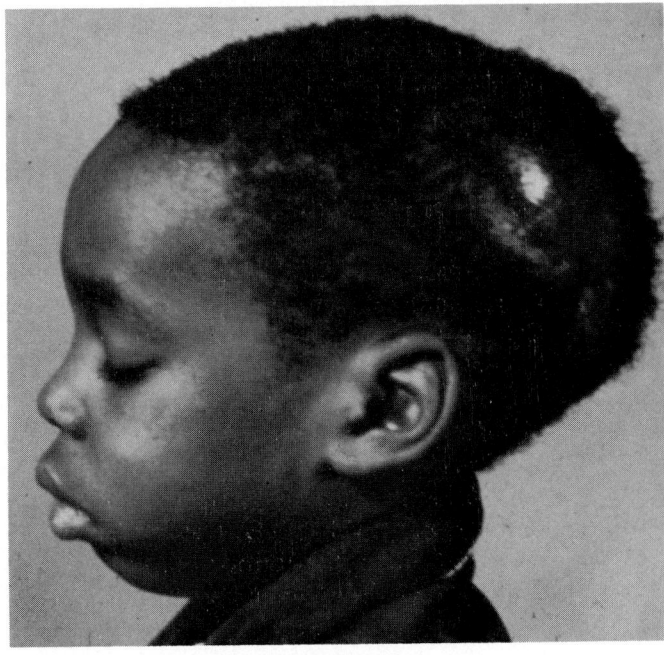

FIGURE 15–6 Blue nevus of the scalp. Total absence of hair over proliferative tumor in a five-year-old child.

growths, such as giant pigmented nevi and Becker's nevus, demonstrate increased terminal hair.

Generalized hypertrichosis can be associated with any central nervous system disorder, such as postencephalitis, multiple sclerosis, and anorexia nervosa. Several congenital abnormalities, including hypertrichosis lanuginosa, Cornelia de Lange syndrome, and the Hurler syndrome, may have related hypertrichosis. Other disorders associated with hypertrichosis include porphyria cutanea tarda, dermatomyositis, acrodynia, and juvenile hypothyroidism. Drug-induced hypertrichosis also occurs secondary to administration of diphenylhydantoin, hexachlorobenzene, testosterone propionate, psoralens, and diazoxide.

Hypertrichosis Lanuginosa

An exceedingly rare disorder, hypertrichosis lanuginosa has two forms: congenital and acquired. Patients have diffuse lanugo hair that is fine and poorly pigmented. The congenital type is inherited and may be associated with a high incidence of infant mortality; the acquired form has been associated with internal malignancies.

IDIOPATHIC HIRSUTISM

The most common form of hirsutism is idiopathic and not associated with any underlying endocrinic or metabolic disorder. Generally, affected persons have a strong family history of hypertrichosis or hirsutism, normal menstrual periods, absence of receding hairline, and no deepening of voice. Pelvic examination reveals normal female genitalia and organs. The pathogenesis of idiopathic hirsutism is assumed to be an increased stimulation of the hair follicles by normal levels of androgen-like hormones.

The treatment of hirsutism is cosmetic and includes cutting the hair with a scissors or razor and applying depilatory agents. Bleaching or electrolysis is occasionally helpful. However, besides being a tedious and expensive process, electrolysis may produce small scars or keloids in the treated area.

SECONDARY HIRSUTISM

Hirsutism secondary to endocrine abnormalities accounts for an exceedingly small percentage of females with excessive body hair (Table 15–7). Evaluation for suspected virilizing and non-virilizing endocrinopathies should include studies of endocrine dysfunction, iatrogenic induction, and tumors of the endocrine system. Hirsutism due to secondary anagen excess and virilization is associated with oily skin, acne, recession of frontal hair, oligomenorrhea, increased musculature, deep voice, and hypertrophy of the clitoris. A minimal laboratory evaluation should include studies of plasma testosterone level, urinary steroids, and plasma cortisol as well as clinical examination for distribution of hair and pelvic examination. For full evaluation, pelvic x-rays, intravenous pyelograms, and angiograms may be indicated. The

TABLE 15-7 CAUSES OF HIRSUTISM

Absence of Virilization and Androgen Excess	Virilization Secondary to Androgen Excess
NORMAL PHYSIOLOGICAL STATES (puberty, pregnancy, menopause); idiopathic cause	ENDOCRINE DISORDERS Adrenal disease Adrenal hyperplasia Adrenal adenomatous carcinoma Cushing syndrome
ENDOCRINE DISORDERS Cushing syndrome ACTH-producing tumors Myxedema Acromegaly	OVARIAN DISEASE Stein-Leventhal syndrome Hyperthecosis Leydig cell hyperplasia Ovarian tumors
IATROGENIC DISORDERS Corticosteroids, systemic ACTH	IATROGENIC DISORDERS Testosterone Anabolic steroids High-dose corticosteroids Progesterone

treatment of secondary hirsutism is identification of the underlying endocrine abnormality followed by appropriate surgical or medical treatment.

REFERENCES

CLASSIFICATION AND PROPERTIES OF HAIR

1. Adachi, K.: The metabolism and control mechanism of human hair follicles. Curr. Probl. Dermatol., 5:37, 1973.
2. Adachi, K., Takaysau, S., Takashima, I., et al.: Human hair follicles: Metabolism and control mechanisms. J. Soc. Cosmet. Chem., 21:901, 1970.
3. Barman, J. M., Astore, I., and Pecoraro, V.: The normal trichogram of the adult. J. Invest. Dermatol., 44:233, 1965.
4. Brown, C. (ed.): The First Human Hair Symposium. New York, Medcom Press, 1974.
5. Butcher, E. O.: Development of the pilary system and the replacement of hair in mammals. Ann. N.Y. Acad. Sci., 53:508, 1951.
6. Chase, H. B.: Growth of the hair. Physiol. Rev., 34:133, 1971.
7. Kobori, T., and Montagna, W. (eds.): Biology and Disease of the Hair. Baltimore, University Park Press, 1975.
8. Montagna, W., and Dodson, R. L.: Hair growth. In: Montagna, W., et al. (eds.): Advances in Biology of Skin. Vol. 9. New York, Pergamon, 1969.
9. Swanbeck, J., Nyren, J., and Juhlin, L.: Mechanical properties of hairs from patients with different types of hair disease. J. Invest. Dermatol., 52:248, 1970.
10. Van Scott, E. J.: Keratinization and hair growth. Ann. Rev. Med., 19:337, 1968.

CONGENITAL AND FAMILIAL ALOPECIA

11. Altman, J., and Stroud, J.: Netherton's syndrome and ichthyosis linearis circumflexa. Psoriasiform ichthyosis. Arch. Dermatol., 100:550, 1969.
12. Chernosky, M. E., and Owens, D. M.: Trichorrhexis nodosa: Clinical and investigative studies. Arch. Dermatol., 94:577, 1966.
13. Comaish, S.: Autoradiographic studies of hair growth and rhythm in monilethrix. Br. J. Dermatol., 81:443, 1969.

14. Coupe, R. L., and Lowry, R. B.: Abnormality of the hair in cartilage-hair hypoplasia. Dermatologica, 101:329, 1970.
15. Damsto, T. J., and Prakken, J. R.: Atrichia with papular lesions: A variant of congenital ectodermal dysplasia. Dermatologica, 108:114, 1954.
16. Hersle, K.: Netherton's disease and ichthyosis circumflexa. Report of a case and a review of the literature. Acta Derm. Venereol., 52:298, 1972.
17. Mackee, G. M., and Rogen, I.: Monilethrix—A clinical and histological study with a report of six cases and a review of the literature. J. Cutan. Dis., 34:444, 1916.
18. Malt, R. A.: Keratin in monilethrix. J. Invest. Dermatol., 44:364, 1968.
19. Muller, S. A.: Alopecia: Syndrome of generic significance. J. Invest. Dermatol., 60:475, 1973.
20. Netherton, E. W.: A unique case of trichorrhexis nodosa—"bamboo hair." Arch. Dermatol., 78:483, 1958.
21. Orentrich, N.: Disorders of the hair and scalp in childhood. Pediatr. Clin. North Am., 18:953, 1971.
22. Owens, D. W., and Charles, M. E.: Trichorrhexis nodosa. Arch. Dermatol., 94:586, 1960.
23. Papa, C., Mills, O. H., and Hansahw, E. M.: Trichorrhexis nodosa. Arch. Dermatol., 106:88, 1972.
24. Porter, P. S., and Lobitz, W. B. Q., Jr.: Human hair: A genetic marker. Br. J. Dermatol., 83:225, 1970.
25. Price, V. H., Thomas, R. S., and Jones, F. T.: Microscopic studies of pili annulati. Proceedings of XII International Congress of Dermatology. Munich, 1967; Berlin, 1968, pp. 786–788.
26. Price, V. H., Thomas, R. S., and Jones, F. T.: Pili annulati. Optical and electron microscopic studies. Arch. Dermatol., 98:640, 1968.
27. Price, V. H., Thomas, R. S., and Jones, F. T.: Pseudo pili annulati. An unusual variant of normal hair. Arch. Dermatol., 102:354, 1970.
28. Solomon, I. L., and Green, O. C.: Monilethrix. N. Engl. J. Med., 269:1279, 1963.
29. Stelly, W. B., and Rawnsley, H. M.: Aminogenic alopecia: Loss of hair associated with argininosuccinic aciduria. Lancet, 2:1327, 1965.

ALTERATIONS OF HAIR GROWTH CYCLE

30. Blackburn, G. L., Bistrian, B. R., Hoag, C., et al.: Hair loss with rapid weight loss. Arch. Dermatol., 113:234, 1977.
31. Bradfield, R. B., Bailey, M. D., and Margen, S.: Morphological changes in human scalp hair roots during deprivation of protein. Science, 157:438, 1967.
32. Crounse, R. G., and Van Scott, E. J.: Changes in scalp hair roots as a measure of toxicity from cancer chemotherapeutic drugs. J. Invest. Dermatol., 35:83, 1960.
33. Ebling, F. J., Hale, P. A., and Johnson, E.: Hormonal influence on hair growth. Proceedings of the Second International Congress of Endocrinology. Amsterdam, Excerpta Medica Foundation, 1965, p. 441.
34. Freinkel, R. K., and Freinkel, N.: Hair growth and alopecia in hypothyroidism. Arch. Dermatol., 106:349, 1972.
35. Goetle, D. K., and Odom, R. B.: Alopecia in crash dieters. JAMA, 235:2623, 1976.
36. Griffiths, W. A. D.: Diffuse hair loss and oral contraceptives. Br. J. Dermatol., 88:31, 1973.
37. Jackson, D., Church, R. E., and Ebling, F. J.: Hair dynamics in female baldness. Br. J. Dermatol., 87:351, 1972.
38. Jenkins, J. S., and Ash, S.: Metabolism of testosterone by human skin disorders of hair growth. J. Endocrinol., 59:345, 1973.
39. Johnson, A. A., Latham, M. C., and Roe, D. A.: Use of changes in hair assessment of protein calorie malnutrition. J. Invest. Dermatol., 68:311, 1975.
40. Kaidbey, K. H.: Hair growth inhibition as a method of screening drugs for local antimitotic activity. J. Invest. Dermatol., 68:80, 1977.
41. Kaufman, J. P.: Telogue effluvium secondary to starvation diet. Arch. Dermatol., 112:731, 1976.
42. Klein, A. W., Rudolph, R. I., and Leyden, J.: Telogen effluvium as a sign of Hodgkin's disease. Arch. Dermatol., 108:702, 1973.
43. Kligman, A. M.: Pathologic dynamics of human hair loss. I. Telogen effluvium. Arch. Dermatol., 83:175, 1961.
44. Martin, C. M., Southwick, E. G., and Maibach, H. I.: Proparanol induced alopecia. Am. Heart J., 86:236, 1973.
45. Muller, S. A., and Winklemann, R. K.: Alopecia areata, an evaluation of 736 patients. Arch. Dermatol., 88:290, 1963.
46. Papa, C. M., and Kligman, A. M.: Stimulation of hair growth by topical application of androgen. JAMA, 191:521, 1965.

47. Papadopoulos, S., and Harden, R.: Hair loss in patients treated with carbimagol. Br. Med. J., 2:1502, 1966.
48. Pecoraro, V., Astore, I., and Barman, J. M.: Cycle of the scalp hair of the newborn child. J. Invest. Dermatol., 43:145, 1964.
49. Price, V. H.: Testosterone metabolism in the skin: Review of its function in androgenic alopecia, acne vulgaris, and idiopathic hirsutism including recent studies with antiandrogens. Arch. Dermatol., 111:1492, 1975.
50. Rawnsley, H. M., and Shelley, W. B.: Salicylate ingestion and idiopathic hair loss. Lancet, 1:567, 1968.
51. Smith, J. C., Weinstein, G. D., and Burr, J. M.: Hair roots of the human scalp in thyroid disease. J. Invest. Dermatol., 32:35, 1959.
52. Sulzberger, M., Witten, V., and Kopf, A.: Diffuse alopecia in women. Arch. Dermatol., 81:108, 1960.
53. Van Sott, E. J., Reinertson, R. P., and Steinmuller, R.: The growing hair roots of the human scalp and morphologic changes therein following amethopterin therapy. J. Invest. Dermatol., 29:197, 1957.
54. Wilburne, M.: Hair loss and pigmentation due to thiouracil derivatives. JAMA, 147:379, 1971.

PHYSICAL AND CHEMICAL DAMAGE

55. Goldsmith, L. A., and Baden, H. A.: The mechanical properties of hair. J. Invest. Dermatol., 50:200, 1971.
56. Harman, R. R.: Traction alopecia due to hair extension. Br. J. Dermatol., 87:79, 1972.
57. Holder, W.: The broken ponytail. Arch. Dermatol., 103:101, 1971.
58. Kligman, A. M.: Facts and fancies on the care of hair and nails. South. Med. J., 55:1001, 1961.
59. Lipnik, M.: Traumatic alopecia from brush rollers. Arch. Dermatol., 84:183, 1961.
60. LoPresti, P., Papa, C., and Kligman, A.: Hot comb alopecia. Arch. Dermatol., 98:234, 1968.
61. Muller, S. A., and Winklemann, R. K.: Trichotillomania: A clinical pathologic study. Arch. Dermatol., 102:129, 1965.
62. Orfanos, C. E., and Mahrle, G.: Human hair and how it changes under cosmetic procedures in vivo. Parfumeric Kostmetick, 52:203, 235, 1971.
63. Papa, C. M., Mills, O. H., and Hanshaw, W.: Seasonal trichorrhexia nodosa. Arch. Dermatol., 106:888, 1972.
64. Savill, A.: The nylon brush. Br. J. Dermatol., 70:296, 1958.
65. Reiches, A. J., and Lane, C. W.: Temporary baldness due to cold wave throglycolate preparations. JAMA, 144:305, 1950.
66. Rudolph, R. I., Klein, A. W., and Decherd, J. W.: Corn row alopecia. Arch. Dermatol., 108:134, 1973.

SCARRING ALOPECIA

67. Altman, J., and Perry, H. O.: The variations and course of lichen planus. Arch. Dermatol., 84:179, 1961.
68. Burnham, T. K., Fine, G., and Neblett, T. R.: Immunofluorescent "Band" test for lupus erythematosus. Arch. Dermatol., 102:42, 1970.
69. Gay Prieto, J.: Pseudopelade of Brocq: Its relationship to some forms of cicatricial alopecia and to lichen planus. J. Invest. Dermatol., 24:323, 1958.
70. O'Leary, P. A., Montgomery, H. and Ragsdale, W. E.: Dermatohistopathology of various types of scleroderma. Arch. Dermatol., 75:78, 1957.
71. Michel, B., Sy, E. K., David, K., et al.: Immunofluorescent patterns in lichen planus. J. Invest. Dermatol., 54:428, 1970.
72. Pascher, F., Sams, C. F., and Pensky, N.: Lupus erythematosus profundus (Kaposi's-Irang), J. Invest. Dermatol., 25:347, 1955.

HIRSUTISM

73. Ettinger, B., Goldfield, E. B., Burrell, K. C., et al.: Plasma testosterone stimulation–suppression dynamics in hirsute women. Am. J. Med., 54:195, 1973.

74. Ettinger, B., von Werder, K., Thenacrs, C. C., et al.: Plasma testosterone stimulation–suppression dynamics in hirsute women. Am. J. Med., 56:170, 1971.
75. Hegedus, S. I., and Schorr, W. F.: Acquired hypertrichosis lanuginosa and malignancy. Arch. Dermatol., 106:84, 1972.
76. Ismail, A. A. A., Davidson, D. W., Kirkham, K. E., et al.: Studies on sex hormone excretion in normal and hirsute women. Acta Endocrinol., 61:283, 1969.
77. Kaiser, I. H., Perry, C., and Yoonessi, M.: Acquired hypertrichosis lanuginosa associated with endometrial malignancy. Obstet. Gynecol., 47:479, 1976.
78. Karp, L., and Herrmann, W. L.: Diagnosis and treatment of hirsutism in women. Obstet. Gynecol., 41:283, 1973.
79. Livingston, S., Petersen, D., and Boks, L. L.: Hypertrichosis occurring in association with Dilantin therapy. J. Pediatr., 47:351, 1951.
80. Lloyd, C. W., Lobotsky, J., Segre, E. J., et al.: Plasma testosterone and urinary 17-ketosteroids in women with hirsutism and polycystic ovaries. J. Clin. Endocrinol. Metab., 26:314, 1966.
81. Maguire, H. C.: Facial hair growth over site of testosterone injection in women. Lancet, 1:864, 1964.
82. McKenna, T. J., Miller, R. B., Liddle, G. W., et al.: Plasma pregnenolone and 17 OH pregnenolone in patients with adrenal tumors, ACTH excess or idiopathic hirsutism. J. Clin. Endocrinol. Metab., 44:231, 1977.
83. Meikle, A. W., Stringhan, J. D., Dolman, L. I., et al.: Plasma 5 alpha androstenediol: An androgen marker of hirsutism in females. Trans. Assoc. Am. Physicians, 89:133, 1976.
84. Muller, S. A.: Hirsutism. Am. J. Med., 46:803, 1969.
85. Strauss, J. S., and Pochi, P. E.: The hormonal control of the pilosebaceous unit. *In:* Kobori, T., and Montagna, W. (eds.): Biology and Disease of the Hair. Baltimore, University Park Press, 1975, pp. 231–245.

16
LUPUS ERYTHEMATOSUS

NANCY L. FUREY, M.D.
and NANCY B. ESTERLY, M.D.

INTRODUCTION

Lupus erythematosus is a complex illness with a variable clinical presentation, prognosis, and response to therapy. Symptoms of the disease may be transitory, expressed as a mild, non-deforming arthritis and dermatitis, or they may be severe, with inflammation of vital organs such as the kidney and brain, eventuating in death. More commonly, patients with LE have a chronic, smoldering, persistent inflammation of several target organs for many years, with periodic remissions and decreasing frequency of exacerbations. The peak incidence of onset of lupus erythematosus is in the third decade of life, but about 15 per cent of cases occur before 20 years of age.[1]

The disease was first described in about 1828 by Biett and named érythémé centrifuge. He apparently did not publish his description but discussed the disase at meetings with colleagues.[2] In 1851, Cazenave wrote that "this disease which Biett first described and named erythema centrifuge is a type of lupus." Cazenave, Biett's pupil, after studying several cases of the disease and noting that the erythematous eruption resulted in severe residual scarring in some patients, felt the disease should be classified as a variety of lupus and coined the name lupus érythémateux.[3] He presented several cases of Biett's "érythémé centrifuge" at a meeting at the Hospital Saint-Louis on June 4, 1851.

The term "lupus," derived from the Latin word for wolf, was used figuratively as early as the 13th century in the works of the Schola Salernitana and in Rogerius to describe a variety of destructive processes that attacked the face and lower legs.[4] It was believed during the Middle Ages that the wolf was a natural enemy of humans. Legends detailed its reputed attack, in which it slashed open the skin and ate the flesh of its living victim. The comparable ravages of such disease processes as skin cancer, cutaneous tuberculosis, and syphilis were all included under the designation of lupus. Dolaeus, in 1684,[4] defined lupus as a destructive process involving the face and attempted to distinguish it from carcinoma. Gradually, the various chronic, non-hereditary, destructive skin diseases were differentiated on the basis of clinical characteristics and etiology, and specific qualifying words were added to the term lupus to distinguish each disease, e.g., lupus vulgaris, lupus pernio, lupus serpiginosus, lupus foliativus, and lupus verrucosus. Cazenave, in coining the term "lupus érythémateux," emphasized the specific erythema of the skin,

...characterized by a redness which disappears with digital pressure, by a tendency to gradually and continuously thin the skin of affected areas, and by eventual cicatrization. Lupus erythematosus presents diagnostically three important points— redness, thinning of skin without ulceration, and different appearances of the same lesions. Thus one may observe, but only very rarely, an urticarial form.... It appears on the forehead, but most particularly on the cheeks. It appears in the form of somewhat raised plaques of variable puffiness which, instead of quickly disappearing like simple urticaria, persist, sometimes for a long time. This form is very limited and when it resolves, it always leaves behind cutaneous atrophy or even cicatrization.[3]

Early dermatologists erroneously credited Hebra with the first description of LE because in 1846 he reported a facial dermatosis that he called "seborrhea congestiva" and compared its configuration to a butterfly with outspread wings.[2] From this brief description, the facial dermatosis cannot be identified as lupus erythematosus with certainty. Subsequently Hebra, "with riper experience, more fully detailed" perceived that Cazenave had named the disease appropriately and adopted this term.[5] Other names such as "erythema lupinosum" (Veiel) and "lupus seborrhagicus" (Volkmann) were proposed, but with the publication in 1875 of the classic volume, *Diseases of the Skin Including the Exanthemata,* the name "lupus erythematosus" became firmly established.[5]

Moriz Kaposi was the first to recognize and record the acute form of LE.

Lupus erythematosus appears in two forms: In the form of characteristic discs— Lupus erythematosus discoides [and] in the form of peculiar, isolated, and aggregated spots—Lupus erythematosus discretus et aggregatus. It, for the most part, develops very slowly, and has a very chronic course, and, under such circumstances, does not exercise any injurious influence whatever on the constitution. Lupus erythematosus may, however, make its appearance and continue its course accompanied by symptoms of a widely diffused or universal, acute or subacute eruption attended by fever, and may then often, by the intensity of the local and constitutional symptoms, affect the whole organism and endanger the patient's existence, or even prove fatal. Lupus erythem. disc. is confined, with scarcely any exception, to the face and head, has a regular and chronic course, and is unattended by any severe complications but may, nevertheless, now and then, be complicated with erysipelas, or with the aggregated form and its acute symptoms....[6]

At the turn of the century, Sir William Osler[7] unequivocably established LE as a multisystem disease.

By exudative erythema is understood a disease of unknown etiology with polymorphic skin lesions—hyperaemia, oedema, and hemorrhage—arthritis occasionally, and a variable number of visceral manifestations, of which the most important are gastrointestinal crises, endocarditis, pericarditis, acute nephritis and hemorrhage from the mucous surfaces. Recurrence is a special feature of the disease and attacks may come on month after month or even throughout a long period of years. Variability in the skin lesions is the rule, and a case may present in one attack the features of an angioneurotic oedema, in a second of a multiform or nodose erythema, and in a third those of peliosis rheumatica. The attacks may not be characterized by skin manifestations; the visceral symptoms alone may be present, and to the outward view the patient may have no indications whatever of erythema exudativum.

Analysis of numerous cases during subsequent decades resulted in expansion of the clinical spectrum of the disease and definition of the pathological changes.[8-10] In 1941, Klemperer and his colleagues[11] introduced the term "collagen disease" to emphasize the characteristic pathological abnormality in the ground substance.

> From the preceding analysis we have seen that the morbid process in lupus erythematosus revolves about a well-defined disturbance of collagen affecting all organs and tissues of the body.... The widespread, frequent and characteristic alteration of collagen together with the special predilection of the injury for the collagen in certain sites (heart, glomeruli, blood vessels, skin, spleen and retroperitoneal tissues) has been seen in no other disease save diffuse scleroderma.

In 1948, Hargraves' discovery of the "LE cell" in bone marrow preparations from patients with LE,[12] and the subsequent modification of the test to demonstrate this phenomenon in serum from these patients, provided the first laboratory marker of the disease. More recently, several circulating antinuclear antibodies have been identified in sera from patients with LE. The less specific but more sensitive fluorescent antinuclear antibody (ANA) test is now routinely used and widely available in clinical laboratories. Extensive application of this test has permitted identification of patients with early and milder forms of the disease and thus has broadened our concepts of the clinical spectrum, course, and prognosis of LE.

In 1971, the American Rheumatism Association published preliminary criteria for the classification of systemic lupus erythematosus (SLE).[13] The criteria were based on data collected from patients with unequivocal LE, probable LE, and classic rheumatoid arthritis as well as from non-rheumatic patients. The data were computer analyzed, and 14 major manifestations of LE were delineated. The report concluded that a diagnosis of LE can be made if a patient demonstrates four of the 14 manifestations (Table 16-1).

These criteria have been used by several clinics[14-17] and are considered helpful guidelines for diagnosis. However, there are LE patients who do not fulfill four criteria on initial presentation but do so only with evolution of the disease and progressive involvement of several organ systems. The criteria rely on data that were collected ten years ago and derived from patients seen only by rheumatologists. These patients tended to have severe disease and positive LE preparations. Critical laboratory data, including serum complement levels, antinuclear antibody patterns, anti-DNA antibody levels, and other serological tests now available, are not included in these criteria.

From a purely dermatological viewpoint, the criteria pertaining to the cutaneous manifestations are inadequate. Only acute facial erythema and the chronic discoid lesion have been included. Subacute, red, scaly lesions without follicular plugging, which can heal with minimal if any scarring, are not recognized. In addition, the classic telangiectatic, red, papular, and infarctive lesions of the palms and fingertips are not included. Oral and nasopharyngeal ulcerations are listed as a separate manifestation, although these lesions are simply an extension of the cutaneous eruption.

Although still useful for educational purposes and for defining organ involvement, the ARA criteria are most important because they represent the first attempt to identify patients with uniform clinical and laboratory manifestations of lupus. Current evaluation of LE patients depends less on finding a biological false positive test for syphilis (criterion number 9) than on the detection

TABLE 16–1 PRELIMINARY CRITERIA FOR CLASSIFICATION OF SLE*

A person shall be said to have systemic lupus erythematosus (SLE) if any four or more of the following 14 manifestations are present, serially or simultaneously, during any interval of observation:

1. *Facial erythema (butterfly rash).* Diffuse erythema, flat or raised, over the malar eminence(s) and/or bridge of the nose; may be unilateral.
2. *Discoid lupus.* Erythematous raised patches with adherent keratotic scaling and follicular plugging; atrophic scarring may occur in older lesions; may be present anywhere on the body.
3. *Raynaud's phenomenon.* Intermittent severe pallor of the fingers, toes, ears, or nose. Requires a two-phase color reaction, by patient's history or physician's observation.
4. *Alopecia.* Rapid loss of large amount of the scalp hair, by patient's history or physician's observation.
5. *Photosensitivity.* Unusual skin reaction from exposure to sunlight, by patient's history or physician's observation.
6. *Oral or nasopharyngeal ulceration.*
7. *Arthritis without deformity.* One or more peripheral joints involved with any of the following in the absence of deformity: *(a) pain on motion, (b) tenderness, (c) effusion or periarticular soft tissue swelling.* (Peripheral joints are defined for this purpose as feet, ankles, knees, hips, shoulders, elbows, wrists, metacarpophalangeal, proximal interphalangeal, terminal interphalangeal, and temporomandibular joints.)
8. *LE cells.* Two or more classic LE cells seen on one occasion or one cell seen on two or more occasions, using an accepted published method.
9. *Chronic false positive reaction to serological test for syphilis (STS).* Known to be present for at least six months and confirmed by TPI or Reiter's tests.
10. *Profuse proteinuria.* Greater than 3.5 gm per day.
11. *Cellular casts.* May be red cell, hemoglobin, granular, tubular, or mixed.
12. *One or both of the following: (a) pleuritis,* (history of pleuritic pain, rub heard by physician, or x-ray evidence of both pleural thickening and fluid), *(b) pericarditis,* documented by EKG or rub.
13. *One or both of the following: (a) psychosis, (b) convulsions,* by patient's history or physician's observation in the absence of uremia and offending drugs.
14. *One or more of the following: (a) hemolytic anemia, (b) leukopenia* (WBC less than 4000 per cu mm on two or more occasions), *(c) thrombocytopenia* (platelet count less than 100,000 per cu mm).

From: Cohen, A. L., Reynolds, W. E., Franklin, E. C., et al.: Preliminary criteria for the classification of systemic lupus erythematosus. Bull. Rheum. Dis., 23:643, 1971.

of positive tests for antibodies to nuclear material, DNA, or more specific tissue antigens. By identifying subpopulations of lupus patients with common symptom complexes and immunological responses, we may be better able in the future to define a common denominator in these patients. Ideally, patients who may be at risk for involvement of vital organs can be identified early, and vigorous and effective therapy can be initiated.

CUTANEOUS MANIFESTATIONS

The dermatological manifestations of lupus may be so characteristic that they are clinically diagnostic of the disease. Skin changes occur in over 70 per cent of patients with systemic lupus erythematosus[18] and occur as the initial manifestation in 20 per cent of patients, second only to arthritis as the earliest sign of the disorder.[19] Skin lesions found in association with LE may be specific or non-specific. The specific cutaneous LE lesions can be classified as chronic (discoid), subacute, and acute. The morphological appearance of the lesions reflects the host response and the severity and duration of the cutaneous

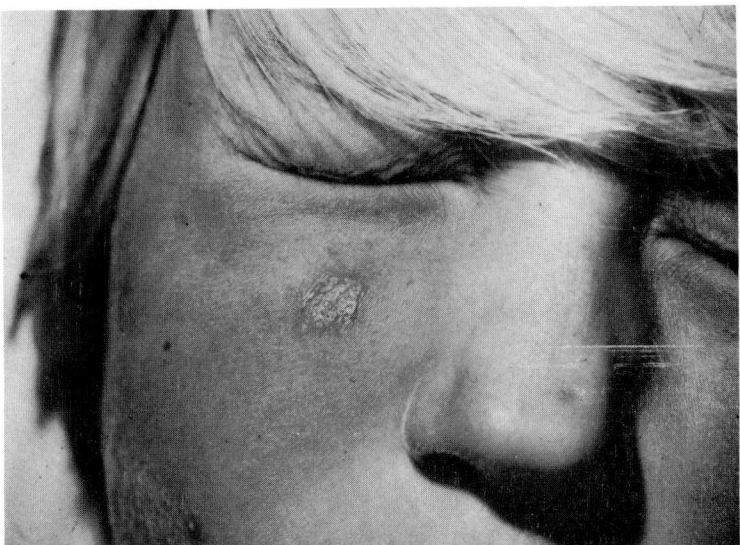

FIGURE 16–1 Early discoid LE plaque demonstrating well-defined border and marked erythema and scaling.

eruption. In general, patients who mount a vigorous cutaneous inflammatory response develop chronic scarring lesions of the skin and have a low incidence of inflammatory response in other organs. On the other hand, those patients who develop only central facial erythema and edema have a higher incidence of severe involvement of vital organs.

Chronic discoid LE lesions begin as simple patches of erythema, evolve into well-circumscribed, red-to-violaceous, scaly, indurated plaques (Fig. 16–1), and eventually heal with atrophy, telangiectasia, and post-inflammatory areas of hyperpigmentation and hypopigmentation (Figs. 16–2 and 16–3). The scales are most often yellowish-gray and thick. On the face and scalp, where the pilosebaceous apparatus is well developed, the scales may plug the dilated follicular openings, giving rise to the descriptive term "carpet-tack scale." With

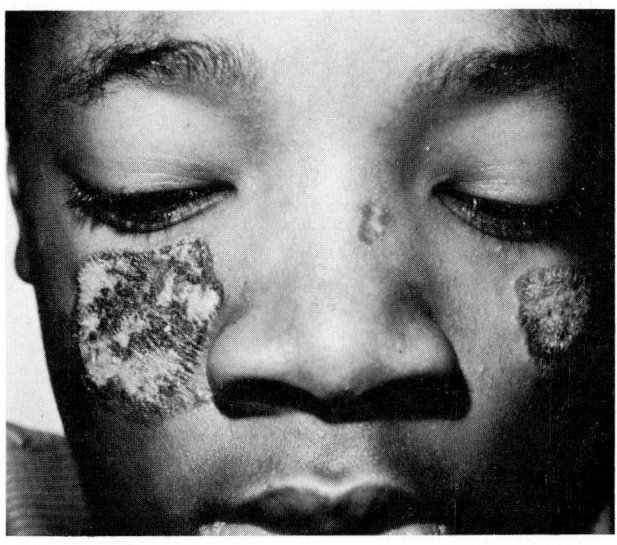

FIGURE 16–2 Chronic discoid LE plaques on cheeks and nose of an adolescent girl.

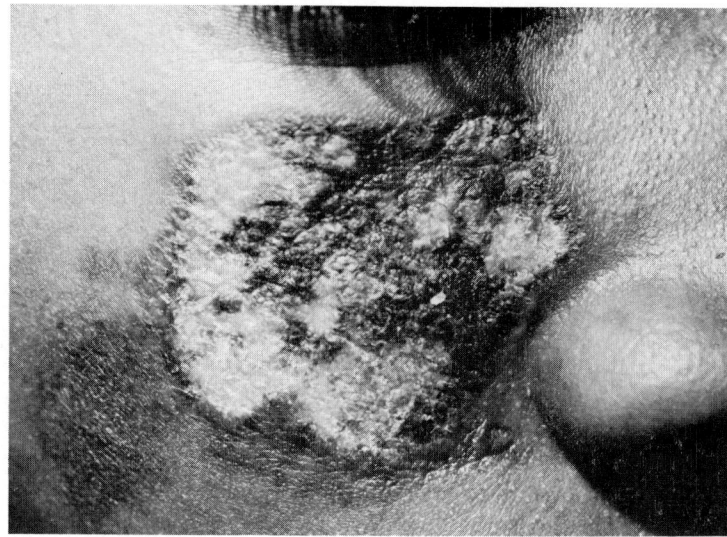

FIGURE 16-3 Closeup of chronic discoid lesion. Note areas of post-inflammatory hyperpigmentation and hypopigmentation with peripheral areas of active inflammation.

chronicity, some lesions may become hypertrophic and elevated, but usually they become atrophic and scarred. A typical discoid LE plaque is a mosaic of changes, owing to the progression of the inflammatory process in some areas and its regression in others. A single lesion may display healed atrophic areas coexistent with an acute process, erythema, scaling, and active inflammation.

Chronic discoid LE lesions occur most commonly on the face and scalp and have a peculiar propensity for the outer ear. Scarring lesions on the inner surfaces of the conchae are virtually diagnostic of discoid lupus. Similarly, when such lesions affect the palms and fingers, they appear as small, patchy, atrophic depressions filled with thick, tenacious scales and surrounded by a halo of bright erythema (Fig. 16-4). Lesions in the mucous membranes of the nasal or

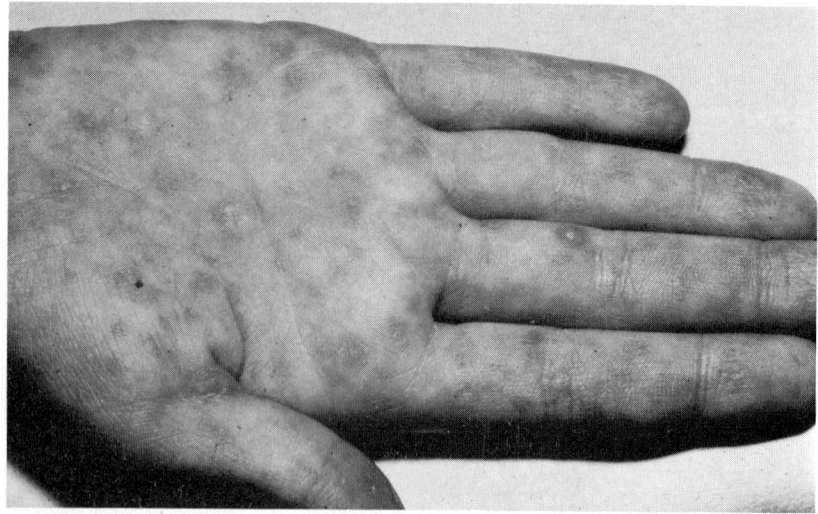

FIGURE 16-4 Multiple erythematous macular lesions and patchy atrophic depressions filled with scales and surrounded by a halo of bright erythema.

oral cavity, where stratum corneum is absent, are complicated by ulceration, particularly if they occur in areas of trauma. Less than 15 per cent of patients with chronic discoid cutaneous LE will have extracutaneous manifestations of SLE or even serological abnormalities of SLE, such as a circulating antinuclear antibody, anti–DNA antibody, or depressed serum complement levels.[20, 21] In a study of 15 patients who had chronic discoid lesions and extracutaneous manifestations of LE, all had a relatively benign course, with no severe renal disease.[21]

At the opposite end of the spectrum, in acute systemic LE, the cutaneous manifestations may be quite varied. The most widely recognized eruption, the acute erythema of the central face or the so-called butterfly rash, is relatively uncommon and occurs in less than 10 per cent of SLE patients.[22] These patients have pronounced redness and edema of the nasal bridge and malar eminences. The entire face may be erythematous, the periorbital area edematous, and the skin over the nose and malar eminences raised and scaly, with a red-violaceous hue and subtle telangiectasia (Fig. 16–5). These patients usually have arthritis, fever, and malaise and have a higher incidence of vital organ involvement. When the eruption is typical, it can be differentiated easily from the eczematous eruption of seborrheic dermatitis, the pustular and papular telangiectatic lesions of acne rosacea, and the erythematous, telangiectatic skin changes of iatrogenic Cushing's disease. However, atypical LE rashes do occur, and a careful evaluation is required to differentiate these more benign conditions.

Subacute cutaneous LE lesions are commonly encountered in SLE and include a variety of inflammatory lesions of moderate intensity (Fig. 16–6). Some patients develop persistent, well-demarcated, erythematous-to-violaceous scaly plaques, which resolve after treatment with no scarring or with only minimal telangiectasia and atrophy. Others have persistent erythematous or violaceous smooth plaques that resemble unremitting urticaria. These also may disappear without residual damage. The lesions most often erupt in sun-exposed areas, i.e., the forehead, cheeks, nose, **V** of the neck, upper arms and dorsa of the hands (Plate IX–A). When these lesions are seen in the early stages of SLE, they often cannot be distinguished from the lesions of early chronic discoid LE

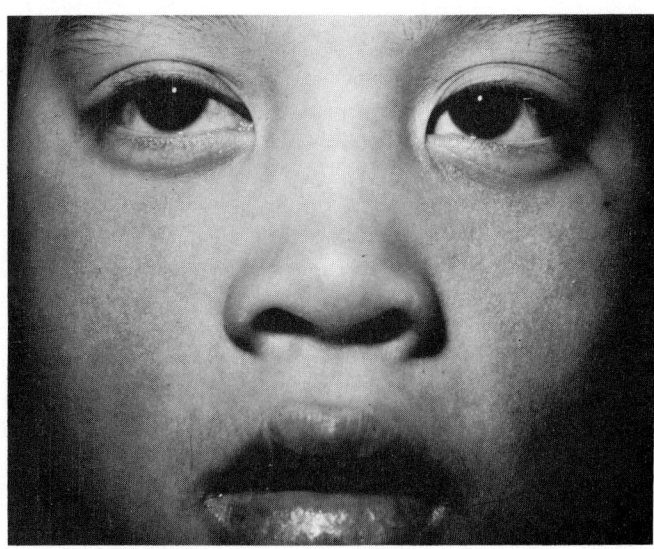

FIGURE 16–5 Acute erythema of both cheeks in a child with systemic LE.

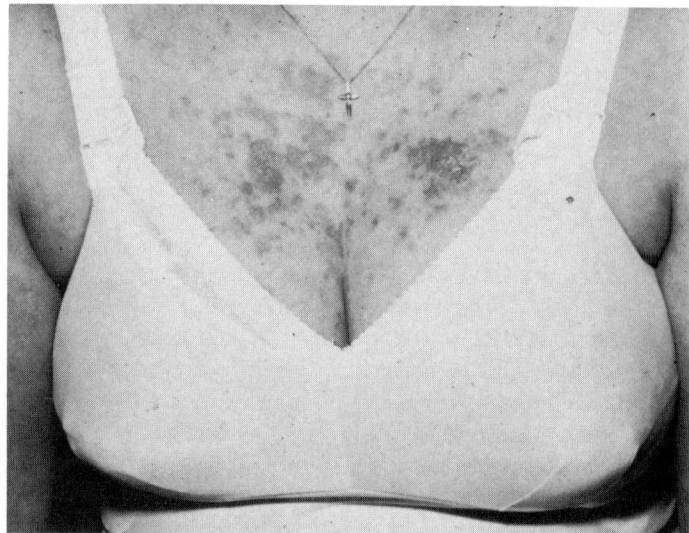

FIGURE 16-6 Subacute erythematous scaling plaques on sun-exposed skin.

(CDLE). Only with complete resolution in a few weeks or months does their subacute character become obvious. The clinical course of the disease in these patients is variable and can be mild or relatively severe.

The underlying systemic vasculitis of SLE is manifested by diverse cutaneous signs. Non-specific urticaria with and without purpura is seen in association with a polymorphonuclear leukocytic vasculitis. Chronic intractable urticaria with arthralgia is occasionally the presenting feature of SLE. Hemorrhagic bullous lesions are rare but when present reflect extensive vasculitis with massive dermal edema.

Some patients display prominent erythema and telangiectasia of the cuticle and proximal nail folds (Plate IX-B). Frequently, these patients also have splinter, subungual hemorrhages and papular telangiectatic lesions on the palmar aspect of the hands and fingertips. Occasionally, with more severe angitis, infarctive fingertip lesions occur. This severe expression of a generalized vasculitis is frequently observed in patients with central nervous system manifestations of LE.[23, 24]

Widespread inflammation of the vascular system is expressed as livedo reticularis and can result in extensive, small, ulcerative lesions, especially of the legs. This purple reticulated discoloration of the lower legs and sometimes the arms and trunk is differentiated from physiological cutis marmorata by its persistence.

Lupus panniculitis (lupus profundus), an unusual manifestation of LE, has a predilection for the subcutaneous tissue of the upper arms and cheeks but may occur on the buttocks, thighs, and trunk as well. Typical lesions are firm, slightly tender, erythematous nodules, which may be smooth or scaly and at times ulcerate and heal with severe atrophic scarring. The nodules are often associated with overlying skin changes of discoid LE. Most of these patients have chronic cutaneous lesions with few systemic manifestations;[25] however, a few patients with widespread systemic disease have been reported.[26-28]

Several types of hair of hair loss can occur in LE. Scarring permanent alopecia is the end result of untreated chronic discoid LE lesions of the scalp. The cosmetic disfigurement may be mild, with only a few small areas of baldness easily covered by surrounding hair, or may be so severe as to involve almost the entire scalp, necessitating the wearing of a hair piece. Subacute lesions will result in patchy, cicatricial alopecia.

There are two forms of non-scarring alopecia. In acute active LE, especially if the patient is febrile, a toxic telogen effluvium may occur, resulting in diffuse thinning of the hair. The scalp is usually erythematous, although it may appear normal. This loss is generally reversible, and hair regrows with remission of the disease.

Another type of hair loss that may be encountered in the LE patient is characterized by the presence of numerous, fine, short hairs of irregular length, especially along the frontal hairline. This finding can be demonstrated in approximately 30 per cent of SLE patients if they are examined carefully.[29] Microscopic examination of these hairs indicates that the short hair, termed "lupus hair," may be caused by growth retardation rather than by breakage.[27] Lupus hair is frequently noted coincidentally with clinical and laboratory evidence of increased disease activity. Recovery of hair growth is usually slow after the activity subsides.

HISTOLOGY OF CUTANEOUS LE LESIONS

In acute, subacute, and chronic cutaneous LE, the primary site of injury occurs near the vessel walls and at the dermal-epidermal junction, as demonstrated by light, immunofluorescent, and immunoelectron microscopic studies.

The early erythematous, edematous, malar rash occurring in patients with acute SLE may not be diagnostic histologically. In the very early stages, the changes may consist only of dilated blood and lymphatic vessels in the upper dermis. There may be small vacuoles along the basal lamina. In biopsy specimens from the fully-developed eruption, the epidermis is atrophic, and there is extensive intracellular edema in the basal cell layer, causing degeneration by liquefaction. Occasionally, lymphedema becomes so severe that intraepidermal or subepidermal vesicles are formed. In the upper dermis, the vessel walls are swollen, with extravasation of leukocytes and erythrocytes and only a sparse infiltrate of lymphocytes. The elastic fibers initially are normal but eventually become fragmented. Collagen bundles appear spongy and become thickened and eosinophilic.

In subacute cutaneous LE lesions, these pathological changes are more pronounced, and in addition to destruction of elastic tissue and collagen, atrophy of sebaceous glands and hair follicles occurs. These histological features correlate with the clinical features of subacute LE lesions in which resolution is variable, with little or no scarring in some cases but with definite mild residual atrophy in others.

Early lesions of chronic DLE may appear similar to subacute LE pathologically. As the lesion progresses, the pathological changes become characteristic and diagnostic, owing to the dense infiltration of lymphocytes along the dermal-epidermal junction and around dermal blood vessels and appendageal structures. There is prominent hyperkeratosis with keratotic plugging of dilated follicular orifices. The malpighian layer is usually atrophic, but there may be areas of acanthosis. A variable degree of degeneration by liquefaction of the basal cell layer is present. At the dermal-epidermal junction, there is a band of para-aminosalicylic acid (PAS)-positive material, unless inflammation has been so intense that only edema and amorphous material remain. In patients with dark skin, incontinence of pigment is characteristic, and the melanin is engulfed by dermal macrophages. The elastic fibers degenerate, and hair follicles, sebaceous glands, and sweat glands atrophy and disappear. The histological changes of old, inactive, healed, scarred lesions of CDLE predictably are not diagnostic. Such lesions cannot be differentiated from other diseases of the skin that terminate in scarring.

In 1963, Burnham and his associates[30] stained frozen sections of LE skin lesions with fluorescein-conjugated anti–human globulin and described the deposition of immunoglobulin along the dermal-epidermal junction (Fig. 16–7). This finding has been repeatedly confirmed[31-33] and can be demonstrated not only in active acute, subacute, and chronic cutaneous LE lesions but also in the clinically uninvolved skin of patients with systemic LE.[34, 35] Patients with discoid LE lesions typically do not have immunoglobulin deposits in uninvolved skin.

In the normal skin of lupus patients with systemic involvement, the deposition of immunoglobulin occurs in a finely granular or stippled pattern.[35] In acute LE lesions, the deposition is more coarsely granular and thready, and there are often deposits in the upper dermis, especially in and around dermal vessels. In subacute and chronic DLE lesions, the staining pattern is more dense and at times can be appreciated as a thick homogeneous band,[36] often with overlying clumps of brightly stained globulin. In lesional and clinically normal skin, both IgM and IgG are frequently found, either alone or together. IgA is found less often and only in conjunction with IgG or IgM. Both classic and

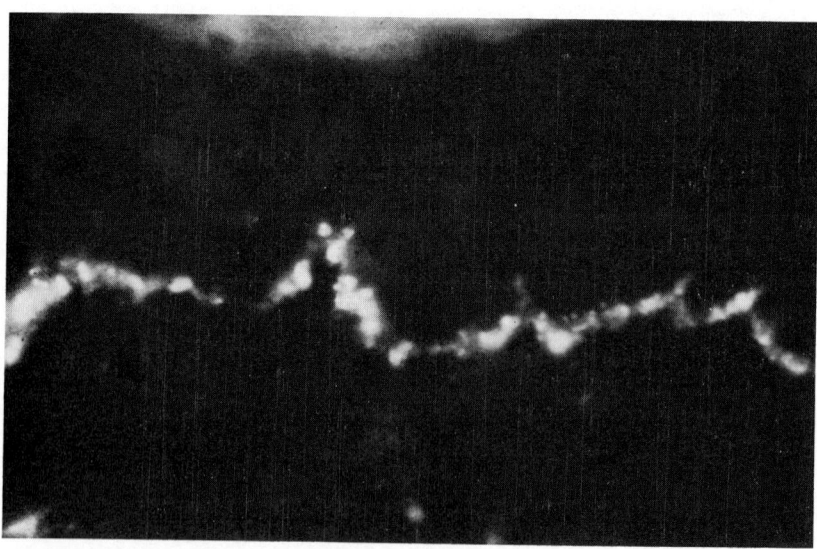

FIGURE 16–7 Direct immunofluorescence of an erythematous scaling plaque showing deposition of immunoglobulin G at the dermal-epidermal junction.

alternate pathway complement components are present in specific LE skin lesions.[37, 38] Early LE lesions may not have deposits of immunoglobulin. Serial biopsies of UV-induced lesions in LE patients have demonstrated a time lag of several weeks between induction of the inflammatory response and detection of subepidermal immunoglobulin.[39]

Immunoelectron microscopic studies of cutaneous LE lesions have demonstrated that the immunoglobulin deposits do not have an affinity for specific subepidermal structures. Immunoglobulin has been found on the basal lamina, extending to the surface of the basal cells, and also as a coating on the collagen fibers in the upper dermis.[40] In SLE lesions, the deposits tend to be more localized to the subepidermal zone and the basal lamina. In CDLE specimens, deposits have been identified also in the mid-dermis.[41]

Examination of lesional skin by immunohistochemical methods is useful diagnostically in patients who have cutaneous lesions that are compatible with but not specific for LE. Such disorders as polymorphic light eruption, seborrheic dermatitis, and drug eruptions can simulate LE both clinically and histologically but are negative when examined by the direct immunofluorescence technique.

The lupus band test is used to evaluate normal-appearing skin from lupus patients for the presence or absence of subepidermal deposition of immunoglobulin. Sun-exposed forearm skin is more likely to be positive than light-protected buttock skin.[42] For diagnostic purposes, a 3 mm punch biopsy of forearm skin is ideal; however, for assessment of prognosis, buttock skin may be preferable. Biopsies from such light-protected sites are more acceptable cosmetically and probably reflect more accurately the extent of cutaneous deposition of immunoglobulin.

Characteristically, patients with chronic discoid skin lesions have a negative lupus band test. Exceptions are seen, however, in the occasional patient with chronic discoid lesions who also has clinical and serological manifestations of systemic disease. Patients with subacute cutaneous lesions do have immunoglobulin deposition, especially in sun-exposed skin. Approximately 50 per cent of patients who satisfy at least four of the ARA criteria for the diagnosis of systemic LE have a positive band test.[43] This test can be useful diagnostically in confirming a diagnosis of SLE in patients without cutaneous lesions.

The positive band test correlates with the presence of antibody to DNA,[42] hypocomplementemia,[44] and lupus nephritis.[45] A higher percentage, approximately 85 per cent, of patients with LE nephritis have a positive band test.[42] The conversion of a lupus band test from negative to positive has been associated with clinical deterioration.[42] There is also evidence that the lupus band test becomes negative following therapy with alkylating agents, when the patient undergoes clinical remission associated with a reduction in DNA antibody titer.[46] Determination of the class of immunoglobulin present can be useful. The finding of only IgM on serial biopsy specimens is indicative of a benign course. There are many patients with IgG who never develop nephritis, but if nephritis is present, the patient usually has IgG alone or in addition to IgM or IgA. The identification of the presence and type of subepidermal deposits of immunoglobulin in uninvolved buttock skin may be useful in the evaluation of selected lupus patients; however, the prognostic significance of the lupus band test is not yet established.

SEROLOGICAL MANIFESTATIONS

ANTIBODIES TO TISSUE COMPONENTS

Patients with active systemic LE develop antibodies to nuclear material. This phenomenon is detectable by the antinuclear antibody (ANA) test, which essentially has replaced the LE cell test because it is more sensitive. The indirect immunofluorescence technique described by Coons and Kaplan in 1957[47] was applied by Friou and other investigators to detect this phenomenon.[48-50] During the 1960's, many investigators[51-57] described multiple morphological patterns of nuclear staining, depending on the tissue substrate used, the type of lupus serum tested, and the attention paid to detail. Most laboratories using human spleen or rat or mouse liver tissue as a source of nuclear antigens recognize three patterns in lupus sera: peripheral, homogeneous, and particulate (sometimes called "speckled" or "thready"). Using sera from patients with scleroderma and occasionally other rheumatic disorders, two more specific patterns are seen: nucleolar and finely speckled. Additional patterns may be recognized if the nuclei are examined with an oil immersion lens.[60] Complicating the laboratory interpretation of staining patterns is the fact that some lupus sera contain a variety of nuclear antibodies and exhibit more than one pattern. The pattern can change with varying dilutions, and sometimes adjacent cells may exhibit different patterns. The individual morphological patterns are presumed to reflect specific antibodies directed toward different antigens within the nucleus.[58-60]

The fluorescent ANA test is the single most useful test for confirming a clinical diagnosis of LE, if it can be properly interpreted. Unfortunately, at the present time the test has not been standardized. Clinical laboratories employ many techniques, including commercial kits, that render the test relatively non-specific. The physician must evaluate the quality and sensitivity of the test as performed in the laboratory before interpreting the results for the patient. Many patients have endured needless anxiety and expense because of an inaccurately or incorrectly interpreted positive ANA test. It should be remembered that a positive test alone is not conclusive evidence for a diagnosis of SLE. Positive tests occur in other rheumatic disorders, such as rheumatoid arthritis and scleroderma, as well as in malignancy and drug reactions. Relatives of SLE patients also may show positive test results.

Ideally, the ANA report should state the substrate used, the titer, and the pattern. In active SLE with murine liver or human spleen, the titer usually exceeds 1:40. The peripheral pattern is characteristic of an SLE patient with antibody to DNA who is at risk for the development of renal disease. The titer of this pattern may reflect disease activity. A particulate or speckled pattern suggests that the patient may have antibodies to extractable nuclear antigens (ENA). Homogeneous patterns are non-specific and are usually significant only in titers greater than 1:160. Nucleolar staining and fine speckles are seen most commonly in scleroderma. Except for the titer of the peripheral pattern, the titer of ANA in a lupus patient does not correlate with severity of disease and is not a useful guide for therapy. Aged, chronically ill patients or patients with malignancy, rheumatoid arthritis, or other hypergammaglobulinemic states may have a positive ANA, but the titer is usually low. A leukocyte-specific antibody may be found in selected patients with rheumatoid arthritis and occasionally in SLE patients if leukocytes are present in the substrate, as in human spleen.[61] This explains why the results of an ANA test may be positive in one laboratory but negative in another and emphasizes the need for standardization of laboratory technique and reporting.

A negative ANA finding virtually excludes the diagnosis of active LE, except in the few reported patients who have an LE-like syndrome associated with anticytoplasmic or antimitochondrial antibodies.[62, 63] The test may also become negative in a patient with complete renal failure.

DNA ANTIBODY

It was recognized as early as 1957[64, 65] that lupus sera reacted with purified DNA. Of all of the laboratory tests available, antibody to DNA seems to reflect disease activity most directly and is probably closely related to the pathogenetic mechanisms. There is appreciable evidence implicating the DNA-anti-DNA complexes in the pathogenesis of lupus nephritis.[66] For this reason, considerable effort has been expended during the last 20 years to devise a sensitive, specific, reproducible, practical test to detect antibodies to double-stranded deoxyribonucleic acid.[67-78] The techniques that have been used most widely are passive hemagglutination,[68-70] Farr DNA binding,[73] solid phase immunoassay,[74] the DNA spot test,[75, 76] and most recently the immunofluorescence test using *Crithidia luciliae* kinetoplasts as a pure DNA substrate.[77, 78]

The presence of antibody to DNA is highly specific for LE. A small percentage of rheumatoid patients have anti-DNA antibody but usually only in low titer.[74] With few exceptions, patients with drug-induced LE syndromes typically do not have antibody to DNA.[79]

DNA antibody is associated with disease activity[81] and is present in high titer in patients with serious systemic disease. High DNA antibody titers are correlated with flares in renal disease as well as with episodes of pleurisy, alopecia, and hemolytic crises.[81-84] The finding of DNA antibody, although an important laboratory marker, should not be considered an indication for instituting more vigorous therapy unless it is associated with a decrease in complement or with clinical evidence of activity. There is no support for the view that early treatment based on the presence of abnormal antibodies prevents the occurrence of problems later. In Fries and Holman's series[85] of DNA-positive patients, significant renal disease followed in only one third of the patients. Anti-DNA antibody is not associated with poor renal outcome but can be used to predict treatable flares. In the same study, an additional one third of patients with DNA antibody continued to be clinically stable in spite of multiple positive tests.

ANTIBODIES TO OTHER NUCLEAR ANTIGENS

Specific antibodies to nuclear antigens extracted from cell nuclei with isotonic buffers have been detected by several techniques.[86-88] The soluble nuclear extract contains several antigens. The Sm antigen[87] has not yet been chemically characterized. It is designated Sm for the first two letters of the name of the patient in whom the antibody was first recognized. A second antigen, designated RNP, has been identified as a ribonucleoprotein.[89] RNP is ribonuclease-sensitive, but Sm is ribonuclease-resistant.

The presence of antibody to Sm antigen is highly specific for SLE,[90] and these patients may have serious renal complications.[90] They do not seem to have any unifying clinical syndrome but commonly have antibodies to DNA and low serum complement levels. Severe anemia also may be more common in the patient with RNAase-resistant, Sm antibody.[59]

The presence of antibody to RNP is associated with a more benign course, with a lower incidence of antibody to DNA, and with a predictably lower incidence of renal disease.[81, 88, 91-93] These patients have been described as having a typical clinical presentation called mixed connective tissue disease (MCTD),[59, 88] suggesting an overlap syndrome of LE, scleroderma, and polymyositis. However, only a minority of patients with antibody to RNP present with tight, swollen hands, Raynaud's phenomenon, and clinical myositis (typical of LE-scleroderma-polymyositis overlap) and are a diagnostic problem.[94, 95] There are also patients with an overlap syndrome who do not have RNP antibody. The majority of patients with RNP antibody who have clinical SLE satisfy at least four of the ARA preliminary criteria for SLE and should be recognized as a subset of LE patients with a particular disease pattern. They frequently have Raynaud's phenomenon, swollen hands, esophageal hypomotility, myositis, and pulmonary disease.[93] The reported cutaneous manifestations are variable. It is significant that these patients have a low incidence of serious renal and central nervous system disease.[93] Except for Raynaud's phenomenon, which is almost always present,[93, 96] the clinical presentation of an RNP-positive patient may vary. The term MCTD is misleading from a clinical standpoint, for it is not just the patient with an overlap syndrome who should be investigated for the presence of antibody to RNP. Clinical observations suggest that a sustained mild course of disease is associated with a consistently higher titer of antibody to nuclear RNP. Conversely, a reduction of antinuclear RNP may be associated with the appearance of anti-DNA and subsequent development of renal disease.[97]

Antibody specific for the nucleolus is found in patients with systemic sclerosis or Raynaud's phenomenon but can be detected in patients with other rheumatic disorders. When it is detected in SLE, it usually coexists with other nuclear antibodies and often indicates that the clinical course will be prolonged and mild, without renal manifestations.[98] The major nucleolar antigen is a nucleolar RNA with a sedimentation coefficient of 7S.[98]

Recently, another antibody to a soluble, acidic nuclear antigen (Ha) has been studied. SLE patients with this antibody have been reported to have a high incidence of the sicca syndrome and have rheumatoid factor.[99]

ANTIBODIES TO CYTOPLASMIC ANTIGENS

In addition to nuclear antibodies, some lupus patients form antibodies to several cytoplasmic antigens,[83, 100] such as mitochondria, lysosomes, ribosomes, and other antigens, such as Ro and La, immunologically but not chemically identified.[95] The biological and clinical significance of these subsets is being investigated. Patients with a lupus-like syndrome who have a negative antinuclear antibody test but who have antimitochondrial antibodies have been described. Such patients may develop recurrent febrile episodes, arthritis, myositis, carditis, pleuritis, and pulmonary infiltrates.[63, 101] Antibodies to a soluble cytoplasmic antigen termed Ro have been detected in a significant number of patients who fulfilled the preliminary criteria for SLE. These patients had a high incidence of photosensitive skin rashes. Eleven patients had no demonstrable antinuclear antibody in their sera but had only anti–Ro cytoplasmic antibody.[102] Moreover, in selected patients the Ro-anti–Ro system appeared to be involved in the pathogenesis of lupus nephritis.[102]

CRYOGLOBULINS

For many years, it has been recognized that proteins in the serum of selected lupus patients precipitate spontaneously in the cold. The cryoprecipitates consist largely of immunoglobulins IgG and IgM and contain varying amounts of complement components.[103] Specific antibody activity, such as antinuclear antibody,[104] DNA antibody,[105] and DNA-anti–DNA immune complexes,[105, 106] have been demonstrated in some of the cryoprecipitates.[105, 106] The presence of cryoglobulins in lupus serum is associated with a high incidence of hypocomplementemia, renal disease, and widespread vasculitis.[103, 107] Complement-dependent cytotoxic activity against normal human lymphocytes has also been detected in lupus cryoprecipitates; however, the lymphocytotoxic activity does not correlate with the severity of the disease.[108]

CIRCULATING IMMUNE COMPLEXES

Substantial evidence implicates circulating DNA-anti–DNA complexes as a major factor in tissue injury, especially of the kidneys. Antibody to DNA appears with signs of clinical activity,[84] and DNA-anti–DNA complexes are found in lupus patients with severe renal disease and acute cerebritis.[109, 110] DNA-anti–DNA complexes have been detected in cerebrospinal fluid in central nervous system lupus.[111] DNA is present along the glomerular basement membrane, and antibody to DNA has been eluted from LE kidneys postmortem.[112, 113] Skin eluates have antinuclear activity and dermal-epidermal deposits contain DNA-anti–DNA complexes.[114, 115] Persistence of serum DNA-anti–DNA complexes is associated with increased morbidity and mortality. Their disappearance correlates with clinical remissions.[110] There is evidence that patients with SLE may have an immunospecific clearance defect, resulting in persisting levels of circulating complexes in selected individuals.[116] Moreover, there are qualitative as well as quantitative differences in circulating immune complexes. Complexes may be complement-fixing or non-complement-fixing.[117] In addition, the size of anti–DNA antibodies may vary. Type I antibodies are bivalent binding antibodies of the IgG class, which have a high avidity and form small, very stable complexes with DNA. Type II antibodies are mainly IgM antibodies with low avidity; they are cross-linking and form large complexes. Thus, qualitative and quantitative variations of immune complexes may account for the highly variable clinical presentation and immunopathology of lupus.

COMPLEMENT LEVELS

Depressed levels of serum complement have been recognized and utilized for many years as a reliable marker for severe SLE, especially LE nephritis.[82, 118, 119] Low total hemolytic complement and high titers of antibody to DNA indicate active disease, especially disease involving the kidney.[120] Although therapy is often based on the results of these laboratory findings, it should be recognized that some patients will have hypocomplementemia with no clinical signs of disease activity. Randomly discovered abnormalities in anti-DNA–antibody and complement levels are of no predictive value, and hypocomplementemia has frequently resolved spontaneously with no recognizable exacerbation of the disease.[121] Serial evaluations of clinical features and laboratory studies should be used to assess disease activity before therapy is altered.

The earliest complement measurements were determined by utilizing the CH50 hemolytic assay, which measures total complement activity. Currently, individual complement components can be measured quantitatively. In active LE, levels of early-reacting components (C1, C4, C2) and late-reacting components (C3 to C9) may be reduced.[122] There also may be a reduction of alternate pathway components.[123] Decreased levels of properdin in selected patients with LE nephritis were found to be due to hypercatabolism rather than to decreased synthesis.[123] Investigations of LE patients with low C3 levels have demonstrated variability in C3 synthesis. Synthesis is sometimes decreased, but hypercatabolism accounts for the low serum level in untreated patients with early active disease.[124, 125]

Congenital deficiency of the second and fourth components of complement is rare but has been described in association with SLE.[126-130] An interesting feature in several of the C2-deficient patients has been the presence of a photosensitive, chronic, cutaneous LE eruption (Plate IX–C).

Low levels of C4 have been reported in the cerebrospinal fluid (CSF) of patients with active CNS lupus.[131] However, some investigators believe that levels fluctuate too widely for CSF C4 to serve as a critical measure of disease activity. Serial determinations may be required from a large series of patients to resolve this controversy. Pleural effusions from lupus patients also have reflected low levels of CH50, C4, and C3, as compared with effusions resulting from other disease processes.[132]

In most hospital laboratories, it is possible to obtain serum C3 levels only by radioimmunodiffusion methods. This test provides a simple, reliable, and accurate assessment of clinical activity. The determination of total hemolytic complement is more difficult and often unnecessary, since C3 levels usually correlate with CH50 values. Exceptions can occur, however; for example, C2-deficient patients with a selective congenital deficiency of complement may have normal C3 levels but decreased total hemolytic complement (CH50) and an absence of C2.

FALSE POSITIVE SEROLOGICAL TEST FOR SYPHILIS

For many years, false positive results in non-treponemal (VDRL) tests for syphilis have occurred in patients with lupus. The frequency of this finding led to the inclusion of this test as one of the ARA criteria for the diagnosis of SLE. The treponemal immoblization test (TPI) was used to identify and distinguish the false positive LE reaction. However, because of the technical difficulties inherent in the TPI test, it has been replaced by the fluorescent treponemal antibody absorption test (FTA-ABS), which is highly specific, sensitive, and less costly to perform. However, false positive FTA-ABS reactions with lupus sera have been encountered frequently.[133, 134] Although these false positive reactions are usually weak or borderline and have an atypical beaded pattern, a strong homogeneous pattern indistinguishable from that of syphilis serum can occur.[135] If the TPI test is unavailable, the inexpensive, quantitative, microhemagglutination test for *T. pallidum* (MHA-TP) can be used in some instances to detect false positive borderline results in FTA-ABS tests. This test is frequently negative or reactive only in low titers with doubtful or positive non-syphilitic FTA-ABS sera.[135]

EXTRACUTANEOUS MANIFESTATIONS

The major extracutaneous manifestations of LE will be discussed only briefly, since the focus of this chapter is the dermatological aspects of the disease. The reader is referred to several monographs and reviews for an in-depth discussion of the systemic findings.[22, 136–141]

Arthritis is the most common initial symptom expressed in LE. Typically, patients have a non-deforming polyarthritis with inflammation of synovial tissues and minimal destruction of cartilage and bone. However, deforming arthritis of the hands with ulnar deviation has become more frequently recognized in a subgroup of patients with longstanding SLE polyarthropathy.[142, 143]

Serositis, with inflammation of the pleural, pericardial, and peritoneal membranes, is also a common manifestation of SLE and is a clinical guidepost of active disease. Pleural effusion, interstitial pneumonitis, focal alveolar hemorrhage, and diffuse pulmonary fibrosis are characteristic complications in the lung. Pericarditis, myocarditis, and endocarditis may occur, rarely with cardiac tamponade and constrictive pericarditis. Scarring of the heart valves with thickening of leaflet tissue can lead to valvular regurgitation and insufficiency. Inflammation of parietal and visceral peritoneum may produce acute abdominal pain. Pancreatitis and ileitis severe enough to require surgical intervention have been reported.

Central nervous system involvement is probably related to immune complex-mediated vasculitis, and IgG, IgM, and C3 deposits have been identified in the choroid plexus of patients with CNS SLE.[144] Cranial nerve disorders, organic psychosis, seizures, status epilepticus, hemiparesis, and intracranial hemorrhage are among the highly variable clinical manifestations. Peripheral neuropathy with sensory deficits is not uncommon, and myelopathy with paraplegia may occur. Psychiatric disorders may be the result of vasculitis, but because mental disturbances may be complicated by the common problem of steroid-induced psychosis or mixed organic and steroid-induced psychosis, their etiology has yet to be defined. Unfortunately, there is no single consistent abnormality of the serum or cerebrosopinal fluid that is diagnostic of central nervous system lupus. Serum complement levels and antibodies to DNA are not a measure of CNS activity. Cerebrospinal fluid IgG levels correlate with serum IgG levels.[145] Isolated determinations of cerebrospinal fluid levels of C4 are not helpful in managing acute CNS problems, although serial determinations may reflect changes in activity. Other complement components have not been adequately evaluated. Cerebrospinal fluid anti-DNA binding may be increased in CNS lupus, and further refinement of technique may make this determination more significant.[145] The usefulness of brain scans has been stressed by some clinicians,[146] but others have found only the flow studies diagnostically helpful, especially if a baseline flow study has been done.[145] Most important in evaluating every LE patient with CNS symptoms is obtaining adequate cultures of cerebrospinal fluid. Unrecognized and potentially treatable meningitis still occurs in patients with SLE.

If lupus nephritis develops, it usually occurs during the first year of active multisystem disease and is less common after five years have elapsed. Definite diagnosis is still based on renal biopsy with light and electron microscopic examination of tissue. Patients with lupus nephritis are generally classified into at least three categories: mild or focal proliferative glomerulitis, severe or diffuse proliferative glomerulonephritis, and membranous glomerulonephropathy.

In focal glomerulitis, the disease is limited to a few glomeruli. The basement membrane is only slightly thickened and at the periphery of a few glomerular tufts there is proliferation of endothelial and mesangial cells with focal necrosis. These patients frequently have microscopic hematuria and proteinuria but seldom develop azotemia and renal insufficiency.

In diffuse glomerulonephritis, there is extensive necrosis of almost all of the glomeruli, with marked proliferation of endothelial and mesangial cells obliterating the capillaries. Electron microscopy demonstrates extensive deposits of immunoglobulin and complement that are predominantly subendothelial and in the basement membrane itself. The deposits have been shown to contain DNA–anti-DNA complexes. These patients may have gross hematuria and proteinuria and can develop azotemia, hypertension, edema, and renal failure.

In membranous glomerulonephropathy, there is marked thickening of the glomerular capillary walls, with very little necrosis or leukocytic infiltration. The deposits of immunoglobulin and complement occur along the capillary epithelium. These patients often have gross hematuria and proteinuria and occasionally hypertension, azotemia, and nephrotic syndrome. In addition, there may be two other types of nephritis, an early form confined to mesangial cells and an interstitial form sparing the glomeruli.

There are many patients with "overlap" disease who may demonstrate focal disease on light microscopy and low-grade diffuse glomerulonephritis on electron microscopy. Even in biopsies classified as membranous glomerulonephropathy, there may be proliferative changes. Serial biopsies of patients with persistent active nephritis also have shown transition from one type to another. There has been controversy about the necessity for renal biopsy, and it is agreed that biopsy is not essential for diagnosis and management of lupus nephritis but is extremely useful as a guide for staging the severity of the diagnosis. Renal function can change rapidly and can be judged most accurately by close clinical observation, serial serological profiles of complement and DNA antibody, urinary excretion of protein, and determinations of creatinine clearance.

Anemia occurs in more than 50 per cent of patients and is the most common hematological abnormalty in active lupus erythematosus. There are multiple causes, immune and non-immune. The most common, the "anemia of chronic disease," is not life-threatening and usually improves as the activity of the disease lessens. This anemia is normocytic and normochromic, with adequate bone marrow iron stores in spite of low serum iron values.[22, 147] There may be associated ferrokinetic abnormalities reflected by altered iron-binding capacity, plasma iron, iron utilization, and poor response to iron therapy.[148] Occasionally, true iron deficiency does exist, owing to occult gastrointestinal blood loss and renal disease. There is some evidence that patients who develop anemia are more likely to deteriorate clinically and experience exacerbation of their renal disease.[22] A positive direct Coombs' test, indicating the presence of immunoglobulin and complement on erythrocyte membranes, is common in lupus patients. However, less than 10 per cent of these patients will have clinically significant hemolysis.[149-151] Drug-induced (methyldopa, penicillin) Coombs' test-positive hemolysis can also be a complicating factor.

Thrombocytopenia occurs in approximately 20 per cent of patients and is usually caused by peripheral destruction of platelets by antiplatelet antibodies.[22] Qualitative defects in thrombocyte aggregation also have been described.[152] Circulating anticoagulants[153] rarely lead to spontaneous hemorrhagic crises but may be significant if invasive diagnostic procedures, such as renal biopsy, are performed. The anticoagulant antibody, usually IgG, is most commonly directed against factors XI, IX, and VIII, and against prothrombin and the prothrombin-converting complex.[153]

The action of antibodies on erythrocytes, thrombocytes, and coagulation factors can usually be reversed by administration of corticosteroids. Splenectomy and immunosuppressive agents are selectively utilized in corticosteroid-resistant patients.

Leukopenia of both granulocytic and lymphocytic lines occurs commonly and is probably caused by a variety of mechanisms. Granulocytopenia can result from peripheral destruction by antigranulocyte antibody[154] and from bone marrow suppression.[155] Qualitative abnormalities of granulocyte function have also been noted.[156, 157] Lymphopenia with marked reduction of the absolute number and alteration of the proportion of thymus-derived (T cell), bone marrow-derived (B cell), and null cells is characteristic of active systemic lupus erythematosus. Patients with active SLE experience a generalized loss of regulatory mechanisms of the immune response, while those with less severe disease have only a moderate impairment. In limited forms of the disorder, such as DLE, immune regulation is generally intact.

The immunological imbalance in SLE is characterized by excessive B cell lymphocyte activity and antibody production[158-160] and impairment of cell-mediated immunity. The absolute number of B-lymphocytes in SLE patients is currently a subject of debate because of the difficulty in obtaining accurate measurements. Circulating immune complexes in SLE serum interfere with the EAC rosette technique,[161] and passive adherence of immunoglobulins to the surface of T cells alter determinations made by the surface immunoglobulin technique.[162] Most investigators report that B cell counts are normal or decreased in SLE[161, 163-165] and may be increased in DLE.[164] However, in active SLE the functional capacity of the B cell population is increased, with greater synthesis of antibody directed against various antigens, especially DNA.[159, 160]

The absolute number of T cell lymphocytes is reduced in patients with SLE[161, 163, 165] and normal in patients with DLE.[164] The T cell population in humans is heterogeneous, composed of cells of varying degrees of maturation with different functional characteristics. A subpopulation of T cells, called suppressor T cells, is capable of regulating bone marrow-dependent B cells by suppressing their capacity to form antibody and secrete immunoglobulins.[166] T cells and monocytes of SLE patients appear to be incapable of suppressing antibody secretion of normal and SLE B cells.[167] This phenomenon may result from a selective depletion or inactivation of suppressor T cells or hyperfunctioning B cells,[167, 168] as has been described in the murine model.[169, 170] The extent of T cell reduction has been shown to correlate with disease activity.[161]

T cell depletion may result from several factors. Lymphocytotoxic antibodies[171-173] and deficient thymic maturation factors[174] have been invoked as possible explanations. Generation of an anti-thymocyte antibody might lead to a premature decrease in thymocyte function.[175] A specific lymphocyte antibody directed against T cells also has been identified.[176] In addition, there may be direct T cell destruction or arrested production caused by a drug or virus capable of inducing LE.

Although there is general agreement that the number of circulating T cells is decreased in active LE, there is disagreement over the intactness of T-lymphocyte function as determined by lymphocyte transformation to specific antigens. Some studies have demonstrated impairment of blast transformation in all patients with active SLE,[177, 178] especially those who were acutely ill.[179, 180] There is less marked impairment in mild SLE and no impairment in DLE.[178] However, contradictory results have been reported in other studies,[165, 181-184] which probably reflect differences in selection of the patients and activity of the disease.

LE patients do have depressed reactions to standard intradermal skin test antigens.[165, 178, 179, 183] Phagocytic function of polymorphonuclear leukocytes and macrophages has been found to be reduced.[165] Depressed cutaneous reactivity could result from defective T cell or macrophage function during antigen processing, with impairment of phagocytosis, constant stimulation of immunogenic molecules, overproduction of autoantibodies, and inhibition of T cell interaction. It has not been determined if depression of cell-mediated immunity is an inherent defect that precedes the disease or is a consequence of it.[185]

PATHOGENESIS

Lupus erythematosus may be regarded as a disease that reflects a dynamic equilibrium between an endogenous or invasive agent and a spectrum of host responses. Much evidence suggests that the mechanisms regulating the immune response are abnormal. The defects may be due to genetic predisposition or to vertical transmission of a chronic Type C viral infection that has altered genetic coding and in turn altered tissue or thymic processing of lymphocytes. This may result in T cell destruction, defective cellular immunity, hyperactive humoral response, circulating immune complexes, and inflammation and destruction of tissue.

Family studies support the concept of a genetic predisposition to lupus, demonstrating an increased prevalence of SLE and serological abnormalities in siblings and first degree relatives.[186-188] A high concordance rate of clinical SLE and serological abnormalities has been documented in monozygous twins.[189] The known close genetic linkage between specific immune response genes,[190] the complement system,[191] and the histocompatibility antigen system in mice suggests by analogy a possible association between the HL-A system and autoimmune disorders in humans. Although there may be a significant incidence of the HL-A1, HL-A8 and HL-A 1,8 phenotypes in specific clinical subgroups of LE, this association has not been firmly established.[192, 194] There have been a few LE patients in whom a genetic deficiency of complement components has been associated with a specific HL-A type.[126, 195]

The relative importance of genetic and environmental factors has not yet been defined. It is reasonable to postulate that the genetic mechanisms that operate in the murine model of SLE,[196, 197] the NZB/W mouse,[198, 199] which permit an endogenous Type C RNA virus infection to take hold, may be similar to mechanisms operating in human subjects. Endogenous Type C viruses have been recovered from NZB mice, and large quantities of a viral envelope glycoprotein have been found in immune deposits in the kidneys of these animals.[200] Type C viruses are oncogenic, with an RNA genome and a viral reverse transcriptase enzyme.[201] They are usually vertically transmitted but can be horizontally transmitted. If a host cell is infected by the virus, the enzyme can transcribe the viral RNA code in DNA, which is then integrated into the host cell genome. A subclass of Type C virus, which is not oncogenic, has been recognized in several animal species, including mice. This virus cannot reinfect cells of the same species but can be propagated on other cell lines (xenotropism).[202, 203]

In humans, evidence for a chronic C-type viral infection is still inconclusive.[199, 204-206] The tuboreticular "virus-like" structures identified several years ago in the tissue of LE patients have been shown to be non-viral. These inclusions probably represent a non-specific response to injury.[207] All attempts at virus isolation from lupus tissue specimens have been negative.[208] However, with immunofluorescence techniques, a Type C viral antigen has been identified in a small percentage of lymphocytes from a few LE patients.[199] Core protein-related antigen was found in the glomeruli of an LE patient,[204] and Type C-like viral antigens have been demonstrated in the tissues of lupus patients.[205] Whether proteins in lymphocytic membranes of normal tissue will cross react with antisera to Type C virus is currently under investigation.[209]

It is possible that a vertically transmitted Type C RNA virus passed to a host with the proper immune response genes and with appropriate modifying factors (hormonal, drug, or physical, e.g., sunlight) could precipitate the clinical expression of the disease. Such a virus could infect thymic tissue, causing destruction of T cells, impairment of suppressor T cells, and emergence of uncontrolled B cell responsiveness. Concurrently, viral envelope components could appear on cell membranes and stimulate a humoral response leading to immune complex formation and further tissue destruction. With massive T cell destruction (direct or autoimmune) and defective cellular immunity, viral replication and expression could be perpetuated. Studies in the murine model of SLE support these concepts.[210-216] Suppressor T cell dysfunction occurs in young NZB/W mice,[213, 214] and thymic hormone activity in these animals is defective.[215] Thymosin treatment of NZB/W mice preserves T cell suppressor function and delays formation of DNA and RNA antibodies.[216]

New Zealand mice, like humans with SLE, have the remarkable ability to develop antibodies to double-stranded DNA. Female NZB/W mice develop higher antibody titers than their male counterparts, have more severe renal disease, and have a shorter life span.[217, 218] The factors permitting response to endogenous DNA are now under investigation. Double-stranded DNA is a poor immunogen in the normal host[219] and can be detected in plasma in a variety of circumstances.[220-223] There are several major sources of DNA and extruded nuclear material in the body. In the marrow, there is continuous production of nucleated red blood cells, with subsequent loss of nuclear material. In the skin, there is continuous production of epidermal cells, which lose their nuclear material during the process of keratinization. There is evidence also that DNA can be efficiently bound in vitro to isolated glomerular basement membranes and to connective tissue in the upper dermis.[224] Collagen binding of DNA may result in the accumulation of DNA-containing immune complexes along the basement membrane collagen of the skin and other tissue.

Since SLE has a predilection for erythropoietically stressed women of childbearing age, and since the disease can be precipitated by ultraviolet light, it has been postulated that the problem may be aggravated by defective DNA discard.[225] There is evidence that DNAase inhibitor levels are high in the serum of SLE patients and in NZB/W mice,[226, 227] suggesting that decreased degradation of normally released DNA may occur in SLE. Similarly, DNA released from keratinizing cells or UV-damaged epithelial cells could bind to basement membrane collagen and act as an "immunoabsorbant" for anti–DNA antibodies. Such factors as increased vascular permeability, decreased levels of C1q (which also binds DNA), and decreased blood DNAase activity would favor this theory.[222]

For at least a century, the adverse effects of exposure to ultraviolet light or sunlight on the cutaneous manifestations of LE have been recognized. Cutaneous lesions can be induced by monochromatic light,[228, 229] and subepidermal deposition of immunoglobulins can be detected subsequent to exposure.[229] Ultraviolet light can transform DNA into an antigenic thymine dimer. When UV-altered DNA is injected into mice, antibodies are produced. After the mice are exposed to sunlight, altered DNA can be demonstrated at the dermal-epidermal junction in a pattern similar to that seen in human cutaneous LE.[230] The effect of ultraviolet light on cellular structures is not limited to the production of thymine dimers; many additional chemical complexes have been described. Accordingly, damage to skin by sunlight or other trauma could result in the production of a variety of altered nuclear macromolecules which, when released in the circulation, could induce antibodies of multiple specificities, such as are found in human SLE.[231]

For a chronic immune complex disease to develop, there must be a constant source of antigen as well as an antibody response and defective clearing of complexes. There must be enough antibody to form immune complexes but not too rapid an elimination of antigen. Thus, an ongoing release of DNA nucleoprotein from tissue damage, or a viral envelope coating of specific cell membranes stimulating antibody formation but not necessarily conferring immunity, could produce immune complex disease of SLE. Additionally, those patients who develop severe immune complex disease, such as nephritis, may be unable to remove complexes efficiently.[116]

If the host also has T cell depletion or dysfunction as a result of viremia (as in the NZB/W mouse), a state of T cell paralysis, loss of suppressor T cell activity, B cell escape, and hyperreactive antibody responses to a variety of antigens could occur. A state of perpetual T cell deficiency and chronic viremia might ensue, until enough immune complex tissue damage occurs to destroy the involved organ. This inability to mount a T cell response to specific antigens (antigenic anergy), with lack of inhibition of B cell function and uncontrolled production of antibodies to further suppress cell-mediated immunity, may account for the widespread tissue accumulation of immune complexes.

If T cell function is partially intact, as in patients with DLE, an appropriate cell-mediated inflammatory response could be mounted, resulting in severe local tissue destruction. With an intact suppressor T cell system, there is no B cell escape and no hyperresponsiveness to DNA and other altered nuclear materials. The indeterminate and subacute forms of LE reflected by non-scarring but persistent inflammatory skin lesions, arthritis, serositis, and mesangial lesions, with no detectable circulating immune complexes or antibody to DNA, may result from a moderate impairment of T cell function and cell-mediated immunity.

In summary, the varying expression of loss of T cell function and cell-mediated response in the subgroups of lupus is reflected by the clinical expression of the disease. An analogous immunological state is recognized in leprosy, in which the antigen is known. Since *Mycobacterium leprae* is a facultative cellular parasite, it cannot be eliminated by humoral antibody but is dependent on cell-mediated mechanisms for removal. Patients infected with *M. leprae* have a spectrum of immune responses, and depending on the antigenic load, can move from one end of the spectrum to the other,[232] from the tuberculoid type seen in patients with functional cell-mediated immunity to the lepromatous type seen in patients with defective cell-mediated immunity.

MANAGEMENT

During the last 20 years, it has become apparent that SLE is more prevalent than was previously recognized and is most often a relatively benign disorder. A recent study of a large stable population, using the ARA criteria for diagnosis of SLE, disclosed an incidence of new cases of 7.6 per 100,000. The projected ten-year survival rate for these patients exceeded 90 per cent. The prevalence of clinically important renal disease was only 11 per cent.[233]

Appreciation of the chronic nature of the disease is probably due in large measure to the detection of early and milder disease by wide application of the antinuclear antibody test. Heightened awareness by practitioners in all medical specialties of the extremely variable presentation of SLE has enlarged the clinical spectrum of the disease. Before 1960, SLE gained its reputation as a rare and vicious disease because only patients with severe forms were recognized. However, patients lacking CNS and renal involvement (80 per cent of all SLE cases) have a chronic, smoldering course with periods of long remission. Some patients have only one or two episodes of active disease followed by complete remission. Ironically, one of the major problems encountered by patients today is overzealous therapy with corticosteroids and immunosuppressants, reflecting the mode of the early 1960's, when the disease was regarded as invariably fatal. Sometimes problems such as sepsis, aseptic necrosis of the hip, and hypertension are encountered, making it difficult to determine whether the disease or the therapy is responsible for the complications.

The management of lupus rests solely on recognition of subtypes of the disease. Because of tremendous individual variation, treatment must be tailored to the particular patient and cannot be extrapolated from the therapy of groups of patients described in the literature. Until multicenter, long-term, prospective studies are available, in which homogeneous populations of patients with lupus have been analyzed from a clinical, immunological and therapeutic standpoint, all estimates of prognosis will be fraught with error. Therefore, no patient should be given a pessimistic outlook.

The prognosis for childhood and adolescent SLE continues to improve. During the early 1960's, the expected course of childhood SLE was considered comparable to that of adult SLE, and with multisystem disease, progressive deterioration of the patient was expected.[234, 235] In 1968, a study comparing the course of SLE in 42 children with the course in 200 adults revealed that the clinical manifestations of the disease were similar, differing only in an increased incidence of hepatosplenomegaly and lymphadenopathy and a significantly poorer prognosis in children.[236] Yet, a recent study of 49 children (under age 20) with SLE demonstrated a ten-year overall survival rate of 86 per cent. Even those patients with diffuse proliferative nephritis and severe renal disease (27 patients) had a 73 per cent ten-year survival.[237]

General supportive measures and specific therapeutic measures must be considered in the care of each patient. Continual education of the patient is probably the single most important aspect of the overall program of management. Every LE patient needs to be informed not only that he or she has lupus, but that there are many forms of the disease, some requiring more careful monitoring and more medication than others. In fact, some patients with mild disease may be advised they need no specific treatment at that time. The adolescent is often quite receptive to learning about the problem, especially if the patient and his or her parents have been influenced by the prejudice of relatives and friends or by televised medical productions that focus on the more dramatic aspects of SLE. The physician should outline the total management program for the patient and his parents, explaining the necessity for regular checkups or even the reason for less frequent checkups, depending on the subtype of LE encountered. If the family is oversolicitous, or the patient is unduly anxious about the disorder, sometimes it is helpful to refer him to one of the many clubs that have been organized to promote education and research and to give emotional support to patients with lupus. The physician who invests time in frank and open discussions with the patient is usually rewarded with active cooperation. Team effort in long-term management permits satisfying interaction between the patient and physician in dealing with a difficult disease.

Lupus patients should be encouraged to modify their life style to achieve an ideal balance between work, play, and rest. Since each patient differs, a fixed number of hours of sleep cannot be recommended. A patient should rest when tired and be as physically active as possible. Regular exercise, especially walking and bicycling, should be encouraged because neither requires special strength or skill, and both permit enjoyment of the outdoors. Strenuous competitive sports should be temporarily restricted for those patients with multisystem activity and those on high-dose steroid or immunosuppressive therapy. Patients should not take unnecessary medications or contraceptive pills.

Direct exposure to the sun should be avoided. All clinicians have seen patients whose initial manifestations of the disease were related to sun exposure, and whose eruptions are limited primarily to sun-exposed skin. Sun exposure can also precipitate other clinical manifestations, such as fever and arthralgia. The experimental evidence relating damage caused by ultraviolet light to DNA release has been discussed earlier. Until the pathogenetic mechanisms of UV-induced LE dermatitis and serositis are clarified, it is prudent for all lupus patients, even those who deny photosensitivity, to avoid direct sun exposure. Sunbathing is a current fad based on the highly questionable cosmetic desirability of being tan, a status symbol of leisure and affluence. Ultraviolet rays are destructive to the dermal fibers of light-complexioned individuals, accelerating aging, and playing a role in the development of skin cancer. Patients should be advised not to take outdoor jobs and to swim and play outdoors after work, when the sun's rays are less intense. If they are outdoors during the day, frequent applications of sunscreens containing para-aminobenzoic acid (PABA) are mandatory. These measures should not be psychologically crippling because they apply to anyone interested in preserving the integrity of the skin.

Most lupus patients can look forward to many functional years and should be encouraged to obtain education and skills that will permit them to lead a productive life. As with any chronic illness, job counseling is particularly important. The physician should note the interests and talents of the patient so that he can offer encouragement and practical advice. Obviously, physically stressful or outdoor labor cannot be encouraged. Patients with Raynaud's phenomenon should be warned against manual work that requires hard use of fingers (e.g., typing). There is no patient who is more time-consuming and difficult to manage than the patient who has been permitted by parents or physicians to indulge in boredom and self-pity.

The most common pitfall in the general management of LE is overtreatment of a patient because of abnormalities revealed by laboratory tests. High sedimentation rates, low complement levels, mild anemia, mild leukopenia, and mild proteinuria are not indications for aggressive therapy if they are not accompanied by clinical symptoms. Far too often, high dosages of steroids have been maintained in anticipation of disease activity, when many times such exacerbations fail to appear or are mild. Indications of impending exacerbation are best appreciated by a careful history and physical examination at each visit. The physical findings of fever, rash, alopecia, pleuritic pain, and weakness are the best indicators of disease instability. The extent of instability can be measured and confirmed by a host of laboratory determinations, but the most significant are the hematocrit, WBC, urinalysis, complement levels, and DNA antibody titers. Periodic laboratory studies are easily obtained and are essential to effective management. In these days of escalating health care costs, it is seldom justifiable to routinely order all available laboratory tests that reflect LE activity. The clinician should order tests appropriate to the type of LE and expand the cost of care only in instances of particular organ involvement, such as LE nephritis, when additional data such as creatinine clearance, 24-hour urinary protein excretion, and levels of serum complement components are desirable. If CNS LE is suspected, a baseline brain scan and spinal fluid examination for IgG, anti–DNA binding, and cultures of cerebrospinal fluid may be indicated, as discussed previously.

Assessing fever in the lupus patient is a special problem. Although a flare in lupus activity commonly causes the fever, it is hazardous to increase steroid therapy before examining the patient for streptococcal pharyngitis, urinary tract infection, bacterial pneumonia, tuberculosis, and subacute bacterial endocarditis. Throat, blood, urine, and sputum cultures should be obtained when indicated. Unusual infections with opportunistic fungi and bacteria also must be considered in the critically ill patient. Sepsis is more emergent than SLE, so it is sometimes justified, even in the absence of identifiable organisms, to treat the patient empirically with a broad-spectrum antibiotic and to institute increased immunosuppressive therapy a few days later if there has been no clinical response.

Patients with chronic scarring discoid skin lesions have a benign clinical course and seldom have multisystem involvement. In a recent analysis of 95 DLE patients, 80 were asymptomatic except for skin lesions, and only three in this group had a positive ANA test.[197] Of the 15 who had other manifestations of LE, 14 had a positive ANA, and three had a positive lupus band test. Two of these patients had membranous glomerulonephritis.[21] The rare coexistence of chronic scarring skin lesions and lupus nephritis has not been studied enough to clarify the immunological status of the affected patients.

Although it is difficult to explain to an adolescent why the chronic scarring type of LE is preferable to other forms of the disease, the physician should try to convey its more favorable long-term prognosis. The skin lesions are never life-threatening, although they can be exceedingly destructive, psychologically crippling, and restrictive of many activities. Efforts should be made to arrest the local spread of lesions without disturbing the general immunological response of the patient, who may be localizing the disease to the skin. Daily administration of systemic steroids for non-disseminated chronic DLE is contraindicated, since high doses for long periods are necessary for control. If there is rapid progression of the lesions, a short-term or alternate day course of oral corticosteroids is occasionally indicated. Intense local therapy with high-potency topical corticosteroids, such as 0.5 per cent triamcinolone acetonide cream or .05 per cent fluocinonide cream or ointment, is administered seven or eight times daily. At night, some areas can be occluded with Saran Wrap held in place by non-irritating paper tape to enhance the local absorption of the steroid. The use of triamcinolone acetonide 0.5 per cent in USP flexible collodion is helpful in sites where occlusive dressings are not practical. Intralesional injection of triamcinolone acetonide can be useful in selected patients. Injections generally are given at three- to four-week intervals to permit assessment of benefits before repeating the treatment. Occasionally, dermal atrophy results but is usually reversible with time. However, non-injected lesions also sometimes involute with atrophy and become indistinguishable from steroid-injected sites.

The use of antimalarials to control the cutaneous and articular manifestations of LE has been limited ever since the numerous reports of ocular toxicity that appeared in the 1960's.[238-242] Chloroquine derivatives accumulate slowly in the tissues of the body and in the retina, causing secondary degeneration of rods and cones.[243] If the macular area is damaged, visual acuity is markedly reduced.

The effectiveness of antimalarials has been well documented.[244] However, there is a high incidence of relapse with discontinuation of therapy; thus, the majority of patients have required repeated courses or long-term maintenance.[245] In selected patients, however, especially those with sudden flare of activity in old lesions accompanied by the development of new ones, it is tempting to offer the benefits of these drugs. Ocular toxicity is rarely encountered in a cooperative patient, if new low-dosage regimens are strictly adhered to and frequent ophthalmological evaluations are performed. Every patient must be required to have a baseline ophthalmological evaluation before initiation of therapy and at three-month intervals thereafter. Protective sunglasses should be worn in direct sunlight, since photoenergy from the skin may intensify the toxic effects. Quinacrine (Atabrine) has a low incidence of ocular toxicity, but most patients find the yellow discoloration of the skin it produces cosmetically unacceptable. All these drugs also have to be monitored carefully to prevent other side effects, such as aplastic anemia and exfoliative erythroderma, which were more common years ago when higher dosages were employed.

Subacute, erythematous, scaly LE skin lesions respond more readily to high-potency steroids than do chronic discoid lesions. Again, fluocinonide cream, ointment, or gel may be applied in a thin film at frequent intervals and covered with Saran Wrap at night when practical.

The erythematous, edematous eruption of the cheeks and bridge of the nose in acute SLE usually responds promptly to the daily high dosages of systemic steroids needed to suppress the extracutaneous activity, and topical application of high-potency steroids often is not required. In fact, the use of these preparations is not advised because many patients continue to treat the residual slight erythema and telangiectasia present in the previously acutely involved area. After several months, these patients may develop a persistent steroid-induced, acneiform eruption that can be very resistant to therapy, requiring administration of low-dosage tetracycline and topical acne preparations for resolution. In addition, long-term topical, high-potency steroid preparations can induce further atrophic changes. Only low- or medium-strength steroid creams, such as 1 per cent or 2.5 per cent hydrocortisone or 0.01 per cent fluocinolone acetonide, should be used to suppress the erythema. Unscented, bland, lubricating skin lotions and creams should be prescribed if the patient complains of pruritus.

The use of appropriate cosmetic foundations and creams can effectively conceal residual damage to the face. An explanation and demonstration of the wide variety of lotions, creams, and gels available to achieve a natural look will usually be accepted even by the teenager who initially resists the idea of cosmetics. For those patients with marked alteration in pigmentation, a water-resistant cosmetic preparation (Cover Mark) can be compounded to blend with their normal skin color. Sometimes, it is very rewarding to realize that the few minutes invested in teaching the mechanics of camouflage can spare the patient some of the agonizing depression associated with the cosmetic problems induced by LE.

It is beyond the scope of this chapter to discuss the management of non-cutaneous aspects of LE except to reemphasize the increasingly good prognosis of all forms of SLE. The arthritic manifestations often can be controlled by the administration of analgesics. Aspirin has been incriminated recently as a cause of toxic hepatitis in LE,[246] but this complication is easily reversible. In more severe arthritis or with LE pleuritis and pericarditis, the more judicious use of steroids and the introduction of alternate day steroid therapy have greatly reduced drug-associated morbidity. In lupus nephritis and vasculitis with CNS manifestations, many regimens are now under investigation. The addition of cytotoxic drugs, cyclophosphamide and azathioprine, with concomitant reduction of steroid dosage, has become a widely accepted therapy, although there are still treatment failures and considerable debate about the effectiveness of such combined programs. But just as it has taken many years to perfect the methods for optimally administering steroids, it may be that more successful regimens will be developed for immunosuppressive agents. A combination of chemotherapy and steroid "pulse" therapy, such as is used in the control of malignancy, may eventually be applicable to LE patients.[140, 248] In selected patients, plasmapheresis,[249] dialysis, and renal transplantation have been used successfully, even with severe and rapid renal deterioration.[250]

Lupus erythematosus may reflect non-specific tissue injury with release of endogenous antigens, such as DNA, which cannot be normally processed by the immunologically crippled host. The host with impaired T cell function (viral-, drug-, or genetically-induced) inappropriately responds with hyperproduction of self-destructive autoantibodies, including anti–T-lymphocyte antibodies,[251] allowing perpetuation of the disease. Lupus patients may have a variety of genetic defects, and there may be multiple inducing agents, including latent or persistent viral agents, to account for the myriad clinical manifestations.

Current research efforts to improve therapy are now being directed toward a restoration of competent host response and a reduction of chronic antigen stimulation. Several immunopharmacological regimens are being used to enhance or suppress functional T and B cells and macrophage populations. Efforts to suppress B cell function in NZB/NZW F_1 mice with the use of L-asparaginase, an immunosuppressive enzyme, have been successful in decreasing circulating levels of anti–DNA antibody and delaying the onset of nephritis. The usefulness of this drug, however, is limited by the appearance of inactivating antibodies.[252] A few recent attempts have been made to improve T cell function. Syngeneic lymphocytes from young mice have been transferred to older mice with T cell defects, resulting in prolongation of life.[253] Administration of thymic hormone (thymosin), however, has not altered the natural course of the disease in New Zealand mice.[254] Nevertheless, in vitro studies with thymosin have shown that it can be effective in restoring T cell function.[216] Further, in viral infections with leukopenia and interference with the differentiation of T cells, thymosin can produce T cells from null cells. It might be postulated that in SLE a lymphokine or thymosin could be used to boost the patient's T cell competence. Pharmocological manipulation of B and T cell populations (killer, memory, suppressor, regulator, and helper cells) may play a major role in combating autoimmune, viral, and malignant disorders in the future.

SLE may not have a single cause or a simple antidote. Future progress in overall management certainly will be facilitated by identification of subtypes of LE patients by specific clinical manifestations and serological markers, such as antibody to DNA, RNP, and Sm antigens, and other antigens yet to be defined. If these subtypes are homogeneous, it will permit a more appropriate selection of pharmacological agents, so that the end result of therapy will be more predictable.

REFERENCES

1. Fries, J. F., and Holman, H. R.: Systemic Lupus Erythematosus: A Clinical Analysis. Philadelphia, W. B. Saunders. 1975, pp. 57–58.
2. Jarcho, S.: Notes on the early modern history of lupus erythematosus. Mt. Sinai J. Med. N.Y., 24:939, 1957.
3. Cazenave, A.: Lupus érythémateux (Erythème centrifuge). Ann. Malad. Peau Syph., 3:297, 1850–1851.
4. Hebra, F., and Kaposi, M.: On Diseases of the Skin, Including the Exanthemata. Vol. 4. London, The New Sydenham Society, 1875, p. 500.
5. Hebra, F., and Kaposi, M.: On Diseases of the Skin, including the Exanthemata. Vol. 4. London, The New Sydenham Society, 1875, pp. 14–47.
6. Hebra, F., and Kaposi, M.: On Diseases of the Skin, Including the Exanthemata. Vol. 4. London, The New Sydenham Society, 1875, p. 27.
7. Osler, W.: On the visceral complications of erythema exudativum multiforme. Am. J. Med. Sci., 110:629, 1895.
8. Libman, E., and Sacks, B.: A hitherto undescribed form of valvular and mural endocarditis. Arch. Intern. Med., 33:701, 1924.
9. Baehr, G., Klemperer, P., and Schifrin, A.: A diffuse disease of the peripheral circulation usually associated with lupus erythematosus and endocarditis. Trans. Assoc. Am. Physicians, 50:134, 1935.
10. Friedberg, C. K., Grass, L., and Wallach, K.: Non-bacterial thrombotic endocarditis associated with prolonged fever, arthritis, inflammation of serous membranes and wide-spread vascular lesions. Arch. Intern. Med., 58:662, 1936.
11. Klemperer, P., Pollack, A. D., and Baehr, G.: Pathology of disseminated lupus erythematosus. Arch. Pathol., 32:569, 1941.
12. Hargraves, M. M., Richmond, H., and Morton, R.: Presentation of two bone marrow elements: The "tart" cell and "LE" cell. Mayo Clin. Proc., 23:25, 1948.
13. Cohen, A. S., Reynolds, W. E., Franklin, E. C., et al.: Preliminary criteria for the classification of systemic lupus erythematosus. Bull. Rheum. Dis., 23:643, 1971.
14. Fernandez-Herliky, I.: Systemic lupus erythematosus. A clinical and prognostic analysis of 120 cases. Lahey Clin. Bull., 21:49, 1972.
15. Lee, T. H., and Rothfield, N. F.: An evaluation of the preliminary criteria for the diagnosis of systemic lupus erythematosus. Arthritis Rheum., 15:532, 1972.
16. Cohen, A. S., and Canaso, J. J.: Criteria for classification of systemic lupus erythematosus–status 1972. Arthritis Rheum., 15:540, 1972.
17. Gibson, T. P., and Debona, G. F.: Use of the American Rheumatism Association's preliminary criteria for the classification of systemic lupus erythematosus. Ann. Intern. Med., 77:745, 1972.
18. Dubois, E. L., and Tuffanelli, D. L.: Clinical manifestations of systemic lupus erythematosus. JAMA, 190:104, 1964.
19. Estes, D., and Christian, C. L.: The natural history of systemic lupus erythematosus by prospectus analysis. Medicine, 50:85, 1971.
20. Scott, A., and Rees, E. G.: The relationship of systemic lupus erythematosus and discoid lupus erythematosus. Arch. Dermatol., 79:422, 1959.
21. Prystowsky, S. O., and Gilliam, J. N.: Discoid lupus erythematosus as a part of a larger disease spectrum. Arch. Dermatol., 111:1448, 1975.
22. Fries, J. F., and Holman, H. R.: Systemic Lupus Erythematosus: A Clinical Analysis. Philadelphia, W. B. Saunders, 1975.
23. Mintz, G., and Fraga, A.: Arteritis in systemic lupus erythematosus. Arch. Intern. Med., 116:55, 1965.
24. Dubin, H. V., and Stawiski, M. A.: Systemic lupus erythematosus resembling malignant atrophic papulosis. Arch. Intern. Med., 134:321, 1974.
25. Tuffanelli, D. L.: Lupus erythematosus panniculitis (profundus): Clinical and immunological studies. Arch. Dermatol., 103:231, 1971.
26. Milner, A. N. P.: Systemic lupus erythematosus with nodular lesions. Report of a case. Br. J. Dermatol., 65:204, 1953.
27. Silva, R. E., and Portugal, H.: A case of lupus erythematosus profundus. Ann. Dermatol. Syphiligr., 82:34, 1955.

28. Pascher, F., Sims, C. F., and Pensky, N.: Lupus erythematosus profundus (Kaposi-Irgang): Report of a case including a comparative study of the histology with that of chronic discoid lupus erythematosus. J. Invest. Dermatol., 25:347, 1955.
29. Alarcon-Segovia David Cetana, J. A.: Lupus hair. Am. J. Med. Sci., 267:241, 1974.
30. Burnham, T. K., Neblett, T. F., and Fine, G.: The application of the fluorescent antibody technique to the investigation of lupus erthematosus and various dermatoses. J. Invest. Dermatol., 41:451, 1963.
31. Cormane, R. H.: "Bound" globulin in the skin of patients with chronic discoid lupus erythematosus and systemic lupus erythematosus. Lancet, 1:534, 1964.
32. Tan, E. M., and Kunkel, H. G.: An immunofluorescent study of the skin lesions in systemic lupus erythematosus. Arthritis Rheum., 9:37, 1966.
33. Kay, D. M., and Tuffanelli, D. L.: Immunofluorescent techniques in clinical diagnosis of cutaneous disease. Ann. Intern. Med., 71:753, 1969.
34. Percy, J. S., and Smyth, C. J.: The immunofluorescent skin test in systemic lupus erythematosus. JAMA, 203:485, 1969.
35. Burnham, T. K., and Fine, G.: The immunofluorescent "band" test for lupus erythematosus. III. Employing clinically normal skin. Arch. Dermatol., 103:24, 1971.
36. Burnham, T. K., Fine, G., and Neblett, T. R.: Immunofluorescent "band" test for lupus erythematosus. Arch. Dermatol., 102:42, 1970.
37. Schrager, M. A., and Rothfield, N.: Clinical significance of serum properdin levels and properdin deposition in the dermal epidermal junction in systemic lupus erythematosus. J. Clin. Invest., 57:212, 1976.
38. Provost, T. T., and Tomasi, T. B., Jr.: Evidence for complement activation via the alternate pathway in skin disease. I. J. Clin. Invest., 52:1779, 1973.
39. Cripps, D. J., and Rankin, J.: Action spectra of lupus erythematosus and experimental immunofluorescence. Arch. Dermatol., 107:563, 1973.
40. Schreiner, E., and Wolff, K.: Systemic lupus erythematosus: Electron microscopic localization of in vivo bound globulins at the dermal-epidermal junction. J. Invest. Dermatol., 55:325, 1970.
41. Wolff-Schreiner, E., and Wolff, K.: Immunoglobulins at the dermal-epidermal junction in lupus erythematosus ultrastructural investigation. Arch. Dermatol. Forsch., 246:193, 1973.
42. Provost, T. T., and Reichlin, M.: Lupus band test (LBT): Correlation of Ig class deposition and serum antibodies to ssDNA, and other nuclear and cytoplasmic autoantigens. Clin. Res., 25:485A, 1977.
43. Tuffanelli, D. L.: Cutaneous immunopathology: Recent observations. J. Invest. Dermatol., 65:143, 1975.
44. Grossman, J., Callerame, M. L., and Condemi, J. J.: Skin immunofluorescence studies on lupus erythematosus and other antinuclear antibody positive diseases. Ann. Intern. Med., 80:496, 1974.
45. Gilliam, J. N., Cheatum, D. E., Hurd, E. R., et al.: Immunoglobulin in clinically uninvolved skin in systemic lupus erythematosus. J. Clin. Invest., 53:1434, 1974.
46. Gilliam, J. N., Hurd, E. R., and Ziff, M.: Immunoglobulin in clinically uninvolved skin in lupus erythematosus: Effect of immunosuppressive therapy. J. Rheumatol., 1(1):4, 1974.
47. Coons, A. H., and Kaplan, M. H.: Localization of antigen in tissue cells. II. Improvements in a method for the detection of antigen by means of fluorescent antibody. J. Exp. Med., 91:1, 1950.
48. Friou, G. J.: Clinical application of lupus serum-nucleoprotein reaction using fluorescent antibody technique. J. Clin. Invest., 36:890, 1957.
49. Holborow, E. J., Weir, D. M., and Johnson, G. D.: A serum factor in lupus erythematosus with affinity for tissue nuclei. Br. Med. J., 2:732, 1957.
50. Holman, H. R., and Kunkel, H. G.: Affinity between the lupus erythematosus serum factor and cell nuclei and nucleoprotein. Science, 126:162, 1957.
51. Beck, J. S.: Variations in the morphological patterns of "autoimmune" nuclear fluorescence. Lancet, 1:1203, 1961.
52. Beck, J. S., Anderson, J. R., Mc Elhinney, A. J., et al.: Antinuclear antibodies. Lancet, 2:575, 1962.
53. Gonzalez, E. N., and Rothfield, N. F.: Immunoglobulin class and pattern of nuclear fluorescence in systemic lupus erythematosus. N. Engl. J. Med., 274:1333, 1966.
54. Rothfield, N. F., and Rodman, G. P.: Serum antinuclear antibodies in progressive systemic sclerosis (scleroderma). Arthritis Rheum., 11:607, 1968.
55. Burnham, T. K., Neblett, T. R., and Fine, G.: The immunofluorescent tumor imprint technique. III. Diagnostic and prognostic significance of the "speckle" inducing antinuclear antibody. Am. J. Clin. Pathol., 50:683, 1968.
56. Ritchie, R. F.: Antinuclear antibodies: Their frequency and diagnostic association. N. Engl. J. Med., 282:1174, 1970.
57. Burnham, T. K., and Bank, P. W.: Antinuclear antibodies. I. Patterns of nuclear immunofluorescence. J. Invest. Dermatol., 62:526, 1974.

58. Tan, E. M., and Kunkel, H. G.: Characteristics of a soluble nuclear antigen precipitating with sera of patients with systemic lupus erythematosus. J. Immunol., 96:464, 1966.
59. Sharp, G. C., Irvin, W. S., May, C. M., et al.: Association of antibodies to ribonucleoprotein and Sm antigens with mixed connective tissue disease, systemic lupus erythematosus and other rheumatic disease. N. Engl. J. Med., 295:1149, 1976.
60. Schur, P. H.: Antinuclear antibodies. N. Engl. J. Med., 282:1205, 1970.
61. Burnham, T. K., and Bank, P. W.: Antinuclear antibodies. J. Invest. Dermatol., 62:526, 1974.
62. Mattioli, M., and Reichlin, M.: Heterogeneity of RNA protein antigens reactive with sera of patients with systemic lupus erythematosus. Arthritis Rheum., 17:421, 1974.
63. Guardia, J., Gomez, J., Martin, C., et al.: Pericarditis, pleural effusion and pneumonitis with transient mitochondrial antibodies. Br. Med. J., 1:370, 1975.
64. Cepellini, R., Polli, E., and Celeda, F.: DNA-reacting factor in serum of a patient with lupus erythematosus diffusus. Proc. Soc. Exp. Biol. Med., 96:572, 1957.
65. Deicher, H. R., Holman, H. R., and Kunkel, H. G.: The precipitin reaction between DNA and a serum factor in systemic lupus erythematosus. J. Exp. Med., 109:97, 1959.
66. Krishnan, C., and Kaplan, M. H.: Immunopathologic studies of LE. II. Antinuclear reaction of globulin eluted from homogenates and isolated glomeruli of kidneys from patients with lupus nephritis. J. Clin. Invest., 46:569, 1967.
67. Seligman, M., Arana, R., and Cannat, A.: The heterogeneity of DNA antibodies in SLE and their clinical significance. In Duthie, J. J. R., and Alexander, W. R. M. (eds.): Rheumatic Diseases. Baltimore, Williams & Wilkins, 1968, pp. 211–224.
68. Jokinen, E. J., and Julkunen, H.: DNA hemagglutination test in the diagnosis of systemic lupus erythematosus. Ann. Rheum. Dis., 24:477, 1965.
69. Levi, M. I., and Poverenny, A. M.: Use of the passive hemagglutination reaction for determining antibodies against deoxyribonucleic acid (DNA). J. Hyg. Epidemiol. Microbiol. Immunol., 9:456, 1965.
70. Koffler, D., Carr, R., Agnello, V., et al.: Antibodies to polynucleotides in human sera: Antigenic specificity and reaction to disease. J. Exp. Med., 134:294, 1971.
71. Sturgill, B. C., Carpenter, R. R., Strauss, A. J. L., et al.: Antibodies in systemic lupus erythematosus and myasthenia gravis which react with thermally denatured DNA-coated bentonite. Proc. Soc. Exp. Biol. Med., 115:246, 1964.
72. Pincus, T., Schur, P. H., Rose, J. A., et al.: Measurement of serum DNA-binding activity in SLE. N. Engl. J. Med., 281:701, 1969.
73. Hughes, G. R. V.: Significance of anti-DNA antibodies in SLE. Lancet, 2:861, 1971.
74. Tan, M., and Epstein, W. V.: A solid-phase immunoassay for antibody to DNA and RNA. J. Lab. Clin. Med., 81:122, 1973.
75. Friou, G. J.: Fluorescent spot test for antinuclear antibodies. Arthritis Rheum., 5:407, 1962.
76. Tan, E. M., and Natali, P. G.: Comparative study of antibodies to native and denatured DNA. J. Immunol., 104:902, 1970.
77. Aarden, L. A., de Groot, E. R., and Feltkamp, T. E. W.: Immunology of DNA. III. *Crithidia luciliae*, a simple substrate for the determination of anti-dsDNA with the immunofluorescence technique. Ann. N.Y. Acad. Sci., 254:505, 1975.
78. Stinal, G., Meingassner, J. G., Swelty, P., et al.: An immunofluorescence procedure for the demonstration of antibodies to native, double-stranded DNA and of circulating DNA-anti-DNA complexes. Clin. Immunol. Immunopathol., 6:131, 1976.
79. Hahn, B. H., Sharp, G. C., Irvin, W. S., et al.: Immune responses to hydralazine and nuclear antigens in hydralazine-induced lupus erythematosus. Ann. Intern. Med., 76:365, 1972.
80. Alarcón-Segovia, D., Fishbein, E., Reyes, P. A., et al.: Antinuclear antibodies in patients on anticonvulsant therapy. Clin. Exp. Immunol., 12:39, 1972.
81. Sharp, G. C., Irvin, W. S., La Roque, R. L., et al.: Association of autoantibodies to different nuclear antigens with clinical patterns of rheumatic disease and responsiveness therapy. J. Clin. Invest., 50:350, 1971.
82. Epstein, W.: Immunologic events preceding clinical exacerbation of systemic lupus erythematosus. Am. J. Med., 54:631, 1973.
83. Quismorio, F. P., and Friou, G. J.: Serologic factors in systemic lupus erythematosus and their pathogenetic significance. CRC Crit. Rev. Clin. Lab. Sci., 639, December 1970.
84. Tan, E. M., Schur, P. H., Carr, R. T., et al.: Deoxyribonucleic acid (DNA) and antibodies to DNA in the serum of patients with systemic lupus erythematosus. J. Clin. Invest., 45:1732, 1966.
85. Fries, J. F., and Holman, H. R.: Systemic Lupus Erythematosus: A Clinical Analysis. Philadelphia, W. B. Saunders, 1975, pp. 112–114.
86. Holman, H. R.: Partial purification and characterization of an extractable nuclear antigen which reacts with SLE sera. Ann. N.Y. Acad. Sci., 124:800, 1965.
87. Tan, E. M., and Kunkel, H. G.: Characteristics of a soluble nuclear antigen precipitating with sera of patients with systemic lupus erythematosus. J. Immunol., 96:464, 1966.
88. Sharp, G. S., Irvin, W. S., Tan, E. M., et al.: Mixed connective tissue disease—An apparently

distinct rheumatic disease syndrome associated with a specific antibody to an extractable nuclear antigen (ENA). Am. J. Med., 52:148, 1972.
89. Mattioli, M., and Reichlin, M.: Characterization of a soluble nuclear ribonucleoprotein antigen reactive with SLE sera. J. Immunol., 107:1287, 1971.
90. Notmann, D. D., Kurata, N., and Tan, E. M.: Profiles of antinuclear antibodies in systemic rheumatic disease. Ann. Intern. Med., 83:464, 1975.
91. Reichlin, M., and Mattioli, M.: Correlation of precipitin reaction and RNA protein antigen and the prevalence of nephritis in patients with systemic lupus erythematosus. N. Engl. J. Med., 286:908, 1972.
92. Prystowsky, S. D., and Tuffanelli, D. L.: Correlation of clinical features and laboratory findings in 30 patients with high titer antibody to ribonucleoprotein (RNP). Clin. Res., 25:286, 1977.
93. Wolfe, J. F., Kingsland, L., Lindberg, D., et al.: Disease pattern in patients with antibodies only to nuclear ribonucleoprotein (RNP). Clin. Res., 25:488A, 1977.
94. Reichlin, M.: Problems in differentiating SLE and mixed connective tissue disease. N. Engl. J. Med., 295:1194, 1976.
95. Reichlin, M., and Mattioli, M.: Antigens and antibodies characteristic of SLE. Bull. Rheum. Dis., 24:756, 1974.
96. Gilliam, J. N., and Prystowsky, S. D.: Mixed connective tissue disease syndrome. Arch. Dermatol., 113:583, 1977.
97. Maddison, P. J., and Reichlin, M.: Quantitation of precipitating antibodies to certain soluble nuclear antigens in SLE. Arthritis Rheum., 20:819, 1977.
98. Miyawaki, S., and Ritchie, R. F.: Nucleolar antigen specific for antinuclear antibody in the sera of patients with systemic rheumatic disease. Arthritis Rheum., 16:726, 1973.
99. Akizuki, M., Moutsopoulos, H. M., Chused, T. M., et al.: Clinical significance of antibodies to a soluble acidic nuclear antigen in systemic lupus erythematosus. Clin. Res., 25:353A, 1977.
100. Schur, P. H., Moroz, L. A., and Kunkel, H. G.: Precipitating antibodies to ribosomes in the serum of patients with systemic lupus erythematosus. Immunochemistry, 4:447, 1967.
101. Maas, D., and Schubothe, H.: Lupus erythematosus-like syndrome with anti-mitochondrial antibodies. Dtsch. Med. Wochenschr., 98:131, 1973.
102. Maddison, P. J., Reichlin, M., and Provost, T. T.: The significance of antibodies to certain cytoplasmic antigens in systemic lupus erythematosus. Clin. Res., 25:485A, 1977.
103. Hanauer, L. B., and Christian, C. L.: Studies of cryoproteins in systemic lupus erythematosus. J. Clin. Invest., 46:400, 1967.
104. Barnett, E. V., Bluestone, R., Cracchiolo, A., et al.: Cryoglobulinemia and disease. Ann. Intern. Med., 73:95, 1970.
105. Winfield, J. B., Koffler, D., and Kunkel, H. G.: Specific concentration of polynucleotide immune complexes in the cryoprecipitates of patients with systemic lupus erythematosus. J. Clin. Invest., 56:563, 1975.
106. Roberts, J. L., and Lewis, E. J.: DNA:Anti-DNA immune complexes in cryoglobulinemic states. Clin. Res., 25:365A, 1977.
107. Gough, W., Lightfoot, R., and Christian, C. L.: Cryoglobulins and complement in immune complex disease. Arthritis Rheum., 17:497, 1974.
108. Zwaifler, N. J., and Bluestein, H. G.: Lymphocytotoxic antibody activity in cryoprecipitates from serum of patients with SLE. Arthritis Rheum., 19:844, 1976.
109. Harbeck, R. J., Bardana, E. J., Kohler, P. F., et al.: DNA:anti-DNA complexes: Their detection in SLE sera. J. Clin. Invest., 52:789, 1973.
110. Bardana, E. J., Harbeck, R. J., Hoffman, A. A., et al.: The prognostic and therapeutic implications of DNA-anti-DNA complexes in systemic lupus erythematosus (SLE). Am. J. Med., 59:515, 1975.
111. Harbeck, R. J., Hoffman, A. A., Carr, R. I., et al.: DNA antibodies and DNA:anti-DNA complexes in cerebrospinal fluid (CSF) of patients with SLE. Arthritis Rheum., 16:552, 1973.
112. Koffler, D., Schur, P. H., and Kunkel, H. G.: Immunological studies concerning the nephritis of systemic lupus erythematosus. J. Exp. Med., 126:607, 1967.
113. Koffler, D., Agnello, V., Thoburn, R., et al.: SLE: Prototype of immune complex nephritis in man. J. Exp. Med., 134:1685, 1971.
114. Landry, M., and Sams, W. M.: Basement membrane antibodies in two patients with systemic lupus erythematosus. Lancet, 1:821, 1972.
115. Landry, M., and Sams, W. M.: Systemic lupus erythematosus. Studies of the antibodies bound to skin. J. Clin. Invest., 52:1871, 1973.
116. Frank, M. M., Jaffe, C. J., Kimberly, R. P., et al.: An immunospecific clearance defect in patients with systemic lupus erythematosus (SLE) related to the levels of circulating immune complexes (IC). Clin. Res., 25:357A, 1977.
117. Kammer, G. M., Glass, D. N., Soter, N. A., et al.: Circulating immune complexes in rheumatic diseases and vasculitis. Clin. Res., 25:361A, 1977.

118. Elliott, J. A., Jr., and Mathieson, D. R.: Complement in disseminated (systemic) lupus erythematosus. Arch. Dermatol., 68:119, 1953.
119. Williams, R. C., Jr., and Law, D. H.: Serum complement in connective tissue diseases. J. Lab. Clin. Med., 52:273, 1958.
120. Shur, P. H., and Sandson, J.: Immunologic factors and clinical activity in systemic lupus erythematosus. N. Engl. J. Med., 278:533, 1968.
121. Lightfoot, R. W., and Hughes, G. R. V.: Significance of persisting serologic abnormalities in SLE. Arthritis Rheum., 19:837, 1976.
122. Gewurz, H., Pickering, R. J., Mergenhagen, S. E., et al.: The complement profile in acute glomerulonephritis, systemic lupus erythematosus and hypocomplementemic chronic glomerulonephritis. Contrasts and experimental correlations. Int. Arch. Allergy Appl. Immunol., 34:556, 1968.
123. Ziegler, J. B., Rosen, F. S., Alper, C. A., et al.: Metabolism of properdin in normal subjects and patients with renal disease. J. Clin. Invest., 56:761, 1975.
124. Sliwinski, A. J., and Zvaifler, N. J.: Decreased synthesis of the third component of complement (C3) in hypocomplementemic SLE. Clin. Exp. Immunol., 11:21, 1972.
125. Fries, J. F., and Holman, H. R.: Systemic Lupus Erythematosus: A Clinical Analysis. Philadelphia, W. B. Saunders Co., 1975, pp. 123–124.
126. Ochs, H. D., Rosenfeld, S. I., Thomas, E. D., et al.: Linkage between the gene (or genes) controlling synthesis of the fourth component of complement and the major histocompatibility complex. N. Engl. J. Med., 296:470, 1977.
127. Agnello, V., de Bracco, M. M. E., and Kunkel, H. G.: Hereditary C2 deficiency with some manifestations of systemic lupus erythematosus. J. Immunol., 108:837, 1972.
128. Wild, H. F., Zvaifler, N. J., Muller-Eberhard, H. J., et al.: C3 metabolism in a patient with deficiency of the second component of complement (C2) and discoid lupus erythematosus. Clin. Exp. Immunol., 24:238, 1976.
129. Day, N. K., Geiger, H., McLean, R., et al.: C2 deficiency: Development of lupus erythematosus. J. Clin. Invest., 52:1601, 1973.
130. Stern, R., Shu, M. F., Fontino, M., et al.: Hereditary C2 deficiency: Association with skin lesions resembling the discoid lesion of systemic lupus erythematosus. Arthritis Rheum., 19:517, 1976.
131. Petz, L. D., Sharp, G. C., Cooper, N. R., et al.: Serum and cerebral spinal fluid complement and serum autoantibodies in systemic lupus erythematosus. Medicine, 50:259, 1971.
132. Hunder, G. G., McDuffie, F. C., and Hepper, N. G. G.: Pleural fluid complement in systemic lupus and rheumatoid arthritis. Ann. Intern. Med., 76:357, 1972.
133. Neblet, T. R., Merriam, L. R., Burnham, T. K., et al.: A source of false-positive fluorescent treponemal antibody (FTA) reactions. J. Invest. Dermatol., 43:439, 1964.
134. Kraus, S. J., Haserick, J. R., and Lantz, M. A.: Fluorescent treponemal antibody-absorption test reactions in erythematosus: Atypical beading pattern and probable false positive reactions. N. Engl. J. Med., 282:1287, 1970.
135. Shore, R. N., and Faricelli, J. A.: Borderline and reactive FTA-ABS results in lupus erythematosus. Arch. Dermatol., 113:31, 1977.
136. Dubois, E. L. (ed.): Lupus Erythematosus. 2nd ed. Los Angeles, University of Southern California Press, 1974.
137. Ropes, M. W.: Systemic Lupus Erythematosus. Cambridge, Harvard University Press, 1976.
138. Baldwin, D. S., Gluck, M. C., Lavenstein, A., et al.: Lupus nephritis. Am. J. Med., 62:12, 1977.
139. Feinglass, E. J., Arnett, F. C., Dorsch, C. A., et al.: Neuropsychiatric manifestations of systemic lupus erythematosus: Diagnosis, clinical spectrum and relationship to other features of the disease. Medicine, 55:223, 1976.
140. Cathcart, E. S.: Current concepts in management of lupus nephritis. Hosp. Practice, 12:59, 1977.
141. Budman, D. R., and Steinberg, A. D.: Hematologic aspects of systemic lupus erythematosus. Ann. Intern. Med., 86:220, 1977.
142. Kramer, L. S., Ruderman, J. E., Dubois, E. L., et al.: Deforming non-erosive arthritis of the hands in systemic lupus erythematosus (SLE). Arthritis Rheum., 13:329, 1970.
143. Aptekar, R. G. Lawless, O. J., and Decker, J. L.: Deforming non-erosive arthritis of the hand in systemic lupus erythematosus. Clin. Orthop., 100:120, 1974.
144. Atkins, C. J., Kondon, J. J., Quismorio, F. P., et al.: The choroid plexus in systemic lupus erythematosus. Ann. Intern. Med., 76:65, 1972.
145. Small, P., Mass, M. F., Kohler, P. F., et al.: Central nervous system involvement in SLE. Arthritis Rheum., 20:869, 1977.
146. Bennahum, D. A., Messner, R. P., and Shoop, J. D.: Brain scan findings in central nervous system involvement by lupus erythematosus. Ann. Intern. Med., 81:763, 1974.
147. Harvey, A. M., Shulman, L. E., Tumulty, P. A., et al.: Systemic lupus erythematosus. Review of the literature and clinical analysis of 138 cases. Medicine, 33:291, 1954.
148. Whittingham, S., Balazs, N. D. H., and Mackay, I. R.: The effect of corticosteroid drugs on

serum iron levels in systemic lupus erythematosus and rheumatoid arthritis. Med. J. Aust., 54(2):639, 1967.
149. Weens, J. H., and Schwartz, R. S.: Etiologic factors in hemolytic anemia. Semin. Hematol., 7:303, 1974.
150. Wasserman, L. R., Stats, D., Schwartz, L., et al.: Symptomatic and hemopathic hemolytic anemia. Am. J. Med., 18:961, 1955.
151. Rosse, W. F.: The antiglobulin test in autoimmune hemolytic anemia. Annu. Rev. Med., 26:331, 1975.
152. Regan, M. G., Lackner, H., and Karpatkin, S.: Platelet function and coagulation profile in lupus erythematosus. Ann. Intern. Med., 81:462, 1974.
153. Lee, S. L., and Miotti, A. B.: Disorders of hemostatic function in patients with systemic lupus erythematosus. Semin. Arthritis Rheum., 4:241, 1975.
154. Boxer, L. A., Greenberg, M. S., Boxer, G. J., et al.: Autoimmune neutropenia. N. Engl. J. Med., 293:748, 1975.
155. Duckham, D. J., Rhyme, R. L., Jr., Smith, F. E., et al.: Retardation of colony growth of in vitro bone marrow culture using sera from patients with Felty's syndrome, disseminated lupus erythematosus (SLE), rheumatoid arthritis, and other disease states. Arthritis Rheum., 18:323, 1975.
156. Clark, R. A., Kimball, H. R., and Decker, J. L.: Neutrophil chemotaxis in systemic lupus erythematosus. Ann. Rheum. Dis., 33:167, 1974.
157. Orozco, J. H., Jasen, H. L., and Ziff, M.: Defective phagocytosis in patients with systemic lupus erythematosus (SLE). Arthritis Rheum., 13:342, 1970.
158. Budman, D. R., Merchant, E. B., Doft, B., et al.: Antibody forming cells in the peripheral blood of patients with active SLE. Arthritis Rheum., 20:110, 1977.
159. Jasin, H. E., and Ziff, M.: Immunoglobulin synthesis by peripheral blood cells in systemic lupus erythematosus. Arthritis Rheum., 18:219, 1975.
160. Budman, D. R., Merchant, E. B., Steinberg, A. D., et al.: Increased spontaneous activity of Ab forming cells in the peripheral blood of patients with active SLE. Arthritis Rheum., 20:829, 1977.
161. Messner, R. P., Lindström, F. D., and Williams, R. C., Jr.: Peripheral blood lymphocyte cell surface markers during the course of systemic lupus erythematosus. J. Clin. Invest., 52:3046, 1973.
162. Lobo, P. I., Westervelt, F. B., and Horwitz, D. A.: Identification of two populations of immunoglobulin-bearing lymphocytes in man. J. Immunol., 114:116, 1975.
163. Scheinberg, M. A., and Cathcart, E. S.: B and T cell lymphopenia in SLE. Arthritis Rheum., 16:566, 1973.
164. Gilliam, J. N., and Hurd, E. R.: Comparison of circulating T and B lymphocytes in discoid versus systemic lupus erythematosus. Clin. Immunol. Immunopathol., 6:149, 1976.
165. Landry, M.: Phagocytic function and cell-mediated immunity in systemic lupus erythematosus. Arch. Dermatol., 113:147, 1977.
166. Miller, J. F. A. P.: T cell regulation of immune responsiveness. Ann. N.Y. Acad. Sci., 249:9, 1975.
167. Abdou, N. I., Sagawa, A., Pascual, E., et al.: Suppressor T cell abnormality in idiopathic systemic lupus erythematosus. Clin. Immunol. Immunopathol., 6:192, 1976.
168. Bresnihan, B., Jason, H. E., and Ziff, M.: Impaired suppressor function of peripheral blood mononuclear cells in systemic lupus erythematosus. Arthritis Rheum., 19:791, 1976.
169. Krakauer, R. S., Waldmann, T. A., and Strober, W.: Loss of suppressor T cell in adult NZB/NZW mice. J. Exp. Med., 144:662, 1976.
170. Barthold, D. R., Kysela, S., and Steinberg, A. D.: Decline in suppressor T cell function with age in female NZB mice. J. Immunol., 112:9, 1974.
171. Glinski, W., Gershwin, M. E., and Steinberg, A. D.: Study of peripheral blood lymphocytes (PBL) in systemic lupus erythematosus (SLE). Clin. Res., 23:291A, 1975.
172. Terasaki, P. I., Mottironi, V. D., and Barnett, E. V.: Cytotoxins in disease: Autotoxins in lupus. N. Engl. J. Med., 283:724, 1970.
173. Mittal, K. K., Rossen, R. D., Sharp, J. T., et al.: Lymphocyte cytotoxic antibodies in systemic lupus erythematosus. Nature, 225:1255, 1970.
174. Scheinberg, M. A., Cathcart, E. S., and Goldstein, A. L.: Thymosin-induced reduction of "null cells" in peripheral blood lymphocytes of patients wth systemic lupus erythematosus. Lancet, 1:424, 1975.
175. Herbert, J., Sadeghie, S., Schumacher, H. R., et al.: Null cells in peripheral blood of normals and systemic lupus erythematosus. Clin. Immunol. Immunopathol., 6:347, 1976.
176. Lies, R. B., Messner, R. P., and Williams, R. C., Jr.: Relative T cell specificity of lymphocytotoxins from patients with systemic lupus erythematosus. Arthritis Rheum., 16:369, 1973.
177. Bitter, T., Bitter, F., Silberschmidt, R., et al.: In vivo and in vitro study of cell-mediated immunity (CMI) during the onset of systemic lupus erythematosus (SLE). Arthritis Rheum., 14:152, 1971.

178. Paty, J. G., Sienknecht, C. W., Torones, A. S., et al.: Impaired cell-mediated immunity in systemic lupus erythematosus (SLE). A controlled study of 23 untreated patients. Am. J. Med., 59:769, 1975.
179. Rosenthal, C. J., and Franklin, E. C.: Depression of cellular-mediated immunity in systemic lupus erythematosus, reaction to disease activity. Arthritis Rheum., 18:207, 1975.
180. Utsinger, P.: Lymphocyte responsiveness in systemic lupus erythematosus. Arthritis Rheum., 19:88, 1976.
181. Horwitz, D. A.: Impaired delayed hypersensitivity in systemic lupus erythematosus. Arthritis Rheum., 15:353, 1972.
182. Block, S. R., Gibbs, C. B., Stevens, M. D., et al.: Delayed hypersensitivity in systemic lupus erythematosus. Ann. Rheum. Dis., 27:311, 1968.
183. Hahn, B. H., Bagby, M. K., and Osterland, C. K.: Abnormalities of delayed hypersensitivity in systemic lupus erythematosus. Am. J. Med., 55:25, 1973.
184. Lockshin, M. D., Eisenhauer, A. C., Kohn, R., et al.: Cell-mediated immunity in rheumatoid diseases: II. Mitogen responses in RA, SLE, and other illnesses: Correlation with T- and B-lymphocyte populations. Arthritis Rheum., 18:248, 1975.
185. Horwitz, D. A., and Cousar, J. B.: A relationship between impaired cellular immunity, humoral suppression of lymphocyte function and severity of systemic lupus erythematosus. Am. J. Med., 58:829, 1975.
186. Masi, A. T.: Family, twin, and genetic studies: A general review illustrated by systemic lupus erythematosus. Population studies of the rheumatic diseases. *In* Bennet, P. H., and Wood, P. H. N. (eds.): Proceedings of the Third International Symposium, New York, 1966. International Congress Series, No. 148. Amsterdam, Excerpta Medica, 1968, pp. 267–284.
187. Leonhardt, E. T. G.: Family studies in systemic lupus erythematosus. Clin. Exp. Immunol., 2:743, 1967.
188. Pollack, V. E.: Antinuclear antibodies in families of patients with systemic lupus erythematosus. N. Engl. J. Med., 271:165, 1964.
189. Block, S. R., Winfield, J. B., Lockshin, M. D., et al.: Studies of twins with systemic lupus erythematosus. Am. J. Med., 59:533, 1975.
190. McDevitt, H. O., and Benacerraf, B.: Genetic control of specific immune responses. Adv. Immunol., 11:31, 1969.
191. Ferreira, A., and Nussenzweig, V.: Genetic linkage between serum levels of the third component of complement and the H-2 complex. J. Exp. Med., 141:513, 1975.
192. Stastny, P.: The distribution of HL-A antigens in black patients with systemic lupus erythematosus (SLE). Arthritis Rheum., 15:455, 1972.
193. Nies, K. M., Brown, J. C., Dubois, E. L., et al.: Histocompatibility (HL-A) antigens and lymphocytotoxic antibodies in systemic lupus erythematosus (SLE). Arthritis Rheum., 17:397, 1974.
194. Goldberg, M. A., Arnett, F. C., Bias, W. B., et al.: Histocompatibility antigens in systemic lupus erythematosus. Arthritis Rheum., 19:129, 1976.
195. Osterland, C. K., Espinosa, L., Parker, L. P., et al.: Inherited C2 deficiency and systemic lupus erythematosus. Studies in a family. Ann. Intern. Med., 82:323, 1975.
196. Howie, J. B., and Helyer, B. J.: The immunology and pathology of NZB mice. Adv. Immunol., 9:215, 1968.
197. Lambert, P. H., and Dixon, F. J.: Genesis of antinuclear antibody in NZB/W mice: Role of genetic factors and of viral infections. Clin. Exp. Immunol., 6:829, 1970.
198. Mellors, R. C., and Huang, C. Y.: Immunopathology of NZB/BL mice. VI. Virus separable from spleen and pathogenic for Swiss mice. J. Exp. Med., 126:53, 1967.
199. Lewis, R. M., Tannenberg, W., Smith, C., et al.: C-type viruses in systemic lupus erythematosus. Nature, 252:78, 1974.
200. Yashike, T., Mellors, R. C., Strand, M., et al.: The viral envelope glycoprotein of murine leukemia virus and the pathogenesis of immune complex glomerulonephritis of New Zealand mice. J. Exp. Med., 140:1011, 1974.
201. Maugh, T. H., II.: RNA viruses: The age of innocence ends. Science, 183:1181, 1974.
202. Levy, J. A.: Xenotropic viruses: Murine leukemia viruses associated with NIH Swiss, NZB, and other mouse strains. Science, 182:1151, 1973.
203. Lerner, R. A., Wilson, C. B., Del Villano, B. C., et al.: Endogenous oncornaviral gene expression in adult and fetal mice: Quantitative, histologic, and physiologic studies of the major viral glycoprotein gp 70. J. Exp. Med., 143:151, 1976.
204. Mellors, R. C., and Mellors, J. W.: Antigen related to mammalian type C RNA viral p30 protein located in renal glomeruli in human systemic lupus erythematosus. Proc. Natl. Acad. Sci. U.S.A., 73:233, 1976.
205. Panen, S., Ondoñez, N. G., Kirstein, W. H., et al.: C-type virus expression in systemic lupus erythematosus. N. Engl. J. Med., 295:470, 1976.
206. Barry, D. W., Schaff, Z., Grimley, P. M., et al.: Morphologic, biologic and cytochemical analysis of intracytoplasmic particles found in cultured fibroblasts from patients with systemic lupus erythematosus. J. Invest. Dermatol., 63:407, 1974.

207. Schaff, Z., Barry, D. W., and Grimley, P. M.: Cytochemistry of tubuloreticular structures in lymphocytes from patients with systemic lupus erythematosus and in cultured human lymphoid cells—Comparison to a myxovirus. Lab. Invest., 29:577, 1973.
208. Phillips, P. E.: The virus hypothesis in systemic lupus erythematosus. Ann. Intern. Med., 83:709, 1975.
209. Markenson, J. A., Phillips, P. E., Brinkman, J. P., et al.: Proteins on T cell membranes from normals and patients with systemic lupus erythematosus (SLE) reactive with antisera to type C viruses. Clin. Res., 25:485A, 1977.
210. de Vries, M. H., and Higmans, W.: Pathological changes of thymic epithelial cells and autoimmune disease in NAB, NZW and (NZB × NZW) F_1 mice. Immunology, 12:179, 1967.
211. Teague, P. O., Friou, G. J., and Myers, L. L.: Antinuclear antibodies in mice. I. Influence of age and possible genetic factors in spontaneous and induced responses. J. Immunol., 101:791, 1968.
212. Brezin, C., Cannot, A., and Sekiguchi, M. M.: The presence of serum antinuclear antibodies in mice thymectomized at birth. Rev. Eur. Clin. Biol., 10:839, 1965.
213. Hardin, J. A., Chused, T. M., and Steinberg, A. D.: Suppressor cells in the graft-vs-host reaction. J. Immunol., 111:650, 1973.
214. Allison, A. C., Denman, A. M., and Barnes, R. D.: Cooperating and controlling functions of thymus-derived lymphocytes in relation to autoimmunity. Lancet, 2:135, 1971.
215. Bach, J. F., Dardenne, M., and Salomon, J. C.: Studies of thymus products. IV. Absence of serum 'thymic activity' in adult NZB and (NZB × NZW) F_1 mice. Clin. Exp. Immunol., 14:247, 1973.
216. Talal, N., Dauphinee, M., Pillarisetty, R., et al.: Effect of thymosin on thymocyte proliferation and autoimmunity in NZB mice. Ann. N.Y. Acad. Sci., 249:438, 1975.
217. Denman, A. M., Denman, E. J., and Holborow, E. J.: Effects of anti-lymphocyte globulin on kidney disease in NZB × NZW F_1 mice. Lancet, 2:841, 1966.
218. Howie, J. B., and Helyer, B. J.: The immunology and pathology of NZB mice. Adv. Immunol., 9:215, 1968.
219. Plescia, O. J., Bruan, W., and Palczuk, N. C.: Production of antibodies to denatured deoxyribonucleic acid (DNA). Proc. Natl. Acad. Sci. U.S.A., 52:279, 1964.
220. Hughes, G. R. V., Cohen, S. A., Lightfoot, R. W., et al.: The release of DNA into serum and synovial fluid. Arthritis Rheum., 14:259, 1971.
221. Steinman, C. R.: Circulating DNA in SLE patients with active vasculitis and/or CNS disease. Arthritis Rheum., 20:136, 1977.
222. Izui, S., Lambert, P. H., and Miescher, P. A.: In vitro demonstration of a particular affinity of glomerular basement membrane and collagen for DNA. J. Exp. Med., 144:428, 1976.
223. Hunter, D., Dilley, J., and Holman, H. R.: Isolation and characterization of DNA, RNA and immune complexes from systemic lupus erythematosus and normal plasma. Arthritis Rheum., 16:554, 1973.
224. Gilliam, J. N.: DNA binding to normal skin connective tissue as a localizing factor for DNA-anti-DNA complexes. Arthritis Rheum., 20:117, 1977.
225. Gabrielsen, A. E.: Lupus erythematosus: A disease of DNA discard? Lancet, 2:1116, 1974.
226. Frost, P. G., and Lachmann, P. J.: The relationship of deoxyribonuclease inhibitor levels in human sera to the occurrence of antinuclear antibodies. Clin. Exp. Immunol., 3:447, 1968.
227. Hadjiyannaki, K., and Lachmann, P. J.: The relation of deoxyribonuclease inhibitor levels to the occurrence of antinuclear antibodies in NZB/NZW mice. Clin. Exp. Immunol., 11:291, 1972.
228. Freeman, R. G., Knox, J. M., and Owens, D. D.: Cutaneous lesions of lupus erythematosus induced by monochromic light. Arch. Dermatol., 10:677, 1969.
229. Cripps, D. J., and Ranken, J.: Action spectra of lupus erythematosus and experimental immunofluorescence. Arch. Dermatol., 107:563, 1973.
230. Natali, P. G., and Tan, E. M.: Experimental skin lesions in mice resembling systemic lupus erythematosus. Arthritis Rehum., 16:579, 1973.
231. Tan, E. M.: Immunopathology and pathogenesis of cutaneous involvement in systemic lupus erythematosus. J. Invest. Dermatol., 67:360, 1976.
232. Turk, J. L.: Leprosy as a model of subacute and chronic immunologic disease. J. Invest. Dermatol., 67:457, 1976.
233. Fessel, W. G.: Systemic lupus erythematosus in the community. Arch. Intern. Med., 134:1027, 1974.
234. Cook, C. D., Wedgwood, R. J. P., and Craig, J. M.: Systemic lupus erythematosus. Description of 37 cases in children and a discussion of endocrine therapy in 32 of the cases. Pediatrics, 26:570, 1960.
235. Jacobs, J. C.: Systemic lupus erythematosus in childhood. Pediatrics, 32:257, 1963.
236. Meislin, A. G., and Rothfield, N.: Systemic lupus erythematosus in childhood. Pediatrics, 42:37, 1968.

237. Fish, A. J., Blau, E. B., Westberg, N. E., et al.: Systemic lupus erythematosus within the first two decades of life. Am. J. Med., 62:99, 1967.
238. Henkind, P., and Rothfield, N. F.: Ocular abnormalities in patients treated with antimalarial drugs. N. Engl. J. Med., 269:433, 1963.
239. Bernstein, H. N.: Chloroquine ocular toxicity. Surv. Ophthalmol., 12:415, 1967.
240. Nylander, U.: Ocular damage in chloroquine therapy. Acta Ophthalmol., 92:, 1967.
241. Voipio, H.: Incidence of chloroquine retinopathy. Acta Ophthalmol., 44:349, 1966.
242. Rees, R. B., and Maibach, H. I.: Chloroquine. A review of reactions and dermatologic indications. Arch. Dermatol., 88:280, 1963.
243. Hodgkinson, B. J., and Kolb, H.: A preliminary study of the effect of chloroquine on the rat retina. Arch. Ophthalmol., 84:509, 1970.
244. Buchanan, R. N., Jr.: Quinacrine in the treatment of discoid lupus erythematosus: A 5-year follow up survey: Results and evaluation. South. Med. J., 52:978, 1959.
245. Christiansen, J. V., and Nielsen, J. P.: Treatment of lupus erythematosus with mepacrine. Results and relapses during a long observation. Br. J. Dermatol., 68:73, 1956.
246. Seaman, W. E., and Plotz, P. H.: Effect of aspirin on liver tests in patients with RA or SLE and in normal volunteers. Arthritis Rheum., 19:155, 1976.
247. Rothfield, N. F.: Immunosuppressive therapy in lupus erythematosus. Ann. Intern. Med., 83:727, 1975.
248. Cathcart, E. S., Scheinberg, M. A., Idelson, B. A., et al.: Beneficial effects of methylprednisolone "pulse" therapy in diffuse proliferative lupus nephritis. Lancet, 1:163, 1976.
249. Jones, J. V., Cumming, R. H., Bucknall, R. C., et al.: Plasmaphoresis in the management of acute systemic lupus erythematosus. Lancet, 1:709, 1976.
250. Sugarman, M., Kamdar, A., Barbarer, B. H., et al.: Reversible renal insufficiency in systemic lupus erythematosus (SLE). Clin. Res., 24:111A, 1976.
251. Auer, T. O., Tomasi, T. B., Jr., and Milgram, F.: Natural thymocytologic autoantibodies in NZB and other strains of mice. Cell. Immunol., 10:404, 1974.
252. Mehta, J., Knotts, L. L., and Hahn, B. H.: Effect of altered lymphocyte function on immunologic disorders in NZB/NZW mice. I. Favorable response to L-asparaginase. Arthritis Rheum., 20:65, 1977.
253. Morton, R. O., Goodman, D. G., Gershwin, M. E., et al.: Suppression of autoimmunity and lymphoid proliferation in NZB mice with steroid-sensitive x-radiation-sensitive syngeneic young thymocytes. Arthritis Rheum., 19:1347, 1976.
254. Gershwin, M. E., Steinberg, A. D., Ahmen, A., et al.: Study of thymic factors. II. Failure of thymosin to alter the natural history of New Zealand mice. Arthritis Rheum., 19:862, 1976.

17 | VASCULAR REACTIVE DISEASES

RAYMOND V. CAPUTO, M.D.
and LAWRENCE M. SOLOMON, M.D.

URTICARIA

Urticaria, probably the most well known yet among the least understood of all dermatological disorders, occurs in 15 to 20 per cent of children in the adolescent age group.[1] Clinically, it appears as transient, discrete, erythematous wheals, which may coalesce and form large edematous patches with raised, advancing, serpiginous borders (Fig. 17-1). A white halo frequently surrounds the border of the patch. Simple urticaria involves only the superficial layers of the dermis. Angioedema is a deeper reaction, manifested as non-pitting edema of both the skin and the mucous membranes (Fig. 17-2); angioedema occurs in association with urticaria more frequently than it does alone.[2]

Acute and chronic urticarias represent a vascular reaction to a multitude of stimuli. The pattern of the eruption does not change regardless of the etiology.

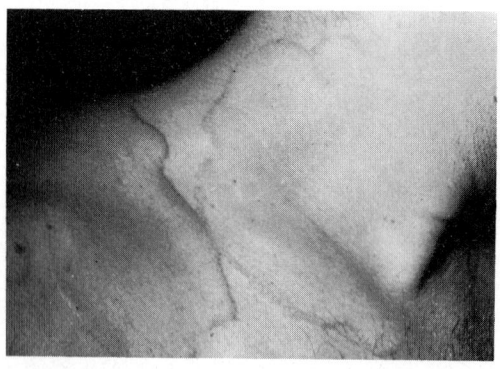

FIGURE 17-1 Urticaria. Wheals form bizarre configurations and change from hour to hour.

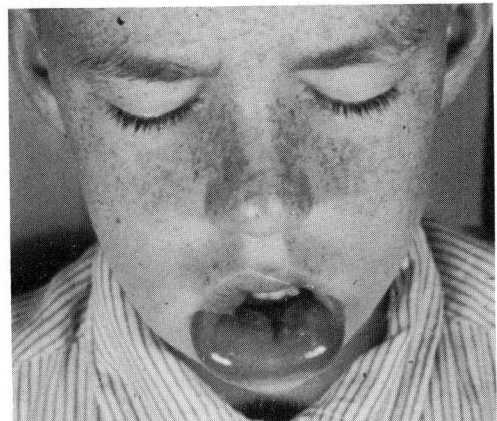

FIGURE 17–2 Angioedema. Youngster had unexplained recurrent acute angioedema of lower lip.

Acute urticaria constitutes 20 per cent of cases; the remaining 80 per cent are usually chronic. In most instances of urticaria, no etiological agent is found.[2] Although acute urticaria seems to be more common in the pediatric and adolescent age groups, the combined incidence of both types correlates with the incidence in adults.[3] Although urticarial reactions do not occur with greater frequency in atopic individuals than in those with normal skin, acute forms seem to be more prevalent in atopic persons.[4]

Table 17–1 lists many of the general causes of urticaria. These may be separated into immunological and non-immunological causes (Table 17–2). According to the classification of Coombs and Gell,[5] Type I hypersensitivity reactions (reaginic IgE antibodies) account for the majority of acute immunologically mediated urticarias[6] and appear to be related to intracellular activity of cyclic AMP (adenosine-3′,5′-monophosphate).[7] Type III reactions, mediated by circulating immune complexes, are the second most common type, producing a serum sickness syndrome with activation of the complement

TABLE 17–1 ETIOLOGICAL CLASSIFICATION OF URTICARIA AND ANGIOEDEMA

Drugs (including Type I and Type III reactions)
Foods
Insect and arthropod bites and stings
Inhalants
Physical urticaria syndromes
  Dermographism
  Pressure urticaria
  Cold urticaria
  Heat urticaria
  Solar urticaria
  Aquagenic urticaria
  Vibratory angioedema
Cholinergic urticaria
Infections
Contact urticaria
Collagen vascular disease
Endocrine causes
Psychogenic urticaria
Idiopathic causes

TABLE 17-2 CLASSIFICATIONS OF URTICARIA AND ANGIOEDEMA ACCORDING TO PATHOGENESIS

Immunological forms
    Reaginic antibodies: Type I
        Drugs
        Arthropod and insect bites and stings
        Inhalants
    Cytotoxic antibodies: Type II
        (e.g., blood transfusion reactions)
    Circulating soluble immune complexes: Type III
        (e.g., serum sickness)

Non-immunological forms
    Cholinergic urticaria
    Urticaria caused by external agents
        Pressure urticaria
        Aquagenic urticaria
        Heat urticaria
        Urticaria pigmentosa
        Vibratory angioedema
    Drugs causing direct histamine release

Both immunological and non-immunological forms
    Physical urticaria syndromes
        Dermographism
        Cold urticaria (familial or acquired)
        Solar urticaria
    Foods
        Immunologically mediated (IgE)
        Non-immunologically mediated
    Contact urticaria
        Immunological forms
        Non-immunological forms

Questionable pathogenesis
    Urticaria associated with systemic internal disease
        Neoplasm
        Collagen vascular disease
        Amyloidosis
        Endocrine disorders
    Urticaria associated with infections (presumed immunological)
    Psychogenic urticaria
    Idiopathic urticaria

system. Type II reactions, mediated by cytotoxic antibodies, are rarely responsible for urticaria; Type IV reactions (delayed or cellular hypersensitivity) do not cause urticaria.[8] Non-immunological forms of urticaria include those caused by drugs that release histamine, cholinergic urticaria, and some types of physical urticaria. All these forms may involve depression of cyclic AMP production.[9]

PATHOGENESIS AND HISTOLOGICAL FINDINGS

In 1927, Lewis[10] described the now classic triple response of cutaneous vessels to histamine: erythema, wheal, and flare. Degranulation of tissue mast cells, whatever the cause, results in local release of histamine and other vasoactive amines, thus producing wheal formation. Localized vasodilatation (erythema) permits transudation of fluid (wheal formation)[11] between the swollen endothelial cells of the superficial vascular plexus; an axonal reflex phenomenon results in the flare.[12] SRS-A (slow-reacting substance of anaphylaxis), serotonin, kinins, and prostaglandins PGE_1 and PGE_2, all of which produce vasodilatation, also have some role in the pathogenesis of the urticarial wheal.[13] Histologically, in addition to edema, one finds superficial perivascular inflammation consisting of lymphocytes, neutrophils, and occasionally eosinophils.[14]

ETIOLOGICAL CLASSIFICATION

Drugs. Of all drugs, penicillin most commonly causes acute urticarial reactions, both Type I, including anaphylaxis, and Type III. Penicillin need not have been systemically administered, since urticaria may result from traces of penicillin in milk and dairy products.[15] Cephalosporin antibiotics, structurally related to the penicillins, may produce cross reactions in up to 15 per cent of penicillin-sensitive individuals,[16] resulting in urticaria. The reader is referred to other sources for a list of additional drugs that cause urticaria.[17,18]

Drug-induced urticaria may result from non-allergic mechanisms. Aspirin (acetylsalicylic acid) is capable of precipitating acute urticaria and also may exacerbate chronic urticaria.[19] Although the exact mechanism remains speculative, a non-immunological basis is postulated, possibly because of the effect of aspirin on prostaglandin metabolism.[20] Certain other drugs (codeine, morphine, quinine, and polymyxin) cause direct release of histamine without involving other mediators.[21]

Food. Urticaria caused by food protein or food additives may be produced by either immunological or non-immunological mechanisms.[8] Acute urticaria, usually mediated by reaginic antibody,[12] most commonly follows ingestion of nuts, fish, eggs, and fresh berries; anaphylaxis is rarely associated with foods.[22] Ingestion of large quantities of crustacean muscle (lobster or crayfish) produces urticaria, probably owing to the direct release of histamine.[21] Food additives, including azo dyes (particularly tartrazine) and benzoic acid preparations, may perpetuate chronic urticaria, particularly in patients with salicylate hypersensitivity.[23,24]

Detection of the cause of chronic food-induced urticaria requires a detailed history and thorough food diary documentation over an extended period of time; in some instances, elimination and readdition diets may be helpful.[25] Food additive sensitivity may be established by azo dye and benzoate provocative tests.[26] Intradermal skin testing is probably not very helpful in individuals with food allergy.

Inhalants. Animal dander, mold spores, pollens, and similar airborne particles are occasionally incriminated in the production of urticaria.[27] Positive intradermal skin reactions to selected antigens in some patients suggest a reaginic mechanism, and treatment with desensitization may be helpful.[28]

Insect and Arthropod Bites and Stings. Stings and bites of *Hymenoptera* species (bees, wasps, hornets, and yellow jackets) and *Arthropoda* species (ants and mosquitoes) can produce generalized urticarial reactions or anaphylaxis. These reactions are mediated either by reaginic antibody or by immune complex processes.[29] Hyposensitization seems to lessen the severity of symptoms upon subsequent exposure.[30]

Papular urticaria (lichen urticatus, prurigo simplex), an extremely pruritic variety, represents a combined immediate and delayed hypersensitivity reaction to insect bites.[31] Indurated lesions, which represent the delayed component, are much more common in younger children[32] and may persist for several months. Histologically, pseudoepitheliomatous hyperplasia associated with a perivascular and periappendageal lymphocytic and eosinophilic infiltrate is found.[33] Topical antipruritic agents such as calamine lotion and systemic antihistamines seem to be the best form of therapy; hyposensitization therapy also has had some success in the management of this condition.[34]

PHYSICAL URTICARIA SYNDROMES

DERMOGRAPHISM

Dermographism (Fig. 17–3) occurs in 1.5 to 5 per cent of the population and is characterized by localized erythema and the appearance of a wheal following firm stroking of the skin with a blunt instrument.[35] Although the mechanism of wheal formation is unknown, histamine does not seem to be the mediator of the vasodilatation.[36] Direct mechanical injury to the blood vessels may render them highly permeable, allowing leakage of plasma.[37] Passive transfer with IgE antibody[35] has been demonstrated in some affected individuals. Treatment with hydroxyzine may be somewhat effective in reducing the size of the wheal.[38]

White dermographism (blanching of the skin at a site stroked firmly by a pointed instrument) represents a phenomenon of altered vascular reactivity. It

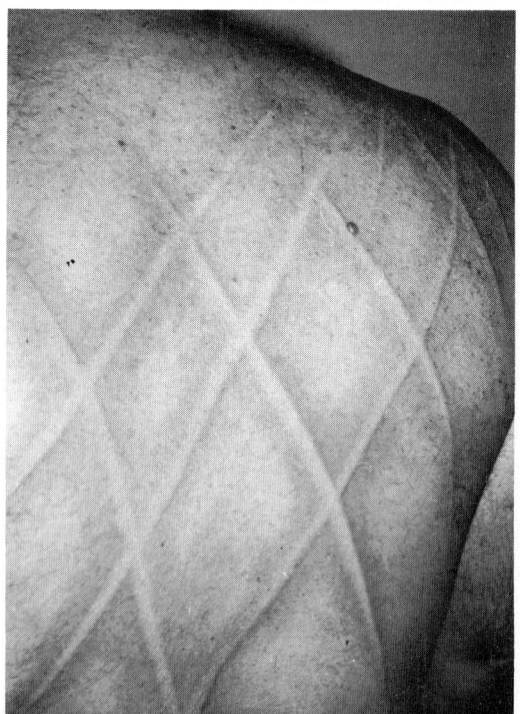

FIGURE 17–3 Dermographism.

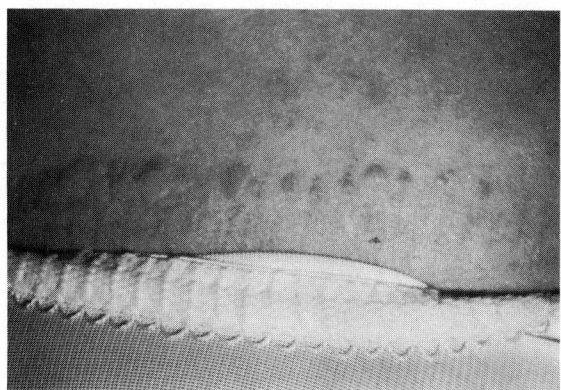

FIGURE 17–4   Pressure urticaria.

is seen in the involved skin of patients with atopic dermatitis as well as in allergic contact dermatitis.[39]

Pressure Urticaria

Pressure urticaria (Fig. 17–4) refers to deep, painful swellings that develop several hours after sustained pressure has been applied to the skin and that may persist for up to 24 hours.[40] Chemical mediators have not been incriminated in this uncommon disorder. Ryan[41] postulated the presence of a fibrinolytic disturbance or Arthus phenomenon due to localized capillary endothelial damage. Although prednisone, in a dosage of 30 mg a day, seems to control the symptoms, the best form of therapy is prevention.[40]

Vibratory Angioedema

Inherited as an autosomal dominant trait, this disorder consists of erythematous and edematous lesions of skin and subcutaneous tissues in response to local frictional or vibratory stimuli. Stimuli of significant intensity may cause a generalized erythema or an erythema associated with headache, suggesting the possibility of histamine release. No dermographism has been demonstrated. Serum C4 and C1 esterase inhibitor levels have been found to be normal. No therapy has proved effective.[42]

Cold Urticaria

The rare familial form of cold-induced urticaria is inherited as an autosomal dominant trait and manifests itself as erythematous burning patches and papules developing within a few minutes or hours of exposure to cold air or water. It is associated with systemic signs, including fever, chills, arthralgia, headache, malaise, and muscle tenderness, as well as with significant leukocytosis.[43] Histologically, an intense polymorphous infiltrate is apparent in the skin.[43] The ice cube test may fail to produce the lesion. Although histamine does not play a role, the presence of leukocytosis suggests other chemotactic

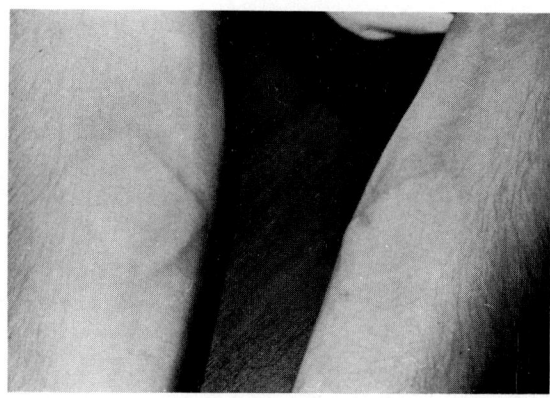

FIGURE 17–5 Cold urticaria induced by ice cubes.

factors and vasoactive substances.[44] No therapy beyond genetic counseling and avoidance of cold is advised.

Acquired cold urticaria develops after application of cold to the skin or mucous membranes but also may be associated with generalized urticaria and systemic signs and symptoms suggestive of histamine release and diffusion.[43] Indeed, higher histamine levels have been demonstrated after affected individuals were exposed to cold.[45] The ice cube test has shown positive results, and passive transfer of IgE has been demonstrated.[44] Cyproheptadine administered prior to cold exposure seems to lessen the severity of attacks.[46]

Secondary cold urticaria, with positive ice cube test results (Fig. 17–5), may also follow an underlying disorder, such as cryoglobulinemia, syphilitic paroxysmal cold hemoglobinuria, cold hemagglutination syndromes,[47] and rarely, cold panniculitis.[48] More often, localized cold urticaria may result in a non-specific manner from tissue injury such as frostbite, burns, or injury at the site of desensitization or infection.

Heat Urticaria

Localized urticaria may develop within minutes at sites of the skin exposed directly to heat; the mechanism of action is unknown, and therapy at present is ineffective.[49] A delayed form exists, in which direct contact with a hot object or prolonged exposure to radiant heat may produce urticaria several hours later.[50]

Solar Urticaria

Harber[51] identified a photosensitive disorder in patients who developed pruritic wheals within minutes of exposure to sunlight and classified it according to the causative wavelength. Although the most frequent manifestation of the condition is an urticarial reaction in the exposed skin, systemic reactions caused by histamine release have been observed following prolonged and intensive exposure to the sun.[52] The mechanism of action is unknown, although the possibility of achieving passive transfer of the condition suggests an immunological basis.[53] Takeshi[54] postulated the presence of an undetected serum photoallergen. Topical application of sunscreens containing para-aminobenzoic acid (PABA) and systemic administration of chloroquine seem to increase tolerance to sunlight in the UVB spectrum.[55, 56] Repeated gradual exposure to sunlight may produce tolerance to light in some of these patients.[57]

Erythropoietic protoporphyria, an inborn error of porphyrin metabolism, sometimes is manifested by solar urticaria.[58] This disease can be distinguished from other forms of solar urticaria by the presence of excessive amounts of protoporphyrins and coproporphyrins in the erythrocytes and stool of affected individuals (see Chapter 6).[59]

Aquagenic Urticaria

Shelley[60] described a peculiar form of urticaria following contact with water, which occurs most frequently in adolescents. It is marked by the development of small, perifollicular, papular, urticarial lesions with surrounding axon reflex erythema. He postulated that the contact of water with sebum produced a toxic substance in some individuals, resulting in local histamine release from the perifollicular mast cells. Exercise and other cholinergic factors do not precipitate this reaction in patients affected by aquagenic urticaria.[61] Administration of antihistamines by mouth seems to lessen the severity of the disorder.

Cholinergic Urticaria

This urticaria may be provoked by exercise, exertion, warming of the body, or emotional distress; it occurs in up to 15 per cent of adolescents and young adults.[62] Small (1-3 mm) wheals with a large surrounding flare appear minutes after the causative stimulus has been applied. The palms and soles are always spared. The central nervous system may mediate this phenomenon through efferent cholinergic sympathetic nerves.[63] Acetylcholine, through some unknown mechanism, may stimulate histamine release and thus cause the lesions. Treatment with hydroxyzine seems to be only slightly effective; fortunately, however, this condition tends to subside spontaneously.

Contact Urticaria

Direct contact of the skin with certain chemicals may result in local urticaria. Non-immunological causes include certain plants (nettles, dogwood leaves, and tumbleweed) and arthropods (caterpillars), which stimulate release of histamine and other vasoactive substances upon contact.[64] Immunological reactions include those producing only urticaria (Stage I), urticaria and angioedema (Stage II), urticaria and asthma (Stage III), and the most severe, urticaria manifested in association with anaphylaxis (Stage IV).[65] Routine closed patch skin tests are usually negative after 48 hours; open patch tests usually produce urticarial lesions within 30 minutes. Because anaphylaxis may result from the test, precautions should be taken in case resuscitation becomes necessary.

INFECTIONS

Various infections may be followed by an urticarial reaction, possibly resulting from an immunological reaction. These include:
1. Acute viral infections, such as hepatitis, infectious mononucleosis, and Coxsackie A9 infections.[8]
2. Bacterial infections, such as urinary tract infections and chronic periodontal and sinus infections.[12]
3. Fungal infections, such as *Candida albicans* and rarely *Trichophyton rubrum*.[66]
4. Parasitic and protozoan infestations, such as those usually associated with eosinophilia (*Ascaris,* hookworm, *Strongyloides,* schistosomes, *Echinococcus, Filaria, Giardia, Amoeba, Trichomonas,* and malaria).[12]

PSYCHOGENIC URTICARIA

Many physicians feel that psychological factors, such as emotional upsets, anxiety, and depression, play some role in precipitating exacerbations of chronic urticaria.[2] The mechanism is unknown. Supportive psychotherapy and hypnosis may be helpful.[17]

MISCELLANEOUS CAUSES

Less common causes of urticaria include: systemic lupus erythematosus, dermatomyositis, juvenile rheumatoid arthritis,[67] Hodgkin's lymphoma, leukemia, other malignant tumors,[12] hyperthyroidism,[68] ovarian abnormalities (autoimmune progesterone urticaria),[69] and amyloidosis associated with deafness (autosomal dominant syndrome).[70]

GENERAL PRINCIPLES OF MANAGEMENT

Most episodes of acute urticaria are self-limiting and require no investigative procedures other than a complete history and physical examination. However if the lesions continue to appear beyond six weeks, one is justified in making appropriate studies to identify a possible underlying disorder.

In general, systemically administered antihistamines are effective only in acute urticaria. Topically applied antihistamines are not effective, since they are poorly absorbed. Chronic urticaria may be treated sequentially with various classes of antihistamines;[6] when one class fails, an antihistamine from another class may be tried. Beta-adrenergic drugs (e.g., epinephrine) are helpful or even life-saving in acute urticaria associated with angioedema,[71] but the side effects and brief action of epinephrine preclude its use for minor chronic exacerbations. Topical steroid preparations are not effective, although topical agents such as calamine lotion may provide temporary relief. Systemic corticosteroids offer rapid symptomatic relief of acute urticaria and angioedema.[6] However, this method should be avoided in treating the chronic form of the disease. The amount of steroid required to suppress the reaction continues to increase as the period of relief becomes shorter.

URTICARIA-LIKE SYNDROMES

SERUM SICKNESS

Serum sickness, occurring seven to 12 days following antigenic stimulation by drugs, vaccines, infections, or insect and arthropod bites and stings, is a syndrome of fever, generalized lymphadenopathy, pruritic urticarial eruption, and arthralgia.[8, 72] Following antigenic exposure, circulating soluble antigen-antibody complexes (Type III reaction) accumulate in the serum. These complexes may be deposited in the joint spaces[73] and in the kidney,[74] producing arthralgia, arthritis, and nephritis. Vasculitis may occasionally be apparent within skin lesions. Although no highly specific laboratory studies are available to identify the disorder, the erythrocyte sedimentation rate usually is increased, and serum complement (CH5O) may be somewhat decreased,[75] owing to activation of both the classic and the alternate pathways of the complement cascade.

Systemically administered antihistamines and analgesics usually control the most disturbing symptoms. However, severe attacks, with high fever, arthritis, and nephritis, may benefit from parenteral administration of corticosteroids.

HEREDITARY ANGIOEDEMA

Hereditary angioedema (HAE) is inherited as an autosomal dominant trait and is manifested by recurrent attacks of non-pitting edema involving the skin, subcutaneous tissue, and mucous membranes, especially in the pharynx and larynx. The gastrointestinal tract may also become involved, with resultant cramping abdominal pain.[76] Common urticaria usually is not present. Attacks of angioedema are often precipitated by direct trauma or emotional stress but may occur spontaneously. Acute laryngeal edema represents an immediate threat to life, accounting for mortality in 30 per cent of patients whose condition had not been recognized.[77]

PATHOGENESIS

Two distinct forms of HAE are recognized at present. In the most common type (85 per cent), the level of C1 esterase inhibitor, an alpha-2 globulin in the serum, is found to be extremely low[78] because of decreased synthesis in the liver.[79] During an attack, levels of C4 and C2, already chronically reduced during asymptomatic periods, are further depleted.[80, 81] In the variant form, normal levels of C1 esterase inhibitor are present, but the inhibitor is apparently non-functional.[82] Postulations based on the work of Jacob and Monod suggest that, in the heterozygote state, the individual may exhibit markedly impaired synthesis of esterase inhibitor or may produce a non-functional inhibitor because both structural genes may be repressed by an abnormal repressor substance.[82] Because of the interaction of the complement system with the coagulation scheme, a deficiency of C1 esterase inhibitor initiates consumption of both the components of the complement cascade and the fibrinolytic constituents[83] of the blood.

TREATMENT

Long-term prophylactic treatment includes the use of anti-fibrinolytic and hormonal agents. Although ε-aminocaproic acid (EACA), an anti-fibrinolytic agent, seems to be effective in reducing the number of attacks, adverse side effects, such as muscle discomfort, elevation of serum muscle enzymes, and possible thrombotic episodes, limit its usefulness.[84] Androgen therapy (methyltestosterone, oxymetholone) also helps to control the disease but causes masculinization in females.[85] This side effect precludes its use in children and young women. Gelfand[86] has reported promising results with danazol, an anabolic androgenic steroid with minimal masculinizing side effects. It not only effectively controls the activity of the disease but also seems to correct the underlying defect by increasing the levels of C1 esterase inhibitor and C4. It may be that danazol acts by derepressing the repressor substance previously mentioned, thus permitting the structural gene to produce the necessary C1 esterase inhibitor protein in adequate amounts.

Preventive measures and short-term therapy of acute episodes consist of the infusion of fresh-frozen plasma before more traumatic procedures are initiated.[87] This provides an immediate source of C1 esterase inhibitor. Epinephrine, corticosteroids, and antihistamines also may be tried during acute episodes, although the response to these agents is not wholly satisfactory.[82] Tracheostomy may be life-saving in severe attacks that are unresponsive to other treatment modalities.

FIGURATE ERYTHEMAS

Because large figurate lesions (cyclic, annular, or serpiginous) may exist side by side with urticaria and angioedema, the figurate erythemas will be discussed briefly and should be included in the differential diagnosis of urticaria.

ERYTHEMA ANNULARE CENTRIFUGUM

Erythema annulare centrifugum is an eruption characterized by persistent, erythematous, ringed, somewhat scaly lesions, which slowly enlarge centrifugally (Fig. 17–6). The cause of this condition is unknown. Most affected individuals are otherwise normal, but Korting[88] believes a search for visceral neoplasms, leukemia, and reticuloendothelioses should be conducted, since they may be associated with the eruption of these lesions. Erythema annulare centrifugum should not be confused with erythema gyratum perstans, very rarely found in the adolescent, which is manifested as large, constantly changing, polycyclic patterns with a "grained wood" appearance.

ERYTHEMA CHRONICUM MIGRANS

Erythema chronicum migrans is a poorly understood subacute dermatitis. It is characterized by a single erythematous papule, which, through central

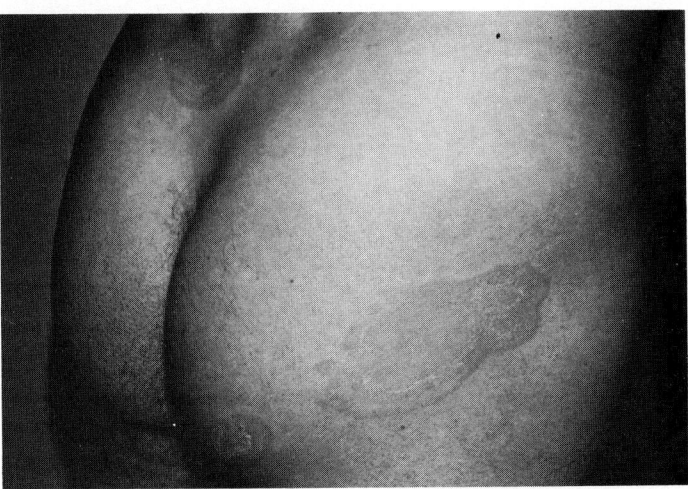

FIGURE 17–6 Erythema annulare centrifugum has a predilection for the bathing suit area and resembles a dermatophyte infection.

clearing and peripheral extension, produces a large, slightly elevated, erythematous, auricular-shaped lesion, reaching 20 to 30 cm in diameter. A burning, prickling, or itching sensation usually is present in the lesion. Fever, headache, regional lymphadenopathy, and even meningitis may accompany the dermatitis.[89]

The mechanism of formation of the lesions is mysterious, but Afzelius[90] believed that a tick bite (*Ixodes ricinus*) may be involved in the pathogenesis. Lennhoff[91] demonstrated the presence of "spirochetal organisms" in histological sections of erythema chronicum migrans, and Degos[92] reported positive microagglutination tests for rickettsial species in the sera of affected individuals. For these reasons, penicillin and tetracycline have been administered to patients, with variable results.[93, 94] Hellerstrom[95] postulated an allergic pathogenesis by showing positive cell-mediated intradermal skin testing to tick extract. Transfer of disease from one individual to another was shown by Binder.[96] The sum of these studies suggests that the causative agent may be a microbiological agent, transmitted by tick bite and mediated by an immunological reaction.

Interest in erythema chronicum migrans has been stimulated by a recent epidemic of arthritis in children and adults in three Connecticut communities.[97] Referred to as "Lyme arthritis," this syndrome is characterized by recurrent attacks of painful arthritis in a few large joints (especially the knees) and skin lesions similar to those of erythema chronicum migrans.

The peak incidence of new cases occurring in familial and geographical clusters is in summer and early fall. Attacks of arthritis last for an average of one week but may persist up to six months. The disease has a sudden onset and tends to be recurrent. In 25 per cent of patients, a single erythematous papule appears somewhere on the body four weeks prior to the onset of joint symptoms. The lesion develops in a manner identical to that of erythema chronicum migrans; it lasts one-and-a-half weeks on the average but may persist throughout the duration of joint symptoms. In some patients there is a history of tick or insect bite. Associated symptoms include fever (38.08 to 38.76°C or 100 to 103°F), malaise, fatigue, headache, burning sensation at the site of the skin lesions, stiff neck, and an additional maculopapular eruption. Unlike juvenile rheumatoid arthritis, Lyme arthritis has no associated iridocyclitis. Treatment, including administration of penicillin, tetracycline, and acetylsalicylic acid, has not affected the course of the disease.

A search for antinuclear antibodies, rheumatoid factor, and lupus erythematosus (LE) cells has repeatedly proved to be fruitless, as have complement fixation and hemagglutination inhibition studies to a variety of agents. However, approximately 50 per cent of patients have been found to have decreased levels of C3 in the serum. IgM and IgG cryoprecipitates have also been demonstrated in the sera of patients during acute episodes, raising the possibility of a circulating immune complex–mediated syndrome.[98]

ERYTHEMA MARGINATUM

Erythema marginatum is a non-pruritic, evanescent rash occurring mainly on the trunk and extremities. It is found in patients suffering from acute rheumatic fever.[99] The lesions vary greatly in size; some start as single, enlarging, erythematous papules, forming large circinate, serpiginous, and annular lesions that migrate from one place to another and are transient in nature (Plate X–A). Although the edges may be slightly elevated, the lesions are not indurated. They can be "brought out" by applying heat to the skin. The lesions usually become apparent after the carditis is established. However, the skin manifestations may precede the onset of clinical evidence of carditis, so that rheumatic fever should be suspected in the presence of an evanescent, erythematous, figurate eruption in a young adult. The presence of one of the other major criteria suggested by Jones (such as carditis, polymigratory arthritis, chorea, or subcutaneous nodules) or two minor criteria (such as arthralgia or fever) strengthens the suspicion of rheumatic fever. Further support may be obtained from laboratory evidence of acute phase reactants, such as increased erythrocyte sedimentation, increased C-reactive protein, increased antistreptolysin O (ASO) titer, or demonstration of group A beta-hemolytic streptococci in bacterial cultures taken from the pharynx.[100] Erythema marginatum is believed to represent a vascular phenomenon reactive to a preceding streptococcal infection.

ERYTHEMA NODOSUM

Erythema nodosum is the result of a vascular reaction in the subcutaneous fatty tissue. The pathomechanism is not known, but a perplexing variety of agents may trigger the reaction. It occurs in approximately 8 per cent of the adolescent population,[101] with a marked predominance in females.[102] A prodromal period of fever, malaise, pharyngitis, chills, myalgia, and arthralgia is more common in young adults than in children.[102]

The disease is characterized by the sudden appearance of several discrete, round or ovoid erythematous patches, primarily on the anterior aspect of the lower legs (Plate X–B), less frequently on the thighs, buttocks, and arms, and rarely on the face. The patches become swollen and painful, and at the end of one week the lesions are indurated and shiny, with ill-defined borders. They are extremely tender to palpation. Several lesions may coalesce to form a large, painful, erythematous area, which may be confused with thrombophlebitis The nodules begin to regress in two to six weeks, undergoing the purplish-blue and yellow discoloration of a resolving bruise. There is usually no suppuration or ulceration. A fine desquamation of the overlying skin usually ushers in the final phase of resolution, and the lesions heal without scarring.[103] New crops of lesions may appear during the resolution phase, but attacks are seldom recurrent.[104] Fine[105] has reported a chronic form of erythema nodosum, lasting for more than eight years. However, the disease is most often self-limiting and does not become chronic.

ETIOLOGY

Infectious agents are the most common cause of erythema nodosum. Table 17–3 lists a number of these as well as other possible causes. Streptococcal infection seems to be the most common mechanism of erythema nodosum in adolescents.[106] Hicks[107] has reported erythema nodosum secondary to *T. rubrum* infection of the feet. Subcutaneous injection of trichophytin skin test in these patients produced erythema nodosum-like lesions in some cases. *T. mentagrophytes* has also been associated with erythema nodosum.[108] Oral contracep-

TABLE 17–3 AGENTS BELIEVED TO CAUSE ERYTHEMA NODOSUM*

Infections	Drugs	Miscellaneous
Bacterial	Sulfonamides	Sarcoidosis
Streptococcus	(especially sulfathiazole)	Discoid lupus
Tuberculosis	Salicylates	erythematosus
Meningococcus	Phenacetin	Polyarteritis nodosa
Chancroid	Bromides	Leukemia
Diphtheria	Iodides	Pregnancy
Leprosy	Penicillin	Rheumatic fever
Syphilis	Oral contraceptives	Ulcerative colitis
Yersinia	BCG vaccine	Granulomatous colitis
Viral		
Herpes simplex		
Psittacosis		
Cat-scratch fever		
Lymphogranuloma venereum		
Fungal		
Histoplasmosis		
Coccidiomycosis		
Blastomycosis		
Trichophyton rubrum		
T. mentagrophytes		
Parasitic		
Ascariasis		

*Adapted from Kibel, M. A.: Erythema nodosum in children. S. Afr. Med. J. Sci., 44:873, 1970, and Pillsbury, D. M., and Shelley, W. B.: Erythema nodosum. *In:* Wintrobe et al. (eds.): Harrison's Principles of Internal Medicine. New York, McGraw-Hill, 1962, p. 1924.

tives are rare causes of this disease,[109, 110] and pregnancy may be the cause of recurrent episodic erythema nodosum.[111] Pinski[112] found erythema nodosum in patients with acute monocytic, chronic lymphocytic, and chronic granulocytic leukemia.

LABORATORY STUDIES AND HISTOPATHOLOGICAL FINDINGS

Although laboratory studies in patients with erythema nodosum tend to produce non-specific abnormalities, an elevated erythrocyte sedimentation rate seems to be a constant feature. The white blood cell count is often elevated, but whether this is directly related to erythema nodosum or to the disease that provoked the reaction is unknown.[113] The ASO titer may indicate recent or remote infection with beta-hemolytic streptococci. Radiographic studies of the chest, especially in those patients with a more protracted prodromal period, may reveal the presence of hilar lymphadenopathy, indicative of sarcoidosis.[114]

Erythema nodosum is essentially a disease of the venous system, involving both the large veins and the venules, particularly those in the adipose tissue. Löfgren[115] reported thrombophlebitis in 40 per cent of his cases, indicating that in some patients the disease may have a deeper component. The classic elements of erythema nodosum are vascular inflammation and the presence of lymphocytic cells in the fat lobule septa.[116] However, a wide spectrum of inflammatory processes exists, including phlebitis and hemorrhage into the septal areas or directly into the fat lobules, true panniculitis, with polymorphonuclear leukocytes replacing an entire fat lobule, and subacute lymphocytic or chronic granulomatous inflammation. Since any of these features may predominate in any area of the hypodermis, an incisional wedge biopsy of the involved skin is recommended for histological examination.[117]

Differential diagnosis of erythema nodosum includes: (1) erythema induratum (or nodular vasculitis), in which caseation necrosis and ulceration are present, (2) Weber-Christian panniculitis, (3) subcutaneous fat necrosis with or without associated pancreatic disease,[118] (4) subacute migratory thrombophlebitis, and (5) traumatic or factitial panniculitis.[119]

THERAPY

Erythema nodosum usually requires no more than palliative treatment. The administration of salicylates may be helpful when the lesions are very painful.[113] Oxyphenbutazone and phenylbutazone also have benefited some patients.[120] Potassium iodide, in a dosage of 900 mg a day, also seems to be fairly effective when compared with other anti-inflammatory agents.[121] Although systemically administered corticosteroids often provide rapid relief of symptoms, their use should be restricted to very severe episodes or to those patients with frequent recurrences.[113] Care must be taken to avoid exacerbating an underlying disease process by giving corticosteroids and also to avoid prescribing aspirin for those patients whose condition may have been caused by aspirin (see Table 17–2). It is generally wise to treat the disease that provoked the reaction in the skin, but since the underlying cause is most often not discovered, this may not be possible.

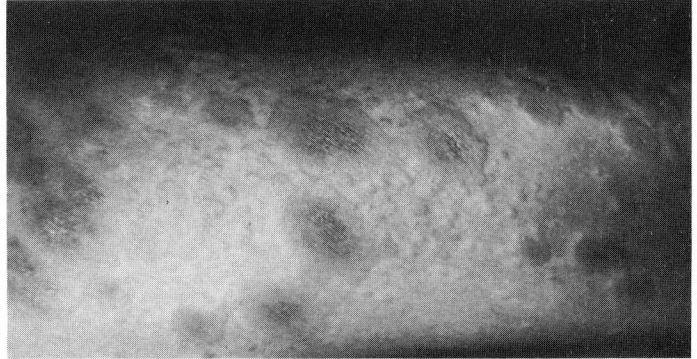

FIGURE 17-7 Erythema multiforme. Beside the target lesions are small papules with a halo of vasoconstriction around the central erythematous raised areas.

ERYTHEMA MULTIFORME

Erythema multiforme commonly affects children, adolescents, and young adults. It represents a vascular reactive phenomenon to a variety of agents. Drugs, infections (bacterial, viral, fungal, and parasitic), collagen vascular disease, foods, contactants, pregnancy, malignancies,[122,123] and inhaled insecticide[124] have been reported to precipitate the eruption, *although most often no cause is detected.* A wide spectrum of symptoms and signs may ensue, from simple urticarial lesions to severe blistering eruptions.[125] Although the causative mechanism is unknown, the available evidence favors an immunological reaction.[126]

CLINICAL COURSE

Erythema multiforme usually appears first as pruritic erythematous urticarial papules, often surrounded by a halo of vasoconstriction (Fig. 17-7). As the individual lesions enlarge peripherally, the center flattens and turns dusky blue-gray, resulting in the formation of the characteristic "target" or

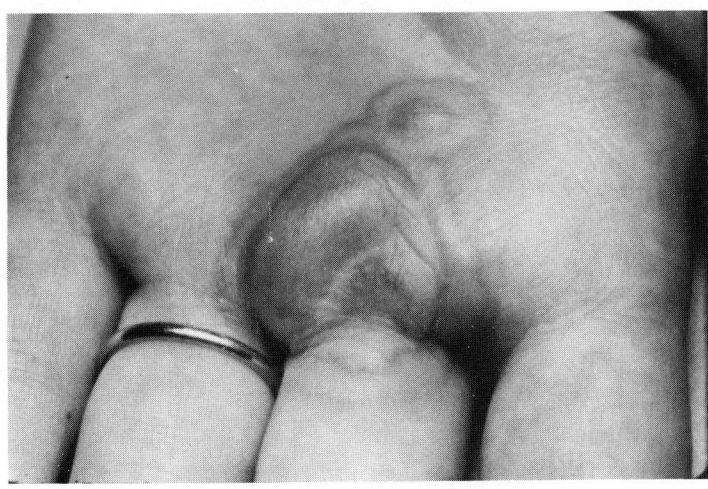

FIGURE 17-8 Erythema multiforme. Lesions on the palm. (Courtesy of Dr. Steven Roberts)

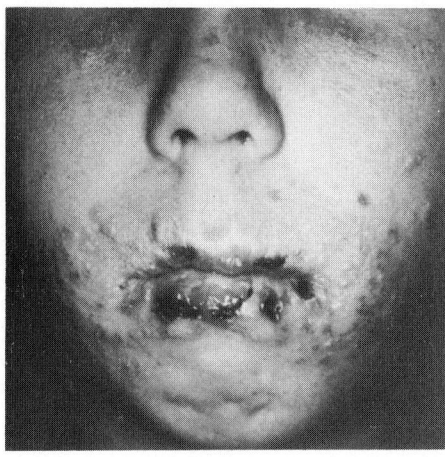

FIGURE 17-9 Stevens-Johnson syndrome (severe erythema multiforme) secondary to recurrent herpes simplex infection. (Courtesy of Dr. Steven Roberts)

"iris" lesion (Plates X–C and D). Concentric rings may form around the target lesion (Plate X–E). New crops of lesions appear at intervals of a few days, so that several different stages may be apparent at the same time. Any part of the body, including the mucous membranes, may be involved, although symmetrical distribution of lesions on the dorsa of hands, palmar and plantar surfaces, and extensor surfaces of the extremities are the most common (Fig. 17–8). Further progression of the lesions causes central bulla formation[127] or even purpuric or ecchymotic areas. The disease is usually self-limited, lasting one to four weeks. Recurrences are common, especially those precipitated by herpes simplex infections, in particular, type II, herpes progenitalis.[128]

A severe blistering variant, Stevens-Johnson syndrome (erythema multiforme exudativum), characteristically involves the mucous membranes and is often associated with high fever, malaise, and eventual prostration (Figs. 17–9 and 17–10). Stomatitis ensues, with hemorrhagic crusting, secondary infection, and keratoconjunctivitis with corneal ulceration and scarring;[129] urethritis and balanitis may further complicate the picture. Rarely, hematuria and nephritis

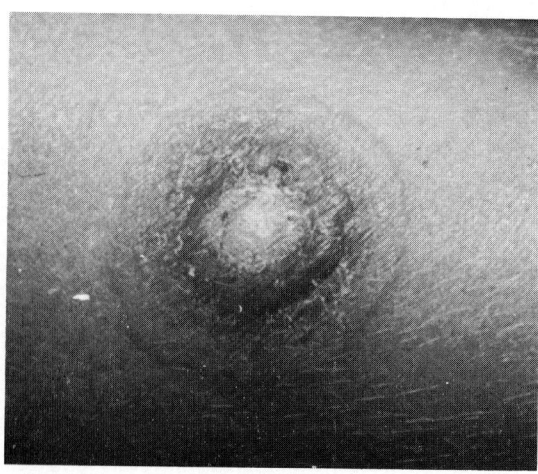

FIGURE 17-10 Target lesion of erythema multiforme with a central blister. (Courtesy of Dr. Steven Roberts)

with progressive renal failure may result and persist for several weeks.[130, 131] The mortality rate of Stevens-Johnson syndrome during the acute stage is about 5 to 15 per cent.[132]

Tissue sections obtained by biopsy in an uncomplicated case contain edema of the superficial dermis, with vacuolar degeneration of the basal cell layer and superficial lymphohistiocytic infiltrate.[127] Necrosis of the basal cell layer, with subsequent overlying epidermal damage, produces the characteristic subepidermal bulla.

DIFFERENTIAL DIAGNOSIS

Once the typical target lesions have become apparent, the diagnosis of erythema multiforme usually suggests itself. However, in the urticarial stage the differential diagnosis is more complex; bullous pemphigoid should be considered. Progression of the latter process toward tense bullae, with characteristic deposition of immunoglobulin (IgG) and complement C3 at the basement membrane zone (demonstrated by direct immunofluorescence preparations), establishes the correct diagnosis.[133] Pemphigus vulgaris may have mucosal involvement similar to that of the Stevens-Johnson syndrome, but the histological and immunofluorescence patterns are distinctly different from those seen in other conditions. Dermatitis herpetiformis is a polymorphous eruption, which may contain a characteristic immunofluorescent pattern of IgA deposition in the basement membrane zone.[134] Both the direct and indirect immunofluorescent tests are negative in erythema multiforme. Toxic epidermal necrolysis, due to Group II, phage type 71 staphylococcal nasopharyngitis (staphylococcal scalded-skin syndrome) and the drug-induced variety (especially phenytoin) should also be considered in the differential diagnosis (see Chapter 8).

TREATMENT

Mild forms of erythema multiforme require only symptomatic therapy with antihistamines and salicylates. The major aim of management is to elicit the precipitating cause. In the Stevens-Johnson syndrome, secondary infection should be prevented by applying frequent compresses and cleansing the encrusted areas. Extensive ulceration, high fever, and resultant fluid loss may be present in the severe forms of the disorder, requiring isolation techniques and intravenous fluid replacement. Hambrick[135] and Shklar[136a] found the systemic administration of corticosteroids ineffective in the treatment of mild erythema multiforme. Rasmussen found systemic corticosteroids to lessen the symptoms, but the duration of the disease was not altered, and more complications ensued.[136b] Most patients have a self-limiting form of the disease, which does not require high-dose corticosteroid therapy. If, however, the patient's condition deteriorates into the more severe form, most physicians, including ourselves, would administer corticosteroids intravenously.

CHRONIC URTICARIA VASCULITIS AND HYPOCOMPLEMENTEMIA

A new, rare clinical syndrome, consisting of chronic urticaria, hypocomplementemia, and vasculitis, has recently been described in association with systemic symptoms. The syndrome seems to be more prevalent in females than in males. The vasculitic component of this condition usually resembles urticaria, in contrast to the purpuric or necrotic lesions more commonly found in other forms of vasculitis.[137]

CLINICAL COURSE

The eruption is usually generalized, with recurrent crops of pruritic erythematous wheals that blanch under pressure. Individual lesions are transient, lasting 24 to 72 hours. Livedo reticularis may also occur,[137] as may angioedema (manifested as painful swelling of the limbs and face) and laryngeal edema.[138] Other prominent features found in several patients[139] include cramping abdominal pain associated with nausea, vomiting and diarrhea, mild glomerulonephritis, and episodic arthralgia and arthritis caused by synovitis involving multiple large joints. Feig[140] has reported multisystem involvement, including myositis, pseudotumor cerebri, and adenopathy.

LABORATORY STUDIES

The most consistent laboratory finding in these patients is an elevated erythrocyte sedimentation rate.[141] During attacks, levels of C1q, C2, C3, and C4 and are decreased, although the properdin pathway components are normal. These findings suggest activation of the classic complement pathway.[142] Soter[141] has reported the occurrence of chronic urticaria and vasculitis with normal complement levels. Serum immunoglobulins show random abnormalities, including elevation of IgG, IgM, or IgA levels[141] and episodic hypergammaglobulinemia E associated with significant eosinophilia.[142] The LE preparation, antinuclear antibody (ANA), and rheumatoid factor tests are characteristically negative. The C1 esterase inhibitor level is normal. Very low concentrations of cryoglobulins may occasionally be found, but these do not rise to the levels found in cryoglobulinemia.[143] Renal involvement may produce hematuria, and the creatinine clearance may be decreased during attacks, suggesting focal nephritis.

HISTOLOGICAL FINDINGS

Skin biopsy specimens reveal necrotizing angiitis, with endothelial swelling, necrosis of blood vessel walls, fibrinoid deposits within the lumen, and a dense polymorphonuclear and lymphocytic infiltration of vessel walls with leukocytoclasis (nuclear dust) and extravasated red blood cells. In addition, papillary dermal edema similar to that found in urticaria may be present, but eosinophils are absent.[137] Direct immunofluorescence of skin lesions has revealed deposits of IgG, IgM, IgA, and occasional IgE,[142] in addition to C3 within the blood vessel walls.

IgE and complement have been identified in the glomerular basement membrane of the kidney in association with a mild membranoproliferative glomerulonephritis.[139]

ETIOLOGY

Geha[142] has postulated that this syndrome may result from hypersensitivity to an unidentified antigen. The multisystem involvement suggests a form of collagen vascular disease,[140] although the negative ANA, LE preparation, and rheumatoid arthritis (RA) latex fixation tests argue against this conclusion. The association of synovial and renal involvement with decreased serum complement levels favors a Type III-mediated or circulating immune complex disease, producing local vascular injury. No chemical mediators have yet been identified in this syndrome.[141]

DIFFERENTIAL DIAGNOSIS

Other skin diseases associated with hypocomplementemia include systemic lupus erythematosus (SLE), mixed IgM-IgG cryoglobulinemia, cutaneous vasculitis associated with rheumatoid arthritis, and occasionally drug reactions.[142] An inability to demonstrate positive LE preparation, ANA, RA factor, and cryoglobulins rules out these diagnostic possibilities. Serum sickness should be considered in the differential diagnosis, although it can usually be identified by a generalized lymphadenopathy and a history of specific antigenic exposure. The elevated sedimentation rate, a characteristic feature of this syndrome, should rule out the diagnosis of urticaria or hereditary angioedema. Henoch-Schönlein purpura (HSP) must also be considered, since it may contain urticarial lesions and leukocytoclastic angiitis in addition to renal, abdominal, and joint symptoms. However, in HSP the skin lesions are usually purpuric, and hypocomplementemia is only rarely seen.[144]

TREATMENT

Although this disease is usually refractory to therapy, a trial of systemic antihistamines is warranted. While the role of systemic corticosteroids seems to be equivocal, Geha[142] has reported improvement of the skin lesions and return of complement levels to normal with prednisone in a dosage of 2 mg/kg/day. However, the mechanism of responsiveness to steroids and the long-term prognosis remain uncertain.

HENOCH-SCHÖNLEIN PURPURA

Henoch-Schönlein purpura (HSP or anaphylactoid purpura) is a leukocytoclastic angiitis and therefore not caused by thrombocytopenia. HSP may be associated with arthralgia, nephritis, and gastrointestinal disturbances, which are manifested in a variable time sequence and in a variety of combinations. HSP is a common disease in pediatric patients but also may be seen in adolescents and young adults. Boys seem to be affected more frequently than girls. The mortality rate of HSP, attributed mostly to renal complications, is about 2 per cent of patients who seek medical help.[145]

ETIOLOGY

Henoch-Schönlein purpura possibly represents a vascular hypersensitivity reaction to a variety of agents, including drugs, viral infections,[146, 147] and insect bites.[148] Streptococcal infection, documented either by culture or by serological studies, has also been incriminated as a cause. A prodromal upper respiratory infection in some patients may point toward a viral etiology.[149] Rogers[150] has even reported a case attributed to cold exposure.

CLINICAL COURSE

Following a mild prodrome, asymptomatic erythematous urticarial papules develop symmetrically on the buttocks, anterior parts of the legs, and posterior areas of the thighs. The trunk and face may also become involved. As the lesions enlarge, they become petechial and eventually coalesce to form ecchymotic patches (Fig. 17–11).

Arthralgia or arthritis, caused by periarticular involvement rather than hemarthrosis, involves the large joints, especially the knees and ankles. The gastrointestinal manifestations include cramping abdominal pain, vomiting, hematemesis, and occult or gross blood in the stool. Intussusception, bowel obstruction, and bowel infarction with perforation occur rarely, but one should keep these complications in mind because of their serious consequences.[151] Renal manifestations occur in two thirds of all cases and potentially produce the greatest morbidity. These vary from asymptomatic microscopic hematuria to a

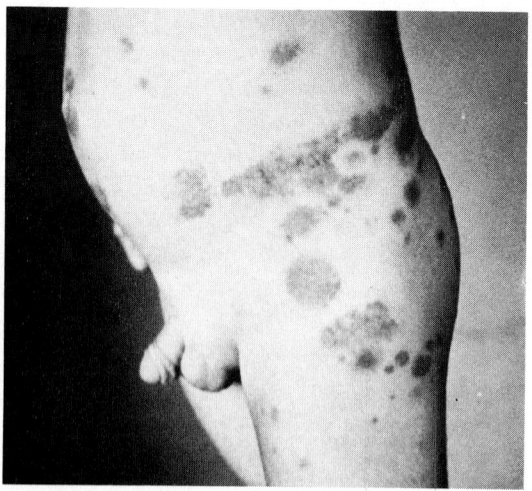

FIGURE 17–11 After a streptococcal infection of his throat, a 14-year-old boy developed Henoch-Schönlein purpura (anaphylactoid purpura) and associated urticarial erythematous lesions with purpura, painful articular swelling, and microscopic hematuria.

nephrotic or nephritic syndrome, with focal proliferative glomerulonephritis possibly progressing to chronic renal failure.[152] Central nervous system involvement fortunately is rare but may result in seizure disorders, paresis, and coma.[153] The duration of the disease is usually four to six weeks, with no sequelae in most patients.

LABORATORY DATA

Hematological studies of the patient's clotting functions, including prothrombin time, partial thromboplastin time, and platelet count, do not show abnormalities in HSP. In contrast to glomerulonephritis following streptococcal infection, serum complement levels are normal. Anemia due to blood loss may be present; the erythrocyte sedimentation rate is usually increased. Examination of the urine may reveal the presence of microscopic hematuria, pyuria, casts, and proteinuria. The stool may contain occult blood. In summary, there are no laboratory tests of the blood specifically indicative of HSP.

HISTOLOGY AND PATHOGENESIS

Biopsy specimens of a purpuric skin lesion contain leukocytoclastic vasculitis consisting of a polymorphonuclear and lymphocytic invasion and necrosis of the blood vessel walls and subsequent thrombus formation. Erythrocytes extravasated into the dermis account for the purpuric component.[14]

Ullman[154] demonstrated the presence of IgG, C3, and fibrinogen at the dermal-epidermal junction and within the vessel walls of involved and uninvolved skin of patients with Henoch-Schönlein purpura, suggesting the presence of an immune complex–mediated disease. Similar deposits have been found in the renal glomeruli and in the rectal mucosa of affected patients.[155] Ansell[156] demonstrated focal areas of vasculitis in the small intestine during crises of abdominal pain. Recently, IgA, C3, fibrin, and fibrinogen have been demonstrated in the purpuric lesions and glomeruli, suggesting that the alternate complement system may also be involved.[157b]

DIFFERENTIAL DIAGNOSIS

Since Henoch-Schönlein purpura can present such a varied picture, many possible diagnoses may have to be considered. These include post-streptococcal acute glomerulonephritis, juvenile rheumatoid arthritis, acute rheumatic fever, polyarteritis nodosa, lupus erythematosus, ulcerative colitis, regional enteritis, and acute intra-abdominal crises in addition to septicemia with disseminated intravascular coagulation. Hypergammaglobulinemic purpura, associated with petechiae on the lower extremities and a polyclonal gammopathy, may also enter the differential diagnosis.[157a]

TREATMENT

Most cases of HSP are mild, requiring no pharmacological therapy. Infectious causes should be sought and treated appropriately when possible.

Salicylates are not the treatment of choice for the joint symptoms, since gastric ulceration and platelet dysfunction may result,[145] confusing the problem and possibly increasing the risk of morbidity. Systemic corticosteroids, such as prednisone 2 mg/kg/day up to 60 mg a day, may provide prompt symptomatic relief of severe joint pain.[149] Although the skin manifestations do not always respond to such therapy, corticosteroids may lessen the severity of abdominal pain and help prevent gastrointestinal catastrophes.[145] In prolonged courses of treatment, Hurley[155] has shown that prednisone (60 mg/m^2/day) in combination with azathioprine (4 mg/kg/day) may be effective in the control of patients wih severe renal damage and nephrotic syndrome.

MUCHA-HABERMANN DISEASE

Mucha-Habermann disease, also known as pityriasis lichenoides et varioliformis acuta, is a self-limited condition characterized by crops of scattered, scaling, papular, and necrotic lesions. About one fifth of all cases occur in the 11 to 20 year age group. Mucha-Habermann disease is a form of vasculitis that in most instances follows a benign, two- to six-month course. The cause is unknown, and no transformation to a more serious form of vasculitis or predisposition to malignant change has been found.[158]

CLINICAL COURSE

Successive crops of red papules and papulovesicles, 2 to 5 mm in size (Fig. 17–12), develop suddenly on the trunk. The lesions may number from five to 10 or be very numerous and widespread, in some cases involving the oral mucosa. Progression of the primary lesion results in central hemorrhagic necrosis and crusting (Fig. 17–13). Superficial scarring follows the healing stage. Most patients experience new lesions for eight to 26 weeks and rarely may have mild systemic symptoms, such as low-grade fever. In most patients, the skin is the only organ affected. Burke[159] has reported a variant of Mucha-Habermann

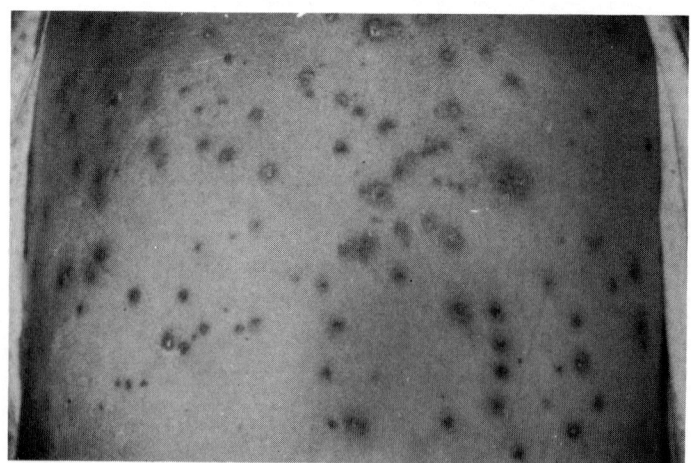

FIGURE 17–12 Mucha-Habermann disease. (Courtesy of Dr. Steven Roberts)

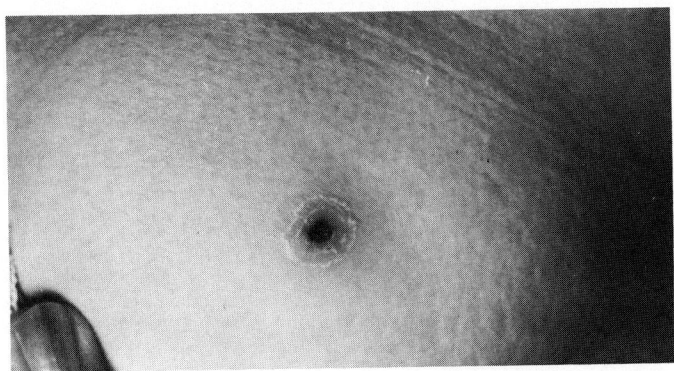

FIGURE 17–13 Mucha-Habermann disease. Ripe lesion with central necrosis. (Courtesy of Dr. Steven Roberts)

disease (Degos type) with a severe febrile course and large ulceronecrotic skin lesions. In the rare severe case, the prognosis is guarded.

The etiology of Mucha-Habermann disease remains elusive. Zlatkov[160] demonstrated positive complement fixation to Toxoplasma in the serum of affected individuals and in intradermal skin tests and postulated that Toxoplasma may play an etiological role. A viral cause has also been suggested but not proved.

Histologically, early lesions contain erythrocytes extravasated into the epidermis, superficial and deep perivascular lymphohistiocytic infiltrate, and overlying parakeratosis. As the individual lesion undergoes superficial necrosis, the epidermis becomes ulcerated. The endothelial cells of the small vessels become edematous, occasionally forming a thrombus; the dermal-epidermal junction becomes obscured, accounting for the lichenoid appearance of the lesion.[161] Direct immunofluorescence studies of the vessels have not been productive,[162] indicating that immune complexes apparently play no role in the development of this disease, in contrast to allergic vasculitis.[163]

DIFFERENTIAL DIAGNOSIS

Varicella may contain numerous lesions in different stages and may be confused with Mucha-Habermann disease. The course of the disease and the absence of multinucleated giant cells in scrapings taken from a vesicle base help to distinguish the two disorders. Papulonecrotic tuberculid, variola, insect bite reaction, and secondary syphilis may be considered, but histological examination of a lesion will help to identify the process.

TREATMENT

Topical and systemically administered corticosteroids, antimalarials, sulfones and isoniazid have not proved to be very efficacious therapy for Mucha-Habermann disease. Shelley[164] has reported successful control with high-dose tetracycline (2 gm a day) in some cases. However, tetracycline should not be used in children under eight years of age because of potential enamel hypoplastic changes in the teeth. Methotrexate in a dosage of 7.5 to 20 mg weekly has brought about improvement in persistent cases, although lesions have recurred with discontinuation of the therapy.[165] Because of its potential for hepatic toxicity and hematopoietic side effects, this drug should be used for Mucha-Habermann disease only in the most unusual circumstances and after careful deliberation.

REFERENCES

1. Sheldon, J. M., Mathews, K. P., and Lovell, R. G.: The vexing urticaria problem. Present concepts of etiology and management. J. Allergy Clin. Immunol., *25*:525, 1954.
2. Champion, R. H., Roberts, S. O. B., Carpenter, R. G., et al.: Urticaria and angioedema: A review of 554 patients. Br. J. Dermatol., *81*:588, 1969.
3. Freeman, G. L., and Johnson, S.: Allergic diseases in adolescents. Am. J. Dis. Child., *107*:549, 1964.
4. Michaelsson, G.: Chronic urticaria. Acta Derm. Venereol., *49*:404, 1969.
5. Coombs, R. R. A. and Gell, P. G. H.: The classification of allergic reactions underlying diseases. *In* Clinical Aspects of Immunology. Oxford, Blackwell, 1963, p. 317.
6. Monroe, E. W., and Jones, H. E.: Urticaria: An updated review. Arch. Dermatol., *113*:80, 1977.
7. Lichtenstein, L. M. and Margolis, S.: Histamine release in vitro: Inhibition by catecholamines and methylxanthines. Science, *161*:902, 1968.
8. Warin, R. P., and Champion, R. H.: Urticaria. Philadelphia, W. B. Saunders, 1974, pp. 26–28.
9. Johnson, A. R., Moran, N. C., and Mayer, S. E.: Cyclic AMP and histamine release in rat mast cells. J. Immunol., *112*:511, 1974.
10. Lewis, T.: The Blood Vessels of the Human Skin and Their Responses. London, Shaw and Sons, 1927.
11. Majno, G., Gilmore, V., and Leventhal, M.: On the mechanism of vascular leakage caused by histamine-type mediators: A microscopic study in vivo. Circ. Res., *21*:833, 1967.
12. Matthews, K. P.: A current view of urticaria. Med. Clin. North Am., *58*:185, 1974.
13. Juhlin, L., and Michaelsson, G.: Cutaneous reactions to kallikrein, bradykinin and histamine in healthy subjects and in patients with urticaria. Acta Derm. Venereol., *49*:26, 1969.
14. Lever, W. F.: Histopathology of the Skin. 5th ed. Philadelphia, J. B. Lippincott, 1975, p. 133.
15. Vickers, H. R.: Dermatologic hazards of the presence of penicillin in milk. Proc. R. Soc. Med., *57*:1091, 1964.
16. Thorburn, R., Johnson, J. E., and Cluff, L. E.: Studies on the epidemiology of adverse drug reactions. JAMA, *198*:345, 1966.
17. Beall, G. N.: Urticaria: A review of laboratory and clinical observations. Medicine, *43*:131, 1964.
18. Freedman, S. O.: Clinical Immunology. New York, Harper & Row, 1971, p. 61.
19. Moore-Robinson, M., and Warin, R. P.: Effect of salicylates in urticaria. Br. Med. J., *4*:262, 1967.
20. Yurchak, A. M., Wicher, K., and Arbesman, C. E.: Immunologic studies on aspirin. J. Allergy Clin. Immunol. *46*:245, 1970.
21. Paton, W. D. M.: Histamine release by compounds of simple chemical structure. Pharmacol. Rev., *9*:269, 1957.
22. Golbert, T. M., Patterson, R., and Pruzansky, J. J.: Systemic allergic reactions to ingested antigens. J. Allergy Clin. Immunol., *44*:96, 1969.
23. Juhlin, L., Michaelsson, G., and Zetterstrom, O.: Urticaria and asthma induced by food and drug additives in patients with aspirin hypersensitivity. J. Allergy Clin. Immunol., *50*:92, 1972.
24. Doeglas, H. M. G.: Reactions to aspirin and food additives in patients with chronic urticaria, including the physical urticarias. Br. J. Dermatol., *93*:135, 1975.
25. Sheldon, J. M., Lovell, R. G., and Mathews, K. P.: A Manual of Clinical Allergy. 2nd ed. Philadelphia, W. B. Saunders, 1967.
26. Warin, R. P., and Smith, R. J.: Challenge test battery in chronic urticaria. Br. J. Dermatol., *94*:401, 1976.
27. Waldbott, G. L. and Merkle, K.: Urticaria due to pollen. Ann. Allergy, *10*:30, 1952.
28. Shelley, W. B., and Florence, R.: Chronic urticaria due to mold hypersensitivity. Arch. Dermatol., *83*:549, 1961.
29. Frazier, C. A.: Cutaneous manifestations of insect allergy. Cutis, *13*:1038, 1974.
30. Barr, S. E.: Allergy to *Hymenoptera* stings. JAMA, *228*:718, 1974.
31. Blank, H., Shaffer, U., Spencer, M. C., and Marsh, W. C.: Papular urticaria. Pediatrics, *5*:408, 1950.
32. Rook, A., and Frain-Bell, W.: Papular urticaria. Arch. Dis. Child., *28*:304, 1953.
33. Massie, F. S.: Papular urticaria: Etiology, diagnosis, and management. Cutis, *13*:980, 1974.

34. Cohan, R. H., and Griffin, G.: Papular urticaria. J. Fla. Med. Assoc., 63:992, 1976.
35. Newcomb, R. W., and Nelson, H.: Dermographia mediated by immunoglobulin E. Am. J. Med., 54:174, 1973.
36. Winkelmann, R. K., Wilhelmj, C. M., and Horner, F. A.: Experimental studies on dermographism. Arch. Dermatol., 92:436, 1965.
37. Ostrov, M.: Dermatographia: A critical review. Ann. Allergy, 25:591, 1967.
38. Matthews, C., Kirby, J. D., James, J., and Warin, R.: Dermographism: Reduction in wheal size by chlorpheniramine and hydroxyzine. Br. J. Dermatol., 88:279, 1973.
39. Uehara, M., and Ofuji, S.: Abnormal vascular reactions in atopic dermatitis. Arch. Dermatol., 113:627, 1977.
40. Ryan, T. J., Shim-Young, N., and Turk, J. L.: Delayed pressure urticaria. Br. J. Dermatol., 80:485, 1968.
41. Warin, R. P., and Champion, R. H.: Urticaria. Philadelphia, W. B. Saunders, 1974, p. 136.
42. Patterson, R., Mellies, C. J., Blankenship, M. L., and Pruzansky, J. J.: Vibratory angioedema: A hereditary type of physical hypersensitivity. J. Allergy Clin. Immunol., 50:174, 1972.
43. Tindall, J. P.: Cold urticaria. Postgrad. Med., 50:133, 1971.
44. Houser, D., Arbesman, C., and Wicher, K.: Cold urticaria: Immunologic studies. Am. J. Med., 49:23, 1970.
45. Beall, G. N.: Plasma histamine concentrations in allergic diseases. J. Allergy Clin. Immunol., 34:8, 1963.
46. Wanderer, A. A., and Ellis, E.: Treatment of cold urticaria with cyproheptadine. J. Allergy Clin. Immunol., 48:366, 1971.
47. Griem, S. F., and Rothman, S.: Cutaneous sensitivity to cold. Am. Pract. Digest Treat., 7:1335, 1956.
48. Solomon, L. M., and Beerman, H.: Cold panniculitis. Arch. Dermatol., 88:987, 1963.
49. Delorme, P.: Localized heat urticaria. J. Allergy Clin. Immunol., 43:284, 1969.
50. Michaelsson, G., and Ros, A.: Familial localized heat urticaria of delayed type. Acta Derm. Venereol., 51:279, 1971.
51. Harber, L. C., Halloway, R. M., Wheatley, V. R., and Baer, R. L.: Immunologic and biophysical studies in solar urticaria. J. Invest. Dermatol., 41:439, 1963.
52. Warin, R. P., and Champion, R. H.: Urticaria. Philadelphia, W. B. Saunders, 1974, pp. 151–152.
53. Sams, W. M.: Solar urticaria: Studies of the active serum factor. J. Allergy Clin. Immunol., 45:295, 1970.
54. Takeshi, H., and Koji, M.: Solar urticaria: Photoallergen in a patient's serum. Arch. Dermatol., 113:157, 1977.
55. Sams, W. M., Epstein, J. H., and Winkelmann, R. K.: Solar urticaria: Investigation of pathogenetic mechanisms. Arch. Dermatol., 99:390, 1969.
56. Epstein, J. H., Vandenberg, J. J., and Wright, W. L.: Solar urticaria. Arch. Dermatol., 88:135, 1963.
57. Harber, L. C.: Solar urticaria. In: Demis, D. J., Crouse, R. G., Dobson, R. L., et al. (eds.): Clinical Dermatology. Vol. 4. New York, Harper & Row, 1974.
58. Reed, W. B., Wuepper, K. D., Epstein, J. H., et al.: Erythropoietic protoporphyria: A clinical and genetic study. JAMA, 214:1060, 1970.
59. Magnus, I. A., Jarrett, A., Prankerd, T., and Rimington, C.: Erythropoietic protoporphyria: A new porphyria syndrome with solar urticaria due to protoporphyrinaemia. Lancet, 2:447, 1961.
60. Shelley, W. B., and Rawnsley, H. M.: Aquagenic urticaria: Contact sensitivity reaction to water. JAMA, 189:895, 1964.
61. Chalamidas, S. L., and Charles, R.: Aquagenic urticaria. Arch. Dermatol., 104:541, 1971.
62. Kounis, N. G., and MacMahon, R. G.: Cholinergic urticaria with systemic manifestations. Ann. Allergy, 35:243, 1975.
63. Herxheimer, A.: The nervous pathway mediating cholinergic urticaria. Clin. Sci. Mol. Med., 15:194, 1956.
64. Goldman, L., Sawyer, F., Levine, A., et al.: Investigative studies of skin irritations from caterpillars. J. Invest. Dermatol., 34:67, 1960.
65. Maibach, H., and Johnson, H.: Contact urticaria. Arch. Dermatol., 111:726, 1975.
66. Weary, P. E., and Guerrant, J. L.: Chronic urticaria in association with dermatophytosis. Arch. Dermatol., 95:400, 1967.
67. Braverman, I. M.: Urticaria as a sign of internal disease. Postgrad. Med., 4:450, 1967.
68. Isaacs, N., and Ertel, N.: Urticaria and pruritus: Uncommon manifestations of hyperthyroidism. J. Allergy Clin. Immunol., 48:73, 1971.
69. Farah, F. S., and Shbaku, Z.: Autoimmune progesterone urticaria. J. Allergy Clin. Immunol., 48:257, 1971.
70. Black, J.: Amyloidosis, deafness, urticaria and limb pains: A hereditary syndrome. Ann. Intern. Med., 70:989, 1969.
71. Bourne, H. R., Lichtenstein, L. M., and Melmon, K. L.: Pharmacological control of allergic histamine release in vitro: Evidence for an inhibitory role of 3',5'-adenosine monophosphate in human leukocytes. J. Immunol., 108:695, 1972.

72. Dixon, F. J., Vasques, J. J., and Weigle, W. O.: Pathogenesis of serum sickness. Arch. Pathol., 65:18, 1958.
73. Cochrane, C.: Mechanisms involved in the deposition of immune complexes in the tissues. J. Exp. Med., 134:75, 1971.
74. Arakawa, M., and Kimmelstiel, P.: The glomerulonephritis of acute serum sickness: A study using light and electron microscopy. Am. J. Clin. Pathol., 54:60, 1970.
75. Shturman-Ellstein, R., and Kohler, P.: More on serum sickness illness and prodromal manifestations of viral hepatitis. J. Pediatr., 89:521, 1976.
76. Gigli, I.: Hereditary angioedema. J. Invest. Dermatol., 60:516, 1973.
77. Donaldson, V. H., and Rosen F. S.: Hereditary angioneurotic edema: A clinical survey. Pediatrics, 37:1017, 1966.
78. Donaldson, V. H., and Evans, R. R.: A biochemical abnormality in hereditary angioneurotic edema: Absence of serum inhibitor of C1 esterase. Am. J. Med., 35:37, 1963.
79. Johnson, A. M., Alper, C. A., Rosen, F. S., and Craig, J.: C1 inhibitor: Evidence for decreased hepatic synthesis in hereditary angioneurotic edema. Science, 173:553, 1971.
80. Ruddy, S., Gigli, I., Sheffer, A. L., and Austen, K. F.: The laboratory diagnosis of hereditary angioedema. Excerpta Med., 162:351, 1967.
81. Austen, K. F., and Sheffer, A. L.: Detection of hereditary angioneurotic edema by demonstration of a profound reduction in the second component of human complement. N. Engl. J. Med., 272:649, 1965.
82. Frank, M. M., Gelfand, J. A., and Atkinson, J. A.: Hereditary angioedema: The clinical syndrome and its management. Ann. Intern. Med., 84:580, 1976.
83. Donaldson, V. H., Ratnoff, O. D., Klemperer, M. R., and Rosen, F. S.: Studies on a peptide from hereditary angioneurotic edema plasma with permeability factor and kinin activity. J. Immunol., 101:818, 1968.
84. Frank, M. M., Sergent, J. S., Kane, M. A., and Alling, D. W.: Epsilon-aminocaproic acid therapy of hereditary angioneurotic edema. N. Engl. J. Med., 286:808, 1972.
85. Spaulding, W. B.: Methyltestosterone therapy for hereditary episodic edema. Ann. Intern. Med., 53:739, 1960.
86. Gelfand, J. A., Sherins, R. J., Alling, D. W., and Frank, M. M.: Treatment of hereditary angioedema with danazol. N. Engl. J. Med., 295:1444, 1976.
87. Jaffe, C. J., Atkinson, J. P., Gelfand, J. A., et al.: Hereditary angioedema: The use of fresh frozen plasma for prophylaxis in patients undergoing oral surgery. J. Allergy Clin. Immunol., 55:386, 1975.
88. Korting, G. W.: Diseases of the Skin in Children and Adolescents: A Color Atlas. Philadelphia, W. B. Saunders, 1969, p. 8.
89. Hellerstrom, S.: Erythema chronicum migrans afzelius with meningitis. Acta Derm. Venereol., 31:227–234, 1951.
90. Afzelius, A.: Erythema chronicum migrans. Acta Derm. Venereol., 2:120, 1921.
91. Lennhoff, C.: Erythema chronicum migrans. Acta Derm. Venerol., 29:310, 1949.
92. Degos, R., Touraine, R., and Arouete, J.: Chronic erythema migrans. Ann. Dermatol. Syphiligr., 89:247, 1962.
93. Hollstrom, E.: Penicillin treatment of erythema chronicum migrans afzelius. Acta Derm. Venereol., 38:285, 1958.
94. Scrimenti, R. J.: Erythema chronicum migrans. Arch. Dermatol., 102:104, 1970.
95. Hellerstrom, S.: Beitrag zur Pathogenese des Erythema Chronicum Migrans Afzelii. Acta Derm. Venereol., 14:517, 1933.
96. Binder, E., Doepfmer, R., and Hornstein, O.: Experimentelle Ubertragung des Erythema Chronicum Migrans von Mensch zu Mensch. Hautarzt, 6:494, 1955.
97. Steere, A. C., Malawista, S. E., Snydman, D. R., et al.: An epidemic of oligoarticular arthritis in children and adults in three Connecticut communities. Arthritis Rheum., 20:7, 1977.
98. Steere, A. C., Hardin, J. A., and Malawista, S. E.: Erythema chronicum migrans and Lyme arthritis: cryoimmunoglobulins and clinical activity of skin and joints. Science, 196:1121, 1971.
99. Canizares, O.: Cutaneous lesions of rheumatic fever. Arch. Dermatol., 76:702, 1951.
100. Stollerman, G. H., Markowitz, M., Taranta, A., et al.: Jones criteria (revised) for guidance in the diagnosis of rheumatic fever (committee report). Circulation, 32:664, 1965.
101. Johnson, C. C., Hanson, N. O., and Good, C. A.: Erythema nodosum: The possible significance of associated pulmonary hilar adenopathy. Ann. Intern. Med., 34:938, 1951.
102. Doxiadis, S. A.: Erythema nodosum in children. Medicine, 30:283, 1951.
103. Scott, T. F.: Erythema nodosum in "hypersensitivity syndromes." Pediat. Clin. North Am., 3:771, 1956.
104. Kibel, M. A.: Erythema nodosum in children. S. Afr. Med. J. Sci., 44:873, 1970.
105. Fine, R. M., and Meltzer, H. D.: Chronic erythema nodosum. Arch. Dermatol., 100:33, 1969.
106. Laurance, B., Stone, D. G. H., Philpott, M. G., et al.: Etiology of erythema nodosum in children. Lancet, 2:14, 1961.

107. Hicks, J. H.: Erythema nodosum in patients with t. pedis and onychomycosis. South. Med. J., 70:27, 1977.
108. Dickey, R. F.: Erythema nodosum caused by *T. mentagrophytes* granuloma. Cutis, 9:679, 1972.
109. Darlington, L. G.: Erythema nodosum and oral contraceptives. Br. J. Dermatol., 90:209, 1974.
110. Kirby, J. F., and Kraft, G. H.: Oral contraceptives and erythema nodosum. Obstet. Gynecol., 40:409, 1972.
111. Daw, E.: Recurrent erythema nodosum of pregnancy. Br. Med. J., 2:44, 1971.
112. Pinski, J. B., and Stansifer, P. D.: Erythema nodosum as the initial manifestation of leukemia. Arch. Dermatol., 89:339, 1964.
113. Weinstein, L): Erythema nodosum. Disease-a-Month, June, 1969, pp. 3--30.
114. Vesey, C. M. R., and Wilkinson, D. S.: Erythema nodosum: A study of 70 cases. Br. J. Dermatol., 71:139, 1959.
115. Löfgren, S.: Erythema nodosum: Studies on the etiology and pathogenesis in 185 adult cases. Acta Med. Scand., 174:9, 1946.
116. Winkelmann, R. K., and Forstrom, L.: New observations in the histopathology of erythema nodosum. J. Invest. Dermatol., 65:441, 1975.
117. Forstrom, L., and Winkelmann, R. K.: Acute panniculitis. Arch. Dermatol., 113:909, 1977.
118. Forstrom, L., and Winkelmann, R. K.: Acute generalized panniculitis with amylase and lipase in skin. Arch. Dermatol., 111:497, 1975.
119. Forstrom, L., and Winkelmann, R. K.: Factitial panniculitis. Arch. Dermatol, 110:747, 1974.
120. Golding, D.: Treating erythema nodosum. Br. Med. J., 4, 560, 1969.
121. Schulz, E. J., and Whiting, D. A.: Treatment of erythema nodosum and nodular vasculitis with potassium iodide. Br. J. Dermatol., 94:75, 1976.
122. Shelley, W. B.: Herpes simplex virus as a cause of erythema multiforme. JAMA, 201:71, 1967.
123. Bianchine, J. R., Macaraeg, P., and Lasagna, L.: Drugs as etiologic factors in the Stevens-Johnson syndrome. Am. J. Med., 44:390, 1968.
124. Bhargava, R. K., Singh, V., and Soni, V.: Erythema multiforme resulting from insecticide spray. Arch. Dermatol., 113:686, 1977.
125. Bedi, T. R., and Pinkus, H.: Histopathological spectrum of erythema multiforme. Br. J. Dermatol., 95:243, 1976.
126. Baer, R.: Perspective: Erythema multiforme–1976. Am. J. Med. Sci., 271:119, 1976.
127. Ackerman, A. B., Penneys, N. S., and Clark, W. H.: Erythema multiforme exudativum: Distinctive pathological process. Br. J. Dermatol., 84:554, 1971.
128. Britz, M., and Sibulkin, D.: Recurrent erythema multiforme and herpes genitalis (Type 2). JAMA, 223:812, 1975.
129. Harley, R. D.: Erythema multiforme. *In* Pediatric Ophthalmology. Philadelphia, W. B. Saunders, 1975, p. 865.
130. Bluefarb, S. M., and Szanto, P.: Erythema multiforme: Associated with acute renal tubular necrosis. Arch. Dermatol., 92:367, 1965.
131. Comaish, J. S., and Kerr, D. N.: Erythema multiforme and nephritis. Br. Med. J., 2:84, 1961.
132. Costello, M. J.: Erythema multiforme exudativum (erythema bullosum malignans-pluriorificial type). J. Invest. Dermatol., 8:127, 1947.
133. Beutner, E. H., Jordan, R. E., and Chorzelski, T. P.: The immunopathology of pemphigus and bullous pemphigoid. J. Invest. Dermatol., 51:63, 1968.
134. Dick, H. M., Fraser, N. G., and Murray, D.: Immunofluorescent antibody studies in dermatitis herpetiformis. Br. J. Dermatol., 81:692, 1969.
135. Hambrick, G. W.: The treatment of erythema multiforme, dermatitis herpetiformis and pemphigus. Mod. Treat., 2:916, 1965.
136a. Shklar, G., and McCarthy, P.: Oral manifestations of erythema multiforme in children. Oral Surg., 21:713, 1966.
136b. Rasmussen, J. E.: Erythema multiforme in children. Response to treatment with systemic corticosteroids. Br. J. Dermatol., 95:181, 1976.
137. Soter, N. A., Austen, K. F., and Gigli, I.: Urticaria and arthralgias as manifestations of necrotizing angiitis (vasculitis). J. Invest. Dermatol., 63:485, 1974.
138. Sissons, J. G. P., Peters, D. K., Williams, D. G., et al.: Skin lesions, angioedema, and hypocomplementemia. Lancet, 2:1350, 1974.
139. McDuffie, F. C., Sams, W. M., Jr., Maldonado, J. E., et al.: Hypocomplementemia with cutaneous vasculitis and arthritis. Mayo Clin. Proc., 48:340, 1973.
140. Feig, P. U., Soter, N. A., Yager, H. M., et al.: Vasculitis with urticaria, hypocomplementemia, and multiple system involvement. JAMA, 236:2065, 1976.
141. Soter, N. A.: Chronic urticaria as a manifestation of necrotizing venulitis. N. Engl. J. Med., 296:1440, 1977.
142. Geha, R., and Akl, K.: Skin lesions, angioedema, eosinophilia, and hypocomplementemia. J. Pediat., 89:724, 1976.
143. Lo Spalluto, J., Dorward, B., Miller, W., Jr., et al.: Cryoglobulinemia based on interaction between a gamma macroglobulin and 7S gamma globulin. Am. J. Med., 32:142, 1962.

144. Kalowski, S., and Kincaid-Smith, P.: Glomerulonephritis in Henoch-Schönlein syndrome. *In:* Kincaid-Smith, P., Mathew, T. H., and Lovell-Becker, E. (Eds.): Glomerulonephritis. New York, John Wiley & Sons, 1973, pp. 1123–1132.
145. Sibler, D.: Henoch-Schönlein syndrome. Pediatr. Clin. North Am., *19*:1061, 1972.
146. Jensen, B.: Schönlein-Henoch's purpura: Three cases with fish or penicillin as antigen. Acta Med. Scand., *152*:61, 1955.
147. Ackroyd, J. F.: Allergic purpura, including purpura due to foods, drugs, and infections. Am. J. Med., *14*:605, 1953.
148. Burke, D. M., and Jellineck, H. L.: Nearly fatal case of Schönlein-Henoch syndrome following insect bite. Am. J. Dis. Child., *88*:772, 1954.
149. Ashton, H., Frenk, E., and Stevenson, C. J.: The management of Henoch-Schönlein purpura. Br. J. Dermatol., *85*:199, 1971.
150. Rogers, P. W., Bunn, S. M., Jr., Kurtzman, N. A., and White, M. G.: Schönlein-Henoch syndrome associated with exposure to cold. Arch. Intern. Med., *128*:782, 1971.
151. Feldt, R. H., and Stickler, G. B.: The gastrointestinal manifestations of anaphylactoid purpura in children. Mayo Clin. Proc., *37*:465, 1961.
152. Koskimies, O., Rapola, J., Savilahti, E., and Vilska, J.: Renal involvement in Schönlein-Henoch purpura. Acta Med. Scand., *63*:357, 1974.
153. Lewis, I. C., and Philpott, M. G.: Neurological complications in the Schönlein-Henoch syndrome. Arch Dis. Child., *31*:369, 1956.
154. Ullman, S., Halberg, P., Jorgenson, F., and Balslov, J. T.: Deposits of immunoglobulins and complement in the dermoepidermal junction of patients with anaphylactoid purpura. Acta Derm. Venereol., *55*:359, 1975.
155. Hurley, R. M., and Drummond, K. N.: Anaphylactoid purpura nephritis: Clinicopathologic correlations. J. Pediatr. *81*:904, 1972.
156. Ansell, B. M.: Henoch-Schönlein purpura with particular reference to the prognosis of the renal lesion. Br. J. Dermatol., *82*:211, 1970.
157a. Jacobs, J. C.: Hypergammaglobulinemic purpura in a child. J. Pediatr., *87*:91, 1975.
157b. Giangiacomo, J., and Tsai, C. C.: Dermal and glomerular deposition of IgA in anaphylactoid purpura. Am. J. Dis. Child., *131*:981, 1977.
158. Marks, R., Black, M., and Jones, E. W.: Pityriasis lichenoides: A reappraisal. Br. J. Dermatol., *86*:215, 1972.
159. Burke, D. P., Adams, R. M., and Arundell, F. D.: Febrile ulceronecrotic Mucha-Habermann disease. Arch. Dermatol., *100*:200, 1969.
160. Zlatkov, N. B., and Andreev, V. C.: Toxoplasmosis and pityriasis lichenoides. Br. J. Dermatol., *87*:114, 1972.
161. Szymanski, F.: Pityriasis lichenoides et varioliformis acuta. Arch. Dermatol., *79*:7, 1959.
162. Black, M. M., and Marks, R.: The inflammatory reaction in pityriasis lichenoides. Br. J. Dermatol., *87*:533, 1972.
163. Braverman, I. M., and Yen, A.: Demonstration of complexes in spontaneous and histamine-induced lesions and in normal skin of patients with leukocytoclastic angiitis. J. Invest. Dermatol., *64*:105, 1975.
164. Shelley, W. B., and Griffith, R. F.: Pityriasis lichenoides et varioliformis acuta: A report of a case controlled by high dosage of tetracycline. Arch. Dermatol., *100*:596, 1969.
165. Cornelison, R. L., Jr., Knox, J. M., and Everett, M. A.: Methotrexate for treatment of Mucha-Habermann disease. Arch. Dermatol., *106*:507, 1972.

18

MISCELLANEOUS DERMATOSES

by LAWRENCE M. SOLOMON, M.D.
with the assistance of
RAYMOND CAPUTO, M.D.
JAMES DAVIS, M.D.
DAVID EVANS, M.D.
MICHAEL GREENBERG, M.D.
CARLOTTA HILL, M.D.
EDWARD KEUER, M.D.
DOLAR KOYA, M.D.
NATHANIEL MORGAN, M.D.
ANITA PEDVIS-LEFTICK, M.D.

Previous chapters in this text have discussed many cutaneous disorders of major importance to the well-being of the adolescent. However, there remain a number of other conditions, which include the following categories:
1. Disorders of epidermal function, including pigmentary and keratinizing dysfunction
2. Spotty (papulosquamous) eruptions
3. Certain vascular disorders
4. Cutaneous problems related to athletic activity.

Each of these categories will be discussed briefly because each is of some significance to the adolescent. Some of these disorders, such as pityriasis rosea, are minor but occur very frequently in this age group. Others, such as dermatomyositis, are serious diseases that affect all age groups and are discussed more fully elsewhere.[104] However, some comments concerning their effect on the adolescent are appropriate. Still other conditions, such as vitiligo, are important by virtue of the cosmetic disfigurement they cause at a time when this aspect of a skin disease may seriously affect the quality of life.

ACANTHOSIS NIGRICANS

Acanthosis nigricans is a non-inflammatory dermatosis manifested by a light brown-to-black, velvety accentuation of normal skin lines in a symmetrical distribution. It may reflect the presence of such diverse processes as obesity, endocrinopathies, genetic syndromes, and skull fracture, but it is not necessarily associated with a disease state.[1] Acanthosis nigricans is clinically and histologically distinct, no matter what the inciting cause, and is itself not a malignant process. It localizes preferentially to the flexor surfaces, axillae, genital region, neck, or any other intertriginous area. On occasion, it may affect the mouth. An early sign may be darkening of the palms, elbows, knees, or the skin over interphalangeal joints, which the patient may mistake for dirt (Fig. 18–1). The transition from affected to unaffected skin is not sharp. Local conditions, such as maceration, excessive sweat, and heat, are aggravating factors in genetically predisposed individuals. Histologically, the lesions are the result of epidermal hyperkeratosis and papillomatosis without inflammation.

Curth[1] first demonstrated the significance of acquired (adult-onset) acanthosis nigricans as a cutaneous marker of internal malignancy. She proposed a classification of this disorder designating "malignant" (adenocarcinoma-associated) and "benign" types. In the adolescent, the most frequent causes of acquired acanthosis nigricans are obesity and endocrine disease.[1-3] There is also a congenital form, usually present at birth or appearing during the first month of life, which may be associated with profound psychomotor retardation. Still another type, familial acanthosis nigricans, has also been studied by Curth.[4]

"Malignant" acanthosis nigricans occurs very rarely in children and adolescents[5] and is associated with adenocarcinoma, Hodgkin's disease,[6] or osteogenic sarcoma.[7] In 60 per cent of the patients studied by Curth,[1] the malignancy and skin lesions were found concurrently. Rarely, the dermatosis improves with palliation of the malignancy and may exacerbate with its recurrence.[8] Lerner[9] has postulated that an unidentified peptide hormone originating in pituitary or neoplastic tissue causes the skin changes.

Obesity in adolescence is a predisposing factor in the development of acanthosis nigricans. In one study,[10] the only major variables were found to be a

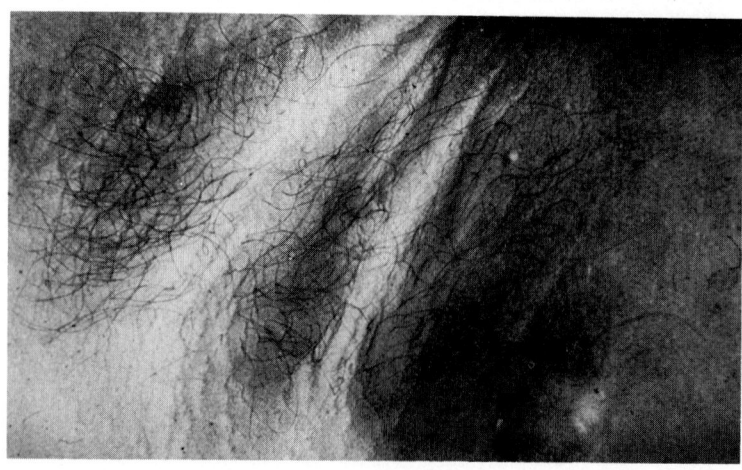

FIGURE 18–1 Acanthosis nigricans.

family history of obesity and preceding significant head trauma. The inability to identify a specific cause of acanthosis nigricans may be due to a lack of sophisticated procedures for measuring subtle changes in endocrine hormone levels or hormone receptor sites. However, massively obese patients with acanthosis nigricans have been found to have abnormal diurnal plasma cortisol levels.[11] Drugs, such as diethylstilbestrol, nicotinic acid, and corticosteroids, have also been said to produce this dermatosis.[3]

Pseudoacanthosis nigricans is a minor variant of the obesity-associated type,[1] which occurs in obese brunettes of both sexes. It will often regress after weight reduction.

DIFFERENTIAL DIAGNOSIS

Localized or generalized nevoid disorders of the epidermis (epidermal nevi or ichthyosis hystrix) may be mistaken in some instances for acanthosis nigricans. The confusion is compounded by the similar histological pictures these disorders may present. Nevoid conditions tend to have a linear distribution that stops at the midline and is asymmetrical, whereas acanthosis nigricans is symmetrically distributed in flexural areas.

Addisonian hyperpigmentation is not associated with textural changes in the skin surface. Erythrasma, which may be present bilaterally in flexural areas, can be diagnosed by the coral-red fluorescence it emits under Wood's light examination.

TREATMENT

Treatment of acanthosis nigricans is usually not very effective, although 0.1 to 0.5 per cent retinoic acid, 10 to 20 per cent urea cream, or 3 to 6 per cent lactic acid cream, applied topically, may provide some palliation.

VITILIGO

Vitiligo is an acquired chronic hypomelanotic disorder of the skin and mucous membranes. The incidence of vitiligo varies with geographical location, ranging from less than 1 per cent to 8 per cent. A recent epidemiological survey of the Isle of Bornholm in Denmark gives the prevalence of vitiligo as 0.38 per cent of a population of 47,033. Howitz and his colleagues[12] found that 11 per cent of new cases of vitiligo occurred in the age group between 10 and 19, but an analysis of 400 cases in patients of Indian descent revealed an incidence of 27 per cent of new cases in the same age group.[13]

In unremitting cases, depigmentation is often slowly progressive over a period of 15 to 20 years. Twenty per cent of persons with vitiligo have affected family members, although a genetic cause has not been proved.

ETIOLOGY

The etiology of vitiligo is unknown. A current hypothesis implicates autoimmune mechanisms, since some autoimmune disorders, such as achlorhydria, pernicious anemia, thyroiditis, insulin-dependent juvenile diabetes mellitus, and halo nevi, have been found in association with vitiligo.[14, 15] Self-destruction of melanocytes that somehow fail to protect themselves against the toxic metabolic intermediates generated during melanogenesis has also been postulated to occur in vitiligo.[16] The toxic metabolite theory is supported by evidence of the production of depigmented patches on the skin after contact with certain phenolic hydrocarbons.

CLINICAL MANIFESTATIONS

In some patients, the onset and progression of vitiligo appear to be related to episodes of physical or emotional stress. The condition may be manifested anywhere on the skin surface as hypopigmented or completely depigmented macules or patches, usually with well-defined borders. In dark-skinned people, the patchy depigmented areas are accentuated by the striking contrast with surrounding normal skin, producing a conspicuous cosmetic problem. This bizarre appearance may be particularly disturbing to the adolescent who is psychologically vulnerable to problems concerning physical appearance. The well-defined borders of depigmentation may appear to scallop the normal, sometimes hyperpigmented, adjacent skin (Fig. 18–2). Occasionally, mild inflammation may be evident at the borders, producing inflammatory vitiligo.[17] As the disease progresses, additional depigmented patches usually develop *in a symmetrical distribution.* Certain areas, such as the face, eyelids, and axillae as well as the pudendal and genital regions, are favored sites of onset. The skin over bony prominences and sites of trauma become vitiliginous as a result of the isomorphic or Koebner phenomenon,* which is also found in psoriasis, lichen planus, and several other skin disorders.[18] For unknown reasons, vitiligo will occasionally develop in a dermatomal or linear distribution pattern.[19]

Partial or complete repigmentation of vitiliginous lesions less than two years old may occur after prolonged sun exposure, particularly in younger individuals. Repigmentation usually develops in a perifollicular pattern, but it also may originate from the sides of the lesions. Complete repigmentation of all involved areas is the exception rather than the rule, and recurrences are common.

In general, the lesions of vitiligo are asymptomatic, although pruritus may be present in the marginal inflammatory type.[17] While sunburn may occur at sites of depigmentation, solar keratoses are not a frequent complication in affected areas. However, the depigmented skin may become rough and leathery after repeated exposure to the sun.

The general health of persons with simple vitiligo is not affected, provided no associated autoimmune disorders, such as pernicious anemia, hypothyroidism, hyperthyroidism, hypoparathyroidism, Addison's disease, diabetes mellitus, and rheumatic disease, are present.[20] The incidence of vitiligo appears to be greater among individuals who have alopecia areata and atopic dermatitis. Oculo-auditory syndromes, such as the Vogt-Koyanagi-Harada syndrome, characterized by uveitis, dysacousia, and patchy hair depigmentation,[21] may

---

*The Koebner phenomenon refers to the predilection of sites of cutaneous trauma to develop the disease.

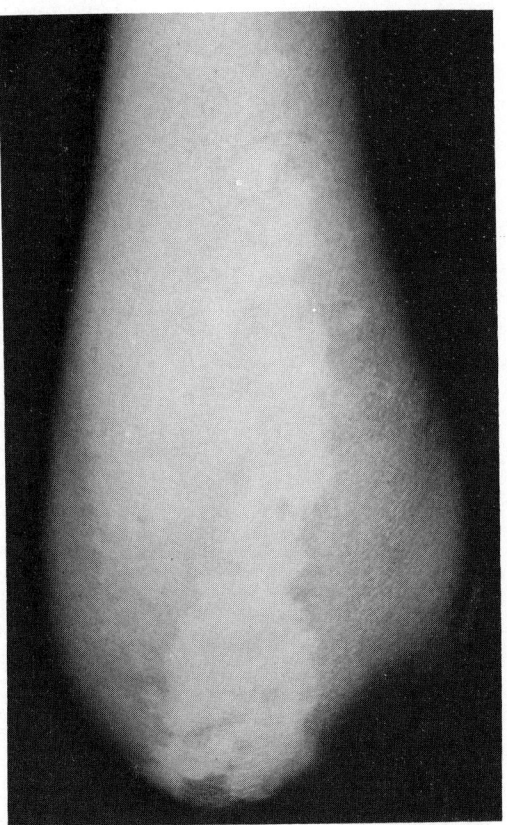

FIGURE 18–2 Vitiligo.

complicate vitiligo. Halo nevi, along with circulating antibodies against the cytoplasm of malignant melanoma cells,[24] may also accompany the lesions.

HISTOLOGICAL FINDINGS

Lesions of vitiligo contain either inactive melanocytes or no detectable melanocytes. A few melanocytes with sparse melanin granules may be found in early lesions. At the hyperpigmented borders of the lesions, the melanocytes often appear large, possessing long dendritic processes filled with melanin granules.[23]

Electron microscopic studies of specimens from the periphery of depigmented lesions disclose subcellular abnormalities in the melanocytes, such as vacuolization of cytoplasm, aggregation of melanosomes, autophagic vacuoles, fatty degeneration, pyknosis, and homogeneous cytoplasmic degeneration. Direct continuities between Schwann cell basal lamina of nerve endings and basal lamina of melanocytes occur in these areas.[24] Melanocytes are absent in specimens obtained from the center of old vitiliginous patches.

TREATMENT

The treatment of vitiligo is lengthy and not very satisfactory. Orally administered psoralens followed by graduated exposure to ultraviolet light

(UVA band) has been found to stimulate some repigmentation in patients with vitiligo of recent onset. Children may respond more rapidly than older persons,[25, 26] but their treatment often requires a prolonged optimistic effort. Kenney[27] considers psoralen-induced repigmentation to be more permanent than that induced by spontaneous resolution. Photographs should be taken prior to beginning therapy, so that the process of repigmentation can be followed accurately.

The use of topical psoralens followed by graduated exposure to sun or black light is a treatment modality under study.[28] However, it is hampered by the difficulty of applying the medication only to the affected areas in order to avoid increasing the contrast between areas of vitiligo and normal skin. The use of potent topical corticosteroids also has resulted in some repigmentation of early lesions.[29] However, the problems of steroid induced atrophy and systemic absorption complicate the long-term treatment of extensive vitiligo when this modality is used.

X-LINKED ICHTHYOSIS

All of the ichthyoses may affect the adolescent, causing considerable discomfort and psychological trauma. However, the skills of diagnosis and management of these hereditary epidermal disorders in the teenager are no different from those required in children or adults,[30, 31] with one exception. That exception is X-linked (sex-linked) ichthyosis, a condition that at birth may have the appearance of other forms of ichthyosis. However, the true diagnosis becomes apparent in adolescence, since it is during the second and third decades that a major marker of the disease, corneal opacities, becomes noticeable by slit lamp examination of the eyes.[32] As the name implies, this condition affects boys primarily, although an affected homozygous female has been described.[33] There is evidence to support the contention that X-linked ichthyosis is related to the Xg blood group.[34]

Deep corneal opacities may be found in almost all affected males and, with less consistency, in carrier females.[35, 36] The opacities are discrete, diffusely located near Descemet's membrane or deep in the corneal stroma. They appear as fine filaments, dots, or coronas which do not affect vision. Lenticular and fundal abnormalities may also rarely occur.

Clinically, X-linked ichthyosis is usually present at birth, very rarely presenting itself in the form of a collodion baby.[37] In the infant and child, one finds a scaly dermatosis affecting the scalp, ears, neck, and flexures, with accentuated involvement of the abdomen, back, front of the legs, and feet (Fig. 18–3). The scales are often large, dark brown and are shed episodically, leaving masses of keratin on bedsheets. The epidermis is found to be hypertrophic on microscopic examination. In the child, these features may not all be present, and in fact they may be barely noticeable until adolescence. X-linked ichthyosis not only is characteristic in the mode of genetic transmission and the nature of the ocular lesions it produces, but according to Wells and Jennings[38] it produces a fairly distinct histological and clinical picture in the skin.

The management of X-linked ichthyosis may be enhanced by appropriate genetic counseling and the topical application of a cream, lotion, or ointment containing concentrations of lactic acid of from 3 to 6 per cent, as tolerated.

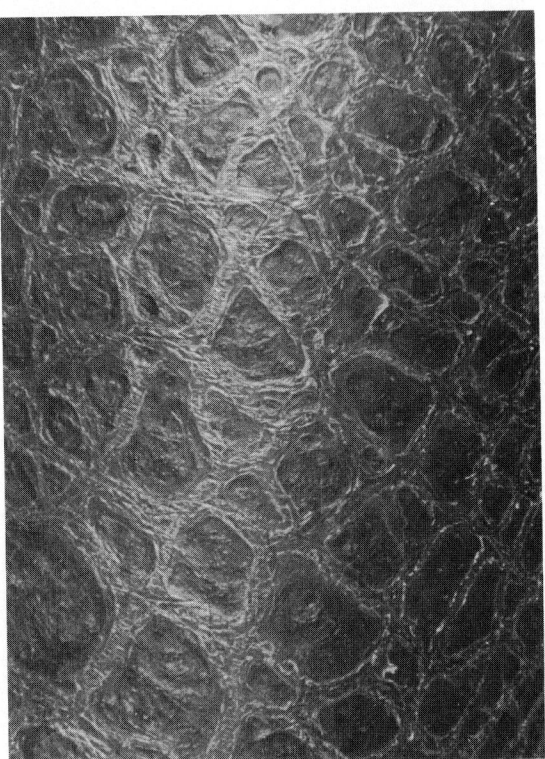

FIGURE 18-3 X-linked ichthyosis.

LICHEN PLANUS

Lichen planus, a unique dermatitis first described by Erasmus Wilson in 1869,[39] consists of violaceous flat-topped papules located on the flexor aspects of the arms, the neck, the legs, and the base of the spine. Changes may also be found on the nails and genitalia and, most characteristically, in the mouth (Plate XI–D). A variable degree of pruritus is usually present. While there are few data on lichen planus in children and teenagers, it was found to account for approximately 1 per cent of new cases registered at dermatological clinics.[40] The disease is quite uncommon in infants, though some patients are affected in childhood.[41-43] There is a higher incidence of childhood lichen planus in tropical regions[44] than in the U.S.A.

ETIOLOGY

The etiology of the eruption is unknown, although infection has been suggested by some authors.[45-47] Familial cases are rare, and the isolated reports of them do not support a genetic basis for the disease. Reduced levels of glucose-6-phosphate dehydrogenase (G6PD) have been found in some lesions of lichen planus,[48] yet red cell G6PD levels do not differ between patients with lichen planus and control subjects.[49] Interestingly, primaquine, quinacrine, tolbutamide, para-aminosalicylic acid (PAS), and thiazides, which are known to cause hemolysis in the red cells of G6PD-deficient patients, have produced an eruption clinically and histologically indistinguishable from lichen planus.[50] Gold, arsenic, quinidine, certain phenothiazines, analgesics,[51] and contact with color film developers have produced similar eruptions. Investigation has also been focused on the epidermis, including the melanocyte, as the primary pathological target.[52, 53] Dermal-epidermal deposition of C1q, C4, and C3 fragments and C5 has incriminated the complement pathway in the process.[54] However, it is possible that this phenomenon is secondary to the pathological changes in the epidermis.

CLINICAL SIGNS

Linear lesions may follow minor trauma to the skin (Koebner phenomenon), and a long streak of lichen planus is particulary common in affected children.[43, 55, 56] Unusual forms of lichen planus[57] include a very itchy hypertrophic (warty) variety involving the lower limbs and an atrophic (parchment-like) variety affecting the scalp.[58, 59] A lacy network of white papules is often found on the buccal mucosa, and rarely the tongue may be involved. The nails are affected in about 10 per cent of adult patients but not children.[60] Severe erosions following the appearance of blisters occur very rarely in the mouth[61] and on the feet.[62]

HISTOLOGICAL FEATURES

Under the light microscope, the lesions of lichen planus are seen to contain hyperkeratosis, hypergranulosis, irregular acanthosis, liquefaction degeneration of the basal layer, and a dermal lymphocytic infiltrate lying close to the adjacent epidermis.[53]

TREATMENT AND PROGNOSIS

Topically applied corticosteroids in emollient bases are helpful in relieving pruritus in most cases. An occlusive dressing, such as Saran Wrap, over the medication is useful for more resistant areas. Some success has also been achieved with the use of topically applied retinoic acid preparations[63] and griseofulvin[64] administered by mouth, but their efficacy must be confirmed by further studies. Intralesionally administered corticosteroids are quite effective in the treatment of hypertrophic lesions. Acute disseminated varieties of lichen planus may require administration of prednisone by mouth in doses of 20 to 30 mg per day. Oral lesions may respond to steroid mouthwashes or, in severe cases, to intralesional steroids or to surgery.

In approximately two thirds of patients, the disease remits within 15 to 18 months.[43, 56] Chronicity is characteristic of the hypertrophic variety and of the oral mucous membrane lesions. Lichen planus has not been found to be associated with any systemic disease, and though instances of epitheliomas arising in the lesions have been reported,[65, 66] the risk is slight.

PITYRIASIS ROSEA

Pityriasis rosea is a self-limited papulosquamous disorder, which occurs most frequently in adolescence.[67] A prodrome of headache, malaise, pharyngitis, and lymphadenitis may precede the onset of the eruption by one to two weeks. A "herald patch" appears first as a single oval area of scaly dermatitis 2 to 5 centimeters in diameter. It may occur anywhere on the body but is most commonly found on the trunk or the proximal extremities. One to two weeks later, a characteristic non-pruritic eruption follows, consisting of oval, fawn-colored scaly macules, whose long axes follow the lines of skin cleavage.[68] The pattern of dermatitis on the trunk often resembles an inverted Christmas tree. The collarette of scale is attached to the lesion peripherally, so that the free edges point toward the center of the macule (Plate XI–B). Although most lesions develop on the trunk, an inverse pattern may occur, with inflammatory papules starting on the wrists and thighs and spreading proximally to involve the trunk. This atypical form of pityriasis rosea may be extremely difficult to diagnose if there is no history of a herald patch having preceded it. Complete clearing of the eruption is usually apparent within six to 12 weeks; unless scratching and infection have supervened, there is no residual scarring.

Although the etiology of pityriasis rosea is unknown, a viral cause seems possible, since the condition occurs in epidemic forms[69] with seasonal clusters[68] and has a prodromal syndrome. Although a causative virus has not been identified, an immune response presumably does occur in affected individuals, because recurrence is very rare, and an increase in IgM-and IgD-bearing B-lymphocytes has been found in the acute stages of the disease.[70]

The histological features of pityriasis rosea are not diagnostic but include intraepidermal microvesicles, focal parakeratosis, and a superficial perivascular lymphohistiocytic infiltrate with mild exocytosis. Overall, the microscopic picture resembles that of eczema. However, erythrocytes extravasated into the dermis or epidermal area, such as those found in Mucha-Habermann disease, have also been described.[71]

DIFFERENTIAL DIAGNOSIS

The herald patch may be mistaken for tinea corporis, but the clinical course and the absence of hyphae in KOH preparations (see Chapter 3) allow one to distinguish between the two conditions. The other papulosquamous disorders, such as psoriasis, seborrheic dermatitis, lichen planus, and secondary syphilis, should also be considered. It may be necessary to leave the diagnosis tentative either until the condition declares itself over a period of weeks or as features of the other disorders appear. A serological test for syphilis is usually included in the initial examination of these patients.

TREATMENT

Pruritus, if it is present, usually responds to topical anti-pruritic lotions and systemic antihistamines. A mild erythema-producing dose of ultraviolet light has been reported to be efficacious in shortening the course of the disease.[72] In teenagers, exposure to ultraviolet light can be most easily accomplished by sending the patient outdoors to sunbathe cautiously. Reassurance that the condition is harmless and clears spontaneously is also helpful.

GRANULOMA ANNULARE

Granuloma annulare is a chronic benign dermatosis of unknown cause, characterized by one or more intracutaneous papules that tend to form ring-like configurations. Granuloma annulare was first described in 1895 by Fox, who referred to it as "ringed eruption on fingers."[73] It was Radcliffe-Crocker[74] who in 1902 gave the disease its present name.

ETIOLOGY

The etiology of granuloma annulare is unknown. For many years it was believed to be related to tuberculosis, yet in a study of 31 cases at the Mayo Clinic between 1916 and 1941, tuberculosis was found in only one patient.
Ultraviolet light, trauma, diabetes mellitus, thyroiditis, and insect bites have all been considered as possible precipitating factors. Attempts to reproduce granuloma annulare using various forms of trauma, including carbon dioxide snow, cantharides extract, and ultraviolet light, have all been unsuccessful.[75] Granuloma annulare, necrobiosis lipoidica, and rheumatoid nodules have all been believed in the past to have similar origins because of their similar histological features. However, the juvenile form of localized granuloma annulare is very rarely associated with systemic disease. The link between generalized granuloma annulare and diabetes mellitus is controversial. Wells and Smith[76] and Dicker and his colleagues[77] found no relationship between granuloma annulare and diabetes mellitus. The data collected by Rhodes and his coworkers[78] and Haim and his associates[79,80] demonstrated a significant relationship between disseminated granuloma annulare and diabetes mellitus. If such an association exists, it is seen only in the generalized form of the disease and primarily in adults, rather than with the single or multiple (10 or so) lesions found in children.
Granuloma annulare may be confused with tinea corporis because both form annular lesions. Granuloma annulare, however, lacks the scaling of tinea infections and usually has papules at the periphery. Other annular lesions to be considered include those of sarcoidosis, syphilis, annular lichen planus, creeping eruption, and insect bites.[79]

HISTOPATHOLOGICAL FINDINGS

The epidermis usually has a normal appearance, while the dermis contains one or several foci of partial or complete collagen degeneration. Lymphocytes, fibroblasts, giant cells, and epithelioid cells are present in the infiltrate. Vascular dilatation with endothelial swelling and mucin deposition within the degenerated collagen[81] complete the findings.

Using immunofluorescent techniques, Dahl and his colleagues[82] found C3 and inflammation in the blood vessels and fibrinogen deposited in the degenerated collagen of biopsy specimens of granuloma annulare lesions. They hypothesized that chronic immune vasculitis could be involved in the pathogenesis of the disorder.

COURSE

Prognosis is not affected by age, sex, or number of lesions. Fifty per cent of cases resolve within two years. Of these, 40 per cent recur, usually at the site of initial involvement. Of these recurrences, 80 per cent resolve within two years.

Wells and Smith[76] compared the course of 125 untreated patients with that of 83 patients who had undergone one or more forms of treatment, including vitamin E, occlusion, carbon dioxide snow, x-irradiation, and trauma to the lesion (biopsy). None of these caused a significant decrease in the rate of resolution of the eruption. Granuloma annulare, however, has been found to resolve during pregnancy and after measles.[83]

Granuloma annulare has been recorded in every age group from seven months of age to 76 years. Females are affected twice as often as males, but 66 per cent of cases begin before the age of 30.[76] Familial cases have been documented but are rare.[84] One of us (LMS) has the impression that granuloma annulare occurs more frequently in atopic individuals.

CLINICAL FINDINGS

The eruption usually begins with a papule or nodule that involutes centrally and extends peripherally to form a ringed structure bordered by individual nodules or papules. The papules or nodules may be yellow, pink, translucent, ivory, or the same color as the surrounding skin. The center of the ring may be either slightly depressed or at the plane of surrounding skin and may have a slightly erythematous or blue hue (Plate XII–C). The lesions may vary from 1 to 5 centimeters in diameter. Fifty per cent of patients have a single lesion,[75] but multiple lesions are common in children. The eruption is often symmetrical, affecting the dorsa of the hands and the forearms in 60 per cent of cases, the feet and legs in 20 per cent, the trunk alone in 8 per cent, and the trunk and an extremity in 5 per cent. It rarely occurs on the palms, soles, scalp, or face. One case reported involvement of the mucous membranes.[76] The legs and feet are more commonly affected in children than in adults.

Atypical forms of granuloma annulare do exist, and these may present with papules, plaques, or nodules. Giant lesions have been observed as well as subcutaneous and disseminated papules. All the atypical forms may develop the characteristic annular lesions of granuloma annulare.[79] Rubin and Lynch[85] described five cases of the subcutaneous form in children, in which subcutaneous nodules were found most frequently on the palms, buttocks, scalp, and legs. Generalized perforating (ulcerating) granuloma annulare is rare but also affects children. The lesions tend to be located on the extremities and become exacerbated in the summer.[86]

TREATMENT

Treatments that have been applied in the past include x-irradiation, liquid nitrogen, ethyl chloride, or Freon spray, intralesional steroid injections, chloroquine, diethylstilbestrol, gold injections, and antihistamines. None of these has been found to curtail the course of the disease.

The treatment that has been consistently found most effective is the intralesional injection of triamcinolone acetonide or the administration of systemic corticosteroids. Sparrow and Abell[87] treated 45 cases of granuloma annulare with either intralesional injections of triamcinolone or saline. In 70 per cent of patients treated with triamcinolone and 40 per cent of those treated with saline, there was resolution of the lesions. Recurrence of lesions followed in 80 per cent of each group, but the new lesions responded rapidly to retreatment. In the disseminate form of granuloma annulare, only systemic steroids may alter the course of the disease.

In most patients with few lesions, the condition is asymptomatic and follows a benign course, so that intervention should not be necessary if the patient acquires an understanding of the process.

LICHEN SCLEROSUS ET ATROPHICUS

Lichen sclerosus et atrophicus is a benign disease of unknown etiology, occurring predominantly in females. It is characterized clinically by distinctive white papules and plaques that show a predilection for the anogenital area. The first clinical description of the condition was offered by Hallopeau in 1887, and five years later Darier described its histological characteristics. About 10 per cent of cases of lichen sclerosus et atrophicus begin before the age of 13,[88] and these occur almost exclusively in females. Only 10 instances have been reported in which prepubertal males were affected.[89] The disease has been found in both sexes in both black and Caucasian children. Very rarely, more than one member of a family may be affected. In adults, lichen sclerosus et atrophicus is typically a disease of menopausal females. In one large series, the female-to-male ratio was estimated to be about 10 to one.[90]

CLINICAL FEATURES

The primary lesions are slightly raised, flat-topped, white, polygonal papules containing tiny dark dots. Individual papules may coalesce to form plaques surrounded by an erythematous border. Purpura, small bullae, and telangiectasias may be seen within plaques in the genital area. Older lesions become atrophic and develop a parchment-like surface with hyperpigmentation at the periphery. Excoriations, maceration, and ulceration may be superimposed on the primary lesions (Plate XII–A).

The lesions may begin asymmetrically but in time usually become symmetically distributed.[91] Although the anogenital area is involved in the majority of cases, lesions may occur anywhere on the body with or without anogenital involvement. In females, anogenital lesions tend to surround both the vulva and the anus, producing an hourglass or figure eight pattern. In uncircumcised males, an annular zone of induration may form on the mucosal surface of the prepuce about the preputial orifice.[92] Lesions may also occur on the glans and shaft of the penis. Extragenital sites of predilection include the upper trunk, neck, axillae, breasts, forearms, and face. Oral mucous membrane lesions have been found in adults. The symptoms produced by genital lesions in girls tend to be less severe than those in women and include pruritus, irritation, burning, soreness, vaginal discharge, dysuria, constipation, pain on defecation, bleeding, and exudation.[90, 93-98] But genital lesions may also be symptomless.[93, 95] In males, dysuria and inability to retract the prepuce may be an early indication of the disease.[92] Extragenital lesions tend to be asymptomatic.

The general health of patients remains good. No abnormalities other than local tissue changes are known to be associated with lichen sclerosus et atrophicus, so that no laboratory studies of body fluids have yielded useful information.

However, lichen sclerosus et atrophicus in girls is frequently associated with vulvovaginitis. Other less commonly associated diseases are morphea,[90] congenital defects of the genitourinary system,[95] recurrent urinary tract infections,[95, 98] and self-induced ulcerations.[90]

The Koebner phenomenon has been well documented in childhood lichen sclerosus et atrophicus. Lesions may develop in surgical scars[94, 96] or in a vaccination site.[100] Reactivation of quiescent disease[96] as well as exacerbation of existing disease[95] may take place following trauma.

HISTOPATHOLOGICAL FINDINGS

The histopathological changes found in lichen sclerosus et atrophicus in children are identical to those seen in adults. The well-recognized features[99] include hyperkeratosis of the superficial epidermis, with plugging of the hair follicles, thinning of the stratum malpighii (sometimes associated with loss of the rete ridges), liquefaction degeneration of the basal layer, edema, homogenization of the collagen in the upper dermis, and a band-like infiltrate of (predominantly) lymphocytes in the mid-dermis.[99]

ETIOLOGY

Although the etiology of lichen sclerosus et atrophicus is unknown, its frequent association with vulvovaginitis and trauma has led some authors to speculate that trauma and local irritation may be provoking factors.[96] On the other hand, the preponderance of cases in females and the frequency of onset at menopause and improvement at puberty suggest that hormonal factors may play some role[101] in the course of the disease.

DIFFERENTIAL DIAGNOSIS

The differential diagnosis of adolescent lichen sclerosus et atrophicus may include guttate morphea, atrophic lichen planus, candidiasis, and irritant or allergic dermatitis.

COURSE AND PROGNOSIS

The course of lichen sclerosus et atrophicus with onset in childhood is chronic and unpredictable.[102] In the majority of youngsters, the disease begins before the age of seven; the youngest patient to be reported was only a few weeks old.[95] Although many patients improve at menarche, some do not, and in others the disease may become worse.[95] The effects of pregnancy also are variable,[90, 93, 95] and anovulatory drugs seem to have a deleterious effect.[90, 95] However, the prognosis of childhood lichen sclerosus et atrophicus is somewhat better than that of adult-onset disease. In adults, involution is uncommon and is usually accompanied by residual atrophy. In contrast, approximately two thirds of children improve or undergo involution during puberty.[90, 95, 98] Involution may be a very slow process, taking place over months or years, and it does not appear to be hastened by any form of treatment. Furthermore, involution in childhood often takes place without residual atrophy.[95] In patients in whom apparent involution has taken place, the disease may be reactivated years later by trauma,[96] pregnancy, and anovulatory drugs.[90]

When anogenital lichen sclerosus et atrophicus persists beyond the pubertal years, complications are frequently seen. In females, atrophy of the clitoris and labia minora (with fusion of the latter) may be seen as well as stricture of the introitus.[90, 98] The possibility of lichen sclerosus et atrophicus being a premalignant condition perhaps has been overstated. Longstanding disease acquired in childhood and persisting into adulthood has in one instance resulted in carcinoma, but this transformation must be extremely rare. More important, there is often confusion at the clinical and histological levels between lichen sclerosus et atrophicus, atrophic lichen planus, and leukoplakia. In such cases, the pathologist's diagnosis may require a second or third opinion and must be buttressed by the clinical evolution of the disease.

TREATMENT

There is no specific treatment for lichen sclerosus et atrophicus. Pruritus usually responds to topical steroids and lubricants.[89, 90, 94, 95, 98] Patients should be instructed in good personal hygiene and avoidance of trauma to the affected area.[93, 98] Circumcision or a dorsal slit operation provides relief in cases of acquired phimosis.[92]

JUVENILE DERMATOMYOSITIS

Since dermatomyositis was first described in 1887 by Unverricht,[103] juvenile and adult forms have been distinguished. When dermatomyositis affects the teenager, it often takes on the juvenile form. Adult dermatomyositis will not be discussed here, since a thorough review can be found elsewhere.[104]

Dermatomyositis most often presents in the child or adolescent with fatigability, muscular weakness, stiffness, and a peculiar heliotrope color of the eyelids (Plate XI–A).[105] There is a slightly higher incidence in females.[106, 107] The etiology of the disease is unclear, but an immunologically mediated vasculitis appears to be present in affected tissues, with deposits of immunoglobulins and complement demonstrable in the vessel walls of muscles.[108] Evidence of lymphocyte-induced muscle injury has also been found.[109]

The diagnosis of dermatomyositis may be made on the basis of clinical symptoms, abnormal electromyographic studies, and increased serum levels of "muscle" enzymes (SGOT, SGPT, aldolase, and creatine phosphokinase or CPK). In the presence of a distinct clinical picture, biopsy of muscle and skin may not add significant information. We perform tissue biopsy only when the diagnosis is obscure. Activity of the disease may be monitored by sequential studies of CPK or aldolase in the serum.

Calcinosis cutis is seen more frequently in the juvenile than in the adult form of dermatomyositis. This may result from the greater amount of muscle destruction found in children with the disease. A study from the Mayo Clinic found that the skin, in 74 per cent of affected children, contained calcifications, as compared with 20 per cent in adults.[110] The calcification occurs most often over the proximal muscles of the shoulder and pelvic girdle. In spite of the disability caused by calcinosis cutis, which tends to ulcerate, the study found that calcinosis cutis signaled an improved survival rate, although it was a poor indicator of recovery of function. Treatment for secondary calcinosis cutis is disappointing. Chelating agents have been found ineffective,[111] while disodium etidronate (EHDP) shows some promise.[105] Surgical removal of calcified tissue may also provide a measure of relief.[112]

The association of the adult form of dermatomyositis with internal malignancy has been well documented.[113] This association is not found in the juvenile form, while another complication, gastrointestinal hemorrhage, occurs in the juvenile form but not usually in adult dermatomyositis.

Systemic steroids have been used with some success to treat childhood and adolescent dermatomyositis. Methotrexate and azathioprine have also shown some effectiveness.[109] We agree with Dubowitz[114] that moderate-dose, short-term treatment schedules, guided by clinical response rather than laboratory enzyme values, is the most reasonable approach to the disease and results in the greatest improvement with the fewest treatment complications. Death may result from gastrointestinal perforation, cardiac failure, palato-respiratory insufficiency,[105] respiratory distress, or cachexia.

THE SCLERODERMAS

Scleroderma, literally "hard skin," is, in reality, a group of diseases of unknown etiology characterized by inflammatory, fibrotic, and degenerative changes in connective tissue, with vascular lesions present in the skin and internal organs. The sclerodermas may be classified as follows:

A. Systemic
   1. Acrosclerosis
   2. Diffuse scleroderma
B. Localized
   1. Morphea
   2. Generalized morphea
   3. Linear scleroderma

a. En coup de sabre
b. Hemiatrophy

Various hypotheses have been offered concerning the cause of the sclerodermas, including infection, abnormal calcium metabolism, neural and vascular abnormalities and autoimmunity. Several pieces of evidence favor immunological involvement: There are serological immunological abnormalities; lymphocytes from affected patients have destroyed fibroblasts cultured from involved tissue;[115] and sclerodermatous changes have been noted in graft versus host reactions. A mutation involving the lymphoid stem cells and X chromosome could account for the preponderance of the disease in females.[115] However, most observers agree that, at present, the cause(s) remain unknown.

SYSTEMIC SCLERODERMA (SS)

According to Rodnan,[116] scleroderma was first described in a 17-year-old girl, recorded by Caulo Curzio in a monograph published in 1753. Yet, the data of Tuffanelli and Winkelmann showed that only 7.2 per cent of 727 cases had onset of the disease in the second decade.[117] Systemic sclerosis, although uncommon in children,[118, 119] is clinically similar to that seen in adults. In the adolescent, as in the adult, scleroderma (in both systemic and localized forms) preferentially attacks females in a ratio of approximately three to one. The clinical course is characterized by slow changes that may occur over weeks or years.[120] In a study of seven adolescents, tightness of the skin was the first symptom noted by four patients, a change in skin pigmentation was the initial symptom in two, and Raynaud's phenomenon in three others[120] (with more than one symptom occasionally present at the outset of disease). In one patient, Raynaud's phenomenon antedated the appearance of recognizable skin changes by six years. Although many of the patients described in the earlier literature probably had either localized scleroderma or scleredema (a more acute and less widespread induration of the skin), three patients described by Cockayne,[121] Dennett,[122] and Langmead[123] appear to qualify as cases of congenital scleroderma.

The natural history of skin lesions in scleroderma is as follows: First, localized erythema and edema occur, with the affected areas slowly becoming firm and waxy and sometimes surrounded by a violaceous halo. These changes are eventually supplanted by atrophy and hypo- or hyperpigmentation.[120] Telangiectasias and subcutaneous calcium deposits may follow and are nine to 10 times more frequent in females (Fig. 18–4).[115]

In children with scleroderma, Raynaud's vasospastic phenomenon is particularly common. Although trophic ulcers and infections of affected digits are not unusual, severe gangrenous changes and autoamputation of the phalanges are less frequent. Obstructive arterial disease is demonstrable by arteriography in 90 per cent of affected individuals.[124] Muscle weakness and atrophy may occur in as many as one third of children with SS.

Roentgenographic abnormalities of the esophagus are present in over 50 per cent of children with scleroderma accompanied by symptoms of esophageal reflux and dysphagia. Cardiac involvement may result from myocardial fibrosis or may arise as a complication of pulmonary hypertension or fibrosis. Renal disease is relatively rare during childhood but if it develops is a major cause of death.[124]

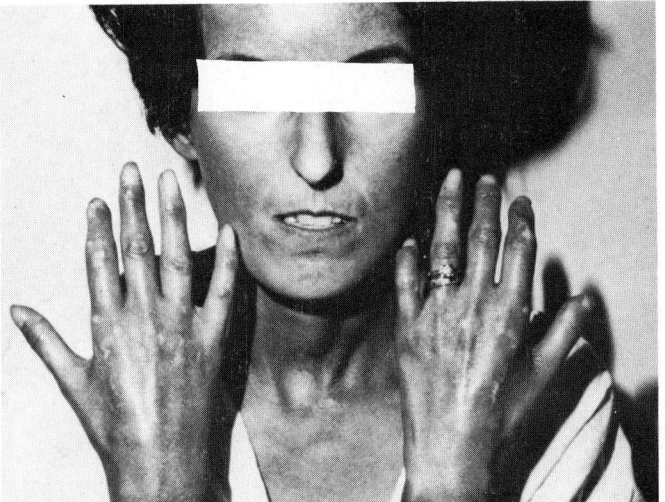

FIGURE 18–4 Scleroderma.

In the early stage, histological findings include thickened collagen, a mononuclear infiltrate between collagen bundles and around vessels, and inflammation of subcutaneous fat with replacement by collagen. In the sclerotic stage, the inflammation subsides, the dermal collagen appears thickened, and the eccrine glands are atrophied and "bound down" by collagen deposition. Occasionally, muscle fibers are vacuolated and separated by edema and by focal infiltrates.[125]

Routine laboratory studies are often non-specific. However, radiographic studies of the gastrointestinal tract and lungs along with pulmonary function studies, urinalysis, serum BUN and creatinine values, and CBC are helpful in detecting early sclerotic changes, anemia, thrombocytopenia, or leukocytosis. Non-specific elevation of gamma globulin was found in four of seven patients in the series of Kornreich.[120] The erythrocyte sedimentation rate, lupus erythematosus (LE) preparations, and tests for rheumatoid factor are generally normal. Antinuclear factors are seldom found in children with scleroderma (in one series,[126] two of 14 patients had significantly elevated titers), but the titers tend to be lower than in patients with systemic lupus erythematosus (SLE). Transaminases may be elevated as a result of muscle damage.

Corticosteroids, salicylates, D-penicillamine,[127] and chloroquine have all been administered with little effect in scleroderma. Surgery likewise has not been particularly helpful in its management. For the extremities, conservative orthopedic measures and physiotherapy may aid in preventing and minimizing contractures and deformity.[120]

The extent of renal, cardiac, and pulmonary involvement dictates the long-term prognosis. In five patients followed by Jaffe and Winkelmann,[119] the disease lasted from two to 21 years. A regression of sclerosis and reduced frequency of Raynaud's phenomenon was noted in some patients. Acrosclerosis (the more common type of systemic scleroderma) was believed to be less severe, less protracted, and accompanied by less extensive sclerosis of the viscera in children than in adults. Four of the seven adolescent patients seen by Kornreich expired, including three with evidence of cardiac and pulmonary complications.

LOCALIZED (FOCAL) SCLERODERMA

The etiology of focal scleroderma, like that of systemic scleroderma, is unknown. First described by Thomas Addison over a century ago,[128] focal scleroderma has been found in patients as young as two weeks. Because it influences growth of the affected area, deformity and malfunction ensue more frequently in children than in adults.[129]

Three types of focal scleroderma were described by Christianson:[130] morphea (including guttate lesions), generalized morphea, and linear scleroderma.

In Christianson's study of 235 cases,[130] 108 lesions were found to be linear, 83 plaque-like, and 44 generalized. The linear lesions were usually single and unilateral, affecting, in order of decreasing frequency, the legs, arms, frontal region (en coup de sabre), and chest.[130] Of the 108 patients with linear lesions, 26 had associated vertebral column anomalies, including spina bifida occulta, sacralization of lumbar segments, and extra lumbar vertebrae. Scoliosis and kyphosis are frequent complications.[131] A sizable number of patients develop unilateral atrophy of one or more extremities, facial hemiatrophy, or contractures of limbs or digits.

Lesions of the plaque type, as opposed to the linear type, are most frequently multiple, asymmetrically located, and bilateral. Affected areas, in order of decreasing frequency, are the thorax, trunk, neck, extremities, and face (Fig. 18–5). Occasionally, adolescents have decreased range of motion at a joint under or near a patch of scleroderma. Although rare, limitation of motion in an area not adjacent to focal patches of involved skin may result from peritendinous fibrosis. Arthralgias are common, affecting about one third of all patients with focal scleroderma.

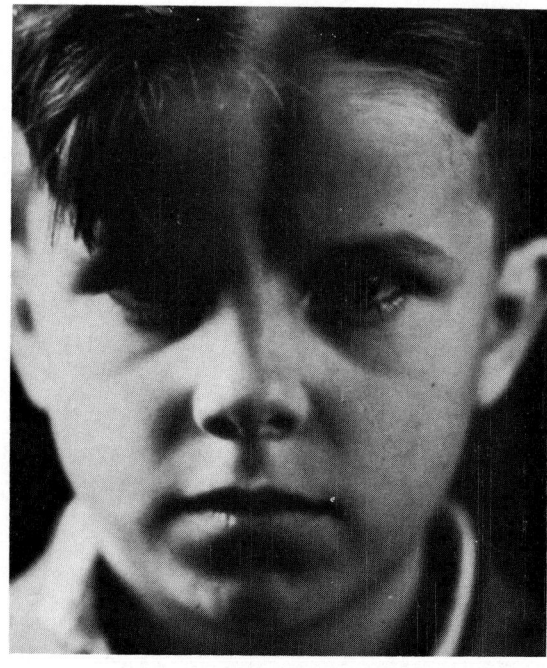

FIGURE 18–5 Morphea.

Complete remissions in focal scleroderma occur, lasting from months to years. However, in one case, recorded activity of the disease was maintained for over 33 years.[132]

PYODERMA GANGRENOSUM

The term "pyoderma gangrenosum" was first suggested by Brunsting, Goeckerman, and O'Leary in 1930[133] and probably represents the same condition given a variety of other names in the past.[134-136] Pyoderma gangrenosum is a severe chronic inflammatory disease of the skin which begins as a painful sloughing ulceration. The affected individual often has a concurrent disease that relates in a mysterious but positive manner to the cutaneous disorder.[133, 137, 138] Pyoderma gangrenosum may precede or follow the onset of the systemic disease.[139, 140] Forty-seven to 60 per cent of cases have been found to be associated with ulcerative colitis.[140, 141] Other gastrointestinal disorders, such as regional ileitis and polyps of the bowel,[142-144] have also been associated with the disorder, as have paraproteinemia, hypogammaglobulinemia, arthritis, empyema, polycythemia vera, and plasmocytic leukemia.[133, 145-152] Secondary anemia is a frequent finding.

While the etiology of pyoderma gangrenosum is unknown, numerous hypotheses have been proposed, including a localized form of the Shwartzman reaction,[153] involvement of proteolytic enzyme in the gut,[154] abnormal intravascular coagulation, altered immunoglobulins, primary vasculitis, and virus.[145] Malnutrition, avitaminosis, and lowered resistance to infection often seem to be predisposing factors. Bacteria isolated from the skin lesions are considered to be secondary invaders.

Pyoderma gangrenosum occurs in both sexes and in all age groups from early childhood to the 70's. The patient is often acutely ill and extremely uncomfortable and may require hospitalization. Some patients have died in the acute toxic stage of the disease. Pyoderma gangrenosum follows a well-defined clinical pattern with some variations, beginning as a crop of small discrete vesicles, pustules, papules, or nodules, surrounded by an inflammatory areola. The initial lesions then soften, ulcerate and extend peripherally in a serpiginous configuration, finally coalescing to form a large ulcer with an overhanging border (Plate XI-C). One or more lesions usually develop on the legs, although any part of the body may be involved. During the most active stage of ulceration, the tender border is well defined by a blue, edematous, boggy margin, measuring 5 to 8 millimeters in width. This border is extensively undermined by necrosis of the subcutaneous tissue.[133] The base of the central ulcer is moist and covered by mucopurulent exudate consisting of pus and necrotic tissue debris. When the general condition of the patient improves and the ulcer begins to heal, profuse granulomatous tissue appears at the edge of the ulcer. Eventually, a thin atrophic scar results.

The histological appearance of pyoderma gangrenosum is not diagnostic.[155] The dermis is necrotic, with mixed acute and chronic inflammatory cells, fibroblasts, foreign body giant cells, and plasma cells. The cellular infiltrate may extend into the subcutaneous fat. Direct immunofluorescent studies have not demonstrated the presence of IgG, IgM, IgA, IgE, or C3.[156]

TREATMENT

The administration of antibiotics has not been consistently effective in halting the progress of ulceration. Local palliative measures include prolonged immersion in a warm bath and the application of wet dressings with silver nitrate solution (0.2 to 0.5 per cent). Local surgery, cauterization, carbon dioxide snow, and x-ray treatment have no practical value in the therapy of pyoderma gangrenosum and may aggravate it. Treatment of any underlying associated disorder is essential to improve the skin lesions. Blood transfusion and correction of anemia also have been found useful. Administration of prednisone in doses of 40 to 80 mg per day (alone or in combination with Dapsone) has led to remission of skin lesions in many instances. Dapsone in a dose of 100 mg daily has brought about improvement in many patients but may induce[156a] side effects, such as anemia, neuropathy, and renal papillary necrosis, when used for prolonged periods.[156b]

NECROBIOSIS LIPOIDICA DIABETICORUM

Necrobiosis lipoidica diabeticorum (NLD) is a chronic progressive cutaneous inflammatory and scarring process characterized by papular or plaque-like lesions. It occurs chiefly, but not solely, on the legs and is seen primarily in females.[157-159] More than 80 per cent of all patients with NLD are Caucasian women, many of whom are diabetic. About 3 per cent of diabetic women have NLD, yet 87 per cent of all patients with NLD have diabetes mellitus.[158, 160] While NLD is seen in all age groups, about 20 per cent of cases begin in adolescence.[158] The course of NLD is similar for diabetic and non-diabetic patients.[157] In some cases, skin lesions precede the onset of diabetes by as much as eight years.[158] NLD may also be associated with an early diabetic state, demonstrable only by impairment of carbohydrate tolerance, evoked by stressing the individual with corticosteroids. The correlation between the course of the eruption and either hyperglycemia or glycosuria is poor,[161, 162] and control of diabetes mellitus with insulin and diet does not seem to influence NLD lesions. The severity and course of NLD does not necessarily parallel that of the coexisting diabetes mellitus.

Minor trauma seems to play a role in inciting the lesion, but the pathogenesis of the disorder remains obscure. Hypotheses concerning the pathogenesis of NLD include (1) primary vascular injury, (2) general disturbance in fat metabolism with local lipid disturbance in the skin, and (3) elevated circulating protein-bound carbohydrates in serum, with arteriole sludging, exudation of plasma, deposition of PAS-positive hyaline material, and eventual vascular occlusion with resulting dermal necrobiosis.[158, 163.]

The lesions are usually asymptomatic, although some patients complain of itching and burning. The lesions most commonly occur on one or both legs and more rarely on the arms, thighs, abdomen, breasts, face, and scalp.[159] The scalp lesions are associated with alopecia. The average number of lesions found is five, but it may vary from one to more than 15. The lesions range in diameter from a few millimeters to several centimeters.

The lesion of NLD often passes through several phases, beginning as a small, red, infiltrated papule that slowly enlarges and takes on a violaceous hue.

The lesion then becomes a slightly raised, firm, yellow plaque which may ulcerate in about one fourth of cases. Eventually, it involutes into a flattened, atrophic, yellowish patch with a scaly red or violaceous infiltrated border (Plate XII–B).[164] Although most lesions evolve into telangiectatic atrophic patches, 15 per cent clear spontaneously.[157, 160] Some lesions are unusual in that they resemble granuloma annulare.

HISTOLOGICAL FINDINGS

The lesions of NLD contain two distinct histological patterns: palisading granulomas and tuberculoid or sarcoid granulomas.[160, 165] A mixture of the two patterns is also seen occasionally.[160]

Palisading granulomas have foci of necrobiosis of collagen and elastic fibers, surrounded by a chronic inflammatory infiltrate focused around blood vessels. Obliterative changes may be seen in small vessels.[159] Varying amounts of phospholipids and free cholesterol may be found in the center of the lesions, associated with degenerated collagen and hemosiderin. Giant cells are also present but sparsely distributed.

Tuberculoid or sarcoid lesions have foci of epithelioid cells and an inflammatory infiltrate composed of lymphocytes, plasma cells, and giant cells of the Langhans' and foreign body types.[159, 160] Some giant cells contain asteroid bodies, which stain like elastic fibers. Very little necrobiotic debris accumulates.[166]

DIFFERENTIAL DIAGNOSIS

The diagnosis of NLD can usually be made clinically, although the lesions may be confused with xanthomas, which are also seen in diabetics and are firm, yellowish papules or plaques occurring on the extensor aspects of the extremities. The finding of intracellular lipids in the foam cells of the xanthomas permits differentiation of the two conditions.

Granuloma annulare is perhaps the one condition most easily confused with NLD, both clinically and microscopically. Granuloma annulare is more prevalent in children and adolescents, and the lesions usually are located on the dorsal aspects of the hands and feet rather than on the shins. However, in atypical cases, the eruptions may be difficult to distinguish.

TREATMENT

The application of topical steroids and the injection of corticosteroids into the lesion, using conventional methods or a jet injector, are of considerable value, particularly if the condition can be treated before the onset of severe atrophy or ulceration.[169] If the lesions respond to treatment, gradual resolution, with transient atrophy, tiny ulcers, and slight hyperpigmentation, is the rule. Surgical excision and grafting have also been advocated as treatment for NLD.[166-168] Recently, fibrinolytic agents[170] as well as stanozolol and nicotinic acid derivatives of inositol have also been studied and suggested as useful treatments for NLD.

SWIMMING POOL GRANULOMA

Atypical mycobacteria, such as *Mycobacterium marinum (M. balnei)*, may be inoculated into the skin through abrasions from swimming in a pool or natural waters, fishing, or cleaning a fish tank.[171, 172] Localized epidemics of cutaneous atypical mycobacterial infections have occurred in Sweden, the United States, and Great Britain, accounting for many of the more than 600 reported cases.[173, 174] The popularity of aquatic sports in adolescence probably explains the high incidence of swimming pool granuloma in this age group.

Mycobacterium marinum is an acid-fast, non-motile bacillus, which is longer and wider than *M. tuberculosis* and often has transverse bands. Aronson[175] first described the tuberculoid granulomas caused by *M. marinum* in the internal organs of salt-water fish found dead in the tanks of the Philadelphia Aquarium. *M. marinum* has a wide range of habitats, living as a saprophyte in water but also able to infect fresh-water and marine fish, other cold-blooded animals, and humans.[176] Growth of the organism in culture usually occurs in two to three weeks at a temperature of 30 to 33° C. Specimens may be obtained by direct scraping or aspiration from pus or biopsy material. Mycobactosel, a Löwenstein-Jensen medium containing antibiotics, is very useful for the isolation of *M. marinum* from contaminated specimens.[176] Cream-colored colonies incubated in the dark will turn bright yellow one day after exposure to light. In contrast to *M. tuberculosis* and *M. kansasii*, *M. marinum* does not grow at 37° C, which may account for the localization of the infection to the acral areas of the body, which are the usual sites of primary inoculation.

CLINICAL MANIFESTATIONS

Yellow or reddish pea-size papules and pustules with surrounding erythema appear 10 days to four weeks after inoculation of the organism from contaminated water or tissue.[177] The lesions tend to occur at points of trauma on the elbows, knees, hands, feet, or nose. The lesions generally enlarge and may develop into verrucous plaques or nodules with ulcerated centers (Fig. 18–6). While single lesions are the rule, multiple lesions distributed in an ascending

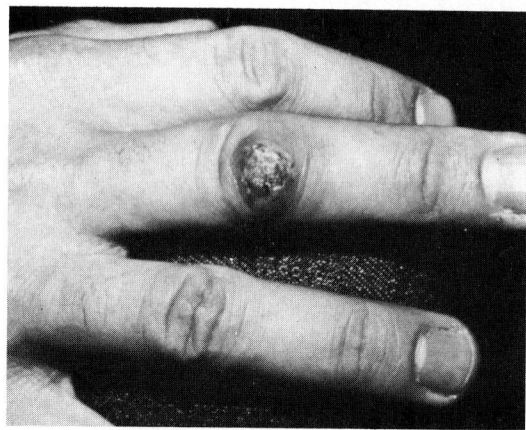

FIGURE 18–6 Inoculation of atypical mycobacterium (*M. marinum*) acquired from cleaning a fish tank.

lymphatic pattern are being recognized with greater frequency and *are highly reminiscent of sporotrichosis (sporotrichoid infection)*.[178, 179] The lesions usually heal with scarring within a few months to two years but have rarely persisted for as long as 27 years.[176, 180] Regional lymphangitis and lymphadenopathy are not common, and the patient's general health is not affected. Most individuals infected with *M. marinum* will react positively to routine skin tests for tuberculosis.[181] The usefulness of specific skin test antigen to *M. marinum* is quite limited because of cross reactions between different mycobacterial antigens, which may result in both false positive and negative reactions.

The differential diagnosis to be considered includes tuberculosis verrucosa cutis, nocardiosis, sporotrichosis, coccidioidomycosis, blastomycosis, histoplasmosis, leishmaniasis, yaws, syphilis, and benign and malignant skin tumors.

HISTOPATHOLOGICAL FINDINGS

Lesions two or three months old may show a non-specific inflammatory pattern with aggregation of neutrophils, monocytes, and macrophages containing the acid-fast organisms.[178] Lesions persisting six months or more usually have a characteristic tuberculoid pattern, with mixed groups of epithelioid cells, small lymphocytes, and scattered giant cells of the Langerhans type. Areas of necrosis occasionally occur centrally in some granulomas. With appropriate stains, acid-fast bacilli may be demonstrated within macrophages. The epidermis may show reactive proliferation with hyperkeratosis, papillomatosis, and acanthosis; an ulcer may also remove the epidermis in the center of the lesion.

TREATMENT

The atypical mycobacterial infections are relatively resistant to streptomycin, isoniazid, para-aminosalicylic acid (PAS), neomycin sulfate, penicillin, chloramphenicol, and thiosemicarbazone.[182, 183] Surgical excision or curettage and electrodesiccation may be attempted to eradicate small lesions. However, recurrences are not uncommon. Superficial radiotherapy has been reported to be successful in some patients.[179] Prolonged locally applied heat also sometimes leads to cure. Recent reports claim that tetracycline or a semi-synthetic derivative of tetracycline (minocycline hydrochloride) may be helpful in vivo, despite in vitro results to the contrary.[183, 184] Preventive measures consist of disinfecting swimming pools and avoiding direct contact with contaminated water by wearing protective gloves when cleaning fish tanks.

KELOIDS

Keloids are elevated fibrotic scars that progressively enlarge in an aberrant pattern. The aggressive scar tissue characteristically extends beyond the confines of the original wound and frequently invades the surrounding tissue with claw-like projections. The claw-like edges of the growth may account for the term "keloid," which is derived from the Greek word for claw ("chele") and the French "chéloide."[185]

Adolescents appear to be more susceptible to keloid formation than other age groups.[186-188] Males and females are equally affected. Keloids are approximately eight times more prevalent in blacks than in Caucasians,[189] but Bernstein[190] believes that Caucasians who reside in the tropics have an increased tendency to develop keloids. Omo-Dare's[188] epidemiological study in the rural western Nigerian town of Igbo-Ora (population 30,000) suggests that the predisposition to keloid formation is inherited as an autosomal recessive trait.

The etiology of the condition remains unknown. Recent investigations[191] on the biology of keloids have shown that the rate of collagen synthesis is greater in keloids than in either hypertrophic scars or normal skin. However, the inhibition of collagen degradation is also significant and possibly more important than the increased rate of collagen synthesis in keloid formation. Activated macrophages, which stimulate fibroblasts to collagen synthesis, may play some role in the pathogenesis of these tumors,[191, 192] but factors accounting for the initiation and sustenance of collagen deposition are far from completely understood.

CLINICAL MANIFESTATIONS

Keloids are firm tumors with shiny, hairless surfaces, which are often pruritic or painful, lobulated, and sessile or pedunculated. Invasive scarring beyond the borders of the original wound is characteristic of keloid and helps to differentiate it from a hypertrophic scar. Whereas the latter may be pruritic, tender, and elevated above the surface of the skin, it does not invade normal skin as the keloid does. Unlike normal scars, which may complete their molding process within one year, keloids may require as long as 20 to 40 years to reach

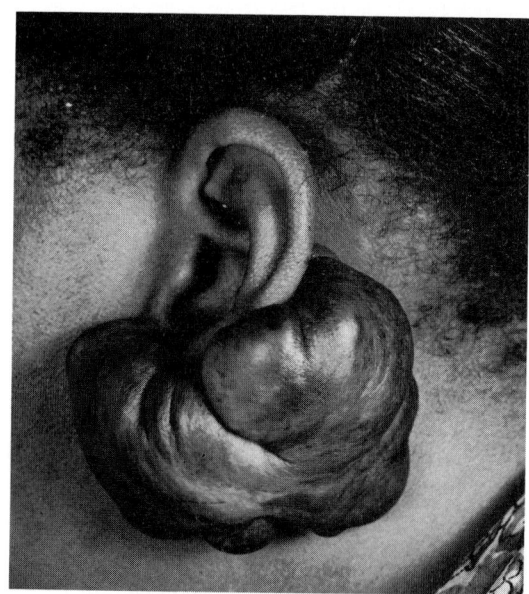

FIGURE 18–7 Keloid. Such lesions may complicate piercing of ears.

maximal growth.[193] Indolent ulceration may occur following trauma or application of heat to the skin overlying these fibrotic tumors. Some body areas, such as the presternal area, neck, face, and helix and lobe of the ear, are particularly disposed to keloid formation. The ear lobe is particularly susceptible to keloids secondary to ear piercing (Fig. 18–7). Sites of predilection are apparently related to the amount of natural tension in the region of the original wound. Increased skin tension in certain areas is related to the draping effect of the skin on the supporting musculoskeletal frame.[194, 195]

HISTOPATHOLOGICAL FINDINGS

Early hypertrophic scars and keloids are indistinguishable from one another on histological examination.[196, 197] Collagen fibers are formed in the granulation tissue during the early fibroblastic stage of wound healing. In keloids and hypertrophic scars, these collagen fibers are arranged in a characteristic whorl-like or nodular pattern.[197] In later stages, the number of fibroblasts and capillaries decreases. The lesions become less cellular, and whorls of hyalinized collagen without encapsulation are found in the dermis.[198] In hypertrophic scars, the nodules of collagen become thinner and straighter, with orientation parallel to the free surface of the skin. Unlike hypertrophic scars, keloids tend to retain their nodular patterns indefinitely.

TREATMENT

The treatment of keloids must be individualized according to the size, location, and duration of the lesion. Keloids tend to recur after excision and the completeness of local excision does not seem to affect the rate of recurrence.[199] However, surgery, followed by properly timed postoperative radiotherapy and intralesional injections of corticosteroids, may improve selected lesions.[186, 195, 200] The inhibition of keloid formation by postoperative irradiation is to be expected, since both proliferating fibroblast and endothelial vascular buds are radiosensitive.[200] Intralesional steroids alone will usually soften or flatten keloids that are less than six months old. The studies of Cohen and his colleagues[201] suggest that the abnormally high rate of collagen synthesis found in keloids of recent onset is not reduced by intermittent intralesional corticosteroid injections. However, their findings do indicate that the rate of collagen degradation is enhanced, possibly through increased collagenase activity.[201]

DERMATOLOGICAL ATHLETIC INJURIES IN THE ADOLESCENT

In previous chapters we have discussed the role of cutaneous injury in exacerbating existing disease. The active teenager may sustain minor injuries to normal skin while participating in athletic events. One of the more common injuries is a contusion, in which dermal or subcutaneous vessels are disrupted. The extravasated blood changes from its initial purplish-red to brown to green and then to yellow before it finally disappears by the process of phagocytosis. Elevation of the affected area and application of ice to reduce inflammation and swelling during the first 24 hours following a contusion should result in marked symptomatic improvement in the bruise and help to differentiate it from erythema nodosum, with which it may be confused.

"Black heel" or calcaneal petechia[202] is a traumatic subepidermal hemorrhage induced by strenuous athletic activity. The lesion usually consists of an irregular bluish-black plaque with surrounding punctate hemorrhages, located on the posterior or posterolateral aspect of the heel[203, 204] just above the border of the thick plantar keratin where the protective calcaneal fat pad diminishes.[202] These lesions are not palpable but are flush with the surface of the skin. "Black heel" is usually a painless condition.[205] On superficial examination, both the patient and physician may worry about the presence of malignant melanoma.[203] However, close inspection of the periphery of the black patch will reveal individual punctate petechial lesions. The overlying skin may be pared with a scalpel to expose the specks of dried blood.

"Black heel" is most often the result of playing basketball, racquet ball, tennis, and volleyball, sports that involve considerable twisting, jumping, and sudden stops. The sudden stop, in which the foot is slammed onto the floor or hard ground, causes a shearing stress[204] and vascular shock effect,[202] producing disruption of the papillary blood vessels. The same process may affect the edge of the palms[205-207] in weight lifters and chinners. Treatment is not required, since the lesions fade spontaneously.

Corns and calluses are areas of thickened stratum corneum resulting from repeated friction or pressure over the involved skin. Only a minimal amount of constant or intermittent pressure is needed to induce excess keratinization. A traumatic blister may develop if friction and pressure are increased beyond certain limits. The blisters are contained in the epidermis and result from necrosis of prickle cells. Talc applied to the hands is effective in preventing the friction encountered by gymnasts and weight lifters. Corns, calluses, and blisters may be caused by improperly fitted athletic shoes. Shoes that are too large permit the foot to slide, while those that are too short may cramp the foot.[208] The callus develops at the site of pressure, usually over the bony prominence of the foot, and discomfort ensues when the callus becomes too thick. To alleviate the symptoms, the keratotic covering may be shaved and 40 per cent salicylic acid plaster applied to the base of the callus. Painful blisters may be punctured and dressed with an antibiotic ointment.

Miliaria results from the exposure of an unacclimatized individual to a hot, humid atmosphere. It may take two forms: Miliaria rubra (prickly heat) appears as tiny red papules that represent rupture of individual eccrine sweat gland ducts by retained sweat, with subsequent inflammatory response in the dermis. Miliaria crystallina also is caused by retention of sweat in the ducts but at a more superficial level, with resulting tiny transparent superficial vesicles. The latter type of miliaria is most commonly a consequence of sunburn, and the vesicles disappear as the injured epidermis desquamates. Loose clothing may help to prevent miliaria, and the most effective treatment is to reduce sweating by applying talc to the skin and placing the individual in a cool, dry environment.

ARTHROPOD BITES

Insect bites are constant hazards of the human environment, and active teenagers are frequent victims. Most often, the bite will result in transient discomfort, pruritus, and a temporary blemish, although an anaphylactic reaction may be a rare complication. In the case of bloodsucking insect bites, it is not the mechanical aspect of the bite that causes the problem but components of the insect's saliva that are injected into the skin. The secretions produce pruritus and contain allergens responsible for local immune reactions.

Mosquito bites may produce an immediate reaction (wheal, erythema, and pruritus) or a delayed reaction (papular lesion with burning pruritus lasting for several hours).[209] Mosquitoes prefer warm, moist skin covered with perfumed products. Preventive measures include wearing light-colored clothing and using an insect repellant. Repellants containing DEET (diethyltoluamide) seem to be the most effective.

Biting midges (gnats) inject no anesthetic, so that the bite is felt and observed immediately. Pruritic welts develop rapidly and may persist for several days. Some lesions may open and weep for a few weeks. These insects emerge at sundown. Commercial repellants seem to be effective in the prevention of midge bites.

Deerflies can be found along woodland trails. Their bite is painful and may result in a pruritic welt. These flies have been known to cause generalized systemic reactions (urticaria, light-headedness, wheezing, and angioedema).[210] Treatment of fly bites involves preventing secondary infection, which is caused by scratching. The involved area should be cleaned with soap and water, followed by application of an antibiotic ointment. Cold compresses may be used for severe edema. Antihistamines may help relieve the itching.

Those who hike in high grass and areas of underbrush may encounter chiggers. In chigger bites, the bright red larvae are the culprits, since they need blood to complete their cycle and develop into mites. The larvae produce secretions that dissolve tissue and penetrate the epidermis to produce irritation and pruritus.[209] Unlike the scabies mite, chiggers are non-burrowing. The initial lesion presents as a small macule which becomes a pruritic urticarial papule within 24 hours. Some bites may become hemorrhagic and persist for several weeks. The lesions, which typically occur at clothing barrier lines, may itch intensely and intermittently for several weeks. To relieve pruritus and prevent secondary infection, calamine lotion and an oral antihistamine may be prescribed. Preventive measures include dusting the skin with powdered sulfur mixed with talc and tucking the pants tightly into the boots while hiking. Clothing should be sprayed from the waist down with an insect repellant containing DEET.

Ticks are found outdoors in many regions and drop from shrubs and weeds onto any warm-blooded creature. They attach themselves to the skin by curved teeth, and the attachment is secured with a cement-like secretion.[209] If one attempts to pull the tick from the skin, the mouth parts may remain in the wound, and toxins may be squeezed into the host. Ticks may be removed by placing a drop of ether or a hot object on the protruding part. Treated tick bites are small red macules that usually vanish quickly, but tick bite granulomas may develop in the following weeks, producing pruritic nodules that resolve very slowly.

The insects that provoke the most frequent serious allergic reactions are the hymenoptera (bees, wasps, hornets, and yellow jackets). It is estimated that up to 20 per cent of the population is allergic to the venom produced by hymenoptera.[210] Most often there is immediate pain, with wheal formation at the site of the sting. If edema extends over an area covering two or more joints, the victim should be considered sensitive to hymenoptera and likely to develop a generalized systemic reaction after a subsequent sting. When possible, the stinger should be gently removed by scraping. Once the stinger is removed, the area should be cleaned with soap and water, followed by the application of ice to relieve pain and swelling. Systemic reactions may include dry cough, abdominal pain, nausea, vomiting, urticaria, angioedema, hoarseness, wheezing, and anaphylactic shock. The reaction may begin insidiously and progress to a severe state within minutes. For mild reactions, inhalation of ephedrine followed by a repeated inhalation in two minutes may relieve symptoms. Antihistamines may also be effective. For severe reactions in the average adolescent, epinephrine 0.3 to 0.5 ml of 1:1000 aqueous solution should be injected subcutaneously every 15 to 30 minutes until symptoms subside. Aminophylline (5.6 mg/kg over 20 to 30 minutes) may also be given intravenously for breathing difficulties. If a maintenance dose is required, aminophylline may be given at the rate of 0.9 mg/kg/hour. Patients who are sensitive to bee venom may benefit from desensitization.[211-213] They should also carry an insect sting kit whenever they are outdoors in warm weather.[214]

FRECKLES (EPHELIDES)

Freckles are red or brown circumscribed macules, usually less than 5 millimeters in size, which are scattered on sun-exposed areas of the skin. They commonly appear in infancy or early childhood in genetically predisposed individuals. Brues[215] found that freckling may be transmitted as an autosomal dominant trait when linked with red or brown hair. Freckles become darker after repeated exposure to ultraviolet radiation, which differentiates them from lentigines. The common freckle is not associated with systemic disorders. However, persons who have extensive freckling and dark hair may be heterozygous carriers of the autosomal recessively inherited disorder xeroderma pigmentosum. Freckling in non-exposed areas, such as the axillae, is highly suggestive of neurofibromatosis.

Histologically, freckles are characterized simply by increased melanin pigmentation in the epidermal cells. Breathnach,[216] using histochemical techniques, found fewer melanocytes per unit area in freckles than in normal adjacent skin. However, the melanocytes in freckles were larger and more dopa-positive than melanocytes in adjacent areas of pale epidermis. Additional ultrastructural studies by Breathnach disclosed that the melanocytes in freckles produced increased numbers of large (greater than $.37\mu$), ellipsoidal melanosomes similar in character to those of dark-skinned individuals. His findings suggest that specific melanocytes, which at birth are potentially capable of producing large melanosomes, are not activated by ultraviolet light irradiation until two to four years of age.[217]

Conservative management of freckles may be accomplished by avoidance of sun exposure and use of sunscreens and cosmetics (e.g., Cover Mark).

REFERENCES

ACANTHOSIS NIGRICANS

1. Curth, H. O.: Significance of acanthosis nigricans. Arch. Dermatol., 66:80, 1952.
2. Winkelman, R. K., Scheen, S. R., Jr., and Underdahl, L. O.: Acanthosis nigricans endocrine disease. JAMA, 174:1145, 1960.
3. Brown, J., and Winkelman, R. K.: Acanthosis nigricans: A study of 90 cases. Medicine, 47:33, 1968.
4. Curth, H. O., and Aschner, B. M.: Genetic studies on acanthosis nigricans. Arch. Dermatol., 79:55, 1959.
5. Curth, H. O.: Cancer associated with acanthosis nigricans. Arch. Surg., 47:517, 1943.
6. Ackerman, A. B., and Lantis, L. R.: Acanthosis nigricans associated with Hodgkin's. Arch. Dermatol., 95:202, 1967.
7. Garrott, T. C.: Malignant acanthosis nigricans associated with osteogenic sarcoma. Arch. Dermatol., 106:384, 1972.
8. Curth, H. O.: Dermatosis and malignant internal tumors. Arch. Dermatol., 71:95, 1955.
9. Lerner, A. B.: On the causes of acanthosis nigricans. N. Engl. J. Med., 281:106, 1969.
10. Hollingsworth, D. R., and Amatruda, T. T.: Acanthosis nigricans and obesity. An endocrine abnormality. Arch. Intern. Med., 124:481, 1969.
11. Demis, J., Crounse, R., Dobson, R., and McGuire, J.: Acanthosis nigricans. In: Clinical Dermatology. Vol. 2, Unit 12–26. New York, Harper & Row, 1975.

VITILIGO

12. Howitz, J., and Rehfeld, J. F.: Serum-gastric vitiligo, and achlorhydric atrophic gastritis. Lancet, 2:1399, 1977.
13. Behl, P. N., and Bhatia, R. K.: 400 cases of vitiligo. A clinico-therapeutic analysis. Indian J. Dermatol., 17:51, 1972.
14. Woolfson, H., Finn, D. A., Mackie, R. M., et al.: Serum anti-tumor antibodies and auto-antibodies in vitiligo. Br. J. Dermatol., 92:395, 1975.
15. Bor, S., Feiwel, M., and Chanarin, I.: Vitiligo and its aetiological relationship to organ-specific autoimmune disease. Br. J. Dermatol., 81:83, 1969.
16. Lerner, A. B.: On the etiology of vitiligo and gray hair. Am. J. Med., 51:141, 1971.
17. Eng, A. M.: Marginal inflammatory vitiligo. Cutis, 6:1005, 1970.
18. Chapman, R. S.: Coincident vitiligo and psoriasis in the same individual. Arch. Dermatol., 107:776, 1973.
19. Jackson, R.: The lines of Blaschko: A review and reconsideration: Observations of the cause of certain unusual linear conditions of the skin. Br. J. Dermatol., 95:349, 1976.
20. Fields, J. P., Fragola, L., and Hadley, T. P.: Hypoparathyroidism, candidiasis, alopecia, and vitiligo. Arch. Dermatol., 103:687, 1971.
21. Weber, S. W., and Kazdan, J. J.: The Vogt-Koyanagi-Harada syndrome in children. J. Pediatr. Ophthalmol., 14:96, 1977.
22. Copeman, P. W., Lewis, M. G., Phillips, T. M., and Elliott, P. G.: Immunological associations of the halo naevus with cutaneous malignant melanoma. Br. J. Dermatol., 88:127, 1973.
23. Lever, W. F., and Lever, G. S.: Pigmentary disorders. In: Lever, W., and Schaumburg-Lever, G. (eds.), Histopathology of the Skin. Philadelphia, J. B. Lippincott, 1975, p. 420.
24. Morohashi, M., Hashimoto, K., Goodman, T. F., Jr., et al.: Ultrastructural studies of vitiligo, Vogt-Koyanagi syndrome, and incontinentia pigmenti achromians. Arch. Dermatol., 113:755, 1977.
25. El-Mofty, A. M., and Nada, M. M.: Vitiligo and its treatment. Aust. J. Dermatol., 15:1, 1974.
26. Sehgal, V. N.: Oral trimethylpsoralen in vitiligo in children: A preliminary report. Br. J. Dermatol., 85:454, 1971.
27. Kenney, J. A., Jr.: Vitiligo treated by psoralens. A long-term follow-up study of the permanency of repigmentation. Arch. Dermatol., 103:475, 1971.
28. Arora, S. K., and Willis, I.: Factors influencing methoxsalen phototoxicity in vitiliginous skin. Arch. Dermatol., 112:327, 1976.
29. Bleehen, S. S.: The treatment of vitiligo with topical corticosteroids, light, and electromicroscopic studies. Br. J. Dermatol., 94(Suppl. 121):43, 1976.

X-LINKED ICHTHYOSIS

30. Frost, P.: X-linked ichthyosis. *In:* Moschella, S. L., Pillsbury, D. M., and Hurley, H. J., Jr. (eds.): Dermatology. Philadelphia, W. B. Saunders, 1975, p. 1064.
31. Cockayne, E. A.: Inherited Abnormalities of the Skin and Its Appendages. London, Oxford University Press, 1933, p. 213.
32. Solomon, L. M., and Esterly, N. B.: The skin and the eye. *In:* Goldberg, M. F. (ed.): Genetic and Metabolic Eye Disease. Boston, Little, Brown, 1974, p. 515.
33. Czorsz, B.: Mschr. Unfalheilk. Medizin, 2:1180, 1928 (as quoted by McKusick, V.: Mendelian inheritance. *In:* Man. 4th Ed. Baltimore, Johns Hopkins University Press, 1975, p. 634.)
34. Kerr, C. B., Wells, R. S., and Sanger, R.: X-linked ichthyosis and the Xg groups. Lancet, *2*:1369, 1964.
35. Jay, B., Blach, R. K., and Wells, R. S.: Ocular manifestations of ichthyosis. Br. J. Ophthalmol., *52*:217, 1968.
36. Lever, R. S., Frost, P., and Weinstein, G.: Eye changes in ichthyosis. JAMA, *206*:2283, 1968.
37. Esterly, N. B.: The ichthyosiform dermatoses. Pediatrics, *42*:990, 1968.
38. Wells, R. S., and Jennings, M. C.: X-linked ichthyosis and ichthyosis vulgaris. Clinical and genetic distinctions in a second series of families. JAMA, *202*:485, 1967.

LICHEN PLANUS

39. Wilson, E.: On lichen planus. J. Cutaneous Dis., *8*:117, 1869.
40. Rook, A., Williams, D. S., and Ebling, F. J.: Textbook of Dermatology, Blakeston, London, 1965, p. 1351.
41. Adamson, H. G.: Three cases of lichen planus in children. Br. J. Dermatol., *32*:1, 1920.
42. Baker, H. W.: Lichen planus in a boy aged 8 years. Proc. R. Soc. Med., *40*:29, 1947.
43. Altman, J., and Perry, H. O.: The variations and course of lichen planus. Arch. Dermatol., *84*:180, 1961.
44. Dostrovsky, A., and Sagher, F.: Lichen planus in subtropical countries. Arch. Dermatol., *59*:308, 1949.
45. Swanbeck, F., and Thyresson, W.: Electron microscopy of intravascular particles in lichen ruber planus. Acta Derm. Venereol., *44*:105, 1964.
46. Thyresson, W., and Moburger, G.: Cytological studies in lichen ruber planus. Acta Derm. Venereol., *37*:191, 1957.
47. Johnson, F. R., and Fry, L.: Ultrastructural observations in lichen planus. Arch. Dermatol., *95*:596, 1967.
48. Cotton, D. W. K., van den Hurk, J. J. M. A., and van den Staak, W. B. J. M.: Lichen planus, an inborn error of metabolism. Br. J. Dermatol., *87*:341, 1972.
49. Cotton, D. W. K., and van den Staak, W. B. J. M.: Letter to the editor. Br. J. Dermatol., *93*:353, 1975.
50. Beutler, E.: Glucose-6-phosphorylase dehydrogenase deficiency. *In:* Stanbury, J. B. et al. (eds.): The Metabolic Basis of Inherited Disease. New York, McGraw-Hill, 1972, p. 1360.
51. Almeyda, J., and Levantine, A.: Lichenoid drug eruptions. Br. J. Dermatol., *85*:604, 1972.
52. Black, M. M., and Wilson-Jones, E.: The role of epidermis in the histopathogenesis of lichen planus. Arch. Dermatol., *105*:85, 1972.
53. Lever, W. F., and Schaumburg-Lever, G. (eds.): Histopathology of the Skin, Philadelphia, J. B. Lippincott, 1975, p. 148.
54. Baart de la Faille-Kuyper, E. J., and Baart de la Faille, H.: An immunofluorescence study of lichen planus. Br. J. Dermatol., *90*:370, 1974.
55. Pinhas, H.: Lichen striatus and lichen planus. J. Invest. Dermatol., *11*:9, 1948.
56. Samman, P. O.: A note on the natural history of lichen planus. Br. J. Dermatol., *68*:176, 1956.
57. Cram, P. L., and Muller, S. A.: Unusual variations of lichen planus. Mayo Clin. Proc., *41*:682, 1966.
58. Prieto, J. G.: Pseudopelode of Brocq: Its relationships to some forms of cicatricial alopecias and to lichen planus. J. Invest. Dermatol., *24*:333, 1955.
59. Ronchese, F.: Pseudopelade. Arch. Dermatol., *82*:338, 1960.
60. Zaias, N.: The nail in lichen planus. Arch. Dermatol., *101*:264, 1970.
61. Shklar, G.: Erosive and bullous oral lesions of lichen planus. Arch. Dermatol., *97*:411, 1968.
62. Cram, D. L., Kierland, R. R., and Winkelmann, R. K.: Ulcerative lichen planus of the feet. Arch. Dermatol., *93*:602, 1966.
63. Gunther, S.: Retinoic acid in the treatment of lichen planus. Dermatologica, *143*:314, 1971.
64. Sehgal, V. N., Graham, G. J. S., and Malik, G. B.: Griseofulvin therapy in lichen planus. A double-blind controlled trial. Br. J. Dermatol., *87*:383, 1972.
65. Fulling, H. J.: Cancer development in oral lichen planus. Arch. Dermatol., *108*:667, 1973.
66. Kronenberg, K., Fretzin, D., and Potter, B.: Malignant degeneration of lichen planus. Arch. Dermatol., *104*:304, 1971.

PITYRIASIS ROSEA

67. Mandal, S. B., and Dutta, A. K.: A clinical study of pityriasis rosea. Indian J. Dermatol., *17*:100, 1972.
68. Perlman, H. H., and Lubowe, I.: Pityriasis rosea in children: A review of the literature. J. Pediatr., *40*:109, 1952.
69. Wile, U. J.: Experimental transmission of pityriasis rosea. Arch. Dermatol., *16*:185, 1927.
70. Roberts, J. L., Kermani-Arab, V., and Leslie, G. A.: Pityriasis rosea: Increased IgM and IgD-bearing B lymphocytes. Clin. Res., *26*(2):103A, 1978.
71. Bunch, L. W., and Tilley, J. C.: Pityriasis rosea: A histologic and serologic study. Arch. Dermatol., *84*:79, 1961.
72. Marshall, J.: Pityriasis rosea: A review of its clinical aspects and a discussion of its relationship to pityriasis lichenoides et varioliformis acuta and parapsoriasis guttata. S. Afr. Med. J., *30*:210, 1956.

GRANULOMA ANNULARE

73. Fox, T. C.: Ringed eruptions of fingers. Br. J. Dermatol., *7*:91, 1895.
74. Crocker, H. R.: Granuloma annulare. Br. J. Dermatol., *14*:1, 1902.
75. Izumi, A. K.: Generalized perforating granuloma annulare. Arch. Dermatol., *108*:708, 1973.
76. Wells, R. S., and Smith, M. P.: The natural history of granuloma annulare. Br. J. Dermatol., *75*:199, 1963.
77. Dicker, C., Carrington, S., and Winkelmann, R. K.: Generalized granuloma annulare. Arch. Dermatol., *99*:556, 1964.
78. Rhodes, E. L., Hill, D. M., Ames, A. C., et al.: Granuloma annulare. Br. J. Dermatol., *78*:532, 1966.
79. Haim, S., Friedman-Birnbaum, R., and Shafrir, S.: Generalized granuloma annulare: Its relationship to diabetes mellitus in 8 cases. Br. J. Dermatol., *83*:302, 1970.
80. Haim, S., Friedman-Birnbaum, R., Haim, N., et al.: Carbohydrate tolerance in patients with granuloma annulare. Br. J. Dermatol., *88*:447, 1973.
81. Lever, F., and Schaumburg-Lever, G. (eds.): Histopathology of the Skin. 5th ed. Philadelphia, J. B. Lippincott, 1975, pp. 214–217.
82. Dahl, M. V., Ullman, S., and Gultz, R.: Vasculitis in granuloma annulare. Arch. Dermatol., *113*:463, 1977.
83. Stanker, L., and Laslic, G.: Generalized granuloma annulare. Arch. Dermatol., *95*:509, 1967.
84. Goolamali, S. K., and Stevenson, C. J.: Granuloma annulare in identical twins. Br. J. Dermatol., *86*:636, 1972.
85. Rubin, M., and Lynch, E. W.: Subcutaneous granuloma annulare. Arch. Dermatol., *92*:416, 1966.
86. Duncan, W. C., and Smith, J. B.: Generalized perforating granuloma annulare. Arch. Dermatol., *108*:570, 1973.
87. Sparrow, G., and Abell, E.: Granuloma annulare and necrobiosis lipoidica treated by jet injector. Br. J. Dermatol., *93*:85, 1975.

LICHEN SCLEROSUS ET ATROPHICUS

88. Rook, A., Wilkinson, D. S., and Ebling, F. J. G.: Textbook of Dermatology. 2nd ed. Philadelphia, F. A. Davis, 1972, p. 1118.
89. Apisarnthanarax, P., Osment, L. S., and Montes, L. F.: Extensive lichen sclerosus et atrophicus in a seven year old boy. Arch. Dermatol., *106*:94, 1972.
90. Wallace, H. J.: Lichen sclerosus et atrophicus. Trans. St. Johns Hosp. Dermatol. Soc., *57*:9, 1971.
91. Montgomery, H., and Hill, W. R.: Lichen sclerosus et atrophicus. Arch. Dermatol., *42*:755, 1940.
92. Foirgrieve, J., and Parker, R. A.: Acquired phimosis in the elderly caused by lichen sclerosus et atrophicus. Br. J. Urol., *31*:74, 1959.
93. Barclay, D. L., Mocey, H. B., Jr., and Reed, R. J.: Lichen sclerosus et atrophicus of the vulva in children. Obstet. Gynecol., *27*:637, 1966.
94. Chernosky, M. E., Derbes, V. J., and Burks, J. W., Jr.: Lichen sclerosus et atrophicus in children. Arch. Dermatol., *75*:647, 1957.
95. Clark, J. A., and Muller, S. A.: Lichen sclerosus et atrophicus in children. Arch. Dermatol., *95*:476, 1967.
96. Kindler, T.: Lichen sclerosus et atrophicus in young subjects. Br. J. Dermatol., *65*:269, 1953.
97. Laymon, C. W.: Lichen sclerosus et atrophicus in childhood. Arch. Dermatol., *52*:351, 1945.

98. Török, E., Orley, J., Gorácz, G., and Daroczy, J.: Lichen sclerosus et atrophicus in children. Mod. Probl. Paediatr., *17*:262, 1975.
99. Lever, W. F., and Schaumburg-Lever, G. (eds.): Histopathology of the Skin. 5th ed. Philadelphia, J. B. Lippincott, 1975, p. 260.
100. Anderton, R. L., and Abele, D. C.: Lichen sclerosus et atrophicus in vaccination site. Arch. Dermatol., *112*:1787, 1976.
101. Lascano, E. F., Montes, L. F., and Mozzini, M. A.: Lichen sclerosus et atrophicus in childhood. Obstet. Gynecol., *24*:872, 1964.
102. Shapiro, L.: Lichen sclerosus et atrophicus: First reported case in a boy. Dermatologica, *136*:155, 1968.

JUVENILE DERMATOMYOSITIS

103. Unverricht, H.: Polymyositis acuta progressiva. Z. Klin. Med., *12*:533, 1887.
104. Braverman, I. M.: Skin Signs of Systemic Disease. Chapter 7. Philadelphia, W. B. Saunders, 1970.
105. Goel, K. M., and Shanks, R. A.: Dermatomyositis in childhood. Arch. Dis. Child., *51*:501, 1976.
106. Banker, B. Q., and Victor, M.: Dermatomyositis of childhood. Medicine, *45*(4):261, 1966.
107. Everett, M., and Curtis, A.: Dermatomyositis. Arch. Intern. Med., *100*:70, 1957.
108. Whitaker, N., Jr., and Engel, W. K.: Vascular deposits of immunoglobulin and complement in idiopathic inflammatory myopathy. N. Engl. J. Med., *286*:333, 1972.
109. Jacobs, J.: Methotrexate and azathioprine treatment of childhood dermatomyositis. Pediatrics, *59*:2:212, 1977.
110. Muller, S. A., Winkelmann, R. K., and Brunsting, L. A.: Calcinosis in dermatomyotisis. Arch. Dermatol., *79*:669, 1959.
111. Hill, R. H., and Wood, W. S.: Juvenile dermatomyositis. Can. Med. Assoc. J., *103*:1152, 1970.
112. Carlson, M., Lindseth, R. E., and Derosa, G. P.: Surgical removal of soft tissue calcifications in dermatomyositis. Arch. Surg., *110*(6):775, 1975.
113. Curtis, A. C., Blaylock, H. C., and Harrell, E. R., Jr.: Malignant lesions associated with dermatomyositis. JAMA, *150*:884, 1952.
114. Dubowitz, V.: Treatment of dermatomyositis in childhood. Arch. Dis. Child., *51*:494, 1976.

SCLERODERMA

115. Rook, A.: Textbook of Dermatology. Oxford, Blackwell Scientific Publications, Oxford, 1972.
116. Rodnan, G. P., and Benedek, T. G.: An historical account of the study of progressive systemic sclerosis (diffuse scleroderma). Ann. Intern. Med., *57*:305, 1962.
117. Tuffanelli, D. S., and Winkelmann, R. K.: Systemic scleroderma. A clinical study of 727 cases. Arch. Dermatol., *84*:359, 1961.
118. Hanson, V., and Kornreich, H.: Systemic rheumatic disorders ("collagen diseases") in childhood: Lupus erythematosus, anaphylactoid purpura, dermatomyositis, and scleroderma. Bull. Rheum. Dis., *17*:435, 1967; *17*:441, 1967.
119. Jaffe, M. O., and Winkelmann, R. K.: Generalized scleroderma in children. Arch. Dermatol., *83*:84, 1961.
120. Kornreich, H. K., Koster, K., and Hanson, V.: The rheumatic diseases in adolescence. Pediatr. Clin. North Am., *20*:911, 1973.
121. Cockayne, E. A.: Congenital and acquired scleroderma in childhood. Br. J. Child. Dis.,*13*:225, 1916.
122. Dennett, R. H.: Scleroderma with myositis fibrosa. Br. J. Child. Dis., *8*:551, 1911.
124. Rudolph, A.: Pediatrics. New York, Appleton-Century-Croft, 1977.
125. Lever, W. F., and Schaumberg-Lever, G. (eds.): Histopathology of the Skin. Philadelphia, J. B. Lippincott, 1975.
126. Kornreich, H. K., Drexler, E., and Hanson, V.: Antinuclear factors in childhood rheumatic diseases. J. Pediatr., *69*:1039, 1966.
127. Moynahan, E. J.: D-penicillamine in morphoea (localized scleroderma). Lancet, *1*:428, 1973.
128. Addison, T.: Medico-Chirurgical Transactions of 1854. Quoted by Fox, T. L.: Note on the history of scleroderma in England. Br. J. Dermatol., *4*:101, 1892.
129. Chazen, E. M., Cook, C. D., and Cohen, J.: Focal scleroderma. J. Pediatr.,*60*:385, 1962.
130. Christianson, H. B., Dorsey, C. S., O'Leary, P. A., et al.: Localized scleroderma: Clinical study of 235 cases. Arch. Dermatol., *74*:629, 1956.
131. Robin, L.: Linear scleroderma: Association with abnormalities of the spine and nervous system. Arch. Dermatol., *58*:1, 1948.
132. Gellis, S. S., Feingold, M., Sussman, S. J., et al.: Focal scleroderma. Am. J. Dis. Child., *123*:465, 1972.

PYODERMA GANGRENOSUM

133. Brunsting, L., Goeckerman, W., and O'Leary, P.: Pyoderma (ecthyma) gangrenosum. Clinical and experimental observations in five cases occurring in adults. Arch. Dermatol. Syph., 22:655, 1930.
134. Brocq, L.: Ann. de dermat. et syph. 6:1, 1916. Cited by Greenbaum, S. S.: Phagedenica geometrica (Brocq). Arch. Dermatol. Syph., 43:775–801, 1941.
135. Brewer, G. E., and Meleney, F. L.: Progressive gangrenous infection of the skin and subcutaneous tissue. Ann. Surg., 84:438, 1926.
136. Cullen, T. S.: A progressively enlarging ulcer of the abdominal wall involving the skin and fat following drainage of an abdominal abscess apparently of appendageal origin. Surg. Gynecol. Obstet., 28:579, 1924.
137. Jankelson, I. R., and Massell, B. F.: Pyogenic skin lesions accompanying chronic ulcerative colitis. Am. J. Dig. Dis., 3:19, 1936.
138. Bargen, J. A.: Chronic ulcerative colitis. Hosp. Med., 11:6, 1975.
139. Apted, J. H., Buntine, D., and Newell, A. C.: Pyoderma gangrenosum. Med. J. Aust., 2:423, 1971.
140. Brandt, L., et al.: Pyoderma gangrenosum associated with regional enteritis. Acta Med. Scand., 201:141, 1977.
141. Korelitz, B., and Sommers, S.: Pyoderma gangrenosum complicating Crohn's disease. Am. J. Gastroenterol., 68:171, 1977.
142. Lazarus, G. S., Goldsmith, L. A., Rocklin, R. E., et al.: Pyoderma gangrenosum, altered delayed hypersensitivity, and polyarthritis. Arch. Dermatol., 105:46, 1972.
143. McGarity, W. C., and Barnett, S. M.: Pyoderma gangrenosum in Crohn's disease: Report of a case. Dis. Colon Rectum, 20:49, 1977.
144. Long, P. T., and Uesu, C. T.: Pyoderma gangrenosum. JAMA, 187:336, 1964.
145. Klaus, S. N.: Pyoderma gangrenosum. In: Dennis, D. J., et al. (eds.) Clinical Dermatology, Vol. I, Sections 5–12. New York, Harper & Row, pp. 1–4.
146. Karltorp, N.: Pyoderma gangrenosum with and without hypogammaglobulinemia. Acta Derm. Venereol., 43:263, 1963.
147. Label, N.: Pyoderma gangrenosum with IgG paraproteinemia in plasmocytoma. Hautarzt, 27:603, 1976.
148. Feuerman, E., and Potruch-Eisenkraft, S.: Pyoderma gangrenosum. A case of polycythemia vera. Bull. Soc. Fr. Derm. Syph., 78:260–261, 1971.
149. Pye, R. S., et al.: Bullous pyoderma as a presentation of acute leukaemia. Clin. Exp. Dermatol., 2:33, 1977.
150. Shore, R. N.: Pyoderma gangrenosum, defective neutrophil chemotaxis, and leukaemia. Arch. Dermatol., 112:1792, 1976.
151. Cramers, M.: Bullous pyoderma gangrenosum in association with myeloid leukaemia. Acta Derm. Venereol., 56:311, 1976.
152. Korany, P. M., et al.: Pyoderma gangrenosum associated with Philadelphia chromosome negative chronic myeloid leukaemia. Dermatologica, 150:360, 1977.
153. Rostenberg, A., Jr.: The Shwartzman phenomenon. A review with a consideration of some possible dermatological manifestations. Br. J. Dermatol., 65:389, 1953.
154. Goldgraber, M. B., and Kirsner, J. B.: Gangrenous skin lesions associated with chronic ulcerative colitis. A case study. Gastroenterology, 39:94, 1960.
155. Perry, H. O.: Pyoderma gangrenosum. South. Med. J., 62:899, 1969.
156. Dantzing, P. I.: Pyoderma gangrenosum. N. Engl. J. Med., 292:47, 1975.
156a. Soto, L. D.: Diaminodiphenylsulfone and steroids in the treatment of pyoderma gangrenosum. J. Dermatol., 9:293, 1970.
156b. Hoffbrand, B. I.: Dapsone and renal capillary necrosis. Br. Med. J., 1:79, 1977.

NECROBIOSIS LIPOIDICA DIABETICORUM

157. Rollins, T. G., and Winklemann, R. K.: Necrobiosis lipoidica granulomatosis; necrobiosis lipoidica diabeticorum in the nondiabetic. Arch. Dermatol., 82:537, 1960.
158. Hildebrand, A. G., Montgomery, H., and Rynearson, E. H.: Necrobiosis lipoidica diabeticorum. Arch. Intern. Med., 66:851, 1940.
159. Wilson-Jones, E.: Necrobiosis lipoidica presenting on the face and scalp: An account of 29 patients and a detailed consideration of recent histochemical findings. Trans. St. Johns Hosp. Dermatol. Soc., 57:202, 1971.
160. Muller, S. A., and Winklemann, R. K.: Necrobiosis lipoidica diabeticorum: A clinical and pathological investigation of 171 cases. Arch. Dermatol., 93:272, 1966.
161. Narva, W. M., Benoit, F. L., and Ringrose, E. J.: Necrobiosis lipoidica diabeticorum with apparently normal carbohydrate tolerance. Arch. Intern. Med., 115:718, 1965.

162. Ellenberg, M.: Diabetic complications without manifest diabetes. Complications as presenting clinical symptoms. JAMA, *183*:926, 1963.
163. Engel, M. F., and Hammack, W. J.: Necrobiosis lipoidica diabeticorum. Arch. Dermatol., *78*:73, 1958.
164. Hitch, J. M.: Necrobiosis lipoidica diabeticorum (Urbach and Oppenheim). Arch. Dermatol., *36*:536, 1937.
165. Mehregan, A. H., and Pinkus, H.: Necrobiosis lipoidica with sarcoid reaction. Arch. Dermatol., *83*:143, 1961.
166. Savitt, L. E.: Favourable response of necrobiosis lipoidica diabeticorum to hydrocortisone suspension. Arch. Dermatol., *71*:506, 1955.
167. Newman, B. A., and Feldman, F. F.: Effects of topical cortisone on chronic discoid lupus erythematosus and necrobiosis lipoidica diabeticorum. J. Invest. Dermatol., *17*:3, 1951.
168. Marr, T. J., Traisman, H. S., Griffith, H. S., et al: Necrobiosis lipoidica diabeticorum in a juvenile diabetic; treatment by excision and skin grafting. Cutis, *19*:348, 1977.
169. Sparrow, L., and Abell, E.: Granuloma annulare and necrobiosis lipoidica treated by jet injection. Br. J. Dermatol., *93*:85, 1975.
170. Rhodes, E. L.: Fibrinolytic agents in the treatment of necrobiosis lipoidica. Br. J. Dermatol., *95*:673, 1976.

SWIMMING POOL GRANULOMA

171. Feldman, R. A., Long, M. W., and David, H. L.: *Mycobacterium marinum:* A leisure-time pathogen. J. Infect. Dis., *129*:618, 1974.
172. Swift, S., and Cohen, H.: Granulomas of the skin due to *Mycobacterium balnei* after abrasions from a fish tank. N. Engl. J. Med., *267*:1244, 1962.
173. Philpott, J. A., Jr., Woodfume, A. R., Philpott, D. S., et al.: Swimming pool granuloma. A study of 290 cases. Arch. Dermatol., *88*:158, 1963.
174. Jolly, H. W., Jr., and Seaburg, J. H.: Infections with *Mycobacterium marinum*. Arch. Dermatol., *106*:32, 1976.
175. Aronson, J. D.: Spontaneous tuberculosis in saltwater fish. J. Infect. Dis., *39*:315, 1926.
176. Winter, F. E., and Runyon, E. H.: Prepatellar bursitis caused by *Mycobacterium marinum (balnei)*. J. Bone Joint Surg., *47*:375, 1965.
177. Chappler, R. R., Hoke, A. W., and Borchardt, K. A.: Primary inoculation with *Mycobacterium marinum*. Arch. Dermatol., *113*:380, 1977.
178. Adams, R. M., Remington, J. S., Steinberg, J., and Seiberg, J. S.: Tropical fish aquariums. A source of *Mycobacterium marinum* infections resembling sporotrichosis. JAMA, *211*:457, 1970.
179. Zeligman, I.: *Mycobacterium marinum* granuloma. Arch. Dermatol., *106*:26, 1972.
180. Izumi, A. K., Hanke, C. W., and Higoki, M.: *Mycobacterium marinum* infections treated with tetracycline. Arch. Dermatol., *113*:1067, 1977.
181. Mollohan, C. S., and Romer, M. S.: Public health significance of swimming pool granuloma. Am. J. Public Health, *51*:883, 1961.
182. Wolinsky, E., Gomez, F., and Zimpfer, F.: Sporotrichoid *Mycobacterium marinum* infection treated with rifampin-ethambutol. Am. Rev. Resp. Dis., *105*:964, 1972.
183. Van Dyke, J. J., and Lake, K. B.: Chemotherapy for aquarium granuloma. JAMA, *233*(13):1380, 1975.
184. Loria, P. R.: Minocycline hydrochloride treatment for atypical acid-fast infection. Arch. Dermatol., *112*(4):517, 1976.

KELOIDS

185. Leider, M., and Rosenblum, M.: A Dictionary of Dermatological Words, Terms, and Phrases. New York, McGraw-Hill, 1968.
186. Inalsingh, C.: An experience in treating five hundred and one patients with keloids. Johns Hopkins Med. J., *134*:284, 1974.
187. Cohen, B. H., Lewis, C. A., and Resnik, S. S.: Wound healing: A brief review. Int. J. Dermatol., *14*:(10):722, 1975.
188. Omo-Dare, P.: Genetic studies on keloid. J. Natl. Med. Assoc., *67*(6):428, 1975.
189. Koonin, A. J.: The aetiology of keloids: A review of the literature and a new hypothesis. S. Afr. Med. J., *38*:913, 1964.
190. Bernstein, H.: Treatment of keloids by steroids with biochemical test for diagnosis and prognosis. Angiology, *15*:253, 1964.
191. Cohen, I. K., and Diegelmann, R. E.: The biology of keloid and hypertrophic scar and the influence of corticosteroids. Clin. Plast. Surg., *4*(2):297, 1977.

192. Leibovich, S. J., and Ross, R.: The role of the macrophage in wound repair. Am. J. Pathol., 78:71, 1975.
193. Brauner, G. J.: Cutaneous diseases in the black races. In: Moschella, S. L., Pillsbury, D. M., and Hurley, H. J. (eds.): Dermatology. Philadelphia, W. B. Saunders, 1975.
194. Borges, A. F., and Alexander, J. E.: Relaxed skin tension lines, Z-plastics on scars, and fusiform excisions of lesions. Br. J. Plast. Surg., 15:242, 1962.
195. Ketchum, L. D.: Hypertrophic scars and keloids. Clin. Plast. Surg., 4:2, 1977.
196. Linares, H. A., Kischer, C. W., Dobrkovsky, M., and Larson, D. L.: The histiotypic organization of the hypertrophic scar in humans. J. Invest. Dermatol., 59:323, 1972.
197. Linares, H. A., and Larson, D. L.: Early differential diagnosis between hypertrophic and nonhypertrophic healing. J. Invest. Dermatol., 62:514, 1974.
198. Lever, W. F., and Schaumburg-Lever, G.: Histopathology of the Skin. 5th ed. Philadelphia, J. B. Lippincott, 1975, p. 577.
199. Cosman, B., and Wolff, M.: Correlation of keloid recurrence with completeness of local excision. Plast. Reconstr. Surg., 50:163, 1972.
200. Levy, D. S., Salter, M. M., and Roth, R. E.: Postoperative irradiation in the prevention of keloids. Am. J. Roentgenol. Radium Ther. Nucl. Med., 127:509, 1976.
201. Cohen, I. K., Diegelmann, R. E., and Johnson, M. L.: Effect of corticosteroids on collagen synthesis. Surgery, 82(1):15, 1977.

DERMATOLOGICAL ATHLETIC INJURIES

202. Crissey, J. T., and Peachey, J. C.: Calcaneal petechiae. Arch. Dermatol., 83:501, 1961.
203. Kirton, V., and Price, M. W.: Black heel. Trans. St. Johns Hosp. Dermatol. Soc., 51:80, 1971.
204. Yaffee, H.: Talon noir. Arch. Dermatol., 104:452, 1971.
205. Ayres, S., Jr., and Mihan, B.: Calcaneal petechiae. Arch. Dermatol., 106:262, 1972.
206. Nabai, H., and Mahregan, A. H.: Black heel. Cutis, 6:751, 1970.
207. Izumi, A. K.: Pigmented palmar petechiae (black palm). Arch. Dermatol., 109:261, 1974.
208. Montgomery, R. M.: Tennis and its skin problems. Cutis, 19:480, 1977.

ARTHROPOD BITES

209. Frazier, C. A.: Insect Allergy. St. Louis, Warren H. Green, 1969.
210. Frazier, C. A.: Insect reactions related to sports. Cutis, 19(4):439, 1977.
211. Mueller, H. L.: Maintenance of protection in patients treated for stinging insect hypersensitivity: A booster injection program. Pediatrics, 59(5):793, 1977.
212. Zeleznick, L. D., Hunt-Kjsobdtka, A. N., Valentine, M. D., et al.: Diagnosis of hymenoptera hypersensitivity by skin testing with hymenoptera venoms. J. Allergy Clin. Immunol., 59(13):2, 1977.
213. Hunt, K. J., Dalentine, M. D., Sabotka, A. K., and Lichtenstein, L. M.: Diagnosis of allergy to stinging insects by skin testing with hymenoptera venoms. Ann. Intern. Med., 85(1):56, 1976.
214. Frazier, C. A.: Emergency first aid for allergic reactions to insect stings or bites. Cutis, 19(6):770, 1977.

FRECKLES

215. Brues, A. M.: Linkage of body build with sex, eye color, and freckling. Am. J. Hum. Genet., 2:215, 1950.
216. Breathnach, A. S.: Melanocyte distribution in forearm epidermis of freckled human subjects. J. Invest. Dermatol., 29:253, 1957.
217. Breathnach, A. S., and Wyllie, L. M.: Electron microscopy of melanocytes and melanosomes in freckled human epidermis. J. Invest. Dermatol., 42:389, 1964.

INDEX

Note: In this index, page numbers in *italics* indicate illustrations; those followed by (t) indicate tables. The abbreviation vs. denotes differential diagnosis.

Acantholytic cell(s), defined, 49
　in pyoderma, 49
Acanthosis nigricans, 434–435, *434*
Acarophobia, 213
Acid, fatty. See *Free fatty acids.*
Acinetobacter, 165
Acinus, glandular, *4*
Acne, 54–77
　course of, 66
　differential diagnosis of, 71–72
　drug-induced, 70, *70*
　ecology of, 58–60
　etiology of, 60–62
　exacerbating factors in, 66–69, 66(t)
　familial predisposition to, 62–63
　in pregnancy, 68
　incidence of, by age and sex, 62
　infantile, 71, *71*
　inflammatory, 64–65
　lesions of, 63–66, *64, 65*
　　distribution of, 63
　　evaluation of, 73
　　inflammatory, 64–65
　　picking at, 68–69
　Mallorca, 70
　microorganisms causing, 59–60
　neonatal, 71, *71*
　nodular, 70
　seasonal changes in, 68
　steroid, 70, *70*
　treatment of, 72–77, 72(t)
　　local, 73–74
　　systemic, 75–76
　"tropical," 67
Acne excoriée des filles, 69
Acne necrotica, 70
Acne rosacea, 70
Acne vulgaris. See *Acne.*
Acrosclerosis, 449
Actinicus, 138
Actinomyces israelii, in cutaneous infection, 297
Actinomycetes, in cutaneous infection, 296–299
Actinomycosis, 297–298
　abdominal, 297
　cervicofacial, 297
　thoracic, 297
Adenoma sebaceum, vs. acne, 72
Adipose tissue, structure and function of, 25–26
Adolescence, stages of, 29–30

Adolescent patient, long-term management of, 38
　physical examination of, 33
　sub-types of, 31
　treatment of, 34–38
　　community resources in, 35
　　family cooperation in, 34
　　plan for, 34
　understanding of, 28–38
Allergen. See *Antigen.*
Allergic contact dermatitis, 108–116
　causes of, 111–112, 111(t), 113(t)
　clinical characteristics of, 103(t), 110–111
　complications of, 114–115
　diagnosis of, 112–113
　　patch testing for, 53, 113–114
　differential diagnosis of, 112–113
　elicitation phase of, 109–110
　involved areas of, 113(t)
　pathogenesis of, 108–110
　sensitization phase of, 108–109
　treatment of, 115–116
　vs. atopic dermatitis, 100, 101(t)
　vs. irritant contact dermatitis, 103(t)
Allergic rhinitis, in atopic dermatitis, 89
Allergy, to light. See *Photosensitivity.*
Alopecia, androgenic, 356, *357*
　congenital, 349–353, *350*
　familial, 349–353, *350*
　hot comb, 358
　in lupus erythematosus, 374–375
　in necrobiosis lipoidica diabeticorum, 452
　in pili torti, 352–353
　in secondary syphilis, *231*
　in tinea capitis, 305
　non-scarring, 347–348, 347(t)
　　causes of, 347, 348(t)
　patterned, 354–356, *355, 357*
　scarring, 347–348, 347(t), 356, 358, 359–361
　　causes of, 347, 348(t)
　　in lichen planopilaris, 359, *360*
　　in lupus erythematosus, 359–360
　　in scalp neoplasia, 361
　　in pseudopelade, 360
　　in scleroderma, 360–361
　traction, 356, 358
Alopecia areata, 354, *355*
Alopecia totalis, 354
Alopecia universalis, 354, Plate VIII-B
American Indians, polymorphous light eruption in, 127
Ampicillin, in gram-negative acne, 76

469

Anagen effluvium, 353–354, 354(t)
Anagen phase, of hair growth, 15, 349
Anaphylaxis, from hymenoptera sting, 460
  and urticaria, 407, 411
Androgens, and alopecia, 356, 357
  and sebum production, 55
  role of, in acne, 61
  in activity of sebaceous gland, 16, 55
Anemia, in lupus erythematosus, 385
  in pyoderma gangrenosum, 451
Anesthetics, topical, and contact dermatitis, 107
Angioedema, 404, 405. See also *Urticaria*.
  causes of, 405(t), 407–408
    immunological, 406(t)
    non-immunological, 406(t)
  hereditary, 413–414
  vibratory, 409
Anogenital region, in lichen sclerosus et atrophicus, 444–445
Antibody(ies), antinuclear, in systemic lupus erythematosus, 378–380
  formation of, in acne, 61
  in syphilis, 239(t)
  streptococcal, screening technique for, 167
  to cytoplasmic antigens, in lupus erythematosus, 380–383
Antidepressant drugs, 36–37
Antigen(s), and delayed hypersensitivity response, 109–110
  cytoplasmic, in lupus erythematosus, 380–383
  HL-A, and lupus erythematosus, 387
    and psoriasis, 145, 150
    and Reiter syndrome, 276
  nuclear, in systemic lupus erythematosus, 378–380
  poison ivy, 111–112
  sensitization to, in contact dermatitis, 108–109
  Rhus, 111–112
Antihistamine(s), in atopic dermatitis, 102
  in urticaria, 412
Antimetabolite drugs, in psoriasis, 158–159
Anxiety, and cutaneous disease, 31
Apocrine glands, 17–18
  development of, 17
  secretion of, 17–18
  structure of, 17
Aquagenic urticaria, 411
Argininosuccinicaciduria, congenital trichorrhexis nodosa in, 352
Arterial disease, in systemic scleroderma, 448
Arthralgia, in focal scleroderma, 450
Arthritis, gonococcal, 287
  in Henoch-Schönlein purpura, 424
  in Reiter syndrome, 277–279
  in systemic lupus erythematosus, 370(t), 373, 383
  psoriatic, 150. Plate V-A
Arthritis-dermatitis syndrome, gonococcal, 285–287, 286
Arthropod bites, 459–460
  causing urticaria, 407
Aspergillosis, 321

Aspergillus fumigatus, in aspergillosis, 321
Aspergillus niger, in aspergillosis, 321
Aspirin, causing urticaria, 407
  in vascular reactive disease, 418
Asteatotic eczema, 105
Asthma, in atopic dermatitis, 89
Ataxia-telangiectasia, 131–132
Athlete's foot, 310–312, *311*, *312*
Athletic cutaneous injury, 457–458
Atopic dermatitis, 87–102, *89*, *90*, *92–94*, 88(t), 95–97(t), 101(t)
  allergic rhinitis in, 89
  asthma in, 89
  atopic disorders associated with, 88–89
  beta-blockade theory of, 99
  blanching phenomenon in, 93–94, *94*
  clinical course of, 89
  clinical features of, 88–95
  complications of, 95–97
  contact irritants in, 93–94
  cutaneous infections in, 95–96, 95(t)
  cutaneous reactions in, 93–94
  diagnosis of, 100, 100(t)
  differential diagnosis of, 88, 88(t), 100, 101(t)
  drug reactions in, 93–94
  emotional stress and, 102
  facial appearance in, *90*
  flexural involvement in, *90*, 91
  hereditary predisposition to, 88, *89*
  immunological defects in, 97–99, 97(t)
  in childhood, *90*, 91
  in infants, 89
  in twins, 88, *89*
  Kaposi's varicelliform eruption in, 188–189
  lesions of, 89–91
    distribution of, 89–91, *90*, *92*, *93*
  molluscum contagiosum in, 201
  ocular complications in, 96
  pathogenesis of, 97–100
  pityriasis alba in, 91
  pruritus in, 89, 94–95
    treatment of, 101–102
  respiratory disorders in, 88–89
  seasonal variation in, 91, 93
  sweating in, 91
  treatment of, 100–102
    dry skin in, 101–102
  vascular phenomena in, 93, 94, *94*
  vs. allergic contact dermatitis, 112
  white line response in, 93–94, *94*
Atopic eczema. See *Atopic dermatitis*.
Atopic triad, 89
Atopy, defined, 88. See also *Atopic dermatitis*.
  in nummular eczema, 116
Atrichia, 351
Autoeczematization, in allergic contact dermatitis, 115–116
Axon reflex, 25

B cell, in systemic lupus erythematosus, 385–387
Bacillus(i), as skin flora, 164

Bacillus subtilis, 164
Bacterial infection(s), 163–183
   in contact dermatitis, 107, 114
   in psoriasis, 145–147, 150, 153
   urticarial response to, 412
   vs. acne, 72
Balanitis, herpetic, 188
   circinata, Plate VI-C
Baldness, 354, 356. See also *Alopecia.*
   male-pattern, 356, 357
Balloon cell nevus, 337
Bamboo hair, 351–352, 350(t), *350*
Barber's itch, 306–307
Basal cell, 8, 9, *9*
   cytoplasm of, *9*
   epidermal layer of, 8, 9, 11
Basal cell carcinoma, nevoid, 125, 333, Plate I-C
   nevus syndrome in, 125
Bathing trunk nevus, 339–341, *340, 341*
Beaded hair, *350,* 351
Becker's melanosis, 331
   nevus, 331
Behavioral responses, maladaptive, to cutaneous disease, 31
Benzoylperoxide, in treatment of acne, 73
Benzyl benzoate, in treatment of scabies, 215–216
Beta-blockade theory, in atopic dermatitis, 99
Beta-carotene, in treatment of erythropoietic protoporphyria, 135
Biopsy, punch. See Punch biopsy.
Bites, arthropod, 459–460
   insect, 459–460
Black dot ringworm, 305, *305*
Blackheads. See *Comedo(nes).*
Black heel, 458
Black light. See *Wood's light.*
Blanching phenomenon, in atopic dermatitis, 93, 94, *94*
   in dermographism, 408–409
Blister, fungus, *41*
Blistering distal dactylitis, 171, *171*
Blood, disorders of, in systemic lupus erythematosus, 385–386
Blood vessels, cutaneous, 23–24
   regulatory functions of, 24
Bloom's syndrome, 130–131
Blue nevus, 343–344, *343,* 361
Bockhart's impetigo, 174
Boil, 175–176
Bone, lesions of, in late congenital syphilis, *242,* 243(t), 243–245, *245,* 251–253, *252*
Boston exanthem, 202(t), 206
Bullous impetigo, 172–174, *173*

Calcinosis cutis, in juvenile dermatomyositis, 447
Callus, 458
Calymmatobacterium granulomatis, 262–263, *265*
Cancer, of cervix, and herpes infection, 186
   of skin, 125

Candida albicans, 44, 165
   in candidiasis, 317, 319, 320
Candidiasis, 44, 317–321, *318, 319,* Plate VII–F
   differential diagnosis of, 320
   identification of by KOH technique, 43–44
   interdigital, 319
      treatment of, 321
   intertriginous, 318
      treatment of, 321
   laboratory findings in, 320
   oral, 317–318
      treatment of, 320
   perianal, 319
      treatment of, 320–321
   vaginal, 318
      treatment of, 320–321
   vs. contact dermatitis, 107, 112
Carbuncle, 175
Carbunculosis, 175–176
Carcinoma, nevoid basal cell, 125, 333, Plate I–C
Carpet-tack scale, in lupus erythematosus, 371
Catagen phase, of hair growth, 15
Cataract formation, in atopic dermatitis, 96
Cell, acantholytic, defined, 49
   basal, 8
      cytoplasm of, *9*
      epidermal layer of, 8, 9, 11
   cornified layer, of epidermis, *8*
   dendritic, 11–14
   granular layer, of epidermis, 8, 9
   Langerhans, 8, 13
   Merkel, 8, 13–14
   multinucleated, in herpes virus infection, 48, *49*
   prickle layer, of epidermis, 8, 9
Cell-mediated immunity, in lupus erythematosus, 386–389
Cell-mediated immunodeficiency, in atopic dermatitis, 98
Cellulitis, 170–171
   clostridial, 177–178
   dissecting, of scalp, and acne, 69–70
   non-clostridial, 178
   treatment of, 171
   vs. erysipelas, 169
Central nervous system, pigmented tumors in, 340
Cervix, cancer of, and herpes infection, 186
Chancre, anal, *225*
   hunterian, *226*
   in female, 225, 227, *226*
   in sulcus coronarius, *225*
   "mixed," 261
   of fourchette, *226*
   of lip, *226*
   of syphilis, 224–228, *225, 226,* 227(t), *259*
      differential diagnosis of, 227(t)
Chancroid, 257–262
   and syphilis, 261
   clinical signs of, 257–261, *258, 259*
   diagnosis of, 261–262
   etiology of, 257
   laboratory tests for, 261–262
   lesion of, 260, *258, 259*

Chancroid (*Continued*)
 "mixed" chancre of, 261
 of cervix, *258*
 of penis, *259*
 treatment of, 262
 ulcerated, *259*
 vs. lymphogranuloma venereum, 271–274(t)
Chemicals, sensitizing, characteristics of, 109(t)
Chickenpox. See *Varicella*.
Chigger bite, 459
Childhood atopic dermatitis, *90*, *91*
Chlamydia, classification of, 268(t)
 in lymphogranuloma venereum, 267
Chocolate, in exacerbation of acne, 66–67
Cholinergic urticaria, 411
Cholinesterases, in cutaneous nerve endings, 25
Choroiditis, in late congenital syphilis, 248
Chromoblastomycosis, 316
Cladosporium carrioni, in chromoblastomycosis, 316
Cladosporium wernecki, in tinea nigra, 301
Clostridia, as skin flora, 164
Clostridial cellulitis, 177–178
Clutton's joints, 244–245, *245*
Cockayne's syndrome, 131
Cold urticaria, 409–410, *410*
Collagen, 20–22
 disease(s) of, defined, 369
 fibrils of, *21*
   formation of, 21
 structure of, 20–21
Collodion baby, 438
Comedo(nes), 63–64, *64*
 production of, 60–61
Complement. See also *Serum complement*.
Complement fixation test, for lymphogranuloma venereum, 275
 for syphilis, 237–238, 239(t)
   false positive reactions in, 240–241
Compound nevus, 335–336, *336*
Condylomata acuminata, 197–198, 281
 in secondary syphilis, 234, *234*
Conjunctivitis, in gonococcal infection, 289
 in Reiter syndrome, 277
Connective tissue, diseases of, 447–451
Contact dermatitis, 102–116, 103(t), 105(t), 109(t), 111(t), 113(t)
Contact dermatitis, allergic. See *Allergic contact dermatitis*.
 clinical features of, 103(t)
 "internal," 115
Contact dermatitis, irritant. See *Irritant contact dermatitis*.
 secondary infection in, 107–108, 114
Contact sensitivity, in atopic dermatitis, 94–95
Contact urticaria, 411
Contactant(s), chemical sensitizing, characteristics of, 109(t)
Contusion, 457–458
Coproporphyria, hereditary, 133
Corneal opacities, in X-linked ichthyosis, 438

Corpuscle, Meissner's, 24–25
 Merkel-Ranvier, 25
 pacinian, 24–25
 Vater-Pacini, 25
Cortex, of hair, 15
Corticosteroids, in treatment of acne, 74, 75, 76, 77
 eczematous dermatitis, 118–119
 in psoriasis, 157–158
 systemic, for allergic contact dermatitis, 115–116
 topical, for allergic contact dermatitis, 115
   for irritant contact dermatitis, 108
Corynebacterium, 163
Corynebacterium acnes, 58–59, 61
Corynebacterium minutissimum, in erythrasma, 294
Corynebacterium tenuis, in trichomycosis axillaris, 295
Cosmetics, in exacerbation of acne, 68
Coup de sabre, 360–361, *360*
Coxsackie virus infection, 205–206, 202(t)
Crotamiton, in treatment of scabies, 214–215
Cryoglobulins, in lupus erythematosus, 381
Cryotherapy, in acne, 75
Cutaneous flora. See *Skin, flora of*.
Cutaneous injury, athletic, 457–458
Cutaneous nerves, 24–25
Cutaneous vasculature, 23–24
Cutis marmorata, vs. systemic lupus erythematosus, 374
Cysts, of acne, 65–66
 pilar, in scalp neoplasia, 361
Cytoplasm, basal cell, *9*
 spinous cell, *10*

Dactylitis, blistering distal, 171, *171*
Deafness, in late congenital syphilis, 249–253
Deerfly bite, 459
Demodex follicularum, in acne causation, 60
Dendritic cells, 11–14
Depression, associated with cutaneous disease, 31
Dermabrasion, in acne, 77
Dermatitis, acute weeping, treatment of, 102
 atopic. See *Atopic dermatitis*.
 chronic, treatment of, 119
 contact. See *Contact dermatitis*.
 vs. eczema, 86
 eczematous. See *Eczematous dermatitis* and *Eczema*.
 fiberglass, 105(t), 106
 nummular, 87, 116–117
 seborrheic. See *Seborrheic dermatitis*.
 "wear and tear," 106
Dermatoglyphic patterns, 7
Dermatomyositis, juvenile, 446–447, Plate XI-A
Dermatophytes, as cause of fungal infection, 40
 culture of, 43
Dermatophytid reaction, 304

Dermatophytoses, 303–314
  classification of, 303–304
Dermatosis(es), miscellaneous, 433–467
  aggravated by sunlight, 138
Dermis, 2, 20–23
  cellular components of, 23
  development of, 20
  papillary layer of, 20
  reticular layer of, 20
  structure of, 20
  tissue of, 3
  vascularization and innervation of, 3
Dermographism, 408–409, 408
Desmosome(s), 9, 11
Detergents, and contact dermatitis, 107
Development, normal, of adolescents, 29–30
Diabetes mellitus, and granuloma annulare, 442
  and necrobiosis lipoidica diabeticorum, 452
Diagnosis, of skin problems, in adolescent, 33–34
Diagnostic procedures, 39–53
Diascopy, in diagnosis of skin lesions, 49, 50
Diet, in acne causation, 66–67
  in treatment of acne, 76
Dihydrotestosterone (DHT), in development of sebaceous gland, 16
Diphtheroids, aerobic, 163–164
  anaerobic, 163–164
  in cutaneous infection, 294–296, 296
Discoid lupus erythematosus, 136, 370–373, 392, 393. See also *Lupus Erythematosus.*
  lesion of, 370–373, 371, 372
    distribution of, 372–373
  management of, 392
Disease, cutaneous, behavioral responses to, 28–29
  depression associated with, 31
  severe and chronic, 37–38
  social and psychological impact of, in adolescence, 30–38
DLE. See *Discoid lupus erythematosus.*
DNA, antibody to, in lupus erythematosus, 377, 379, 381
  excision and repair of, in xeroderma pigmentosum, 126
Donovania granulomatis, 262–263, 265
Dopa, in melanin formation, 12
Drugs, antidepressant, 36–37
  antimetabolite, in psoriasis, 158–159
  antimicrobial, in acne, 75–76
  antiviral, 185, 190
  "caine," and contact dermatitis, 107
  causing acanthosis nigricans, 435
  causing erythema nodosum, 417(t)
  causing urticaria, 407
  hormonal, in treatment of acne, 69, 76
  in exacerbation of acne, 69
  photosensitizing, 137–138
  psychotropic, for adolescent patient, 36–37
  reaction to, in atopic dermatitis, 93–94
  stimulant, for adolescent patients, 36
Dry skin, in atopic dermatitis, 91, 101–102
  in irritant contact dermatitis, 105, 107

Durand-Nicolas-Favre disease, 267–275. See also *Lymphogranuloma venereum.*
Dysplasia, ectodermal, 349–351, 349, 350, 350(t), Plate VIII–A
  anhidrotic, 350(t)
  hidrotic, 350(t)

Ear, herpes infection in, 194–195
  involvement of, in late congenital syphilis, 249–253
  in vitiligo, 436–437
  piercing of, and keloid formation, 457
Eccrine glands, 18–19
ECHO virus infection, 202(t), 206
Ecthyma, 168
Ectodermal dysplasia, 349–351, 349, 350, 350(t), Plate XIII–A
  anhidrotic, 350(t)
  hidrotic, 350(t)
Ectothrix infection, 43
Eczema, 86–119
  acute, 87
  asteatotic, 105
  atopic. See *Atopic dermatitis.*
  chronic, 92
  clinical features of, 87
  defined, 86
  discoid, 87, 116–117
  dyshidrotic, 117
  histological features of, 87
  inflammatory process in, 87
  nummular, 87, 116–117
  of hand and foot, 118, 118(t)
  subacute, 87
  topical therapy for, 118–119
  vs. dermatitis, 86
Eczema herpeticum, in atopic dermatitis, 95
Eczema vaccinatum, in atopic dermatitis, 95
Eczematous dermatitis, 86–119. See also *Eczema.*
Elastic fiber, 21
  function and structure of, 22–23
  in papillary dermis, 22
Elbows, psoriasis of, 148, Plate III–D
Embryogenesis, cutaneous, 1
Emotional stress, in cutaneous disease, 34–36
  in exacerbation of acne, 62, 68–69
  in psoriasis, 150–151, 153–154, 159–160
  in vitiligo, 436
Endocrine disease, and acanthosis nigricans, 434
Endothrix infection, 43
Enterovirus infection, 205–206
Enzymes, oral, in treatment of acne, 77
Ephelides, 460–461
Epidermal-melanin unit, 11
Epidermal nevus syndrome, 333–334
  developmental abnormalities in, 333–334
  mental retardation in, 333–334
Epidermis, 2, 8–14
  dendritic cells of, 11–14
  detail of, 2
Epidermodysplasia verruciformis, 196

Epidermophyton floccosum, in cutaneous infection, 308, 310, 312
Epithelioid nevus, 338, Plate VI–D
Erysipelas, 168–170, *169*
  vs. erysipeloid, 177
Erysipeloid, 176–177
Erythema annulare centrifugum, 414, *415*
Erythema chronicum migrans, 414–416
Erythema gyratum perstans, vs. erythema annulare centrifugum, 414
Erythema marginatum, 416, Plate X–A
Erythema multiforme, 419–421, *419, 420,* Plate X–C, D, and E. See also *Stevens-Johnson syndrome.*
  and herpes infection, 189–190
Erythema multiforme exudativum. See *Stevens-Johnson syndrome.*
Erythema nodosum, 416–418, 417(t), Plate X–B
Erythemas, figurate, 414–416
Erythrasma, 294–295, Plate VII–A
  diagnosis of, by Wood's light, 45, 46, Plate I–B
  vs. acanthosis nigricans, 435
Erythroderma, congenital ichthyosiform, vs. ichthyosis hystrix, 329
  exfoliative, 96
  in allergic contact dermatitis, 115
Erythromycin, in treatment of acne, 76
Erythropoietic porphyria, 133–134
Erythropoietic protoporphyria, 134–135, *134*
  and solar urticaria, 411
Esophagus, disorders of, in systemic scleroderma, 448
Estrogens, in treatment of acne, 55, 68, 76
  and sebaceous gland function, 55
Examination, KOH. See *KOH examination.*
Exanthem, Boston, 202(t), 206
Exanthems, diseases caused by, 201–206, 202(t)
  clinical findings on, 202(t)
Exfoliative erythroderma, 96
  in allergic contact dermatitis, 115
Eye, gonococcal infection of, 288–289
  herpes infection of, 187, 189, 194
  involvement of, in atopic dermatitis, 96
    in erythema multiforme, 420
    in late congenital syphilis, 247–249
    in nevus of Ota, 342, *343*
    in vitiligo, 436–437
    in X-linked ichthyosis, 438
Eyelashes, pediculosis of, 218–219, *218*

Face, appearance of, in atopic dermatitis, 90
  psoriasis of, 148, Plates II–B, III–B
Family–physician relationship, in treatment of adolescent patient, 32
Fasciitis, necrotizing, 178–179
Fatty acids. See *Free fatty acids.*
Favus, 305
Fibers, elastic, *21, 22,* 22–23
Fiberglass dermatitis, 105(t), 106
Fibroblasts, in dermis, 23
Flat wart, vs. acne, 72

Flora, of skin. See *Skin, flora of.*
Fluorescence, in diagnosis of fungal infections, 45–46
Fingernail(s). See *Nail(s).*
Follicle, of hair, 15
Follicular psoriasis, 148, 153
Folliculitis, 174–175, *174*
  gram-negative, 59–60
  in tinea barbae, 306
  ostia, 174
Fonsecaea compactum, in chromoblastomycosis, 316
Fonsecaea pedrosi, in chromoblastomycosis, 316
Foods, causing urticaria, 407
Foot, athlete's, 310–312, *311, 312*
  eczema of, 115, 118(t)
  fungal infection of, 295–296, *296,* 310–312, *310, 311*
  immersion, 106
  involvement of, in erythema multiforme, 420
    in granuloma annulare, 443
  psoriasis of, 148–149
Freckles, 460–461
Free fatty acid(s), in acne, 58, 60–61
  in sebum, 56
FTA-ABS test, false positive reactions in, 241
  in diagnosis of syphilis, 228, 239(t), 241, 242
Fungal infections, 293–325, Plates VII–A to F
  actinomycetes, 296–299
  classification of, 293–294
  dermatophyte, 303–314
  diphtheroid, 294–296, *296*
  examination for, 40–45
  of foot, 295–296, *296,* 310–312, *310, 311*
  of hair shaft, 295, 302–303, *304–306*
  of hand, 312
  of nail, 312–313
  opportunistic, 317–321, *318, 319*
  subcutaneous, 314–316
  superficial, 299–303
  urticarial response to, 412
  vs. acne, 72
Fungus blister, 41
Fungus, examination for, 40–45
  identification of, by KOH examination, *42*
  species of, as skin flora, 165
Furuncle, 175
Furunculosis, 175–176
Fusospirochetosis, in granuloma inguinale, 266

Gamma benzene hexachloride, in treatment of scabies, 213–214
Gangrene, hemolytic streptococcus, 178
  progressive bacterial synergistic, 179
Garment nevus, 339–341, *340, 341*
Gastrointestinal tract, involvement of, in juvenile dermatomyositis, 447
  in pyoderma gangrenosum, 451
Genitals, lesions of, differential diagnosis of, 227(t)
  psoriasis of, 149
  syphilitic chancre of, 226, 227(t)

Genital herpes, 188
Genital warts, 197–198
Giant cell, multinucleated, in herpes virus infection, 48, 49
Gingivostomatitis, in herpes infection, 187
Glabrous skin, 7
Glands, apocrine. See Apocrine glands.
　eccrine, 18–19
　of acini, 4
　of the skin, 4
　sebaceous. See Sebaceous gland.
Glomerulitis, focal, in systemic lupus erythematosus, 384
Glomerulonephritis, diffuse, in lupus erythematosus, 384
Glomerulonephropathy, membranous, in systemic lupus erythematosus, 384
Glomus (glomera), in cutaneous vessels, 24
　in nail bed, 20
Gonococcal infection, 279–289. See also Gonorrhea.
　disseminated, 285–289, 286.
　in children, 288
　ocular, 288–289
Gonorrhea, 279–289. See also Gonococcal infection.
　anorectal, 284–285
　complications of, 282–284, 283
　etiology of, 279–280
　in females, 282–284, 283
　in males, 280, 282, 281, 283
　pharyngeal, 285
　treatment of, 288(t)
Gram-negative organisms, in acne, 59–60
　in gram-negative folliculitis, 59–60
Granular cell layer, of epidermis, 8, 9
Granulocytopenia, in systemic lupus erythematosus, 385
Granuloma, in necrobiosis lipoidica diabeticorum, 453
　swimming pool, 454–455
Granuloma annulare, 442–444, Plate XII–C
　vs. necrobiosis lipoidica diabeticorum, 453
Granuloma inguinale, 262–267
　cicatricial, 265
　complications of, 266
　diagnosis of, 266
　etiology of, 263
　hypertrophic, 265, 265
　laboratory tests for, 266
　lesion of, 263–265, 264, 265
　manifestations of, 263–264
　nodular, 263, 264
　treatment of, 266–267
　ulcerovegetative, 263, 265
　vs. lymphogranuloma venereum, 271–274(t)
Gray patch syndrome, in tinea capitis, 304–305
Green nail syndrome, 180
Ground substance, in dermis, 23
Gummata, in late congenital syphilis, 241, 242
Günther's disease. See Erythropoietic porphyria.
Guttate psoriasis, 145, 148, 153, Plate II–A

Hair, 15–16
　bamboo, 351–352, 350(t), 350
　beaded, 350, 351
　classification of, 347, 349
　disorders of, 347–366
　　physical and chemical trauma in, 352
　　evaluation of, 347–348
　examination of, 347–348
　follicle, 5, 15
　　development of acne lesions in, 58
　growth cycle of, 5, 15–16, 349
　　alterations in, 353–356
　infected, 41, 43
　　diagnosis of, 45, 46
　lupus, 375
　properties of, 15–16, 347, 349
　pubic, pediculosis of, 217–219
　ringed, 353, 350
　shaft of, 5
　structural abnormalities of, 349–353, 350(t), 350
　terminal, 15
　twisted, 352–353, 350(t), 350
　vellus, 15, 15
Hair dryers, in alopecia, 358
Hair shaft, fungal infection of, 295, 302–303, 304–306
　physical and chemical damage to, 356–369
　terminal, structure of, 16
Hair straightening, and alopecia, 358
Hair transplantation, in alopecia, 356
Halo nevus, 338–339, 339
　in vitiligo, 437
Hand, eczema of, 118, 118(t)
　fungal infection of, 312
　housewives', 92
　in lupus erythematosus, 372, 372, Plate IX–B
　involvement of, in erythema multiforme, 420, 419
　in granuloma annulare, 443
　psoriasis of, 148–149, Plates II–E, IV–B
Hand lens, 39, 40
Hartnup disease, 129–130, 129
Hearing loss, in late congenital syphilis, 249–253
Heart, involvement of, in systemic lupus erythematosus, 383
　in systemic scleroderma, 448, 449
Heat, in exacerbation of acne, 67
Heat urticaria, 410
Hemolytic streptococcus gangrene, 178
Hemophilus ducreyi, 257, 260
Hennebert's sign, 253
Henoch-Schönlein purpura, 423–426, 424
Hepatitis, in secondary syphilis, 235–236
Herald patch, of pityriasis rosea, 441
Herpes genitalis, vs. lymphogranuloma venereum, 271–274(t)
Herpes gladiatorum, 187
Herpes simplex infection, 185–190
　and cervical cancer, 186
　and Kaposi's varicelliform eruption, 189
　chronic, 190
　diagnosis of, by Tzanck smear, 48
　disseminated infection in, 186–187

Herpes simplex infection (*Continued*)
  in genitals, 188
  neonatal, 186, 188
  primary, 187–189
  primary cutaneous inoculation, 187
  recurrent, 189–190
  treatment of, 190
  virus causing, 186
Herpes simplex virus (HSV), 185–190, *186*
  Type I vs. Type II, 186–190
Herpes zoster, 193–195, *194*
Hertoghe's sign, of secondary syphilis, *231*
Hidradenitis suppurativa, and acne vulgaris, 69–70
  vs. furunculosis, 175
Higoumenakis' sign, 243–244
Hirsutism, 361–363
  causes of, 363(t)
  idiopathic, 362
  secondary, 362–363
    endocrine abnormalities in, 362–363
Histamine, response to, in urticaria, 406
History-taking, in photodermatosis, 139–140
  in treatment of adolescent patient, 32
HL-A antigens, and lupus erythematosus, 387
  and psoriasis, 145, 150
  and Reiter syndrome, 276
Hormones, causing acne, 61–62
  in sebum production, 55
  in treatment of acne, 69, 76
Hospitalization, of adolescent patient, 37–38
Hot comb alopecia, 358
Housewives' hand, *92*
Hutchinson's incisors, 245–247, *246*
Hutchinson's triad, *246*
Hydration, of skin, in atopic dermatitis, 101–102
  in chronic dermatitis, 119
  in irritant contact dermatitis, 105–106, *107*
Hydroxykynureninuria, vs. Hartnup disease, 130
Hydroxyurea, in treatment of psoriasis, 159
Hymenoptera sting, allergic reaction to, 460
Hyperpigmentation, of acne, in blacks, 65
Hypersensitivity response, delayed, 109–110
  in scabies, 213
  light-induced, 124
Hypertrichosis, 361–362
  nerve involvement in, 362
Hypertrichosis lanuginosa, 362
Hypha(e), of tinea, 42–43, *43*
Hypocomplementemia, in systemic lupus erythematosus, 382

Ichthyosis, X-linked, 438, *439*
Ichthyosis hystrix, 329, *330*
  vs. acanthosis nigricans, 435
  vs. nevus unius lateris, 329
"Id" reaction, 304
Ilven, 328–329, *329*
Immersion foot, 106
Immune complexes, circulating, in systemic lupus erythematosus, 381
Immunity, cell-mediated, in lupus erythematosus, 386–389

Immunization, for rubeola, 203
Immunofluorescence tests, for lupus erythematosus, 376–377, 378
Immunoglobulins, in atopic dermatitis, 97–98
  deposition of, in lupus erythematosus, 376–377, *376*
Immunological defect in ataxia-telangiectasia, 131
  in atopic dermatitis, 97–99, 97(t)
  in lupus erythematosus, 385–386
  in scleroderma, 448
  in vitiligo, 435–436
Impetigo, Bockhart's, 174
  bullous, 172–174, *173*
Impetigo contagiosa, 166–168, *166*
Indians, American, polymorphous light eruption in, 127
Infantile acne, 71, *71*
  atopic dermatitis, 89
Infants, telogen effluvium in, 356
Infection(s), bacterial. See *Bacterial infections.*
  causing erythema nodosum, 417(t)
  cutaneous, in atopic dermatitis, 95–96, 95(t), 96(t)
  ectothrix, 43, *44*. See also *Fungal infections.*
  endothrix, 43
  fungal. See *Fungal infections.*
  gonococcal. See *Gonococcal infections, Gonorrhea.*
  pyogenic. See *Pyogenic infections.*
  streptococcal, and psoriasis, 145–147, 153
  viral. See *Viral infections.*
  vs. acne, 72
  yeast, 44, 317–321, *318, 319*
    examination for, 40–45
Inflammatory process, in eczema, 87
Infundibulum, of hair follicle, cellular components of, 57–58
Insect bites, 459–460
  as cause of urticaria, 407
Insect sting, 460
Insecticides, chlorinated, and porphyria, 133
Interferon, 185
Intradermal nevus, 335–336
Iodine, in treatment of acne, 69
Iris lesion, of erythema multiforme, 419–420, *420*
Iron, excessive, in acquired porphyria, 133
Irritant contact dermatitis, 103(t), 104–108
  causes of, 104–106, 105(t)
  clinical characteristics of, 104
  complications of, 107
  diagnosis of, 106–107
  differential diagnosis of, 106–107
  dry skin and, 105
  excessive moisture and, 105–106
  treatment of, 107–108
  types of, 105(t)
  vs. allergic contact dermatitis, 103(t), 107
  vs. atopic dermatitis, 100, 101(t)
Itching. See *Pruritus.*

Job's syndrome, 99
Jock itch, 308–309, *309*
Joints, involvement of, in late congenital syphilis, 244–245, *245*

Junctional nevus, 335–336, *336*
Juvenile dermatomyositis, 446–447, Plate XI–A
Juvenile melanoma, benign, 338, Plate VI–D
Juvenile paresis, and sensorineural hearing loss, 251

Kaposi's varicelliform eruption, 95, 188–189
Keloid(s), 455–457, *456*
Keratinocytes, 8, 9, 11
  migrations of, 9, 11
Keratitis, and recurrent herpes simplex, 189
  interstitial, in late congenital syphilis, 248–249, *248*
Keratinocytic nevus, 327–334, 327(t)
Keratoconjunctivitis, in herpes infection, 187, 189
Keratohyaline granule, formation of, 9
Keratolysis, pitted, 295–296, *296*
Keratosis pilaris, vs. acne, 71–72
  and monilethrix, 351
Kerion, 305
Kidney, involvement of, in Henoch-Schönlein purpura, 424–425
  in impetigo contagiosa, 167
  in lupus erythematosus, 377, 379, 384
  in secondary syphilis, 236
  in Stevens-Johnson syndrome, 420–421
  in systemic scleroderma, 448, 449
Knees, psoriasis of, 148, Plate III–E
Koebner phenomenon, in lichen sclerosus et atrophicus, 445
  in lichen planus, 440
  in psoriasis, 146(t), 147, 153, Plates II–B, to E
  in vitiligo, 436
KOH examination, for fungal identification, 41–44, *42, 43, 44, 45*
KOH preparation, *42*

Labyrinthitis, meningo-neural, 249, 251
Langerhans' cell, 8, 13, 14, *14*
Larynx, papillomas of, 198
Late congenital syphilis, physical signs of, 243–245, 243(t)
Lentigines, vs. freckles, 460
Leptomeningeal melanosis, 340
Lesions, of acne, 63–66, *64, 65*
  picking at, 68–69
  skin. See *Skin lesions*.
Leukemia, and erythema nodosum, 418
Leukoderma acquisitum centrifugum, 338–339, *339*
Leukopenia, in systemic lupus erythematosus, 385
Lice. See *Pediculosis*.
Lichen planopilaris, 359–360
Lichen planus, 439–440, Plate XI–D
Lichen planus tropicus, 138
Lichen sclerosus et atrophicus, 444–446, Plate XII–A
  prognosis of, 446
  in children, 446
Lichen simplex chronicus, 117–118

Lichen urticatus, 408
Lindane, in treatment of scabies, 213–214
Lip, lesions of, differential diagnosis of, 227(t)
  syphilitic chancre of, 226, 227(t)
Livedo reticularis, in systemic lupus erythematosus, 374
Liven, 328–329, *329*
Liver, involvement of, in secondary syphilis, 235–236
Lungs, involvement of, in atopic dermatitis, 88–89
  in systemic lupus erythematosus, 383
  in systemic scleroderma, 448, 449
Lupus band test, 377
Lupus erythematosus, 136, 367–403. See also *Discoid lupus erythematosus* and *Systemic lupus erythematosus*.
  and scarring alopecia, 359, 360
  and serological test for syphilis, 382–383
  and Type C virus, 386–387
  anemia in, 385
  antimalarial therapy in, 392–393
  cell factor in, 369
  diagnostic tests for, 369, 376–377, 378
  DNA antibody in, 377, 379, 381
    tests for, 379
  extracutaneous manifestations of, 383–386
  familial incidence in, 386–387
  fever in, 392
  hair loss in, 374–375
  immunoglobulin deposition in, 376–377, *376*
  lesions of, 370–377, Plates IX–A to C
    classification of, 370–371
    differential diagnosis of, 373
    histology of, 375–377
  management of, 389–394
  nerve involvement in, 382, 383–384
  pathogenesis of, 386–389
  serological manifestations of, 378–383
  serum patterns in, 378
  steroid therapy in, 393
  ultraviolet light in, 388–391
  vs. lichen planopilaris, 359–360
Lupus hair, 375
Lupus nephritis, 377, 379, 384
Lupus panniculitis, 374
Lupus profundus, 374
Lupus vulgaris, diascopy in diagnosis of, 49
Lyme arthritis, and erythema chronicum migrans, 415–416
Lymphadenitis, in chancroid, 260–261
Lymphadenopathy, in secondary syphilis, 234
Lymphatic vessels, in dermis, 24
Lymphogranuloma inguinale, 267–275. See also *Lymphogranuloma venereum*.
Lymphogranuloma venereum, 267–275
  constitutional symptoms of, 270
  diagnosis of, 270–275, 271–274(t)
  differential diagnosis of, 271–274(t)
  etiology of, 267
  inguinal syndrome in, 268, 270
  laboratory tests for, 275
  lesion of, 268, *269*
  manifestations of, 268–270, *269*
  rectal syndrome in, 270
  treatment of, 275

Lymphopathia venereum, 267–275. See also *Lymphogranuloma venereum.*
Lymphopenia, in systemic lupus erythematosus, 385

Maceration of skin, and contact dermatitis, 105–106
Macrophage(s), in dermis, 23
Malignancy, in acanthosis nigricans, 434
  in nevocytic nevus, 337
Mallorca acne, 70
Mast cells, in dermis, 23
Measles, 203, 204, Plate VI-A
Medulla, of hair, 15
Meissner's corpuscle, 24–25
Melanin, 11–13
  production of, 12–13
    disorders associated with, 132
Melanin-epidermal unit, 11
Melanization, stages of, *13*
Melanocytes, *1*, 8, 11–12, *12*
Melanocytic nevus, 341–344
Melanoma, benign juvenile, 338, Plate VI-D
  malignant, vs. benign juvenile melanoma, 338
    vs. halo nevus, 338–339
    vs. nevocytic nevi, 337
Melanosis, Becker's, 331
  leptomeningeal, 340
  neurocutaneous, 340
Melanosomes, 12–13, *13*
Meleney's ulcer, 179
Meningoencephalitis, in herpes infection, 187
Menkes' kinky hair syndrome, 350(t), 353
Menses, in exacerbation of acne, 68
Merkel cell, 8, 13–14
Merkel-Ranvier corpuscles, 25
Methotrexate, in treatment of psoriasis, 158–159
Micrococcaceae, as normal skin flora, 164
  in acne causation, 59
Micrococci, as normal skin flora, 164
Micro-immunofluorescence (micro-IF) test, for lymphogranuloma venereum, 275
Microsporum audouini, in tinea capitis, 45, 304–306
Microsporum canis, in tineas, 45, 304–306, 307, 308
Midge bite, 459
Miliaria crystallina, 458
Miliaria rubra, 458
Minimal erythema dose (MED), 140
Mite(s), in pathogenesis of acne, 60
  of scabies, 46–47, *47*, 211
    burrow of, *46*
Mixed porphyria, 132
Molluscum contagiosum, 199–201, *199*
  Tzanck smear in diagnosis of, 48–49
Mongolian spot, 341–342
Monilethrix, *350, 351*
Morphea, 450, *450*
  of scalp, 360–361, *360*
Mosaic wart, 197
Mosquito bite, 459

Mouth, herpes infection of, 187
  involvement of, in lichen planus, 439, Plate XI-D
Mucha-Habermann disease, 426–428, *426, 427*
Mucormycosis, 321–322
Mucous patch, syphilitic, 233, Plate VI-B
Mulberry molar, 247, *247*
Muscles, involvement of, in juvenile dermatomyositis, 446, 447
  in systemic scleroderma, 448
Mycelium(a), 42–43, *43*
Mycetoma, 297
  nocardiosis, 299
Mycobacterium(a), infection by, 454–455
Mycobacterium balnei, 454
Mycobacterium marinum, 454
Mycotic infections. See *Fungal infections.*

Nail(s), *6*, 19–20
  disorders of, 20
  dystrophic, *349*
  infection of, fungal, 312–313
    candidal, 319–321, *319*
    scraping of, *41*
  involvement of, in systemic lupus erythematosus, 374, Plate IX-B
  matrix of, *6*, 19
  psoriasis of, 149, Plate IV-A
Necrobiosis lipoidica diabeticorum, 452–453, Plate XII-B
Necrolysis, toxic epidermal, 172–173
Necrotizing fasciitis, 178–179
Negro(es), acquired trichorrhexis nodosa in, 352
  hyperpigmentation of acne in, 65
  keloid in, 456
Neisseria gonorrhoeae, 279–280, 279(t), *281, 282*
Neisseria species, fermentation patterns of, 279(t)
Neonatal acne, 71, *71*
  herpes infection, 188
Neoplasia, of scalp, nevus in, 361
  pilar cysts in, 361
  scarring alopecia in, 361, *361*
Neoplasms, in xeroderma pigmentosum, 125–126
Nephritis, in impetigo contagiosa, 167
Nephrosis, in secondary syphilis, 236
Nerves, cutaneous, 24–25
  involvement of, in herpes zoster, 195
    in Henoch-Schönlein purpura, 425
    in hypertrichosis, 362
    in lupus erythematosus, 382, 383–384
    in secondary syphilis, 236, 241
Netherton's syndrome, 351–352, 350(t), *350*
Neurofibromatosis, and freckling, 460
Neurosyphilis, 236, 241
  congenital, 241
Nevil, 328–329, *329*
Nevocytic nevus. See *Nevus, nevocytic.*
Nevoid basal cell carcinoma, 125, Plate I-C

Nevus(i), 326–346
  balloon cell, 337
  bathing trunk, 339–341, *340, 341*
  Becker's, 331
  blue, 343–344, *343, 361*
    cellular, 342–343
    common, 343–344, *343*
  compound, 335–336, *336*
  congenital giant pigmented hairy, 339–341, *340, 341*
  defined, 326
  epidermal, syndrome in. See *Epidermal nevus syndrome.*
    vs. acanthosis nigricans, 435
  epithelioid, 338, Plate VI-D
  etiology of, 326
  garment, 339–341, *340, 341*
  halo, 338–339, *339*
  in neoplasia of scalp, 361, *361*
  intradermal, 335–336
  junctional, 335–336, *336*
  keratinocytic epidermal, 327–334, 327(t)
    treatment of, 330
  melanocytic, 341–344
  nevocytic, 334–341
    clinical appearance of, 335–336
    compound, 335–336, *336*
    excision of, 336–337
    histopathology of, 335–336
    intradermal, 335–336
    junctional, 335–336, *336*
    life cycle of, 335
    malignant change in, 337
    treatment of, 336–337
  nevus cell. See *Nevus, nevocytic.*
  of Ito, 342
  of Ota, 341, 342–343, *343*
  organoid, 331–333, *332*
  spindle cell, 338, Plate VI-D
  Spitz's, 338, Plate VI-D
  Sutton's, 338–339, *339*
  types of, 327, 327(t)
  verrucous epidermal, 327–329, *328, 329*
    linear, 327–329, *328*
      inflammatory, 328–329, *329*
      localized, 327–328
Nevus cell, origin of, 334–335
Nevus comedonicus, 331, *332*
Nevus sebaceus, etiology of, 333
  in scalp neoplasia, 361
  of Jadassohn, 331–333, *332*
Nevus unius lateris, 328, *329*
Nickel sensitivity, and allergic contact dermatitis, 112
Nicotinamide, deficiency of, in Hartnup disease, 129
Nocardia asteroides, in nocardiosis, 298
Nocardia brasiliensis, in nocardiosis, 298
Nocardiosis, 298–299
Nodular acne, 70
Nodular scabies, 216, *216*
Nodules, of acne, 65–66
Norwegian scabies, 217
Nummular eczema, 87, 116–117
  vs. atopic dermatitis, 100, 101(t)

Obesity, and acanthosis nigricans, 434–435
Ocular-genital-synovial syndrome. See *Reiter syndrome.*
Odland bodies, 9, 11
Onychia, candidal, 319–320, *319*
  treatment of, 321
Onychomycosis, 312–313, *313*
Organoid nevus, 331–333, *332*
Osteolysis, in secondary syphilis, 235, *235*
Osteomyelitis, syphilitic gummatous, 251–253, *252*
Ostia folliculitis, 174
Otitis externa, acute, 180

Pacinian corpuscle, 24–25
Pain, in psoriasis, 149–150
Papilloma(s), laryngeal, 198
Papovavirus, in development of warts, 196
Papules, of acne, 64–65
Paronychia, candidal, 319–320
    treatment of, 321
  herpetic, 187
Patch testing, in allergic contact dermatitis, 53, 113–114
  in urticaria, 411
  photo, 140
Patient, adolescent. See *Adolescent patient.*
Patient-physician relationship, 30–34
Pediculosis, 217–221
  of eyelashes, 218–219, *218*
Pediculosis capitis, 219–220
Pediculosis pubis, 217–219
Pellagra, *129*
  vs. Hartnup disease, 129–130
Pelvic inflammatory disease, and gonorrhea, 283–284
Pemphigus, 49
Pemphigus foliaceus, 138
Penicillin, causing urticaria, 407
  in treatment of pyodermas, 168, 170, 171, 173, 176, 177, 178, 179
    of venereal disease, 250(t), 253, 287, 288(t)
Periderm, 8
Perihepatitis, gonococcal, 284
Periostitis, of temporal bone, 251–253
Petechia, calcaneal, 458
Phagocyte function, defective, in atopic dermatitis, 99, 96(t)
Pharyngitis, and psoriasis, 145, 153
  gonococcal, 285
Phialophora verrucosa, in chromoblastomycosis, 316
Photo testing, in diagnosis of polymorphous light eruption, 128
Photoallergy, defined, 124
  drug-induced, 137–138
Photodermatoses, 123–141
  clinical management of, 139–141
  medical history in, 139–140
  physical examination in, 140
  treatment of, 140–141
Photoprotection, 138–139

Photosensitivity, 124–140
    drug-induced, 137–138
    plant-induced, 137–138
Photosensitization, systemic, 137
    topical, 137–138
    treatment of, 138
Phototoxicity, defined, 124
    drug-induced, 137–138
    tests for, 140
Phthiriasis palpebrarum, 218, *218*
Phycomycosis, 321–322
Phytophotodermatitis, 137
Piedra, 302–303
    vs. trichomycosis axillaris, 295
Piedraia hortae, in black piedra, 302–303
Pili annulati, 353, *350*
Pili torti, 350(t), *350,* 352–353
    in Menkes' kinky hair syndrome, 353
Pilosebaceous unit, 7, 57–58
Pimples. See *Skin lesions.*
Pitted keratolysis, 295–296
Pityriasis alba, in atopic dermatitis, 91
Pityriasis lichenoides et varioliformis acuta, 426–428, *426, 427*
Pityriasis rosea, 441–442, Plate XI–B
    vs. contact dermatitis, 106
Pityrosporum orbiculare, 165
    in acne, 59
    in tinea versicolor, 299
Pityrosporum ovale, in acne, 59
Plantar wart, 197
Poikiloderma congenitale, 132
Poison ivy antigens, 111–112
Polymorphous light eruption (PMLE) 127–128, *128*
    familial predisposition to, 127
    vs. contact dermatitis, 106
Pompholyx, 117
Porcupine man, 329
Porphyria, 132–135
    acquired, 133
    drug-induced, 133
    laboratory tests for, 140
    mixed, 132
    variegate, 132
Porphyria cutanea tarda, 132
    detection of, by Wood's light, 46
Potassium hydroxide examination. See *KOH examination.*
Poxvirus, in molluscum contagiosum, 200
Pregnancy, acne in, 68
    erythema nodosum in, 418
    herpes infection in, 188
    rubella in, 205
    syphilis in. See *Syphilis, late congenital.*
    varicella in, 192
Pressure urticaria, 409, *409*
Prickle cell layer, of epidermis, 8, 9
Prickly heat, 458
Proctitis, gonococcal, 284–285
Proctocolitis, in lymphogranuloma venereum, 270
Progressive bacterial synergistic gangrene, 179
Proteus, as skin flora, 165
Protoporphyria, erythropoietic, 134–135, *134*

Protoporphyrin, 134
Prurigo simplex, 408
Pruritus, in atopic dermatitis, 89, 94–95
    in eczema, 87
    in psoriasis, 149
    in varicella, 192
Pruritus ani, 319
Pseudoacanthosis nigricans, 435
Pseudofolliculitis, 175
Pseudopelade, 360
Pseudomonas, causing pyogenic infections, 179–180
    infection, of toe webs, 180
Pseudopili annulati, 353
Psoralens, and photosensitivity, 137–138
Psoriasis, 143–162, Plates II–A to V–C
    age of onset in, 144
    and skin trauma, 146(t), 147, 153
    arthritis in, 150, Plate V–A
    biopsy in, 152
    diagnosis of, 151–152
    differential diagnosis of, 147–149
    distribution pattern in, 148
    effects of, on major life decisions, 152
    emotional stress in, 150–151, 153–154, 159–160
    fissures in, 149–150
    follicular, 148, 153
    genital involvement in, 149
    guttate, 145, 148, 153, Plate II–A
    histopathological changes in, 152, Plate V–C
    infection in, 150, Plate IV–D
    inheritance of, 144–145
    itching in, 149
    Koebner phenomenon in, 146(t), 147, 153, Plates II–B to E
    laboratory studies for, 153
    lesions of, 147–149, Plates II–A to V–B
    of elbows and knees, 148, Plates III–D and E
    of face, 148, Plates II–B, III–B
    of nails, 149, Plate IV–A
        treatment of, 157
    of palms and soles, 148–149, Plate IV–B
    of scalp, 147–148, Plate III–A
        treatment of, 157
    of trunk, 148, Plates II–C, III–C
    pain in, 149–150
    perianal involvement in, 149
    pharyngitis and, 145, 153
    precipitating factors in, 145–147, 146(t), 153
    prevalence of, 143–144
    prognosis in, 152
    seasonal factor in, 155
    signs of, 147–149
    sites of, 147
    streptococcal pharyngitis and, 145–147, 153
    supportive therapy in, 159–160
    symptoms of, 149–151
    tonsillectomy in, 153
    treatment of, 152–160
        intralesional, 157–158
        systemic, 158–159
        topical, 154–157
        ultraviolet light in, 155–156
    vs. pityriasis rosea, 441

Psychiatric treatment, in adolescent cutaneous disease, 35–36
  in serious or chronic disease, 38
Psychogenic urticaria, 412
Psychotropic drugs, for adolescent patient, 36–37
Puberty, psychological and social effects of, 29–30
Pubic hair, pediculosis of, 217–219
Punch biopsy, 50–52
  equipment for, 50, *51*
  in histopathological diagnosis, 50
  technique of, 50–52, *51, 52*
Purpura, anaphylactoid, 423–426, *424*
  Henoch-Schönlein, 423–426, *424*
Pyoderma(s), 165–183. See also *Pyogenic infections.*
  acantholytic cells in, 49
Pyoderma gangrenosum, 451–452, Plate XI–C
Pyogenic infections, 163–183
  anaerobic, 176–179
  caused by *Pseudomonas,* 179–180
  microaerophilic, 176–179
  staphylococcal, 172–176
  streptococcal, 166–171

Radiation, solar, and skin disorders, 123–140
Radiation therapy, in acne, 77
Radioisotope precipitation (RIP) test, for lymphogranuloma venereum, 275
Ramsay Hunt syndrome, in herpes zoster, 194
Raynaud's phenomenon, in scleroderma, 448, *449*
Reagin tests, in late congenital syphilis, 242
Reflex, axon, 25
Reiter syndrome, 276–279, *277,* Plate VI–C
Resorcinol, in treatment of acne, 73, 74
Retinoic acid, in treatment of acne, 73–74
Rheumatic fever, and erythema marginatum, 416
Rhinitis, allergic, in atopic dermatitis, 89
Rhus antigen, 111–112
Ringworm. See *Dermatophytoses.*
Rothmund-Thomson syndrome, 132, Plate I–D
RPR test, in diagnosis of syphilis, 228, 238, 239(t)
Rubella, 203–205
Rubeola, 203, *204*

Saber shin, 244
Salicylates, causing urticaria, 407
  in vascular reactive disease, 418
Salpingitis, gonococcal, 284
Sarcoptes scabiei, 47, 210, *211*
Scabies, 209–217, *210, 211, 216*
  animal-transmitted, 216–217
  bacterial complications in, 212
  causative mite of, 46–47, *47,* 210, *211*
    burrow of, *46*

Scabies (*Continued*)
  classic, 209–210
    diagnosis of, 210
    lesion of, 209–210, *210, 216*
    transmission of, 211–212
    treatment of, 210–216
      hygienic measures in, 212
      in household members, 211–212
      in sexual partners, 211–212
  crusted, 217
  drugs for, 210–216
    dosage of, 211
  epidemics of, 209
  examination for, 46–47
  hypersensitivity response in, 213
  nodular, 216, *216*
  Norwegian, 217
  variant forms of, 210, 216–217
  vs. atopic dermatitis, 100, 101(t)
Scalded skin syndrome, 172, *173*
Scalp, inflammatory disorders of, 358–359
  neoplasia of, 361, *361*
    scarring alopecia in, 361, *361*
  pediculosis of, 219–220
  psoriasis of, 147–148, Plate III–A
  scaling of, in atopic dermatitis, 91
Scars, in inflammatory acne, 66
  in keloid, 456–457
  post-rhagadic, in late congenital syphilis, 243, *244*
Scleroderma, 447–451, *449*
  female preponderance in, 448
  focal, 450–451
  linear, 450
  localized, 450–451
    of scalp, 360–361, *360*
  systemic, 448–449, *449*
  types of, 447–448
Sebaceous gland, 16–17, 54–58
  development of, 16
  distribution of, 54
  function of, 57
  innervation of, 55
  structure of, 16–17, 54–55
  synthesizing activity of, 56
Seborrheic dermatitis, 117
  vs. atopic dermatitis, 100, 101(t)
  vs. contact dermatitis, 106, 112
  vs. tinea versicolor, 301
Sebum, 56–57
  collection methods for, 56–57
  composition of, 17, 56
    factors affecting, 57
  excretion rate of (SER), and acne, 60–61
  function of, 57
  production of, 55
    factors affecting, 57
    feedback mechanism in, 56
    in acne, 63
  secretion of, 16–17
Sensitization phase, in allergic contact dermatitis, 108–109
Septicemia, *Pseudomonas,* 179–180
Serositis, in systemic lupus erythematosus, 383
Serum complement deficiency, in lupus erythematosus, 136, 382

Serum sickness, urticaria in, 413
Sexual habits, and acne, 69
Skin, appendages of, 14–20
    cancer of, 125
    dry, in atopic dermatitis, 91, 101–102
        in irritant contact dermatitis, 105, 107
    examination of, 39
    flora of, 163–165
    function of, 7–26
    glabrous, 7
    glands of, 4
    hairy, 7
    structure of, 7–26
Skin lesions, in atopic dermatitis, 91
    morphology of, in atopic dermatitis, 91
    of acne, 63–66, *64, 65*
    severity of, and treatment patterns, 30
    pellagrinous, *129*
    squeezing of, 37
SLE. See *Systemic lupus erythematosus.*
Solar radiation, and skin disorders, 123–140
Solar urticaria, 135–136, 410–411, Plate I-E
Sore throat, and psoriasis, 145–147, 153
Specimens, selection of, for mycological study, 40–41
    skin, in punch biopsy, *52*
Spina bifida occulta, in focal scleroderma, 450
Spindle cell nevus, 338, Plate VI-D
Spine, involvement of, in focal scleroderma, 450
Spitz's nevus, 338, Plate VI-D
Sporotrichosis, 314–316
    fixed cutaneous, 314
    lymphocutaneous, 314
    mucocutaneous, 314–315
Sporothrix schenckii, in sporotrichosis, 314, 315
Staphylococci, as normal skin flora, 164
    causing pyogenic infections, 172–176
Staphylococcus aureus, as transient skin flora, 164
    causing pyogenic infection, 165, 172
    in psoriasis, 150, Plate IV-D
Staphylococcus epidermidis, 164
    in etiology of acne, 59
Staphylococcus saprophyticus, 164
Steroid acne, 70, *70*
Steroid therapy, in allergic contact dermatitis, 116
    in atopic dermatitis, 101–102
    in granuloma annulare, 444
    in herpes zoster, 195
    in juvenile dermatomyositis, 447
    in lichen planus, 440
    in lupus erythematosus, 393
    in necrobiosis lipoidica diabeticorum, 453
    in psoriasis, 156–157
Stevens-Johnson syndrome, 420–421, *420*
Stimulant drugs, in treatment of adolescent patient, 36
Stings, insect, 460
Stomatitis, aphthous, vs. enterovirus infection, 205
Stratum corneum, 8
Stratum germinativum, 8

Stratum lucidum, 8
Stratum malpighii, 8
Streptococcal antibodies, screening technique for, 167
    infections, and psoriasis, 145–147, 153
Streptococci, as cutaneous flora, 164
    causing pyogenic infections, 166–171
Streptococcus pyogenes, 165
Streptozyme, 167
Stress, emotional. See *Emotional stress.*
Subcutaneous tissue, 25–26
Sulfur, in treatment of acne, 74
    in treatment of scabies, 215
Sun damage, prevention of, 138–139
Sunburn, and psoriasis, 155–156
    prevention of, 138
Sunlight, aggravating dermatoses, 138
    and lupus erythematosus, 388, 391
    and skin damage, mechanism of, 123–124
    and skin disorders, 123–140
    in treatment of vitiligo, 437–438
Sunscreens, 138–139
Surgery, in treatment of acne, 74–75
Sutton's nevus, 338–339, *339*
Sweating, apocrine, 17
    eccrine, 19
    in atopic dermatitis, 91
Swimming pool granuloma, 454–455
Sycosis barbae, 174–175
Sycosis vulgaris, 174–175
Syphilis, 222–256
    acquired, 224–241
        early, 224–228
            laboratory tests for, 227–228, 237–241
            relapse in, 236–237
        secondary. See *Syphilis, secondary.*
    and chancroid, 261
    antibodies produced in, 239(t)
    chancre of, 224–228, *225, 226,* 227(t). See also *Chancre of syphilis.*
    classification of, 223(t)
    congenital. See *Syphilis, late congenital.*
    diagnosis of, 237–241
        darkfield microscopy in, 237
    etiology of, 222–224
    late congenital, 241–253
        deafness in, 249–253
        dental malformations in, 245–247, *246, 247*
        epiphyseal enlargement in, 244
        eye disease in, 247–249
        facial signs of, 243
        osteomyelitis in, 251–253, *252*
        post-rhagadic scarring in, 243, *244*
        scaphoid scapulae in, 244
        serological reactions in, 242
    latent, 237
    neural involvement in, 236, 241
    secondary, 228–237
        bone involvement in, 235, *235*
        clinical manifestations of, 228–237, *228–232,* 233(t), *234, 235*
        condylomata lata in, *234,* 234
        constitutional symptoms of, 234–237
        cutaneous eruption in, 228–233, *228–232,* 233(t)

Syphilis (*Continued*)
  secondary, differential diagnosis of, 235
    headache in, 235
    kidney involvement in, 236
    lesions of, 228–234, *228–232, 234,* 235
    liver involvement in, 235–236
    lymphadenopathy in, 234
    mucous patch of, 233, Plate VI-B
  tests for, 237–341
    complement fixation, 237–238, 239(t)
    flocculation, 237–238, 239(t)
    non-treponemal antigen, 237–238, 239(t), 240
    reactive reagin, 237–238, 239(t)
    serological, 227–228, 237–241, 239(t)
      false-positive reactions in, 240–241
      in lupus erythematosus, 382–383
    treponemal antigen, 238–242, 239(t)
  treatment of, 250(t)
Syringocystadenoma papilliferum, in nevus sebaceus, 333
Systemic lupus erythematosus, 136, 367–403. See also *Lupus erythematosus.*
  antinuclear antibody in, 378–380
  arthritis in, 370(t), 373, 383
  blood disorders in, 385–386
  butterfly rash of, 373
  diagnostic criteria for, 369–370, 370(t)
  heart involvement in, 383
  immunological defects in, 385–389
  lesion of, 373–375, *373, 374,* Plates IX-B, IX-C
    distribution of, 373–374
  lung involvement in, 383
  nail involvement in, 374, Plate IX-B
  prognosis of, 390
  renal disease in, 384
  serositis in, 383
  serum complement levels in, 382
  vasculitis in, 374

T cell, in systemic lupus erythematosus, 385–389
Tabes dorsalis, juvenile, and sensorineural hearing loss, 251
Tar preparations, for atopic dermatitis, 102
  for psoriasis, 156
Teeth, malformations of, in late congenital syphilis, 245–247, *246, 247*
Telangiectasias, in ataxia telangiectasia, 131–132
Telogen effluvium, 355–356, 355(t)
  neonatal, 356
Telogen phase, of hair growth, 15
Tenosynovitis, gonococcal, 287
Terminal hair, 15
Tetracycline, in treatment of acne, 73, 75–76
  in pregnancy, 75–76
Thrombocytopenia, in systemic lupus erythematosus, 385
Thrombophlebitis, vs. erythema nodosum, 417, 418
Thrush, 317–318
  treatment of, 320

Tick bite, 459–460
Tinea(s), classification of, 40
  hyphae of, 42–43, *43*
  vs. contact dermatitis, 106–107, 112
Tinea barbae, 306–307
Tinea capitis, 304–306, *305,* 359, Plates VII-B, VIII-D
  diagnosis of by Wood's light, 45
Tinea corporis, 307–308, Plates VII-C, D, E
  vs. atopic dermatitis, 100, 101(t)
  vs. granuloma annulare, 442
  vs. pityriasis rosea, 441
Tinea cruris, 308–309, *309*
  in adolescence, 40
Tinea manuum, 312
Tinea nigra, 301–302
Tinea pedis, 101(t), 310–312, *310, 311, 312*
  in adolescence, 40
Tinea unguium, 312–313, *313*
Tinea versicolor, *45,* 299–301, *300, 301*
  identification of by KOH technique, 43–44
Tissue, adipose, 25–26
  of dermis, *3*
  of nail, *6*
  subcutaneous, 25–26
Toenail(s). See *Nail(s).*
Toes, *Pseudomonas* infection of, 180
Tonofibril, 9, *10, 11*
Topical agents, in exacerbation of acne, 68
  in treatment of acne, 73–75
Topical steroids. See *Steroid therapy.*
Toxic epidermal necrolysis, 172–173
TPHA test, in diagnosis of syphilis, 228, 239(t), 241
TPI test, in diagnosis of syphilis, 228, 239(t)
Traction alopecia, 356, 358
Tranquilizers, use of, with adolescent patients, 36
Treponema pallidum, 222, 224, *224*
  identification of, 237
Treponemal antigen tests, in late congenital syphilis, 242
Triamcinolone, in psoriasis, 157
Trichomycosis axillaris, 295
Trichophyton mentagrophytes, in cutaneous infection, 306, 307, 308, 310, 312, 313
Trichophyton rubrum, in cutaneous infection, 307, 308, 310, 312, 313
Trichophyton tonsurans, in tinea capitis, 45, 304–306
Trichophyton verrucosum, in tinea barbae, 306
Trichorrhexis invaginata, 351–352, 350(t), *350*
Trichorrhexis nodosa, 352, 350(t), *350*
  acquired, 352
  congenital, 352
  vs. trichorrhexis invaginata, 351
Trichosporon beigelii, in piedra, 302–303
Trichotillomania, 358, Plate VIII-C
Tropical acne, 67
Tropocollagen molecule, 20–21
Trunk, psoriasis of, 148
Tryptophan, deficiency of, in Hartnup disease, 129
Tryptophanuria, congenital, vs. Hartnup disease, 130

Twins, atopic dermatitis in, 88, *89*
  psoriasis in, 145
Tzanck smear, 48–49
  in diagnosis of bullous disease, 48
  of viral infections, 48

Ulcer, Meleney's, 179
Ulceration, in pyoderma gangrenosum, 451
Ultraviolet light, and skin damage, 123–124
  See also *Sunlight*.
  in lupus erythematosus, 388, 391
  in treatment of acne, 74
    psoriasis, 155–156
    vitiligo, 437–438
Ultraviolet light booth, in treatment of
  psoriasis, 155–156
Urethritis, in Reiter syndrome, 277
Uroporphyrin I, 133
Urticaria, 404–417. See also *Angioedema*.
  acute vs. chronic, 405
  anaphylaxis in, 407, 411
  aquagenic, 411
  as response to infection, 412
  causes of, 405(t), 407–408
    immunological, 405–406, 406(t)
    non-immunological, 405–408, 406(t)
  cholinergic, 411
  chronic, vs. acute, 405
    vasculitis in, 422–423
  cold, 409–410, *410*
  contact, 411
  drug-induced, 407
  food-induced, 407
  from arthropod bites, 407
  from inhalants, 407
  from insect bites, 407
  heat, 410
  histological findings in, 406–407
  in systemic diseases, 412
  management of, 412
  papular, 408
  patch testing in, 411
  pathogenesis of, 406–407, 406(t)
  physical syndromes in, 408–412
  pressure, 409, *409*
  psychogenic, 412
  solar, 135–136, 410–411, Plate I–E
  wheal of, 404, *404*

Vaccination, for measles, 203
  for rubella, 205
Vagina, candidal infection of, 318, 320–321
Varicella, 191–193, *192*
  vs. Mucha-Habermann disease, 427
Varicella-zoster infections, 191–195, *192*
  differential diagnosis of, 191, 193
Variola, vs. varicella, 193
Vascular reactive diseases, 404–432
Vasculature, cutaneous, 23–24

Vasculitis, in juvenile dermatomyositis,
  446–447
  in systemic lupus erythematosus, 374
Vasoconstriction, in atopic dermatitis, 93, 94,
  94
Vater-Pacini corpuscles, 25
VDRL test, false positive reactions in, 240–241
  in diagnosis of syphilis, 228, 238, 239(t),
  240–241
Vellus hair, 15, *15*
Venereal disease, causative agents of, 223(t)
  incidence of, 222
  non-syphilitic, 257–292. See also *Syphilis*.
Verruca(e). See *Warts*.
Verruca plana, vs. acne, 72
Verruca plana juvenilis, 197
Verruca vulgaris, 197, *194*
Verrucous nevus, 327–329, *328, 329*
Vibratory angioedema, 409
Viral infections, 184–208
  Coxsackie, 202(t), 205–206
  drugs for, 185, 190
  ECHO, 202(t), 206
  treatment of, 185
  urticarial response to, 412
Virion, 184
Virus, structure of, 184
Vitamin A, in treatment of acne, 77
Vitiligo, 435–438, *437*
  clinical manifestations of, 436–437
  etiology of, 435–436
  histological findings in, 437
  treatment of, 437–438
Vogt-Koyanagi-Harada syndrome, in
  vitiligo, 436–437
Vulva, elephantiasis of, in lymphogranuloma
  venereum, *269*
Vulvovaginitis, herpetic, 188
  in lichen sclerosus et atrophicus, 445

Wart(s), *194*, 195–199
  age factor in, 195–196
  clinical appearance of, 197–198
  common, *194*, 197
  digitate, 197
  filiform, 197
  flat, 72, 197
  genital, 197–198
  mosaic, 197
  plantar, 197
  transmission of, 197
  treatment of, 198–199
Wassermann test, false positive reactions in,
  240–241
  for syphilis, 238, 239(t)
"Wear and tear" dermatitis, 106
Wet dressings, in treatment of eczematous
  dermatitis, 118–119, 119(t)
White dermatographism, in atopic
  dermatitis, 93, *94*
White line response, in atopic dermatitis,
  93–94, *94*

"Winter itch," 105
Wood's light, 45–47, 140
   in diagnosis of tinea capitis, 45, Plate I–A

Xanthoma, vs. necrobiosis lipoidica
   diabeticorum, 453
Xeroderma pigmentosum, 125–127
   and freckling, 460
   neoplasms in, 125–126

Xerosis. See *Dry skin*.
X-ray therapy, in treatment of acne, 77

Yeast infection, 44, 317–321, *318, 319*
   examination for, 40–45